MATERNITY NURSING

An Introductory Text
sixth edition

MATERNITY NURSING

An Introductory Text
sixth edition

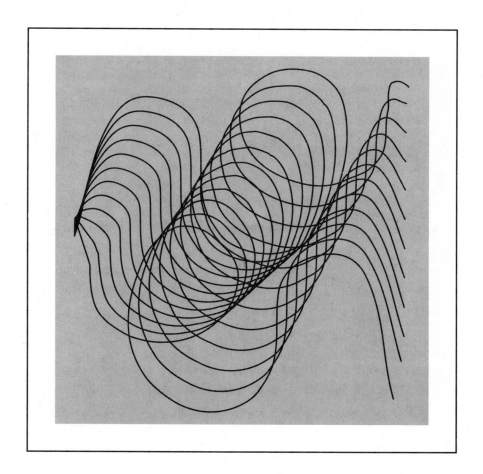

ARLENE BURROUGHS, MEd, RN

Assistant Professor, Maternal-Child Nursing
College of Nursing, University of Illinois at Chicago

W. B. SAUNDERS COMPANY
Harcourt Brace Jovanovich, Inc.

Philadelphia / London / Toronto / Montreal / Sydney / Tokyo

W. B. SAUNDERS COMPANY
Harcourt Brace Jovanovich, Inc.

The Curtis Center
Independence Square West
Philadelphia, Pennsylvania 19106

Library of Congress Cataloging-in-Publication Data

Burroughs, Arlene.

Maternity nursing.—6th ed. / Arlene Burroughs.

p.   cm.

ISBN 0–7216–3313–7

Rev. ed. of: Bleier's maternity nursing. 5th ed. /
Arlene Burroughs. 1986.

Includes bibliographical references and index.

1. Maternity nursing.   I. Burroughs, Arlene. Bleier's
  maternity nursing.   II. Title.   [DNLM: 1. Obstetrical
  Nursing.   2. Pediatric Nursing.   WY   157 B972m]

RG951B87 1992   610.73'678—dc20

DNLM/DLC   91–25731

Here is the latest edition of this book together with the language of the translation and the publisher.

German (4th Edition)—F. K. Schattauer Verlag, Stuttgart, West Germany
Spanish (5th Edition)—McGraw-Hill, Interamericana, Mexico City, Mexico

Editor: Ilze Rader
Developmental Editor: Miriam McCauley
Designer: Bill Donnelly
Production Manager: Ken Neimeister
Manuscript Editors: Deborah Klenotic and Amy Norwitz
Illustrator: W. B. Saunders Staff
Illustration Coordinator: Peg Shaw
Indexer: Ellen Murray
Cover Designer: Ellen Bodner-Zanolle

MATERNITY NURSING (Sixth Edition)   ISBN 0–7216–3313–7

Printed in the United States of America.

Last digit is the print number: 9   8   7   6   5   4   3   2

To Linda Delort, an invaluable co-worker,
during the recent two-year period when I was Acting Department Head,
Maternal Child Nursing, College of Nursing, University of Illinois at Chicago

PREFACE

Maternity Nursing: An Introductory Text (6th ed.) is a continuation of Bleier's *Maternity Nursing*. It is written in a concise, easily understandable style that presents not only basic theoretical content but also the clinical applications necessary to equip students to provide competent, effective, scientific, and technical care.

Content from the previous edition has been critically scrutinized, then updated, expanded, or deleted. Two new chapters have been added, "Sexually Transmitted Diseases," emphasizing the acquired immunodeficiency syndrome (AIDS), and "Women's Health Care," which includes breast cancer and endometriosis. Information on substance abuse, including cocaine, is found in the chapter on health care during pregnancy. Recognizing the need and desire of families to assume more responsibility for their own health, strong emphasis has been placed on the nurse's role as teacher in health promotion and self-care during the childbearing years.

Numerous summary tables, illustrations, and photographs have been carefully selected to enhance certain content and enrich student learning. Learning objectives are listed at the beginning of each chapter. Suggested activities and clinical situations followed by multiple choice questions are found at the ends of chapters to reinforce learning and encourage clinical decision-making skills. Numerous care plans are found throughout the text to assist students in the application of the nursing process to patient care. The nursing care plans are based on the diagnostic components approved by NANDA. Key Points in Education highlight essential elements of self-care that nurses need to teach clients.

The content of the text has been reorganized, with the first six units presenting the entire normal childbearing cycle. Unit seven focuses on complications and their potential impact on the woman, fetus, newborn, and family. The appendix tabulates, in alphabetical order, indications and effects of common drugs used in maternity care.

This text is a product of a deep conviction that nurses have a unique challenge and opportunity to educate and provide health care that influences the health and well-being of women, infants, and families during the childbearing years.

ACKNOWLEDGMENTS

Many individuals have contributed to the preparation of this book by their encouragement and support, and I am most grateful to them. I thank the many friends, colleagues, and students who gave invaluable suggestions in the development of the manuscript.

Sincere thanks go to Carol Howley, MSN, RN, Assistant Professor, Department of Maternal Child Nursing, Indiana University, and to Emma Nemivant, MSN, RN, Instructor, Department of Maternal Child Nursing, University of Illinois at Chicago.

I wish to thank the practical nursing instructors who reviewed portions of the manuscript; their constructive comments and insights were greatly appreciated. Thanks go to

L. Shayne Bryant, RN
Department of Practical Nursing
Chauncey Sparks State Technical College
Eufaula, Alabama

Gloria Clocklin, MSN, RN
Department of Practical Nursing
Northern Michigan University
Marquette, Michigan

Judy Conlin, RN
Practical Nursing Program
BOCES
Orleans and Niagara County Educational
    Center
Sanborn, New York

JoAnn Dever, BSN, MSNEd, RN
Department of Practical Nursing
Indiana Vocational Technical College
Fort Wayne, Indiana

Linda G. Hancock, BSN, RN
Department of Practical Nursing
Thomas Technical Institute
Thomasville, Georgia

Susan Ihlenfeldt, RN
Department of Practical Nursing
Front Range Community College/Larimer
    County Center
Fort Collins, Colorado

Marjorie T. Livengood, MEd, RN
Department of Practical Nursing
Athens Area Technical Institute
Athens, Georgia

Mary Patricia Norrell, BSN, RNC
Department of Practical Nursing
Indiana Vocational-Technical College
Columbus, Indiana

Connie Rose, MS, RN
School of Practical Nursing
Northern Wyoming Community College
Gillette, Wyoming

Maureen M. Solomon, RN
Department of Practical Nursing
J.F. Drake State Technical College
Huntsville, Alabama

Ruth A. Stagg, BSN, RN
Department of Practical Nursing
T.H. Harris Technical Institute
Opelousas, Louisiana

Sincere appreciation goes to Ilze Rader, Senior Nursing Editor, for her wisdom and encouragement in the preparation of this book, and a special thanks to Miriam McCauley, Developmental Editor, for her invaluable counseling, consistent support, and understanding. Others at W. B. Saunders Company that need to be mentioned for their commitment to this project include Marie Thomas, Ken Neimeister, Amy Norwitz, Debbie Klenotic, and Dave Nazaruk.

I am grateful to Nancy Fleming, CMN, PhD, Lynn Gipson, Barbara Kazmeir, Mary Jean Chaykin, and my sister Joyce Griffin for allowing me to use their photographs. Also, I wish to express my appreciation to the University of Illinois Hospital and to several families who have made their unique contribution to the original photographs in this text.

Contents

UNIT I

SOCIAL AND BIOLOGICAL DETERMINANTS OF CHILDBEARING

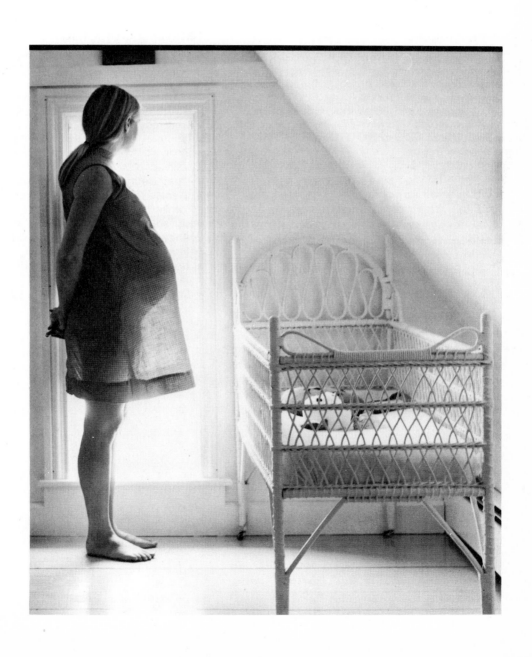

CHAPTER 1 _____

Chapter Outline

Goals of Maternity Care
Trends in Maternity Care
    Current available facilities
    Statistics important to maternal and infant care
Providers of Maternity Care
The Experience of Pregnancy
Current Family Trends
    The traditional family
    The stepfamily and the blended family
    The single female parent
    The single male parent
    The adolescent parent
Health Care and Culture
The Nursing Process and Maternal and Infant Care

Learning Objectives

Upon completion of Chapter 1, the student should be able to
- List the goals of maternity care.
- Name three different kinds of health care personnel who may provide maternity care.
- Name current maternity care facilities.
- Define birth rate, neonatal mortality, perinatal mortality, and maternal mortality.
- Describe the impact of pregnancy on the family.
- Identify family styles that differ from the traditional family.
- List some problems that the single parent experiences and suggest ways the parent might deal with them.
- Name the special problems of the adolescent parent.
- Describe four components of the nursing process.

MATERNITY CARE, FAMILY, AND PREGNANCY

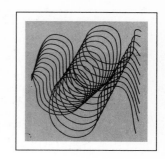

Maternity nursing is the care given by the nurse to the expectant woman (and significant other) during pregnancy, labor, birth, and the postpartum (postbirth) period. In addition, maternity nursing includes the care of the fetus and, after birth, of the newborn infant. Maternity nursing is unique in that for 9 months of pregnancy, during birth, and after birth, the caregiver's attention is focused almost equally on two people, the expectant mother and the fetus/newborn infant. The maternity nurse is in an ideal position to assess the health of the patient and family, conduct health promotion, provide instruction for health care, and offer support during the maternity cycle.

In principle and practice, maternity nursing emphasizes the integrity of the family unit and considers childbearing to be a normal physiological process. In efforts to make pregnancy, labor, birth, and the postpartum period safe, comfortable, and satisfying to the patient and family, great emphasis is placed on the teaching role of the nurse and the physician. *Wellness* is the overriding concern, with symptoms and complications being treated when they occur. The nursing process (discussed in The Nursing Process and Maternal and Infant Care) is applied to provide effective patient care.

Goals of Maternity Care

The ultimate aim of maternity care is for the expectant woman's pregnancy, labor, and birth to be as uneventful (normal) as possible. An additional goal is the well-being of the newborn infant. More specific aims of maternity nursing are as follows:

- To help the expectant woman view

pregnancy, labor, and birth as normal physiological processes.
- To provide adequate support to make pregnancy a positive, gratifying experience.
- To provide adequate instruction to the expectant woman during pregnancy, labor, and birth.
- To be sensitive to the expectant woman's social and economic needs.
- To assist in early detection of a woman's deviation from the norm during the maternity cycle.

Trends in Maternity Care

CURRENT AVAILABLE FACILITIES

A growing number of health care consumers are requesting that their childbirth experience occur in "natural" surroundings. These expectant parents believe that home-like surroundings make the birth more pleasant. They feel that the traditional, structured hospital environment is strange and creates undue anxiety.

Rather than promoting the practice of home births, many hospitals have instituted *alternative birth settings* or centers. In these hospital settings, the woman is offered the protection of medical and skilled nursing care; however, she can give birth to her infant in an attractive *birthing room*. The husband (or significant other) is encouraged to be with the mother during the birthing process. In addition, sibling visitation is encouraged. If the birth is uneventful, the woman and infant may go home within 12 to 24 hours. If a birthing room is not available, usually the mother is allowed to

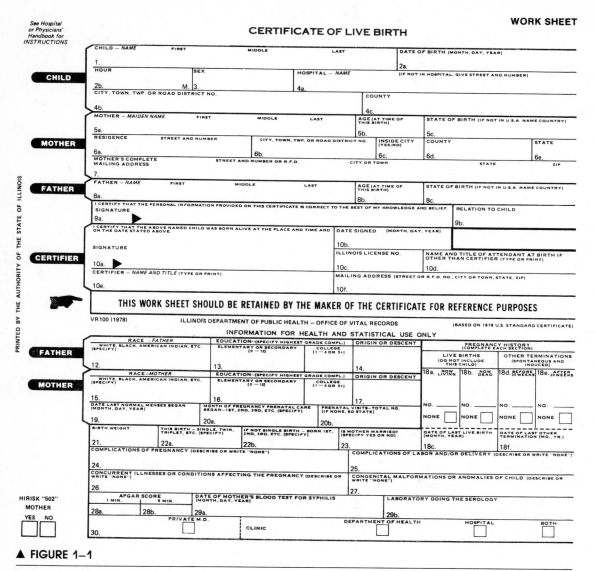

▲ FIGURE 1–1

Original certificate of live birth.

hold her baby soon after birth to encourage the bonding process between mother and infant. Also, *rooming-in* is available in many hospitals to facilitate mother–infant bonding/attachment and acquaintance of family members with the infant.

STATISTICS IMPORTANT TO MATERNAL AND INFANT CARE

It is important for health professionals to obtain information about the way maternity care is given and the outcome of maternal and infant care. One way to accomplish this is to look at statistics. In the United States, it is a legal requirement in all 50 states and the District of Columbia to have a birth certificate completed for every live-born baby. The birth certificate (Fig. 1–1) is registered locally, and a report is sent to the National Office of Vital Statistics in Washington, D.C. This birth certificate provides legal proof of age and citizenship. In addition, data from these records are used to gather information for statistical studies concerning the year-to-year birth rate, maternal mortality rate, and infant perinatal mortality rate. This information makes it possible to compare the outcomes of pregnancies of different states and countries. The following statistics are used:

- Birth rate—The number of births per 1000 population.
- Neonatal mortality rate—The number of deaths, either at birth or during the first 28 days of life, per 1000 live births.
- Fetal mortality rate—The number of fetal deaths among fetuses weighing more than 500 g per 1000 live births.
- Perinatal mortality rate—The number of deaths among fetuses weighing more than 500 g and within the first 28 days of life per 1000 live births. The leading cause of perinatal mortality is low birth weight, with most such infants delivered before term.
- Maternal mortality rate—The number of maternal deaths that occur as a direct result of the reproductive process per 100,000 live births. The three leading causes of maternal mortality in the United States are hemorrhage, infection, and pregnancy-induced hypertension.

Providers of Maternity Care

Expanding knowledge has created new specialties within medicine and nursing. Although midwives have been attending births for centuries, today the *nurse midwife* is a registered professional nurse who has completed a program of advanced study and clinical experience approved by the American College of Nurse Midwives and has passed a certification test. The nurse midwife is qualified to provide continuous and complete care to the expectant woman throughout her pregnancy, labor, and birth. She also cares for the mother and infant in the postbirth period (Fig. 1–2). This comprehensive care is given when the mother's progress is normal and uncomplicated. If not directly present, the physician must be in communication with the midwife during care.

The *obstetric/gynecologic nurse practitioner* is a registered nurse who has completed advanced education that meets individual states' criteria for state licensure and certification at the nurse practitioner level. She cares for the woman during the maternity cycle; however, she does not conduct the delivery of the infant. Care is aimed at health maintenance.

The *maternity clinical specialist* is a registered nurse who has completed an advanced program in maternity care at the master's level. The major emphases in this program are health education, counseling, and assisting the family with the parenting role.

The physicians who participate in maternal and infant care include the following: The *obstetrician* specializes in maternity and gynecological care. He or she cares for the woman with a normal or complicated pregnancy. The *family practice physician* renders care to the family as the need for medical care arises. This may include care of the pregnant woman and her family. The *pediatrician* specializes in the care of infants and children. The pediatrician is often present when complications are expected in the newborn. A *neonatologist* is a subspecialist in pediatrics. He or she specializes in the care of high-risk neonates (newborns), many of whom are of low birth weight and/or preterm.

The Experience of Pregnancy

Pregnancy, including birth, is perhaps the most emotional and dramatic experience of a woman's life. The impact on the woman and her family is tremendous. Because of the mobility and changing cultural patterns of our society, pregnancy is often experienced without the support of family and friends. Current medical and nursing literature reflects the modern experience of pregnancy: the focus has widened from the purely physical aspects to a much more comprehensive view that includes the psychological and social aspects of pregnancy.

Although pregnancy can be an experience full of anticipation and excitement, it can also be a time of stress and abrupt change in life-style for expectant parents. Pregnancy can challenge the current role of each family member. Because pregnancy often evokes feelings, both joyful and perplexing, that have never been experienced before,

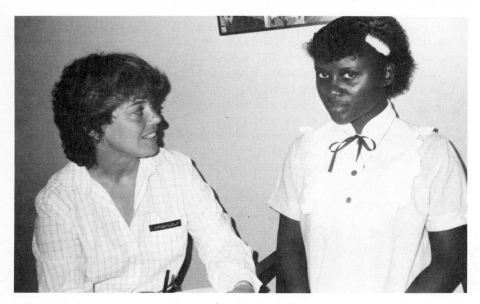

▲ FIGURE 1–2

Nurse midwife caring for pregnant adolescent.

the best of relationships or marriages may be challenged.

Despite the fact that pregnancy can be emotionally stressful, the major emphasis in prenatal evaluation traditionally is physical. Little attention is given to the developmental and emotional stages, to the behaviors characteristic of pregnancy, or to how the couple is interpreting or coping with the experience. The reasons for this are numerous and include the health professional's own inadequacy and lack of perception in dealing with these issues, as well as the pregnant woman's desire to avoid giving the impression that she and the father of the baby are having problems. Maternity nurses as well as other health professionals need to expand the scope of their health care services.

It is important that caregivers recognize that socioeconomic needs, education, and religious beliefs all affect care during pregnancy and birth. Factors that encourage or discourage adequate maternity care include age, whether the woman is single or married, family support, and education. For example, the average young pregnant woman who has not completed high school is not likely to begin her prenatal care until about the middle of her pregnancy. Therefore, it is important for the caregiver to assess the personal and family history in the initial phase of maternity care.

Current Family Trends

The characteristics of the families in our own experience often do not reflect the characteristics of the families of others. Also, family life in various cultures shows great differences.

A family can be defined as two or more persons who are united by blood, marriage, or adoption. A family also can be defined as persons who interact with each other as a unit. Common to the family unit, regardless of whether the participants are married, is the fact that they relate to each other in some way, with specific patterns of behavior.

THE TRADITIONAL FAMILY

In the traditional family, the father, mother, and children live together, often with the father as the main wage earner and the mother as the homemaker (Fig. 1–3). Several factors have been responsible for the changes we are now seeing in the family unit. The changes in women's roles have been caused by changes in economics and societal values. Young women frequently delay marriage and, after commitment to a partner, choose to work on their own career. They may

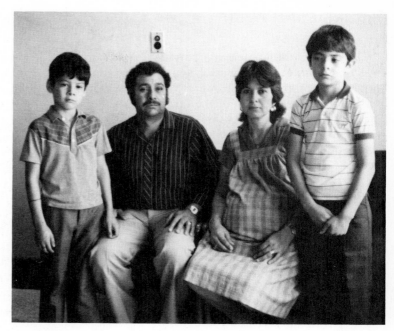

▲ **FIGURE 1–3**

A traditional family: mother, father, and children.

prefer to bear children early in life, or they may wait until they are older, and have established their own identity in the work force. Also, because of the high cost of living, couples may feel it wise to have two wage earners in the family.

THE STEPFAMILY AND THE BLENDED FAMILY

The stepfamily and the blended family (reconstituted family) consist of a wife and husband, one or both of whom have been previously married and who bring to their marriage one or more children from their previous marriage. Later they frequently have children together.

THE SINGLE FEMALE PARENT

Today, single parents are a fast-growing group in our society. The single-parent family is one in which there is one head of the family as a result of a decision to remain unmarried, divorce, abandonment, or death of the spouse. Because less

stigma is now attached to birth out of wedlock, more unwed mothers are choosing to keep their children. At least 5 million American families are headed by a single parent. Today, the number of traditional families—mother, father, and children—is decreasing, and the number of single-parent families is increasing. This arrangement puts additional strain on available health resources and increases use of services. Hence, more single-parent families are at risk for inadequate care. Child care centers are increasing in number but do not meet the need for the large number of single parents.

The single female parent commonly finds herself in difficult circumstances. She often feels alone. Frequently, she seeks health care late in pregnancy. It is particularly important for this single parent to receive nonjudgmental support from health professionals who care for her. Most important, the expectant mother needs to be made aware of all available resources. If she is going to continue to be sexually active but remain single, she should be offered adequate instruction in contraception. This instruction should be given at her level of understanding.

THE SINGLE MALE PARENT

The feelings of single male parents are still not well documented. However, it is known that more single fathers are voicing interest in and concern for their children. Many of the fathers want to be included in childbearing and childrearing. The single male parent may have a better economic status and more options for child care and living quarters than the single female parent. He may employ a caretaker to come to the home or may use child care facilities.

The degree to which single male parents want to be involved varies. Some only want the baby to have their last name. Others wish to share in all the responsibilities of parenting. It is important to work out ways to include the father when possible.

THE ADOLESCENT PARENT

The adolescent parent has a compound problem: coping with adolescence and parenthood. Moreover, the adolescent parent usually is single and has limited financial assistance. The number of adolescents (ages 12 to 19 years) in need of maternity care is increasing. Whereas the birth rate among married persons has consistently dropped in the United States in the past 10 years, the birth rate among unmarried adolescents has almost doubled.

Complicating adolescent pregnancy is the increased risk of medical and social complications in this group owing to delayed prenatal care, poor nutrition, and inconsistency in following instructions about health care. In addition, teenage anatomy is often not well developed for childbirth. In general, an adolescent pregnancy presents an increased chance of perinatal mortality.

Many adolescent girls decide to keep their babies instead of having an abortion or placing them for adoption. With an adequate support system, some adolescent mothers are capable of mothering; however, others need help in child care. Assistance with decision making is needed for a pregnant adolescent's role as a mother and for the prevention of future pregnancies.

Health Care and Culture

Nurses need to be aware of differences in patients' cultural backgrounds in order to develop individualized care plans for them. A woman's cultural background influences her attitudes, values, and beliefs about health care and illness. Most nurses and other health care workers in the United States tend to hold the values and beliefs of middle-class Americans. Therefore, it is important for nurses to recognize and tolerate behavior that differs from their own. Nurses should ask themselves certain basic questions: Do I have the right to judge the patient's behavior as incorrect and seek to change her behavior? Should the patient make the ultimate decision about health care? A major guideline in deciding whether to incorporate a culturally influenced behavior into the care plan is to assess whether it is harmful or helpful in coping with health or illness. For example, if the patient's religious belief includes eating a vegetarian diet, it should be supported. The appropriate nursing intervention is to provide advice about the necessary proteins for an adequate diet without changing the patient's life-style. Efforts should be made to support the patient's own nonmedical value system. History taking, including the patient's religion and cultural background, should be part of the initial prenatal record.

Communication between the nurse and the patient is important. If the patient does not speak English in a predominantly English-speaking community, an interpreter should be used. This could be accomplished by asking a family member to be present during each prenatal visit and while the patient is in labor. This practice would reduce anxiety due to misunderstandings about the prescribed nursing and medical management.

The Nursing Process and Maternal and Infant Care

The *nursing process* is a five-step method that enables the nurse to make responsible decisions regarding the appropriate care for a particular patient. Facts, observations, and theoretical knowledge are all used to make problem-solving decisions in each step. The five steps of the nursing process are as follows:

1. Assessment
2. Analysis
3. Planning
4. Implementation
5. Evaluation

Assessment Phase. In the assessment phase, the nurse collects pertinent subjective and objective information about the health status of the patient. These data consist of observations made by the nurse and information obtained from the patient and her family. The physical, social, and psychological aspects of the patient's health are assessed through history taking, an interview, physical examination, and laboratory tests. The initial assessment by the nurse becomes the baseline data base, which is updated or changed as more information is obtained. Decisions can be made regarding the patient's deficits or potential deficits in her health status.

Analysis Phase. Formation of a nursing diagnosis is accomplished through the interpretation or analysis of the gathered data. Analysis involves judgment and decision making. Problems that can be managed through nursing interventions are

---

NURSING CARE PLAN 1–1

EFFECTS OF FAMILY AND SOCIAL INFLUENCES ON PREGNANCY

Potential Problems and Nursing Diagnoses

1. Knowledge deficit related to expectations and composition of the family.

2. Self-esteem disturbance related to being pregnant and single.
3. Ineffective coping related to inadequate support system.
4. Knowledge deficit related to the patient's values and dietary needs.

5. Knowledge deficit related to pregnant adolescent's need for prenatal care.
6. Impaired communication because of inability to speak English.

Nursing Interventions

Identify and evaluate factors that influence family relationships, such as age, whether patient is married or single, education, and financial support.

Acknowledge the potential negative feelings of being pregnant and single.

Encourage verbalization about the support of significant others during the pregnancy.

Recognize that the patient's values are important in teaching. Suggest ways to incorporate essential proteins that are acceptable to her as a vegetarian.

Educate pregnant adolescent about the need for early prenatal care.

An interpreter should be provided when the caregiver and patient cannot communicate with each other because of a language barrier.

Expected Outcomes

1. Patient recognizes the need for financial support during the pregnancy because of being single, with a limited income.
2. Patient verbalizes negative feelings of self-worth. She agrees to include the social worker in the health care team.
3. Patient verbalizes lack of family support during this pregnancy.
4. Patient identifies foods to include in a vegetarian diet that provide the essential proteins for adequate nutrition.
5. Patient acknowledges need for interpreter to be with her.

selected, categorized, and placed in order of priority. Problems that need attention by other health care professionals are referred to the appropriate individuals. Making the nursing diagnosis is a very important step in the process, because the resultant care plan is based on what the nurse perceives to be the patient's problems and needs. The nursing diagnosis must involve a problem that falls within the boundaries of nursing practice.

Planning Phase. Specifying the expected outcomes or the goals of care serves to direct the nursing care plan. In determining the goals or outcomes, the nurse should consult the patient, if possible. Nursing interventions necessary to achieve the goals are identified. These goals should be specific, individualized, and measurable and should list a desirable amount of time for achievement.

Implementation Phase. Nursing interventions are directed toward increasing the wellness of the patient. This phase consists of actions or interventions taken by the nurse to achieve the desired outcomes or goals. They may be additional observations; measures to bring about healing or to promote comfort; instructions to correct or prevent health problems; and nursing measures to promote health. Nursing interventions should assist the patient in self-care.

Evaluation Phase. In the evaluation phase, the nurse determines whether progress has been made toward the expected outcomes and, if necessary, modifies the care plan accordingly. The nurse must evaluate the effects of an intervention by comparing the expected outcome with the outcome actually observed. This may result in a reassessment and adjustment in the care plan. By refocusing on other identified problems, the care plan may be improved.

Nursing care plans, and sometimes several nursing diagnoses, appear in many of the chapters of this book to aid the student in caring for mothers and infants. Nursing Care Plan 1–1 is presented on page 9.

References

Carlson, J. H., Craft, C. A., McGuire, A. D., & Popkess-Vawter, S. (1991). Nursing Diagnosis: A Case Study Approach. Philadelphia: W. B. Saunders Company.

Degenhart-Leskosky, S. M. (1989). Health education needs of adolescent and nonadolescent mothers. *Journal of Obstetric, Gynecologic, and Neonatal Nursing* 18:238–243.

Dickason, E. J., Schult, M. O., & Silverman, B. L. (1990). *Maternal-Infant Nursing Care.* St. Louis: C. V. Mosby.

Dormire, S. L., Strauss, S. S., & Clarke, B. A. (1989). Social support and adaptation to the parent role in first-time adolescent mothers. *Journal of Obstetric, Gynecologic, and Neonatal Nursing* 18:327–337.

Kim, M. J., McFarland, G. K., & McLane, A. M. (1989). *Pocket Guide to Nursing Diagnoses.* St. Louis: C. V. Mosby.

Ladewig, P. W., London, M. L., & Olds, S. B. (1990). *Essentials of Maternal-Newborn Nursing,* 2nd ed. Redwood City, CA: Addison-Wesley Nursing.

Moore, M. L. (1989). Recurrent teen pregnancy: Making it less desirable. *American Journal of Maternal-Child Nursing,* 14(2):104–108.

Steffen, G. E. (1988). Quality medical care. *Journal of the American Medical Association* 260:56–61.

Stevens, K. A. (1988). Nursing diagnoses in wellness childbearing settings. *Journal of Obstetric, Gynecologic, and Neonatal Nursing* 17:329–335.

SUGGESTED ACTIVITIES

1. Explain how pregnancy affects the family.
2. Summarize, in written form, the single, pregnant adolescent's special needs.
3. Identify the overall aims of current maternity care.
4. List three different vital statistics used to compare the outcome of pregnancies in the United States with the outcome in other countries.
5. List and explain the various components of the nursing process.

REVIEW QUESTIONS

A. Select the best answer to each multiple-choice question.

1. A family can be defined in all of the following ways EXCEPT
   A. Two or more persons who are united by blood, marriage, or adoption
   B. Persons interacting with each other as a unit, whether single or married
   C. Two people who know each other
   D. Mother, father, and son

2. The single-parent family includes those
   A. Unmarried by choice
   B. Divorced or abandoned
   C. Whose spouse is dead
   D. All of the above

3. Which of the following contributes the least to the rate of infant mortality?
   A. The mother's educational level
   B. The mother's age
   C. Availability of or distance from health facility
   D. The mother's ethnic origin

4. In the United States, the adolescent pregnancy rate is
   A. At a status quo
   B. Increasing
   C. Decreasing

5. Legally, a birth certificate must be completed and reported on every birth in
   A. About half of the states
   B. About two-thirds of the states
   C. All 50 states and the District of Columbia
   D. All 50 states

6. The birth certificate is an important document because it is legal proof of
   A. Age
   B. Citizenship
   C. Place of birth
   D. Residence

7. In the nursing process, the nursing history is taken during which phase?
   A. Assessment
   B. Nursing diagnosis
   C. Evaluation
   D. Implementation

8. In the nursing process, the nursing diagnosis is formed during which phase?
   A. Assessment
   B. Analysis
   C. Planning
   D. Evaluation

CHAPTER 2 _____

Chapter Outline

The Female Reproductive System
    External reproductive organs
    Internal reproductive organs
    Pelvis
    Endocrine system and reproduction
The Male Reproductive System
    External reproductive organs
    Internal reproductive organs
    Endocrine system and reproduction

Learning Objectives

Upon completion of Chapter 2, the student should be able to

- Identify the female external reproductive organs.
- Explain the functions of the acini cells and the lactiferous ducts.
- Describe the functions of the ovaries.
- Explain the development of a mature ovum.
- Describe the location and size of the uterus.
- Name the functions of the uterus.
- Name the functions of the vagina.
- Describe the three phases of the menstrual cycle.
- Identify the four bones that make up the pelvis.
- Name the two divisions of the pelvis and explain which one is more important.
- Name the male external organs of reproduction.
- Trace the pathway of the sperm from the testes to the outside of the body.
- Discuss the location and function of the prostate gland.
- Compare the size of the sperm with the size of the ovum, and describe the sperm's appearance.
- Name the functions of the male hormone testosterone.

THE REPRODUCTIVE SYSTEMS

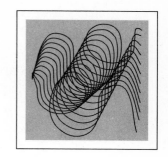

Human reproduction is a complex and fascinating process. The male and female reproductive systems functioning together produce a new life. In order to understand how human reproduction is possible, knowledge of the structural features and functions of various organs is needed.

The Female Reproductive System

EXTERNAL REPRODUCTIVE ORGANS

Vulva

The female external reproductive organs consist of the mons pubis, covered with pubic hair; two paired folds of tissue called the labia majora and labia minora, which surround a space called the vestibule; the vagina opening; the perineum; the sensitive clitoris; and glandular structures (Fig. 2–1). Collectively these structures are known as the vulva.

Mons Pubis

The mons pubis is formed at the upper margin of the symphysis pubis and is shaped as an inverted triangle. Its location is over the two pubic bones of the pelvis. This structure is composed of fatty tissue lying beneath the skin and, from puberty on, is covered with hair. The mons pubis protects from injury the delicate tissue that it surrounds.

Labia Majora and Labia Minora

The labia majora are two folds of fatty tissue that form the lateral boundaries of the vulva. They are covered with skin and hair on the outer aspect and are smooth and moist on the inner aspect, where the openings of numerous small glands are found. The labia majora are analogous to the scrotum in the male. Just inside the labia majora are two smaller folds of skin call the labia minora.

When the labia majora are separated, the labia minora are exposed. The labia minora are soft folds of skin that are rich in sebaceous glands. The labia minora are moist and are composed of erectile tissue containing loose connective tissue, blood vessels, and involuntary muscles. The functions of the labia minora are to lubricate and waterproof the vulvar skin and to provide bactericidal secretions.

Clitoris

The clitoris is a small, sensitive structure that, like the penis, is composed of erectile tissue, nerves, and blood vessels; it is covered at its tip with very sensitive skin. It exists primarily for female sexual enjoyment. Partially hidden at the upper end of the labia, the clitoris frequently appears as the opening to an orifice and may be mistaken for the opening to the urethra.

Vestibule

The vestibule is a boat-shaped depression enclosed by the labia minora and is visible when the labia minora are separated. The vestibule contains

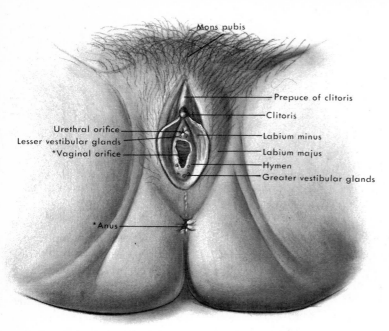

Mons pubis

Prepuce of clitoris

Clitoris

Urethral orifice

Lesser vestibular glands

*Vaginal orifice

Labium minus

Labium majus

Hymen

Greater vestibular glands

*Anus

*The clinical perineum lies between these two openings.

▲ **FIGURE 2–1**

Female external genitals. (From Dienhart, C. M. (1979). *Basic Human Anatomy and Physiology*, 3rd ed. Philadelphia, W. B. Saunders Company.)

the vaginal opening, or *introitus*, which is between the external and internal genitals. At the introitus there is a perforated fold of pink mucous membrane called the *hymen*. The hymen may be broken by the use of tampons, strenuous physical activity, or sexual intercourse.

The vestibule contains the openings of six structures that drain into it: the urethra, Skene's ducts (two), the vaginal orifice, and Bartholin's glands (two). Bartholin's glands are located on each side of the vagina. These glands secrete a yellowish mucus that acts to lubricate the vagina, particularly during sexual arousal. Skene's glands are located just inside the urethra and are part of the vestibule. When a nurse is preparing to do a catheterization, it is this area of the vestibule that is cleansed.

Perineum

The perineum is the region of the genital area that lies between the vulva and the anus. Because of its location, it plays an important role in the birth process. It is composed of the levator ani muscles and fascia, the deep perineal muscles, and the external genitalia muscles. These muscles function as supports to the pelvic organs. The pudendal arteries, veins, and nerves supply the muscles, fascia, and skin of the perineum. At the time of the birth of a baby, an anesthetic (a local or a pudendal block) may be injected into the pudendal nerves so that an incision called an *episiotomy* can be made into the perineum to prevent it from becoming torn (lacerated).

Breasts

The breasts, or mammary glands, are generally considered glands of reproduction because of their functional relationship to reproduction, that is, to secrete milk for the infant. The process is called *lactation*. The two breasts are situated on the anterior wall of the chest. Each breast is divided into a number of lobes (15 to 20) composed of glandular tissue and fat. The glandular tissue can be visualized as a tree-like structure. Beginning at the nipple are 10 to 20 branch-like structures called *lobes*. Branching off from each lobe are 20 to 40 lobules; each lobule branches further, dividing into 20 to 80 sac-like structures called *alveoli*. These sac-like structures have a lining that contains tiny secretory cells called *acini*, which secrete the various components of milk. Surrounding the alveolar cells are contractile cells called *myoepithelial cells,* which contract the alveolus and eject milk or a milk component into the reservoir called the *lactiferous ducts.* It is from these ducts that the infant, by sucking, gets milk through the nipple.

During pregnancy, estrogen inhibits milk secretion. After the expulsion of the placenta there is an abrupt decline in estrogen and progesterone levels. This allows a hormone called *prolactin* to be released from the anterior pituitary gland when the infant sucks. Prolactin stimulates the acini cells to produce milk. Infant sucking also effects the release of *oxytocin* from the posterior pituitary. Oxytocin stimulates the contraction of the myoepithelial cells, which causes the ejection of milk from the alveoli into the ductal system (see Chapter 13).

Both the nipple and the areola, a pigmented area surrounding the nipple, darken during pregnancy. Within the areola are sebaceous glands called *Montgomery's tubercles* which are thought to secrete a substance that lubricates the nipples, protecting them when the infant suckles (Fig. 2–2).

The size of the breasts depends on the amount of fatty tissue deposited in the breasts. Size does not indicate the amount of milk the breasts will produce.

INTERNAL REPRODUCTIVE ORGANS

The internal female organs of reproduction are the ovaries, the fallopian (uterine) tubes, the uterus, and the vagina (Fig. 2–3).

Ovaries

The ovaries are two small, almond-shaped organs located in the upper part of the pelvic cavity, one on each side of the uterus. They have two main functions: the development and later expulsion of the *ovum* (egg), and the secretion of the hormones. Ovaries contain 1 to 2 million ova at birth. By puberty, the ova number approximately 400,000.

During the reproductive years, the ovaries act in concert with the uterus. During the follicular phase of the menstrual cycle, the follicles in the ovary are in various stages of maturity. Once a

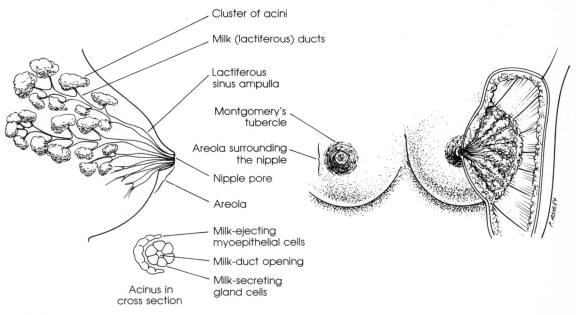

Cluster of acini

Milk (lactiferous) ducts

Lactiferous sinus ampulla

Montgomery's tubercle

Areola surrounding the nipple

Nipple pore

Areola

Milk-ejecting myoepithelial cells

Milk-duct opening

Milk-secreting gland cells

Acinus in cross section

▲ **FIGURE 2–2**

Position and anatomy of mammary glands and milk-producing structures and ducts.

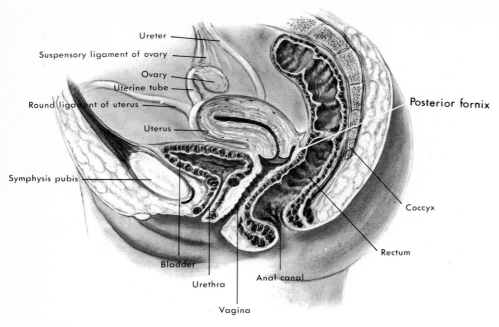

▲ **FIGURE 2–3**

Female internal reproductive organs. (From Dienhart, C. M. (1979). *Basic Human Anatomy and Physiology*, 3rd ed. Philadelphia, W. B. Saunders Company.)

month a mature ovum, called a *graafian follicle,* produces the midcycle spurt of estrogen necessary for ovulation to occur. The ovum ruptures and is expelled. This process is called *ovulation.* Ovulation usually occurs 14 days before the beginning of the next menstrual period. After ovulation, the cells of the ruptured follicle increase in size and form a yellow body called the *corpus luteum.* The corpus luteum also produces estrogen, as well as larger amounts of progesterone, beginning the luteal, or second, phase of the menstrual begins. The hormone progesterone prepares the lining (endometrium) of the uterus for pregnancy. During pregnancy, progesterone suppresses ovulation.

Fallopian Tubes

The two fallopian tubes (uterine tubes) attached to each side of the upper body of the uterus are small, thin, muscular structures, approximately 4 inches (10 cm) long. The tubes carry the ovum from the active ovary to the uterus by the action of cilia or hair-like projections in the lining of the tubes and by peristaltic action. There is no direct connection between the ovaries and the fallopian tubes. Extending from the ends of the uterine tubes are small, finger-like projections called *fimbriae.* Their movements sweep the ovum into the tube, after which the ovum travels to the uterus. It takes about 5 days for the ovum to travel the 4 inches from the ovary to the uterus. Fertilization of ovum by the sperm normally takes place in the outer third of the fallopian tube.

Uterus

The uterus is a hollow, pear-shaped, muscular organ. It is approximately 1 inch (2.5 cm) thick, 2 inches (5 cm) wide, and 3 inches (7.5 cm) long in a nonpregnant woman. During pregnancy, the uterus can stretch and enlarge considerably. The weight of the nonpregnant uterus is 2 oz; this increases to about 2 lb during the 9 months of pregnancy. During pregnancy, the uterus increases in vascularity, which allows sufficient blood supply for its growth. After pregnancy, it returns almost entirely to its former size and shape.

The uterus is situated in the middle of the pelvic cavity between the bladder and the rectum. The supportive ligaments maintain the position of the uterus. The ligaments allow the upper portion of the uterus to move freely. The two important ligaments are the round ligaments and the broad ligaments. During pregnancy these ligaments become stretched, frequently causing backache.

The uterus is divided into three parts. The *body* (corpus) is the main portion of the uterus. The *fundus*, the upper rounded portion, lies above the opening of the fallopian tubes. The *cervix*, the lower portion, projects into the vagina.

The uterus is made up of three layers. The *perimetrium*, the serous outer layer, is continuous with the peritoneum and helps suspend the uterus. The middle layer, the *myometrium*, is a thick, muscular layer. The inner layer, the *endometrium*, is a mucous membrane layer. During menstruation and after delivery, the cells of the endometrium (called *decidua* during pregnancy) are sloughed off. The myometrium contains muscle fibers that run in all directions (Fig. 2–4). It is able to thin out, pull up, and open the cervix, so the fetus can be pushed out of the uterus. The chief characteristic of the cervix, the part of the uterus that dips into the vagina, is its elasticity. In addition, it provides lubrication for the vaginal wall, acts as a bacteriostatic agent, and provides an alkaline environment to shelter the sperm from the acidic vagina.

The functions of the uterus are as follows:

1. Menstruation—The uterus sloughs off the endometrium or lining of the uterus.
2. Pregnancy—The uterus supports the fetus and allows the fetus to grow.
3. Labor and birth—The uterine muscles contract and the cervix dilates during labor to expel the fetus.

Vagina

The vagina is a curved tube leading from the uterus to the external opening of the reproductive organs at the vestibule. It lies between the bladder and the rectum. It consists of muscle and connective tissue and is lined with mucous membrane,

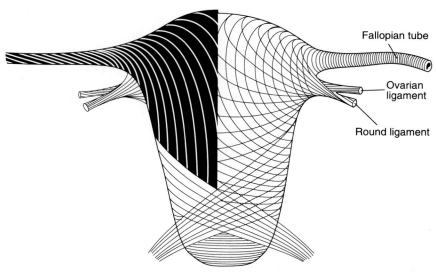

Fallopian tube

Ovarian ligament

Round ligament

▲ FIGURE 2–4

Uterine muscle layers. Note the directions of interlacing myometrial muscle fibers, including external longitudinal bands and internal circular arrangement.

which contains many folds called *rugae*. These folds allow the vagina to stretch during childbirth.

The functions of the vagina are as follows:

1. The excretory duct of the uterus through which the uterine secretions and menstrual flow escape.
2. The female organ of copulation (sexual intercourse).
3. Part of the birth canal.

PELVIS

The female bony pelvis has the unique functions of supporting and protecting the pelvic contents as well as forming a relatively fixed passage through which the baby moves during birth. Its size and shape, therefore, are very important factors in the mechanisms of labor and birth.

Bony Pelvic Structure

The pelvis is made up of four bones: the two innominate bones (hip bones), the sacrum, and the coccyx. The pelvis resembles a basin or bowl—its sides are the innominate bones, and its back is composed of the sacrum and coccyx. The four bones are lined with fibrocartilage and held tightly together by ligaments. The bones are joined in front by the symphysis pubis and in the back by the sacroiliac joints and the sacrococcygeal joint.

The innominate bones result from the fusion of the ilium, the ischium, and the pubis (Fig. 2–5). The two ilia form the upper part of the pelvis, known as the *false pelvis*. The *ischial spines*, sharp projections that form the posterior border of the ischium, are important landmarks and represent the shortest distance of the pelvic cavity. The spines can be palpated during a vaginal examination and are used to determine how far the baby's head has descended into the birth canal. The ischium is a heavy bone below the ilium that forms the lower part of the innominate bone. Its protuberance, the *ischial tuberosity*, is the part on which the body rests while in a sitting position. The pubis is the part of the innominate bone that forms the front of the pelvis. It consists of two pubic bones that unite to form a joint called the *symphysis pubis*, a rounded arch under which the baby's head must pass as it emerges from the birth canal.

Pelvic Divisions

The pelvic cavity is divided into the false and true pelvis. The false pelvis is the portion above the pelvic brim (upper portion) and has little obstetric significance. However, it does serve to support the growing uterus during pregnancy and directs the baby's head into the true pelvis near the end of pregnancy.

Pelvic Measurements

The bony circumference of the true pelvis is made up of the sacrum, the coccyx, and the lower part of the innominate bones. This area is very important because its size and shape must be adequate for passage of the baby during labor and birth. For convenience, three imaginary flat surfaces crossing the pelvis have traditionally been described: the plane of the pelvic inlet (Fig. 2–6), the plane of the least dimensions (midpelvis), and the plane of the outlet (Fig. 2–7).

A clinical measurement used to predict pelvic size is the *diagonal conjugate*. The diagonal conjugate is the distance from the lower margin of the symphysis pubis to the sacral promontory (Fig. 2–8). The examiner measures this diameter by placing two fingers in the woman's vagina and touching the sacral promontory. The minimal acceptable distance for most women is 10 cm. This procedure is part of the prenatal examination and may be uncomfortable for the patient. The woman should be prepared before the pelvic examination and should be given the necessary information and support.

The diameter of the midpelvis (bordered posteriorly by the sacrum, laterally by the ischial spines, and anteriorly by the symphysis pubis) can be measured only by x-ray. Because x-ray is potentially hazardous to the fetus, its use has declined. It may still be used to ascertain a cephalopelvic disproportion, although usually a cesarean section (without x-ray) is done when cephalopelvic disproportion is suspected.

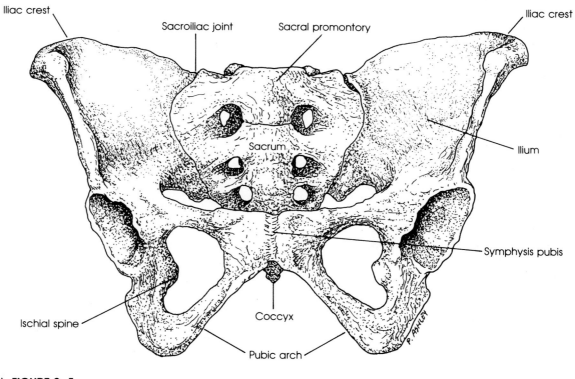

Iliac crest

Sacroiliac joint

Sacral promontory

Iliac crest

Sacrum

Ilium

Symphysis pubis

Ischial spine

Coccyx

Pubic arch

▲ **FIGURE 2–5**

Female pelvis, anterior view.

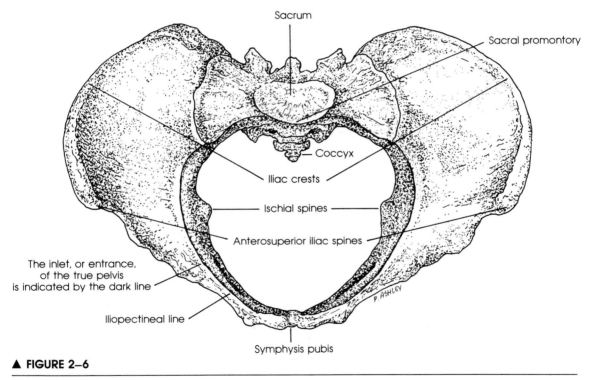

Sacrum

Sacral promontory

Coccyx

Iliac crests

Ischial spines

Anterosuperior iliac spines

The inlet, or entrance,
of the true pelvis
is indicated by the dark line

Iliopectineal line

Symphysis pubis

P. ASHLEY

▲ **FIGURE 2–6**

The inlet of the female pelvis.

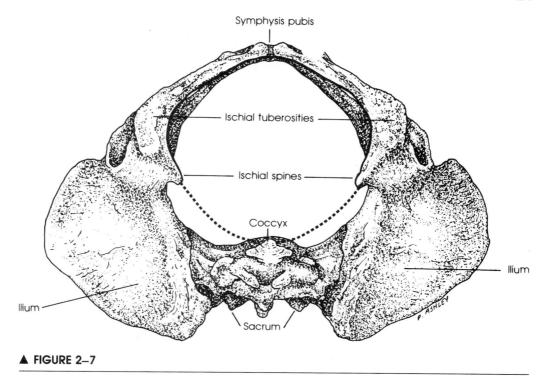

▲ **FIGURE 2–7**

The outlet of the female pelvis. (The outlet, or exit, of the true pelvis is indicated by the dark solid and broken line.)

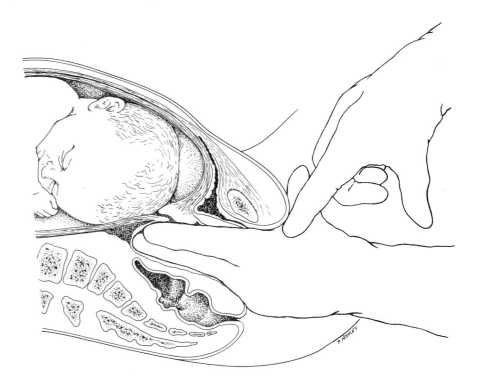

▲ **FIGURE 2–8**

Measuring the diagonal conjugate.

The outlet is a clinical measurement made by palpating the distance between the ischial tuberosities. This diameter is shortened when the pubic arch is narrow; therefore, the pubic arch is assessed for curvature of the sacrum and coccyx. This assessment may supply significant information about the overall shape of the pelvis.

Types of Pelves

The variations of the pelvis have been classified by Caldwell and Moloy. The four basic pelvic types are (a) the *gynecoid* or normal female-type pelvis, which is round; (b) the *android* or male-type pelvis, which has a heart-shaped outlet; (c) the *anthropoid*, which has a long anteroposterior outlet; and (d) the *platypelloid*, which has a wide transverse outlet. The gynecoid pelvis is adapted for the function of childbirth. Its inlet, cavity, and outlet are in better proportion; the pubic arch is wide; and the coccyx is more movable than in the android pelvis (Fig. 2–9).

ENDOCRINE SYSTEM AND REPRODUCTION

A woman's reproductive life has a definite beginning and ending: it begins at puberty and ends at menopause. Puberty is when reproduction becomes possible and other events such as breast development, growth of pubic and axillary hair, and menstruation occur. During the female reproductive years, cyclic changes occur in the ovaries and the uterus. These changes can be considered as two interrelated cycles: the menstrual cycle and the ovarian cycle.

Normal Menstrual Cycle

The menstrual cycle is a predictable event that normally occurs monthly. The typical monthly menstrual cycle is influenced by follicle maturation, ovulation, and corpus luteum formation and ends with menstrual bleeding. The changes that occur in the uterus are dependent on the changes occurring simultaneously in the ovaries. In this unique pattern of events, the development of endometrium occurs at the precise time of the month that the ovum develops in maturity.

For convenience, the menstrual cycle may be divided into five phases: the menstrual phase, the proliferative phase, the secretory phase, the ischemic phase, and the menstrual phase again (Fig. 2–10).

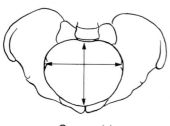

Gynecoid

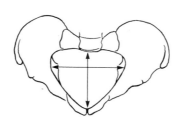

Android

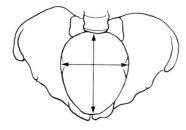

Anthropoid

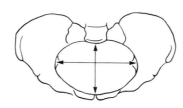

Platypelloid

▲ FIGURE 2–9

Four basic types of pelves (Caldwell-Moloy classification).

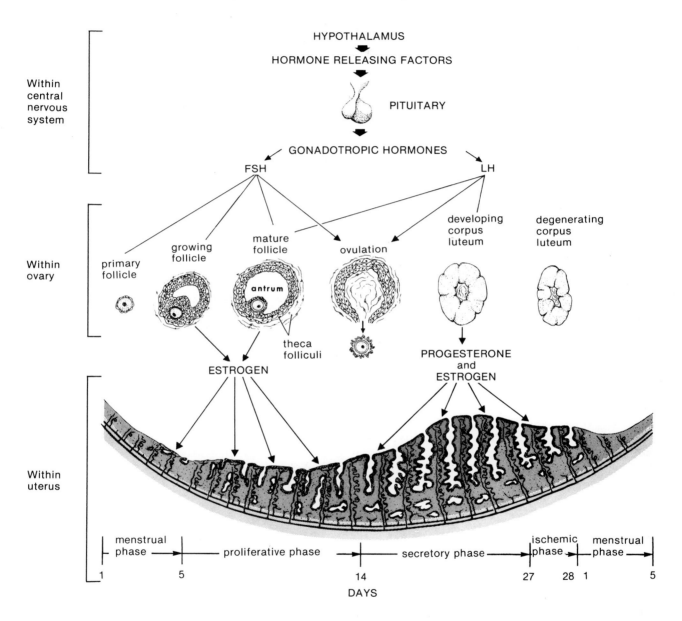

▲ FIGURE 2–10

Female reproductive cycle. FSH, follicle-stimulating hormone; LH, luteinizing hormone. (Adapted from Moore, K. L. (1989). *Before We Are Born,* 3rd ed. Philadelphia, W. B. Saunders Company.)

The *menstrual phase* is counted as 1 to 5 days of the cycle. The first day of menstruation is the beginning of the menstrual cycle. Some of the endometrial cells are sloughed off and discarded, and other cells of the endometrium begin to regenerate. Menstruation typically occurs at 28-day intervals and lasts 3 to 5 days. Estrogen levels are low during this part of the cycle, and the cervical mucus is scanty.

The *proliferative phase* (days 6 to 14) begins when the endometrial cells enlarge. Blood vessels become more prominent and dilated. The endometrium increases in thickness and gradually reaches its peak just before the time of ovulation. The cervical mucus is more prominent as the estrogen level increases. The cervical mucus becomes more watery and alkaline, making the cervical mucosa more favorable to spermatozoa. At ovulation, the mucus is stretchy and forms a ferning pattern. The proliferative phase coincides with the follicular phase of the ovarian cycle.

During the *secretory phase* (days 15 to 26) some estrogen is secreted, but the phase is dominated by progesterone secretion. Progesterone causes the endometrial cells to become thicker, dilated, and tortuous. The coiling of spiral vessels becomes intensified. The endometrial glands (cells) secrete fluids that contain an increased amount of glycogen in preparation for the fertilized ovum.

If fertilization of the ovum does not occur, the *ischemic phase* (days 27 to 28) begins. The corpus luteum begins to degenerate, resulting in a fall in both estrogen and progesterone secretion. Vascular changes occur, including the rupture of small blood vessels and the constriction of spiral arteries, causing a deficiency of blood necessary for the endometrium. Small pools of blood soon form and break through the endometrial surfaces. This indicates the beginning of another menstrual phase.

Ovarian Cycle

The ovarian cycle has two phases: the follicular phase and the luteal phase in a 28-day cycle.

During the *follicular phase* (days 1 to 14) the development of the ovarian follicles occurs. It is influenced by follicle-stimulating hormone (FSH) secreted by the anterior pituitary gland. The function of FSH is to stimulate ovarian follicles to grow, develop, and produce estrogen. Each follicle contains an ovum. Only one ovum is designed to mature fully each month and to leave the ovary. In other words, once a month a mature ovum, called a graafian follicle, produces the midcycle spurt of estrogen that causes luteinizing hormone (LH) to be released from the anterior pituitary gland. The mature ovum then ruptures and is discharged from an ovary. This process is called *ovulation*.

Ovulation usually occurs 14 days before the beginning of the next menstrual cycle. The timing of ovulation is important because the ovum must be fertilized by a sperm within 1 to 2 days after it is expelled from the ovary, if pregnancy is to take place (Fig. 2–11).

The *luteal phase* (days 15 to 28) begins about the 15th day of the cycle. After the rupture of the graafian follicle and the release of the ovum, the cells of the empty follicle become larger and fill with the corpus luteum. Under the influence of LH, the corpus luteum begins to produce increased amounts of estrogen and progesterone. The increased progesterone level suppresses the growth of other follicles in the ovary.

If fertilization of the ovum (conception) does not occur, the size of the corpus luteum decreases. At this time, the LH level becomes so low that it can no longer support the corpus luteum. As the corpus luteum degenerates, its secretion of estrogen and progesterone rapidly decreases. As a result, the endometrium (lining of the uterus) starts to shed, menstrual flow starts, and a new cycle begins (see Fig. 2–10).

FACTS ABOUT THE FEMALE REPRODUCTIVE CYCLE

MENSTRUAL CYCLE

- *Menstrual phase (days 1–5)*

- Menses lasts from 3 to 5 days in a 28-day cycle.

Proliferative phase (days 6–14)

- Estrogen level increases and peaks just before ovulation.
- Cervical mucus becomes favorable to sperm

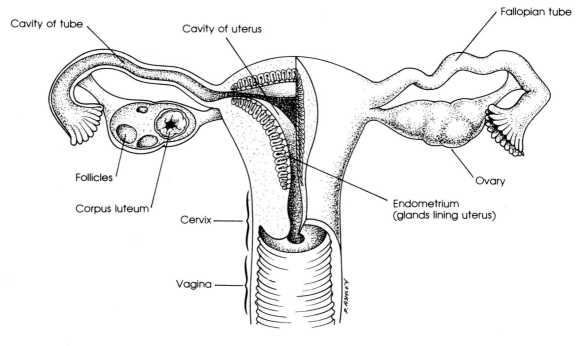

▲ **FIGURE 2–11**

Ovulation: release of the ovum from the follicle.

at time of ovulation: becomes watery and alkaline and shows ferning pattern.
- At time of ovulation basal body temperature rises.

Secretory phase (days 15–26)

- Estrogen is present, but progesterone dominates.

Ischemic phase (days 27–28)

- Corpus luteum degenerates; estrogen and progesterone levels fall.
- Blood breaks through endometrial surfaces, indicating the beginning of another menstrual phase.

OVARIAN CYCLE

- *Follicular phase (days 1–14)*
- Ovum (follicle) develops to maturity.
- This occurs under the influence of FSH and LH.

- The mature ovum ruptures (ovulation) and is expelled.
- Ovulation is triggered by a surge of LH induced by the high level of estrogen.

Luteal phase (days 15–28)

- Corpus luteum develops and produces increased levels of estrogen and progesterone, which suppresses growth of other follicles in the ovary.

The Male Reproductive System

The reproductive system of the male includes the testes, glands, and ducts, which are internal structures, and the penis and scrotum, which are external structures (Fig. 2–12).

1. The sex gland of the male is the testes.
2. The male sex hormone is testosterone.
3. The male sex cell is the sperm.

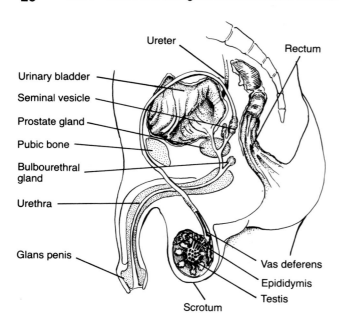

▲ FIGURE 2–12

Male reproductive organs.

EXTERNAL REPRODUCTIVE ORGANS

Penis

The penis is the male organ of copulation, and it is also part of the urinary system. The penis is made up of three columns of erectile tissue covered by thin skin that is freely movable. Two of the columns, the *cavernous bodies,* contain blood spaces, which when empty cause the penis to be limp (flaccid). When psychic or sexual stimulation occurs, these spaces fill with blood, and the penis becomes engorged (swollen), considerably enlarged, and erect. The third column of erectile tissue, the spongy layer, lies beneath the cavernous bodies. Through it passes the urethra from the bladder. The head of the penis is composed of an enlarged portion of spongy tissue, which forms a cap called the *glans penis.* Covering the glans is the loosely fitting skin, called the *prepuce,* or *foreskin.* The foreskin is sometimes removed by circumcision, for hygienic, religious, or cultural reasons.

Scrotum

The scrotum is the pigmented pouch that lies beneath the penis and outside the abdominal cav-

ity. It is divided into two sacs, each sac containing one testis (testicle), the epididymis, and a portion of the spermatic cord. Because the sperm require a temperature slightly lower than body temperature for development and maintenance, when the body temperature is high the muscles of the scrotum relax, dropping the testes away from the body. When exposed to low temperatures the scrotum becomes wrinkled.

INTERNAL REPRODUCTIVE ORGANS

The internal male reproductive organs consist of the testes, epididymis, vas deferens, seminal vesicles, prostate gland, and bulbourethral glands (Cowper's glands). The spermatic cords are internal supporting structures (see Fig. 2–12).

Testes

The testes are two oval-shaped glands about 2 inches long and 1 inch wide. They correspond to the ovaries of the female. Each testis contains specialized tissue arranged in coiled tubes called *seminiferous tubules* where the *spermatozoa* are produced. Between the small tubes is a small group of cells that produce the male sex hormone *testosterone*. This hormone is responsible for the masculine characteristics of the male body. Some of the seminal fluid, or *semen*, in which the spermatozoa (sperm) are transported is also produced in the tubules in the testes.

Epididymis

The testes open into the epididymis, a small coiled tube that is 20 feet long if stretched to its full extent. The mature sperm enter the epididymis, become motile there, and pass through it to reach the vas deferens.

Vas Deferens

The vas deferens, a duct about 18 inches long, is a continuation of the epididymis. It ends by joining the duct of the seminal vesicle to form the ejaculatory duct. The peristaltic activity of the muscles is responsible for the passage of the sperm along the vas deferens to the ejaculatory duct. The vas deferens, the nerves, and the lymphatic and blood vessels form the spermatic cord.

Ejaculatory Duct

The ejaculatory duct is found at the base of the prostate gland and opens into the prostate portion of the urethra. It ejects sperm and seminal fluid into the urethra.

Seminal Vesicles

The seminal vesicles are two sac-like structures at the base of the urinary bladder. Their glandular lining produces a thick, milky secretion that forms much of the ejaculated semen. This secretion is thought to provide nourishment and protection for the sperm. The ducts of the seminal vesicles join the vas deferens to form the ejaculatory ducts, which empty into the urethra.

Prostate Gland

The prostate gland is a chestnut-sized structure that surrounds the urethra, just below the urinary bladder. During ejaculation, it contracts along with the vas deferens and seminal vesicles. It adds a thin, milky, alkaline fluid to the semen. The alkalinity of the fluid is important to fertilization. It helps neutralize the relatively acidic fluid of the vas deferens and the acid of female vaginal secretions. Therefore, it enhances sperm motility and life span.

Bulbourethral Glands (Cowper's Glands)

The bulbourethral glands are about the size of a pea and are situated beneath the prostate gland on each side of the urethra. These glands secrete mucus into the urethra to serve as a lubricant and supply alkaline fluid to the semen.

ENDOCRINE SYSTEM AND REPRODUCTION

As in the female, many changes occur in the male at puberty. At approximately 10 years of age, the testes, prostate gland, seminal vesicles, and penis begin to enlarge as part of the general adolescent growth spurt. Pubic hair, axillary hair, hair on the upper lip, and an enlarged larynx appear. By age 15 years (range 9 to 17), boys are physically able to produce and ejaculate sperm.

Pituitary Gland

During puberty, the pituitary gland begins to release FSH and LH (interstitial cell–stimulating hormones). FSH helps the production of spermatozoa. LH acts on the interstitial cells of Leydig of the testes to release androgens, the most significant of which is testosterone.

Testosterone

Testosterone has several functions. It is responsible for the development of the penis, scrotum,

NURSING CARE PLAN 2–1

NORMAL PHYSIOLOGICAL FUNCTIONS OF THE FEMALE AND MALE REPRODUCTIVE ORGANS

Potential Problems and Nursing Diagnoses

1. Knowledge deficit related to the pattern of hormonal function and development and release of the ovum.

2. Knowledge deficit related to the normal function of the uterus.

3. Knowledge deficit related to physiology of the menstrual cycle.

4. Knowledge deficit related to the close proximity of the vagina to the rectum.

5. Knowledge deficit related to where sperm are produced.

6. Anxiety related to inaccurate perceptions of the functions of female reproductive system.

Nursing Interventions

Explain how the secretion of FSH and LH are necessary for the development and release of the ovum.

Educate patient regarding the physiological functions of the uterus, including its ability to enlarge to meet the demands of the growing fetus.

Educate patient regarding endometrial (uterine lining) changes that occur before menstruation.

Explain the proximity of the vagina to the rectum. Discuss potential contamination and the importance of good female hygiene (stroking downward from the vagina toward the rectum).

Explain that sperm are produced in the male's testes.

Explain the normal functions of the female reproduction system and clarify inaccurate information.

Expected Outcomes

1. Patient demonstrates an understanding of the development and release of the (female) ovum.

2. Patient verbalizes an understanding of the uterus's ability to enlarge to accommodate the growing fetus.

3. Patient demonstrates an understanding of the endometrial changes that occur before menstruation.

4. Patient verbalizes an understanding of why it is important to stroke downward from the vagina toward the rectum to avoid rectal contamination.

5. Patient verbalizes an understanding of where, in the male reproductive system, sperm are produced.

6. Patient identifies some misconceptions in the functions of the female reproductive system.

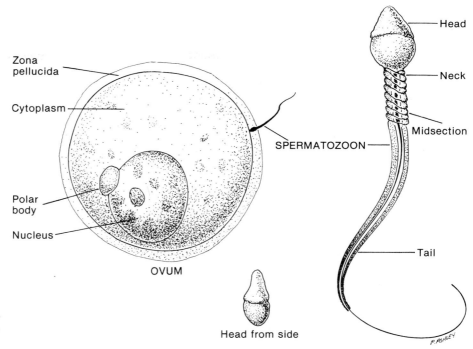

Zona
pellucida

Cytoplasm

Polar
body

Nucleus

OVUM

SPERMATOZOON

Head

Neck

Midsection

Tail

Head from side

P. ASHLEY

▲ **FIGURE 2–13**

Female and male reproduc-
tive cells.

prostate gland, and seminal vesicles. It is essential to the development of male sex characteristics. Under the influence of testosterone, the bones and muscles become thicker and longer. It causes enlargement of the larynx, which results in a lower voice for the male.

Spermatogenesis

The formation of sperm (spermatogenesis) begins at puberty and continues throughout life. A sperm's fertile life is estimated to be 24 to 48 hours. Sperm are much smaller than ova. Sperm cells resemble tadpoles, with oval heads and long tails (Fig. 2–13). During each ejaculation, about 300 million sperm are deposited into the vagina. Only one sperm penetrates and therefore fertilizes the ovum. Immediately after one sperm enters the

ovum, a physiological change takes place in the outer surface of the ovum that prevents entry of additional sperm. Presumably, this change occurs in response to a substance released from the cytoplasm of the ovum.

References

Creasy, B. K., & Resnik, R. (1989). *Maternal-Fetal Medicine: Principles and Practice*, 2nd ed. Philadelphia: W. B. Saunders Company.

Danforth, D. N., & Scott, J. R. (1986). *Obstetrics and Gynecology*, 5th ed. Philadelphia: J. B. Lippincott.

Dickason, E. J., Schult, M. O., & Silverman, B. L. (1990). *Maternal-Infant Nursing Care*. St. Louis: C. V. Mosby.

Fehring, R. J. (1990). Methods used to self-predict ovulation: A comparative study. *Journal of Obstetric, Gynecologic, and Neonatal Nursing* 19:223–237.

Ladewig, P. W., London, M. L., & Olds, S. B. (1990). *Essentials of Maternal-Newborn Nursing*, 2nd ed. Redwood City, CA: Addison-Wesley Nursing.

SUGGESTED ACTIVITIES

1. Using diagrams, explain the function of the female and male reproductive organs.
2. Describe the anatomy of the breasts and their development in preparation for lactation.
3. Explain the processes of menstruation and ovulation.

REVIEW QUESTIONS

A. Select the best answer to each multiple-choice question.

1. The external female reproductive organs include
   A. Vulva
   B. Labia majora and labia minora
   C. Bartholin's glands
   D. All of the above

2. The internal organs of the female include
   A. Uterus, fallopian tubes, and ovaries
   B. Uterus, vagina, and clitoris
   C. Uterus, labia majora, and clitoris
   D. Ovaries, uterus, and Bartholin's glands

3. The female perineum consists of
   A. The area between the vulva and the rectum
   B. The area from the vulva to the urethra
   C. All the structures between the symphysis pubis and the anus
   D. The labia majora and the labia minora

4. Collectively, the external female organs are referred to as the
   A. Labia majora
   B. Clitoris
   C. Cervix
   D. Vulva

5. The release of the mature ovum from the female ovary is called
   A. Menstruation
   B. Primordial follicle
   C. Conception
   D. Ovulation

6. The female organ of sexual excitation is the
   A. Labia minora
   B. Clitoris
   C. Uterus
   D. Vagina

7. The average female menstrual cycle is
   A. 24 days
   B. 28 days
   C. 30 days
   D. 38 days

8. Hormones secreted by the anterior pituitary gland that regulate ovarian activity are
   A. Estrogen and progesterone
   B. Prolactin and progesterone
   C. Follicle-stimulating hormone and luteinizing hormone
   D. Corpus luteum and estrogen

9. Vaginal menstrual bleeding lasts
   A. 3 days
   B. 3 to 5 days
   C. 3 to 7 days
   D. 7 to 10 days

10. The size of breasts
    A. Indicates the amount of milk that can be produced
    B. Has no relationship to the amount of milk produced
    C. Mainly is due to an increase in connective tissue
    D. Is due to the large number of acini cells

11. The male internal reproductive organs include
    A. Scrotum and testicles
    B. Vas deferens and epididymis
    C. Glans penis and testicles
    D. Prepuce and glans penis

12. The sex hormone responsible for male sex characteristics is
    A. Prolactin
    B. Testosterone
    C. Estrogen
    D. Progesterone

13. Compared with the female ova, the male spermatozoa are
    A. Much larger
    B. About the same size
    C. Much smaller
    D. A little smaller

14. The number of spermatozoa deposited into the vagina at each ejaculation is
    A. 1
    B. 100,000
    C. 300,000
    D. 300 million

15. The number of spermatozoa that penetrate and fertilize the ovum is
    A. 1
    B. 2 to 5
    C. 5 to 10
    D. 10 to 15

16. The female clitoris is composed of erectile tissue, as is found in which male organ?
    A. Scrotum
    B. Penis
    C. Vas deferens
    D. Epididymis

17. A mature ovum, called a graafian follicle, is released from the ovary by an increase in the pituitary hormone called
    A. Follicle-stimulating hormone (FSH)
    B. Prolactin
    C. Luteinizing hormone (LH)
    D. Progesterone

18. A clinical measurement of the pelvis to ascertain its adequacy is
    A. Measurement of the diagonal conjugate
    B. Measurement of the midpelvis
    C. Measurement of the ischial spines
    D. None of the above

19. There are four basic types of pelves, and the significance of comparing them is that the female-type pelvis is most adapted for childbirth. The female type is called
    A. Android pelvis
    B. Platypelloid pelvis
    C. Gynecoid pelvis
    D. Anthropoid pelvis

B. Choose from Column II the phrase that most accurately defines the term in Column I.

I

  1. Acini cells _____
  2. Fundus _____
  3. Testes _____
  4. Testosterone _____
  5. Fertilization _____
  6. Fallopian tube _____
  7. True pelvis _____
  8. Areola _____
  9. Endometrium _____
 10. Prostate gland _____
 11. Montgomery's tubercles _____

II

A. Sex hormone responsible for male sex characteristics
B. Secrete substance to lubricate nipples during infant suckling
C. Upper part of the uterus
D. Mucous-membrane lining of the uterus
E. Correspond to ovaries in female
F. Secretes a thin, milky, and alkaline fluid during ejaculation
G. Pigmented area around nipple
H. Place where union of sperm and ovum occurs
I. Area fetus must pass during birth
J. Milk-producing cells of the alveoli of breasts
K. Union of sperm and ovum

CHAPTER 3

Chapter Outline

Sexual Roles at Life Stages
    Prenatal sex roles
    Sex roles in infancy
    Sex roles during preschool years
    Sex roles during preadolescence
    Sexual behavior during adolescence
Sexual Response of the Male
    Male sexual response cycle
Sexual Response of the Female
    Female sexual response cycle
Problems That Affect Female Sexuality
    Vaginismus
    Dyspareunia
    Aging
Infertility
    Infertility in the female
    Infertility in the male
Implications for Nurses

Learning Objectives

Upon completion of Chapter 3, the student should be able to
- Explain sexual roles at different life stages.
- Describe adolescent behavior and sexuality.
- Describe the male sexual response cycle.
- Describe the female sexual response cycle.
- Explain female infertility.
- Explain male infertility.
- Identify problems encountered in female sexuality.
- Discuss nursing assessment of human sexuality.

Human Sexuality

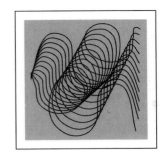

An individual's sense of identity, or self-image, changes throughout life. Therefore, a person's awareness of his or her body is quite different during childhood, preadolescence, adolescence, early adulthood, late adulthood, and old age. Sexuality is one of the most important determinants of human behavior. Many, if not most, aspects of sexual life are determined by values, customs, attitudes, and sexual drives. Although expressions of sexual behavior are molded by personality, they are also modified by hormones.

Discussing views of sexuality is often difficult because many people regard sexuality as something that should not be discussed. In the 1950s, Kinsey and his associates described many sexual practices. In 1966, Masters and Johnson elaborated on sexual needs. Some of their findings are mentioned in this chapter.

Sexual Roles at Life Stages

PRENATAL SEX ROLES

Biological sex in an individual is established at the moment of conception. At about 12 weeks, male and female external genitalia are differentiated. The male embryo develops testes that secrete testosterone, which determines "maleness." The female embryo develops ovaries that are hormonally less active during fetal life than after birth. Later, the sexual behavior of the female is influenced mainly by ovarian hormones—estrogen and progesterone—that affect psyche and sexual behavior.

SEX ROLES IN INFANCY

Infancy is filled with experiences that make the body aware of pleasure. Infants are frequently observed touching and exploring their bodies. They also learn to be comfortable in doing so. An infant's positive experiences are reinforced when parents are comfortable with and accept them.

SEX ROLES DURING PRESCHOOL YEARS

During the preschool years, the child's sexual identity (image) is important to his or her development. Practically speaking, sexual identity is accomplished by absorbing life-styles, attitudes, and mannerisms of people who surround the child. The child's experiences with adults and with other children and the child's feelings about lasting relationships with a member of the opposite sex are very significant.

SEX ROLES DURING PREADOLESCENCE

The preadolescent tends to like to play with other preadolescents of the same sex before interacting comfortably with preadolescents of the opposite sex. Sexual identification usually progresses more smoothly and the child tends to feel more secure when both mother and father (or significant other) are kind, loving people.

If one parent does not have a high degree of nurturing capacity, it may be difficult for the child to identify with that parent. This may perpetuate a poor parent role model. If the male maintains a passive role as a father, relinquishing authority to a more assertive or aggressive mother, the son may have difficulty identifying with the father. In this instance, the female's more assertive, aggressive, and decisive role may be more appealing to the son.

According to the results of Kinsey's studies, 25% of each sex has experienced homosexual or heterosexual play by the age of 12 years. About three-fourths of boys experience orgasm through masturbation before puberty. Homosexual play in childhood, however, does not appear to be associated with the development of homosexuality in adulthood.

During later childhood, further steps lead to heterosexuality: emotional attachment to some member of the opposite sex, preference for companionship of the opposite sex, and, finally, dating the opposite sex. By the time of puberty, heterosexuality usually is well established.

SEXUAL BEHAVIOR DURING ADOLESCENCE

During early adolescence, it is common for young people to have strong ties to members of their own sex. Adolescents are trying to understand who they are before they are ready to interact with individuals of the opposite sex.

Later, increased sexual drives become obvious and difficult to control. Self-understanding through education and role models is important during this period.

For young men, ejaculation serves as a symbol of sexual maturity; menstruation does the same for young women. The frequent erections of the penis in the male adolescent may embarrass him. Masturbation is frequently a source of sexual release, although it may provoke guilt and anxiety. The frequency of masturbation is much lower in females than in males. At this time, society encourages females to be sexually stimulated by the opposite sex and not to act on their own sexual desires and needs.

Petting is the common form of sexual behavior during late adolescence. During the adolescent period, boy–girl relationships are generally encouraged by their peers. Frequently, these relationships lead to heavy petting and sexual intercourse. Because many adolescent girls do not use birth control measures, they become pregnant.

Possible reasons why adolescents do not use birth control include a failure to believe they might get pregnant, lack of knowledge about the methods, disapproval by their family, and lack of resources.

Society is ambivalent about offering contraceptive advice to adolescents because of a fear that this will appear as approval of premarital coitus. Yet society, in general, does not approve of adolescent pregnancies. Health care professionals must learn to discuss sexuality with teenagers and must be aware of the intense pressure placed on adolescents to become sexually active against their own judgment and wishes. Adolescents should be well informed about the chances of impregnation during sexual intercourse and about the responsibilities that come with pregnancy. Adolescents should also be informed about the risk of contracting sexually transmitted diseases through sexual activity.

Sexual Response of the Male

Sexual arousal in males may be due to a variety of stimuli, such as verbal, tactile, visual, olfactory, or lingual, and is often accompanied by some degree of sexual fantasy. Nerve impulses causing greater blood supply to the penis result in an erection. Continued stimulation of the glans penis produces an increased accumulation of nerve impulses. At this point, ejaculation becomes inevitable; muscles then contract, which causes a discharge of semen, accompanied by a general as well as local pleasurable sensation referred to as the orgasm.

There is considerable variation in the threshold at which the ejaculatory event occurs. This is true among individuals and for the same individual at different times. If the male threshold is low, for a variety of possible reasons, premature ejaculation may occur. When premature ejaculation persists, impotence or the inability to achieve or sustain an erection may result. Impotence is often due to psychological causes. Also, it can be caused by some organic condition. The finding of impotence is increased in many men as they get older, particularly in those over 60 years of age. In addition, it can be related to some medications. The majority of men, however, retain sexual ability through old age.

MALE SEXUAL RESPONSE CYCLE

The response to sexual stimulation, identified by Masters and Johnson, follows a pattern of four phases: excitement, plateau, orgasm, and resolution (Fig. 3–1).

Excitement Phase

The excitement phase develops from a source of physical or mental stimulation. The penis responds first to higher centers in the brain and then to reflex nerves in the spinal cord. Vasocongestion occurs in the blood spaces of the penile shaft. This response causes an enlargement and erection of the penis and an elevation of the testes. The muscles of the hands, feet, and rectum may contract, which is frequently followed by a generalized body flush or rash called the "sex flush." The heart rate, respiratory rate, and blood pressure rise. Diversion by fear, loud noises, and other psychosensory stimuli may interfere with erection. Some men are more sensitive to distractions during this phase than others.

Plateau Phase

The plateau phase is reached just before orgasm. A high level of sexual tension is maintained during the plateau phase. Full distention of the penis occurs by continued vasocongestion (increased blood supply to the penis). Heart rate, respiratory rate, and blood pressure continue to increase.

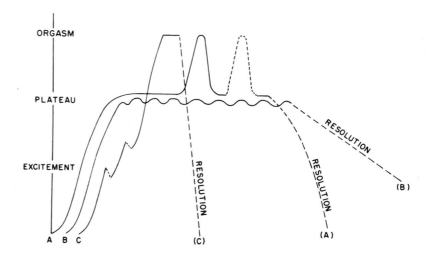

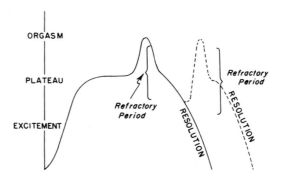

▲ FIGURE 3–1

Top. Cycle of female sexual response. A. Reaction pattern with single or multiple orgasms. B. Reaction pattern without orgasm. C. Reaction pattern without distinct plateau. **Bottom.** Cycle of male sexual response. (From Masters, W. H., & Johnson, V. E. (1966). *Human Sexual Response*, Boston, Little, Brown.)

Some men learn to prolong this phase for the purpose of enjoyment.

Orgasmic Phase

The orgasmic phase develops involuntarily from the recurring contractions of the muscles of the penis and deep perineum, causing a forceful ejaculation of seminal fluid in three or four contractions. These contractions may be followed by some minor, irregular contractions felt by the male as pleasurable sensations.

Resolution Phase

The resolution phase usually occurs in two stages. In the initial stage, called the refractory period, the penis reduces 50% in size. During the state of resolution, the external and internal organs return to a latent state. For both males and females, the four phases of the sexual response take about 30 minutes.

Sexual Response of the Female

The achievement of a satisfactory experience, including orgasm, during sexual intercourse is to a large extent a learned behavior, and, unlike the inevitable ejaculatory response of the male, the response of the female is easily inhibited by emotional, physical, and environmental influences. In other words, the woman's sexual attitudes, state of well-being, and cultural background, as well as the behavior of her sexual partner, all play a role in her achieving all four phases of sexual activity. Under ideal circumstances, the sexual capacity of the female is greater than that of the male. With continued stimulation, multiple orgasms are common in many women. Females can maintain the capacity for sexual response through old age.

The failure of a woman to achieve sexual arousal is somewhat misunderstood, because essentially any woman can be brought to the orgasm phase with effective and appropriate stimulation.

FEMALE SEXUAL RESPONSE CYCLE

The female sexual response follows the same typical pattern as the male's four phases: excitement, plateau, orgasm, and resolution (see Fig. 3–1).

Excitement Phase

The excitement phase develops from physical and psychic stimulation. Vasocongestion causes the clitoris to increase in size. Also, blood supply to the labia minora and labia majora increases. Discoloration of the labia occurs. A mucoid fluid appears on the vaginal walls as lubrication. The nipples become erect, and the breasts may enlarge slightly. There are elevations in heart rate, respiratory rate, and blood pressure.

Plateau Phase

During the plateau phase, the female clitoris swells and retracts under the clitoral sheath; the lower part of the vagina enlarges and lengthens. The uterus draws up in a "tenting effect" that produces additional space near the cervix. Sudden skin redness or the "sex flush" appears. These changes are pleasurable sensations to the woman.

Orgasmic Phase

At the time of orgasm, there is a vigorous contraction of muscles in the pelvic area. The uterus contracts strongly, and the clitoris, vagina, and rectum pulsate rhythmically. Respiration and heart rates continue to rise, and there may be widespread perspiration. During this phase, the woman experiences the peak of her pleasurable sensations.

Some women need to be more assertive about what gives pleasure to them and what turns them off. A sex history, identification of the cause, and education of the couple are important steps in the management of the problem of a woman's inability to have an orgasm. Early social and cultural training that establishes inhibition toward sex can be the cause. With the alleviation of anxiety, anger, and guilt, a high percentage of women become orgasmic (able to have an orgasm).

Resolution Phase

As the resolution phase proceeds, the uterus relaxes. This relaxation allows the cervix to dip into the pool of seminal fluid deposited by the male. During the resolution phase, the external and internal genital organs return to a latent state. The woman usually feels very relaxed and contented. Often, she will have the desire to sleep.

Problems That Affect Female Sexuality

VAGINISMUS

Vaginismus is usually a psychophysical condition in which the muscles surrounding the vagina become spastic and involuntarily contract, closing the vagina and thus preventing penile entrance. This condition may be the result of fear of childbirth, painful intercourse, or deep anger toward the partner.

If there is pain caused by scar tissue, surgery may be indicated. More frequently, however, the treatment consists only of educating the couple and decreasing anxiety.

Another approach involves introducing probes of graduated sizes into the vagina until it is sufficiently dilated to make the entrance of the penis possible.

DYSPAREUNIA

Dyspareunia, or painful sexual intercourse, may occur for many reasons, including infection, vaginal scarring, clitoral irritation, insufficient vaginal lubrication, fatigue, and fear or other psychological problems. The problems should be corrected with appropriate treatment.

AGING

Aging does cause specific changes in the female sexual response cycle, but it does not necessarily impair it. In general, each phase of the sexual response is slowed in the older woman. There is less vaginal lubrication, vasocongestion, and tension. The clitoris will continue to function as a transformer of impulses, and there seems to be little or no reduction in sensitivity. The changes in the female coincide with menopause.

In the male, the sexual drive usually diminishes after 60 years of age. There is a steady increase in the appearance of relative impotence (inability to maintain an erection) after the age of 50 years. The majority of men retain some sexual responses throughout old age.

Infertility

Any couple who seeks medical assistance to accomplish pregnancy deserves attention, regardless of the duration or potential extent of the problem. Not all such couples require a full-scale assessment. Anxiety about inability to become pregnant, rather than physical reasons, may be the only problem. As a general rule, a more detailed infertility study may be deferred until after 1 year of ordinary effort to achieve pregnancy. According to the American Fertility Society, a couple in the childbearing age group that has unprotected intercourse for a period of 1 year and does not conceive may be considered infertile. For this couple, an infertility examination is appropriate.

An important part of nursing care for the infertile couple is emphasizing and teaching self-care. Stress reduction techniques, such as exercise and relaxation techniques, may be helpful. Also, the couple should be encouraged to maintain or improve their overall health. The caregiver should realize that couples who want to bear children need support and education in their decision making. The nurse must be able to listen to the couple's feelings and acknowledge their sensitivity to and perhaps anger at the perceived loss of the childbearing capacity.

INFERTILITY IN THE FEMALE

Before medical tests are performed, the woman as well as the man should have a thorough history taken and a thorough physical examination performed. The woman's history should include her age, age at menarche (start of menstruation), and any menstrual and gynecological disorders. Present illnesses should also be included. Laboratory tests such as blood count, serology, urinalysis, and thyroid function should be included. The couple should be interviewed together and separately regarding their pattern of sexual behavior. Attitudes toward sexual intercourse may be determined during these interviews.

The causes of female infertility are as follows:

- Ovarian function is abnormal.
- The uterus does not prepare for implantation.
- Cervical mucus is unfavorable to sperm transport.
- Tubes are obstructed.
- Tubal function is abnormal (tubes are unable to transport ovum to uterus).

Anovulatory cycles are present in approximately 15% to 29% of infertile women. This is mainly associated with below-normal levels of the hormones necessary for the ova to mature. When these levels are below normal, an anovulatory cycle or infrequent ovulation results. Drugs such as clomiphene citrate (Clomid) may be prescribed to stimulate the secretion of follicle-stimulating hormone and luteinizing hormone (LH), hormones necessary for ovulation (see Appendix on Drugs). "Fertility drugs" occasionally produce multiple births, such as twins and triplets.

Endometrial biopsies are done to assess the influence of progesterone on the uterus. An inadequate progesterone level results in an inadequate luteal phase. This causes a lack of endometrial preparation (the uterine lining does not build up) for the ovum to implant in the uterus. Estrogen assay, midcycle measurement of estrogen at time of ovulation, and LH assay to determine the time of ovulation are diagnostic tests used to assess endometrial changes.

The changes in cervical mucus are important in infertility assessment. Cervical mucus is receptive to spermatozoa at or near the time of ovulation and impedes their penetration at other times. The cervix and its mucus also act as a sperm reservoir and protect the sperm cells from the hostile environment in the vagina. The principal constituent of cervical mucus is a carbohydrate-rich glycoprotein of the mucus, which is an indirect indication of estrogen production. This causes a *ferning* pattern seen in the ovulatory period. To be receptive to the sperm, the cervical mucus must be clear, thin, watery, and profuse. The spinnbarkheit test assesses the consistency and fern-like pattern of the cervical mucus (see Chapter 15).

A basic test of ovulatory function is the *basal body temperature* (BBT) recording, which aids in the identification of the occurrence of ovulation. The woman should record her BBT at the bedside immediately upon awakening. When ovulation occurs, there is a surge of LH, stimulating the corpus luteum to produce progesterone which causes a slight rise (0.5°C to 1.0°C) in the BBT. Progesterone is thermogenic, leading to a slight temperature increase during the second half of the menstrual cycle. The BBT provides an indirect indication of whether the luteal phase is adequate for maintenance of the uterine lining should implantation occur (see Fig. 15–4).

Pathological findings in the uterus, ovarian tubes, and ovaries are significant. Congenital deformities, tumors, endometriosis, and an incompetent cervix (a dilated internal cervical os) all may prevent development of the ovum, implantation of the ovum, or the ability to keep the fetus in the uterus. Ultrasonography is used to detect abnormalities.

A major cause of infertility in the female is tubal blockage caused by congenital defects or adhesions formed from infection or surgery. The Rubin test is used to assess for tubal blockage. Tubal blockage is diagnosed using carbon dioxide insufflation, in which gas is injected into the uterus to see if the tubes are open. If the tubes are open, the gas will pass into the abdominal cavity, and the woman will feel shoulder pain due to the irritation of gas against her diaphragm. Because the Rubin test has a relatively high rate of false-negative and false-positive results, its use has diminished. Hysterosalpingography, a fluoroscopy examination that assesses tubal patency, is frequently used. It is performed immediately after menstruation and in the absence of infection.

Surgical treatment (tuboplasty) is indicated only when other causes of infertility have been ruled out. Microsurgical techniques for tubal pathology are improving and are used with limited success.

The success depends on the extent of the tubal abnormality (see Chapter 15).

In spite of medical advances in the treatment of infertility, 5% to 10% of all couples who are medically healthy remain childless. These couples may choose in vitro fertilization. This method involves aspirating ripe ovarian follicles during a laparoscopy and fertilizing the egg with the male partner's semen. The fertilized egg is then placed in the woman's uterus to grow and develop into a viable fetus. Ethical and religious problems surround in vitro fertilization, and the method is costly. It is therefore unlikely to become a common procedure for all women who are infertile.

INFERTILITY IN THE MALE

The man, like the woman, should have a complete physical examination. This examination would include an assessment of the male genital organs for abnormalities.

Semen Analysis

The most common factors in male infertility are sperm production, motility, and basic structure. The male must be able to produce healthy, motile sperm in sufficient quantity and quality. In many instances the cause of infertility is a low sperm count or deficiency. Infertility in men is defined as a sperm count of less than 60 million/mL with inactive or irregular sperm or semen. Also, when the semen does not contain sufficient amounts of the enzyme that acts to dissolve the corona radiata, a layer of cells surrounding the ovum, the penetration of the sperm into the ovum is prevented. A low or absent sperm count can be caused by

NURSING CARE PLAN 3–1
HUMAN SEXUALITY

Potential Problems and Nursing Diagnoses	Nursing Intervention
1. Knowledge deficit related to sexual behavior at different stages of life.	Explain common sexual behavior during infancy, preschool, preadolescent, adolescent, and adult life.
2. Knowledge deficit related to the sexual response cycle.	Explain the physiological changes that occur during the four phases of the sexual response cycle for both the male and female. Explore patient's deficit in knowledge regarding sexuality.
3. Sexual dysfunction related to sexual concerns.	Provide a climate in which patient can openly discuss his or her sexual concerns. Encourage patient to describe any sexual problems (e.g., vaginismus, dyspareunia, or aging).
4. Anxiety related to infertility.	Provide a climate in which patient can openly express his or her concerns about infertility. Use terminology the patient understands in discussing factors that can cause infertility.

Expected Outcomes
1. Patient verbalizes an understanding about sexual behavior at different stages of life.
2. Patient verbalizes increased knowledge about human sexuality.
3. Patient identifies personal sexual conflicts.
4. Patient identifies and discusses specific concerns about infertility.

increased temperature, as occurs in males with undescended testicles or in males whose employment requires long exposure to high temperature.

It is preferable for semen collection to be performed after 2 to 5 days' abstinence from intercourse. If possible, semen should be collected in a wide-mouth container by either masturbation or coitus interruptus. A condom should not be used for semen collection, because most condoms are treated with spermicidal chemicals that interfere with sperm viability. The specimen should be kept at room or body temperature and examined within 1 hour.

Implications for Nurses

Because human sexuality is an important part of life from birth to death, questions about sexual behavior, sexual inhibitions, and sexual education should be of concern to nurses.

Nurses will first need to feel secure about their own sexuality before giving advice to patients. Understanding sexual values, attitudes, cultural factors, misconceptions, and myths facilitates a fuller knowledge of the sexual behavior of males and females. Sexual history should be part of the health history taken by medical and nursing personnel. Whenever appropriate, nurses should include instruction about human sexuality as part of a patient's care plan (see Nursing Care Plan 3–1). It is advisable to include instruction about sexually transmitted diseases when discussing human sexuality. Prevention of sexually transmitted diseases is of utmost importance to all people, but particularly those in the reproductive age group.

References

Fogel, C. I., & Lauver, D. (1990). *Sexual Health Promotion.* Philadelphia: W. B. Saunders Company.

Ladewig, P. W., London, M. L., & Olds, S. B. (1990). *Essentials of Maternal-Newborn Nursing,* 2nd ed. Redwood City, CA: Addison-Wesley Nursing.

Lowry, L. W., & McGinnis, D. G. (1989). Intergenerational education in human sexuality. *American Journal of Maternal-Child Nursing* 14:341–345.

Masters, W. H., & Johnson, V. E. (1966). *Human Sexual Response.* Boston: Little, Brown.

Starn, J., & Paperny, D. M. (1990). Computer games to enhance adolescent sex education. *American Journal of Maternal-Child Nursing* 15:250–253.

SUGGESTED ACTIVITIES

1. Describe, in writing, the development of an individual's sexual roles from infancy through adulthood.
2. Explain the female and male basic sexual responses that occur during coitus.
3. List three factors that adversely affect female sexuality.

REVIEW QUESTIONS

A. Select the best answer to each multiple-choice question.

1. The order of sexual response, according to Masters and Johnson, is as follows:
   A. Resolution, excitement, plateau, orgasm
   B. Excitement, orgasm, plateau, resolution
   C. Resolution, excitement, orgasm, plateau
   D. Excitement, plateau, orgasm, resolution

2. *Dyspareunia* is a term that refers to
   A. Painful intercourse
   B. Vaginismus
   C. Infertility
   D. Vasocongestion

3. The changes in cervical mucus are important in an infertility assessment. The cervical mucus is most receptive to the sperm at the time of ovulation when it
   A. Has a fern-like pattern
   B. Has an oval pattern
   C. Is thick and yellow
   D. Is scant and watery

4. The major cause(s) of female infertility is/are
   A. Abnormal ovarian function
   B. Cervical mucus unfavorable to sperm transport
   C. Tubal obstruction
   D. All of the above

B. Choose from Column II the phrase that most accurately defines the terms in Column I.

I	*II*
1. Preadolescent _____	A. Surge in the sex drive
2. Adolescent _____	B. Tends to play with same sex
3. Dyspareunia _____	C. Surgical severance of vas deferens
4. Vaginismus _____	D. Involuntary muscle contraction of surrounding muscles of vagina
5. Infertility _____	E. Painful coitus
6. Vasectomy _____	F. Inability to produce offspring

C. Choose from Column II the female sexual response that most accurately defines the terms in Column I.

I	*II*
1. Excitement phase _____	A. Uterus relaxes and external organs return to quiet state.
2. Plateau phase _____	B. Clitoris swells and retracts. Sudden skin flush occurs.
3. Orgasmic phase _____	C. Vigorous contraction of muscles in pelvic area. Rhythmic contraction of uterus, clitoris, and vagina.
4. Resolution phase _____	D. Vasocongestion causing clitoris to increase in size. Mucoid fluid lubricates vaginal walls and nipples become erect.

D. Choose from Column II the male sexual response that most accurately defines the terms in Column I.

I	*II*
1. Excitement phase _____	A. Penis reduces in size and internal organs return to latent state.
2. Plateau phase _____	B. Recurring contractions of muscles of penis occur, causing a forceful ejaculation.
3. Orgasmic phase _____	C. Vasocongestion occurs, causing enlargement and erection of penis.
4. Resolution phase _____	D. Full distention of penis occurs, with increased heart rate and respiratory rate.

UNIT II

DEVELOPMENT OF THE BABY

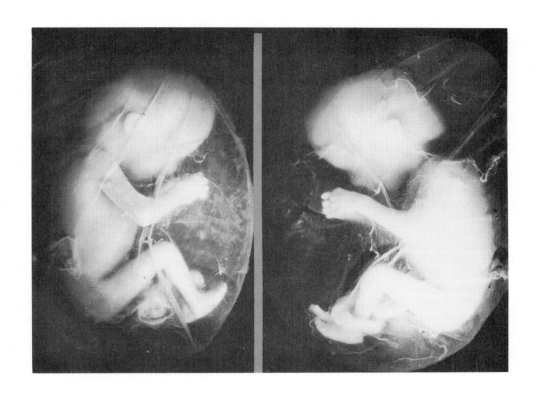

CHAPTER 4

Chapter Outline

Progressive Development of the Embryo and Fetus
    Genetic development
    Fertilization
    Implantation
    Multiple pregnancy
    Fetal membranes and amniotic fluid
    Placenta
    Umbilical cord
Circulation
    Embryonic circulation
    Fetal circulation
    Circulatory changes after birth
Development of the Embryo/Fetus
Function of Fetal Systems
    Circulatory system
    Respiratory system
    Endocrine system
    Gastrointestinal system

Learning Objectives

Upon completion of Chapter 4, the student should be able to

- Identify the number of chromosomes in each human body cell.
- Explain when and how the sex of an individual is determined.
- Describe what happens to the ovum after fertilization.
- Describe how and where implantation takes place.
- List four of the functions of the amniotic fluid.
- Identify the placenta and its functions.
- Describe the makeup of the umbilical cord.
- Describe fetal circulation and name three unique fetal circulatory structures.
- Compare the differences between fetal circulation and circulation after birth.
- Compare the appearance of the fetus at various stages of development.
- State that time period when the fetus is most vulnerable to congenital malformations.
- Describe the sequence of development of the fetal systems.
- Describe when and why the fetus is able to exist outside the uterus.

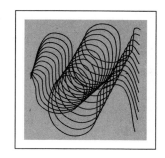

FETAL DEVELOPMENT

Progressive Development of the Embryo and Fetus

At birth, the human body consists of many millions of cells; however, early in development, an individual consists of only one cell, a fertilized ovum containing the individual's blueprint for characteristics such as the color of eyes, hair, and skin.

GENETIC DEVELOPMENT

Each body cell contains within its nucleus specific particles called *chromosomes* (Fig. 4–1). Within these chromosomes are minute structures called *genes*. Genes are the basic unit of heredity. They contain long, chain-like molecules called DNA (deoxyribonucleic acid) and RNA (ribonucleic acid), which carry all the information needed to build each individual cell of the body. Each gene carries a specific trait, that is, each gene is coded for a specific trait, such as blue eyes or black hair.

There are two types of cells within the human body: (a) somatic cells, which are found throughout the body (for example, eye, nerve, and fingernail), and (b) germ or sex cells (gametes). Sex cells are formed in the male and female gonads. The gametes do not mature until puberty.

Chromosomes

The human body cells normally contain 46 chromosomes, or 23 pairs of chromosomes. Of the 46 chromosomes, 44 (22 pairs) are autosomes (or body chromosomes) and 2 (1 pair) are sex chromosomes. In the female, the two sex chromosomes are alike and are designated as XX. In the male, the two sex chromosomes differ in size and shape

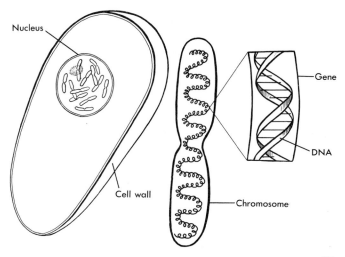

▲ FIGURE 4–1

Chromosomes within the nucleus of a cell.

and are known as XY. The Y chromosome is slightly smaller than the X chromosome.

The number of chromosomes in body cells stays at 46, even though the cells are constantly replacing themselves by the process of division called *mitosis*. Mitosis is preceded by exact duplication of the DNA content in the nucleus, so that the two cells that result from the division will contain the same number and kinds of chromosomes that the one cell contained before dividing.

In the production of germ cells, a different process, called *meiosis*, or *reduction division*, occurs. During meiosis, the number of chromosomes in ova and sperm is reduced to half of 46, or 23 chromosomes (Fig. 4–2). Traits are inherited from both parents, because each sex cell carries half of the chromosomes. If the number of chromosomes in the ovum and sperm did not reduce by half, the new cell resulting from fertilization would have 92 chromosomes, 46 from the sperm and 46 from the ovum. This would not be a normal number of chromosomes.

Sperm and Ova

The schedule for human sex cell formation differs between the two sexes. Spermatozoa production begins at puberty and continues throughout a male's lifetime. Thus, sperm cells are produced continuously and in plentiful supply.

The female, however, is born with all of the cell structures in the ovary from which ova are formed; these structures are called oogonia. At birth, oogonia have begun the first division of meiosis, at which time they are called *oocytes*. The meiotic process is suspended between the time of birth and the time of each ovulation. At the time of ovulation, usually one ovum develops to maturity or is ''ripe.''

Each *spermatogonium* (cell that originates in the male seminal tubule and divides into sperm) produces four functioning sperm. Each oogonium produces only one mature ovum and three smaller structures called *polar bodies*, which have no function and disintegrate during meiosis. The number of sperm produced far exceeds the number of ova produced.

The second meiotic division, which is mitotic in type, occurs after the ovum is in the fallopian tube and is completed after the sperm has penetrated the ovum. The fertilized ovum (when sperm and ovum have fused) is called the *zygote*.

FERTILIZATION

Fertilization usually takes place in the outer one third of the fallopian tube. Approximately 300 million spermatozoa are deposited into the vagina at ejaculation, and many of these make their way up the uterus to the fallopian tube. At this time,

MEIOSIS

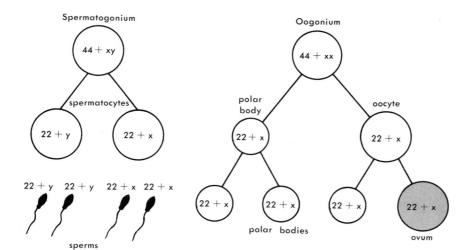

▲ **FIGURE 4–2**

Diagram of meiosis, or cell division of the sex cells, which reduces the number of chromosomes in sperm and ovum by one-half.

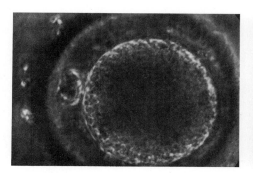
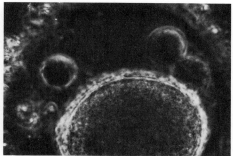

▲ **FIGURE 4–3**

Left. Living human ova with first polar body lying in space (beginning to subdivide). **Right.** Ripe ova, said to be artificially fertilized and showing all three polar bodies; unsuccessful spermatozoa can be seen. (From Arey, L. B. (1974). *Developmental Anatomy*, 7th ed. Philadelphia, W. B. Saunders Company.)

the ovum that the sperm will encounter is surrounded by a membrane called the *corona radiata*. It is assumed that before fertilization can take place, this membrane must be dissolved. This task appears to be accomplished by the enzyme *hyaluronidase*, which is secreted by the multitude of sperm swarming around the ovum. After a single sperm enters the ovum, a chemical signal that seems to warn "no further admittance" prevents the entry of more sperm (Fig. 4–3).

The ovum is able to be fertilized for about 24 to 48 hours after extrusion from the ovary, whereas the sperm is capable of fertilizing the ovum for longer than 48 hours after entering the female genital tract.

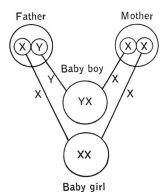

▲ **FIGURE 4–4**

Sex determination at the time of conception.

Sex Determination

The twenty-third pair of chromosomes is the sex chromosome, either XX (female) or XY (male). The sex of an individual is determined by the type of spermatozoa that fertilizes the ovum. Fertilization by an X-bearing sperm produces an XX zygote, which develops into a female. Fertilization by a Y-bearing sperm produces a XY zygote, which develops into a male (Fig. 4–4). Hence, it is the father rather than the mother whose gamete determines the sex of the embryo.

IMPLANTATION

The ovum is fertilized in the outer one third of the fallopian tube. At fertilization, the nucleus of the sperm and the nucleus of the ovum fuse into a single nucleus. The fertilized ovum then begins a series of divisions while traveling down the tube toward the uterus. The *blastocyst*, as the fertilized ovum is now called, does not increase in bulk during this period but simply divides into two cells, then four, then eight, and so on. By the time it reaches the uterus, the blastocyst consists of 16 or more cells. These cells, referred to as the *morula* because they resemble a mulberry, will have differentiated into two types. The inner mass consists of embryonic cells (and later becomes the embryo), and the outer layer is the *trophoblast*, which later contributes to the formation of the placenta. About

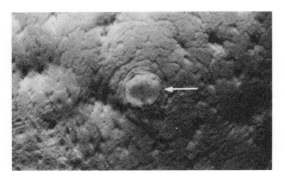

▲ FIGURE 4–5

Photograph of the endometrial surface showing implantation of a human embryo of about 12 days; the implanted conceptus causes a small elevation (arrow). (From Hertig, A. T., & Rock, J. (1941). *Contributions to Embryology, 29:*127. Carnegie Institution, Washington, D.C.)

the fifth day after fertilization, the trophoblast attaches itself to the endometrium (lining of the uterus) (Fig. 4–5). This process is called *implantation*. Normally, the implantation site is in the upper portion of the uterus.

The cells of the trophoblast secrete certain enzymes that permit them to invade the prepared endometrium (during pregnancy, the endometrium is referred to as decidua). During implantation, trophoblastic cells provide nutrition for the embryo from nutrients carried in the maternal blood.

While on its way to the uterine cavity, the unattached blastocyst is immune to many factors. In contrast, during the stages of development that immediately follow implantation, the embryo is extremely sensitive. Thus, after implantation, ter-atogenic agents (drugs, viruses, and radiation) may exert profound effects on the embryo.

From the time of implantation until the eighth week of development, this new human being is called an *embryo*. From the eighth week until birth, it is called the *fetus*.

MULTIPLE PREGNANCY

A multiple pregnancy is one in which more than one fetus develops in the uterine cavity at the same time. When twins result from the splitting of one fertilized egg, they are called identical twins. If two ova are fertilized by two sperm, fraternal, or nonidentical, twins will result (Fig. 4–6). The use of fertility drugs has increased the incidence of multiple pregnancy (twins, triplets, and quadruplets).

Embryonic Cell Differentiation

Soon after implantation, the embryonic mass differentiates into three distinct layers of cells. These layers, from which all organs and tissues evolve, are the *ectoderm, mesoderm,* and *endoderm* (Table 4–1).

The differentiated cells stay attached to the trophoblast by means of the body stalk, which later forms the umbilical cord. Small spaces appear between the inner cell mass and the invading trophoblast. These spaces soon form the *amniotic cavity.* This hollow space will eventually surround the developing embryo and fetus like a protective, transparent capsule.

TABLE 4–1. STRUCTURES DERIVED FROM THE THREE GERM CELL LAYERS

ECTODERM	MESODERM	ENDODERM
Skin	Muscles	Digestive system
Nervous system	Bones	Respiratory tract
Special sense organs:	Connective tissue	(except nose)
Eyes	Circulatory system	
Ears	Reproductive organs	
Nose and mouth	Urinary system	

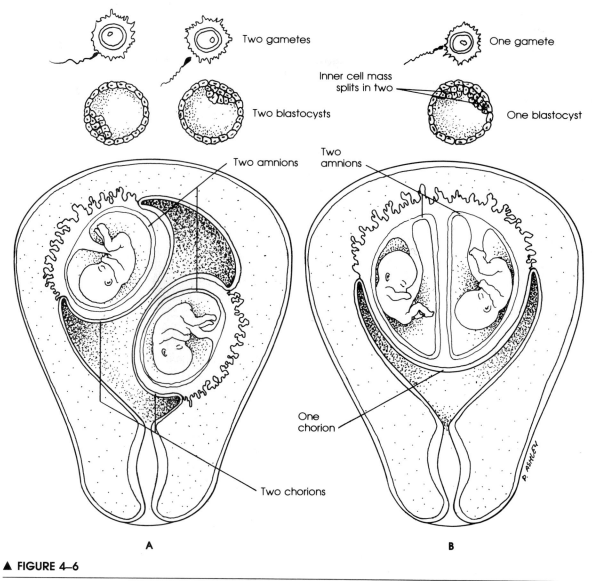

Two gametes

Inner cell mass splits in two

One gamete

Two blastocysts

One blastocyst

Two amnions

Two amnions

One chorion

Two chorions

P. ASHLEY

A   B

▲ **FIGURE 4–6**

A. Formation of nonidentical (fraternal) twins. **B.** Formation of identical twins.

FETAL MEMBRANES AND AMNIOTIC FLUID

Soon after implantation, two membranes form around the embryo. The two membranes are in close contact with each other. The outer membrane is called the *chorion* (previously the trophoblast, which becomes covered with a growth of rootlike projections called *villi*), and the inner membrane is called the *amnion*. As the fetus grows, the membranes stretch to form the amniotic sac, or bag of waters (Fig. 4–7).

The amniotic sac contains a watery liquid called *amniotic fluid*. This fluid consists of 98% water and contains traces of protein, glucose, fetal lanugo (hair), fetal urine, and vernix caseosa (a cheesy material that covers the fetal skin). Examination of the amniotic fluid for diagnostic purposes (amniocentesis) is discussed in Chapter 8.

Chorionic villi   Amniotic sac

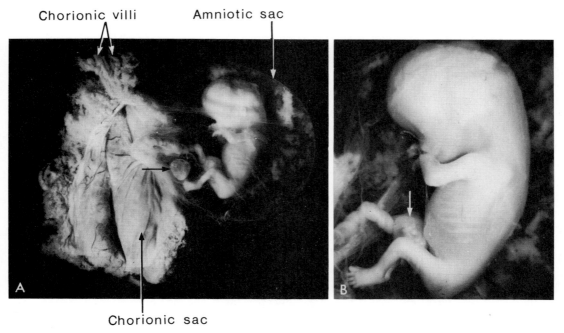

Chorionic sac

▲ **FIGURE 4–7**

A 9-week fetus in the amniotic sac exposed by removal from the chorionic sac. The remnant of the yolk sac is indicated by an arrow in the center. (From Moore, K. L. (1974). *Before We Are Born.* Philadelphia, W. B. Saunders Company.)

The origin of amniotic fluid is not completely known. Initially, most fluid appears to be derived from the maternal blood. Later, the fetus also makes a contribution by excreting urine into the amniotic fluid. Normally, some amniotic fluid is swallowed by the fetus and subsequently absorbed by the gastrointestinal tract. An excess of amniotic fluid is associated with malformations of the fetal central nervous system, for example, anencephaly and hydrocephaly.

The amniotic fluid is neutral to slightly alkaline (pH 7.0 to 7.25). Although the amount of amniotic fluid present at term varies, about 1 L is average. The presence of more than 2 L is called *hydramnios.*

The amniotic fluid serves several purposes. The embryo/fetus, suspended by the umbilical cord, floats freely in the amniotic fluid. This buoyancy permits symmetrical growth and musculoskeletal development of the embryo/fetus. The amniotic fluid also prevents adherence of the amnion's membrane to the embryo/fetus, cushions the embryo/fetus against jolts or impacts the mother may

receive, and maintains a constant temperature for the embryo/fetus.

FUNCTIONS OF THE AMNIOTIC FLUID

*   Allows the embryo/fetus to move about freely
*   Prevents the amnion from adhering to the embryo/fetus
*   Cushions the embryo/fetus against injury from external sources
*   Maintains a constant temperature for the embryo/fetus
*   Provides fluid and nourishment for the embryo/fetus

PLACENTA

By the end of the first month of pregnancy, the placenta has developed sufficiently to supply oxygen and nourishment to the fetus. In addition, the fetus's waste products are eliminated through it. Until about the fourth week, circulation and nourishment are gained by the embryo from the yolk sac (Fig. 4–7). Thereafter, a connection is made between vessels developing in the chorion and those growing out from the fetus through the body stalk to establish fetoplacental circulation.

The placenta develops partly from the invading trophoblast and partly from the endometrium of the uterus. By 10 days, the blastocyst is found buried in the endometrium. The trophoblast enlarges, and spaces for it develop. These spaces join one another, and the trophoblast changes to finger-like projections called villi, which later are called *chorionic villi*. Fetal blood vessels grow into each villus. Maternal blood, on the other hand, empties into the intervillous spaces. Thus, the cell layers of the chorion and the fetal blood vessels themselves are the placental "barrier" between fetal and maternal blood. Substances move across this barrier by diffusion or active transport.

The placental villi can be likened somewhat to the roots of plants submerged in a bowl of water in that they absorb nourishment from the water that surrounds them.

Maternal blood, rich in oxygen and nutrients, reaches the chorionic villi via the uterine arteries. Carbon dioxide and waste products from the fetus are returned through the placenta to the mother's blood.

The placenta's main activities are metabolism, transfer of nourishment and wastes, and endocrine secretion. All are essential for maintaining pregnancy and promoting normal fetal development.

Gases such as oxygen, carbon dioxide, and carbon monoxide easily cross the placental membrane by simple diffusion. Interruption of oxygen transport for even a few minutes will endanger fetal survival. Nutrients vary in their ability to cross the placenta. Water is rapidly and freely exchanged between mother and fetus. Vitamins, glucose, and electrolytes freely cross the placenta. Maternal antibodies can enter the fetus by way of the placenta. However, the placenta is selective in its transfer of immune bodies. Some passive immunity is conferred to the fetus against such diseases as diphtheria. Most drugs cross the placenta freely; some cause congenital malformations (see Appendix B).

In addition to serving as an organ for the exchange of oxygen and waste products, the placenta serves as an endocrine gland. During pregnancy, hormones necessary to maintain pregnancy—estrogen, progesterone, and human chorionic gonadotropin—are secreted by the placenta.

At the end of pregnancy, the placenta is flat and round, about 8 inches (20 cm) in diameter and about 1 inch (2.5 cm) thick; it usually weighs about one-sixth of the baby's weight. The maternal side of the placenta (Duncan's placenta), attached to the uterus, is rough, irregular, and made up of many subdivisions called *cotyledons*. The fetal side (Schultze's placenta) is shiny because of the adherence of the two membranes: The chorion (the outer membrane) and the amnion (the inner membrane) form the sac containing the fetus and the amniotic fluid. The umbilical cord is normally inserted into the central area of the fetal side (smooth side) of the placenta.

UMBILICAL CORD

The lifeline linking the fetus with the placenta is the umbilical cord. It runs between the umbilicus (navel) of the fetus and the placenta. Within the cord are two umbilical arteries and one umbilical vein. Surrounding and protecting the blood vessels is a thick substance called *Wharton's jelly.*

In contrast to the usual pattern of circulation, the umbilical arteries carry nonoxygenated blood and the umbilical vein carries oxygenated blood. Blood from the fetus flows through the umbilical arteries to the placenta, where it gives up carbon dioxide and other waste products. The umbilical vein carries oxygen and nutrients from the placenta to the fetus.

Circulation

EMBRYONIC CIRCULATION

The developing ovum derives nutrition first from its own cytoplasmic mass and then from the decidua (the thickened lining of the uterus) by the activity of the trophoblastic cells. At about the fourth week, the embryo gains circulation and nourishment from the yolk sac. After the fourth week, a connection is made between vessels developing in the chorion and those growing out from the fetus through the body stalk, and fetoplacental circulation is established.

FETAL CIRCULATION

The fetus obtains oxygen through the placenta, rather than using its lungs. Because the placenta is also the source of nutrients for the fetus, it does not need its own liver to serve as a nutrition station. Consequently, three structures route most of the circulated blood past the fetal lungs and liver. These structures or shunts are (a) the *ductus arteriosus,* which is a vessel that connects the pulmonary artery with the aorta, thereby allowing the blood to bypass the lungs; (b) the *foramen ovale,* which is an interatrial shunt; and (c) the *ductus venosus,* which allows most of the blood to bypass the liver.

Because the fetus's source of oxygen is the placenta and not the fetal lungs, blood rich with oxygen and nutrients flows through the umbilical vein. Blood from the umbilical vein enters the *portal venous system* (which drains blood from the fetal intestines and other digestive organs); some of this mixed blood is then moved (shunted) quickly through the liver, bypassing the usual path to the liver by way of a special fetal structure, the ductus venosus.

From the ductus venosus, the blood enters the inferior vena cava and continues its journey toward the heart. Much of the blood is directed preferentially through the right atrium to the left side of the heart through the foramen ovale (a small hole between the two atria of the heart—an interatrial shunt). Therefore, the relatively oxygen rich blood (recently from the placenta) flows from the left atrium to the left ventricle and out the ascending aorta to the fetal head (to the oxygen-needing fetal brain).

As the blood returns from the fetal head, it has a relatively low oxygen content. Thus, most of the superior vena cava blood is efficiently directed to pass through the right atrium into the right ventricle and out the pulmonary artery. A small amount of the blood then goes through the somewhat nonfunctional lungs, nourishing the developing lung tissue. The ductus arteriosus allows 85% to 90% of pulmonary artery blood to bypass the lungs and therefore begin its course down the descending aorta toward the placenta for reoxygenation (Fig. 4–8).

STRUCTURES IN FETAL CIRCULATION

- PLACENTA and VESSELS. Vessels necessary for oxygenation and exchange of waste products.
- UMBILICAL VEIN. One vein that carries oxygenated blood from the placenta to the fetus.
- UMBILICAL ARTERIES. Two arteries that carry deoxygenated blood from the fetus to the placenta.
- FORAMEN OVALE. Opening between the right and left atria of the heart.
- DUCTUS ARTERIOSUS. Fetal blood vessel connecting the pulmonary artery and the aorta.
- DUCTUS VENOSUS. Fetal blood vessel connecting the umbilical vein with the inferior vena cava.

CIRCULATORY CHANGES AFTER BIRTH

Important circulatory adjustments occur at birth when the circulation of fetal blood through the placenta no longer exists and the lungs must start to function. The foramen ovale, the ductus arteriosus, the ductus venosus, and the umbilical vessels are no longer needed. Occlusion of the placental circulation causes an immediate fall in blood pressure in the inferior vena cava and the right atrium. Aeration of the lungs produces a dramatic fall in pulmonary vascular resistance, a marked increase in pulmonary blood flow, and a progressive thinning of the walls of the pulmonary arteries. Because of the increase in pulmonary blood flow, the pressure in the left atrium rises above that in the right atrium, which functionally closes the foramen ovale. Later, anatomical closure results from tissue proliferation, and adhesions develop. The ductus arteriosus constricts at birth and becomes the ligamentum arteriosus. Anatomical closure of the ductus arteriosus normally occurs

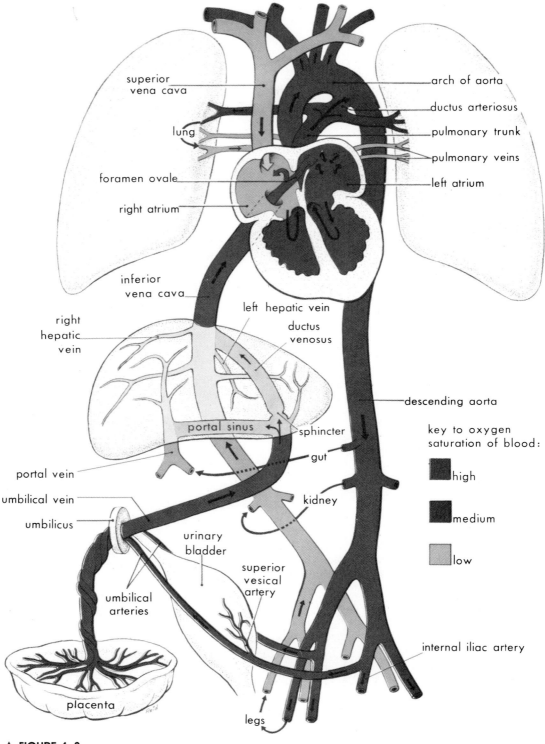

▲ FIGURE 4–8

Fetal circulation. The shading indicates the oxygen saturation of the blood, and the arrows show the course of the fetal circulation. Note that there are three shunts that permit most of the blood to bypass the liver and the lungs: the ductus venosus, the foramen ovale, and the ductus arteriosus. (From Moore, K. L. (1989). *Before We Are Born,* 3rd ed. Philadelphia, W. B. Saunders Company.)

by the end of the third postnatal month. The ductus venosus functionally closes, and blood flows freely through the liver. The fetal vessels constrict immediately after birth, often before the cord is cut.

CIRCULATORY CHANGES AFTER BIRTH

- UMBILICAL VESSELS. The umbilical vessels are cut; in order to receive oxygen the infant must use the lungs.
- LUNGS. Aeration occurs, blood is circulated through the lungs.
- PATTERN OF BLOOD FLOW. Blood flow pattern changes to that of a mature circulation (as the infant begins to breathe).
- CIRCULATION TO LUNGS. As the infant inflates the lungs, pressure is released on the lungs' blood vessels.
- LINE OF LEAST RESISTANCE. As the blood vessels open in the lungs, blood is no longer diverted through ductus arteriosus; rather, following the line of least resistance, blood enters the lungs.
- INCREASED PRESSURE. The change in blood flow increases pressure in the left atrium, which causes the foramen ovale to close.
- HEART FUNCTIONS WITH TWO SEPARATE PUMPS. The right side of the heart receives nonoxygenated blood and pumps it to the lungs. The oxygenated blood is directed to the left side of the heart, where it is pumped through aorta to other parts of the body.
- DUCTUS ARTERIOSUS. The ductus arteriosus functionally closes; therefore nonoxygenated blood cannot mix with oxygenated blood.
- DUCTUS VENOSUS. The ductus venosus functionally closes and the blood flows through the portal system (the liver).

Development of the Embryo/Fetus

During the first 8 weeks the cells divide rapidly and develop different functions. The formation of the organs begins during this time, which is called *organogenesis*. The development of the embryo is most easily disturbed during the organogenesis period. At this time teratogenic agents are most likely to produce malformations. The product of conception is called an *embryo* until the eighth week (or the end of the seventh week) of gestation and thereafter is called a *fetus*. As soon as the fetus is born, it is called a *newborn infant*.

4 Weeks (First Lunar Month). Although at 4 weeks the embryo is only half the size of a pea and still delicate, the heart and brain are beginning to be formed. Already the embryo has a well-defined head region, with the beginning formation of eyes, ears, mouth, and nose, as well as small buds that will eventually become arms and legs. At this early stage of development, the brain is beginning to divide into sections. The development of the embryo is cephalocaudal; that is, it generally proceeds from the head to the tail.

During the next 28 days, the embryo grows to be about 1⅛ inches long. Because of the rapid development of the brain, the head is very large compared with other parts of the embryo. External genitalia appear, but sex cannot be differentiated (Fig. 4–9).

8 Weeks (Second Lunar Month). During the second month, the embryo becomes more recognizably human. The eyes, nose, mouth, and tongue emerge more clearly. The limbs (extremities) grow longer, and buds appear at the ends of them that will later form the fingers and toes.

In the early stages the brain and spinal cord grow more rapidly than the rest of the body. The brain develops from the outer layer of cells, which forms the *neural tube*. Part of this neural tube forms the spinal canal, and part of it forms the brain.

12 Weeks (Third Lunar Month). The ossification centers appear in most of the bones, and the teeth begin to form under the gums. The length of the fetus is 2½ to 3½ inches (6.3 to 8.8 cm), and the weight is 0.5 to 1 oz (14 to 28 g). The kidneys and bladder begin to develop, and secretion of small amounts of urine occurs. At 12 weeks, the external genitalia are more prominent and show signs of male or female characteristics.

16 Weeks (Fourth Lunar Month). The fetus looks like a miniature baby with pink skin, but the head is still large (Fig. 4–10). It is 6 inches long

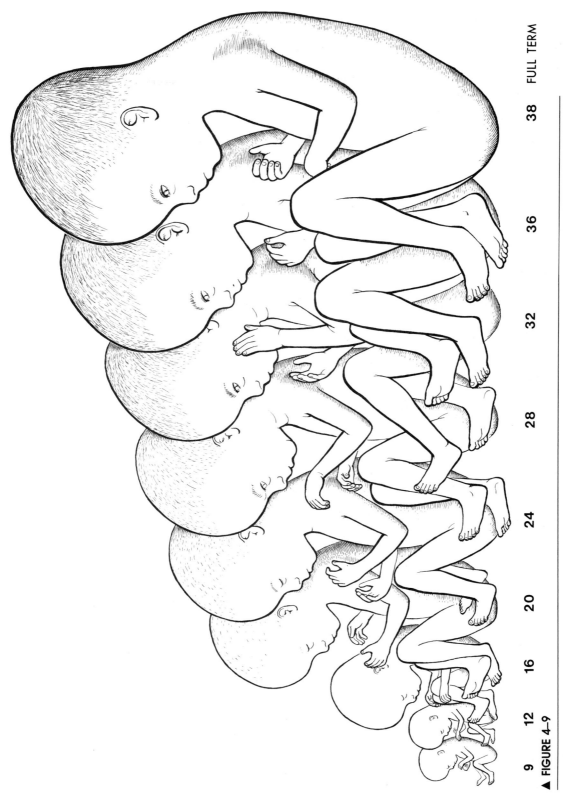

| 9 | 12 | 16 | 20 | 24 | 28 | 32 | 36 | 38 | FULL TERM |

▲ FIGURE 4–9

An embryo becomes a fetus around the end of the seventh week; by this time all beginning structures are present. (From Moore, K. L. (1974). *Before We Are Born.* Philadelphia, W. B. Saunders Company.)

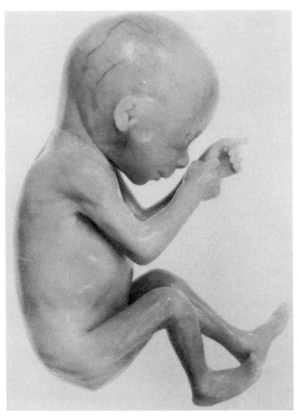

▲ **FIGURE 4–10**

Photograph of a 17-week fetus. Because the skin is very thin, scalp vessels are clearly visible. Movements of the fetus should be felt by the mother. (From Moore, K. L. (1989). *Before We Are Born*, 3rd ed. Philadelphia, W. B. Saunders Company.)

(15.2 cm), weighs 6 oz (170 g), and has formed fingers and toes. The heart muscles are developed. The heartbeat can be heard by using an electronic instrument called the *Doppler amplifier device*. *Meconium* (a thin, dark green to black substance) begins to be present in the bowels.

20 Weeks (Fifth Lunar Month). The fetus is about 8 inches long (20.3 cm) and weighs 10 oz (284 g). A fine downy hair called *lanugo* is seen on the body, and there is some hair on the head. Because of the lack of fat deposits, the skin is very wrinkled. Fetal movements (called *quickening*) are felt by the mother, and the heartbeat can be heard with a stethoscope.

24 Weeks (Sixth Lunar Month). The fetus is 12

inches long (30.4 cm) and weighs 1.5 lb (680 g). A white cheesy material, called the *vernix caseosa,* appears on the skin. This substance protects the skin of the fetus while it is submerged in the amniotic fluid. If the fetus is born at this time, it has a slight chance of survival.

28 Weeks (Seventh Lunar Month). The fetus is approximately 14 inches long (35.4 cm) and weighs more than 2 lb. The eyes have lids that open and close and also brows and lashes. If born, the fetus can survive with life-support systems in the intensive care unit.

32 Weeks (Eighth Lunar Month). The fetus is about 16 inches long (40.6 cm) and weighs more than 3 lb. The fetus has the appearance of a little old man because of the lack of fat deposits under the skin.

36 Weeks (Ninth Lunar Month). The fetus is about 18 inches long (45.6 cm) and weighs more than 5 lb. The fetus appears somewhat plump. The fingernails reach the fingertips. If born at this time, the fetus is able to survive.

40 Weeks (Tenth Lunar Month). The fetus is 20 inches long (50.6 cm) and weighs about 7 lb (3200 g). The soft lanugo hair has almost disappeared, except on the shoulders and upper back. The vernix caseosa is mainly seen in the folds and creases of the skin. The fetus is ready to be born.

42 Weeks (Tenth Lunar Month). The fetus that goes past 42 weeks' gestation is termed *postterm* or *postmature* (overdue). The postterm baby typically has long nails, an abundance of hair on the head, a diminished amount of vernix caseosa, diminished adipose tissue, and dry skin. This postmature infant is at risk for developing life-threatening problems. Because of the increased chance for a stillbirth, medical or surgical intervention is carried out to save the infant's life.

Function of Fetal Systems

A concise, and perhaps too simple, discussion of fetal systems is included here to underscore the significance of maternal nutrition to the fetus; to further illustrate the development of the fetus from early fetal life until birth; and to explain why insults, such as drugs and diseases, can cause injury to the developing fetus in various stages of life (Fig. 4–11).

There is no question that the mother's body must provide adequate oxygen to the fetus and must be able to remove all of the fetus's waste products. If the mother's body did not perform these tasks, the fetus would not survive.

Adequate nutrition intake by the mother assures the fetus of proper nutrients, such as glucose, which is necessary for the fetus's utilization of oxygen. Carbohydrates received by the fetus from the mother are stored in the fetal liver, muscles, and heart as glycogen. The amount of glucose needed by the fetus increases steadily throughout pregnancy. When the mother is malnourished, the infant is likely to be small. More important, the brain of the infant often weighs less than it should. It is possible that the smaller size of the fetal brain affects brain functioning in later life.

For the first 26 weeks of gestation, most of the fetal weight gain is due to accumulation of protein and amino acids, which are necessary for body cells to build and grow. They also assist the fetus in returning carbon dioxide and nitrogen to the maternal circulation.

The fetus draws on the mother's body for most nutrients. However, the mother and fetus adapt to each other during pregnancy.

CIRCULATORY SYSTEM

The circulatory system is the first system to become functional. The development of the heart begins at 18 days, when a pair of heart cords can be distinguished. By the end of the third week, the blood begins to circulate. Pulsations can be visualized during ultrasonography. During the sixth to eighth weeks, the heart and great vessels develop; it is at this time that most congenital malformations appear.

RESPIRATORY SYSTEM

The lungs begin to form early, and by the twenty-fourth day some buds have appeared that eventually form the bronchial tree. Between 20 and 24 weeks, two types of epithelial cells are differentiated. A fatty substance (surfactant) is produced by one type of epithelial cell. This fatty substance keeps the air sacs from sticking together when, immediately after birth, an infant must breathe alone. At about 35 weeks, the lungs have reached maturity with enough surfactant to allow an infant to live with minimal respiratory difficulty.

ENDOCRINE SYSTEM

The first endocrine gland, the thyroid, begins to develop about 1 to 2 weeks after conception. Thyroid hormone production continues to increase until term or 40 weeks' gestation. Certain drugs given to the mother for hyperthyroidism may affect the infant.

Fetal Pancreas. The buds of the fetal pancreas are seen about the seventh week of gestation. Insulin can be obtained from the fetus by the twelfth week. The placenta is relatively impermeable (selective) to insulin, so it is necessary for the fetus to supply its own. Infants of diabetic mothers release insulin when stimulated by the mother's high glucose level. Fetal production of insulin is one factor that makes the control of diabetes more difficult during pregnancy.

Fetal Pituitary Gland. Females have a greater secretion of follicle-stimulating hormone than do males during fetal life. By the eighth week, the males testes are evident. They secrete testosterone, which appears to aid the early development of the external genitalia.

GASTROINTESTINAL SYSTEM

The fetus swallows amniotic fluid by 4 months' gestation. In spite of this, at birth the newborn, particularly the premature newborn, has a tendency to allow fluid to get into the lungs rather than swallowing it.

Liver. At 4 weeks, the liver ducts are visible. At about 20 weeks, the liver is the major source of hemoglobin for the fetus. A disorder such as hemolytic disease can be confirmed by an increased amount of bilirubin in the amniotic fluid. Conversion of bilirubin from the fat-soluble form to the water-soluble form occurs in the liver. In the fetus, elimination occurs via the placenta. In

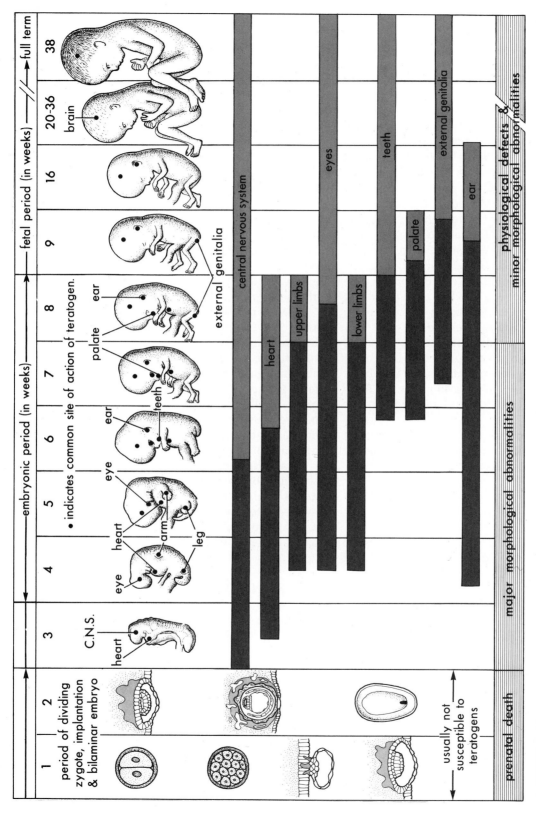

▲ FIGURE 4–11

The sensitive or critical periods in human development. Darker areas show highly sensitive periods; lighter areas show periods that are less sensitive to teratogens. CNS, central nervous system. (From Moore, K. L. (1974). *Before We Are Born.* Philadelphia, W. B. Saunders Company.)

order for fetal bilirubin to clear the placenta, it must remain unconjugated and bound to albumin. This step requires that the bilirubin bind to an enzyme called *glucuronyl transferase*. This enzyme is relatively deficient in the fetus and full-term infant. Therefore, after birth, jaundice in the newborn is common. The danger of an elevated bilirubin level in the blood is that it may lead to brain and nervous tissue damage.

Summary

In summary, the fetal systems develop in an orderly fashion. By the end of the seventh week, the beginnings of all the major organs and systems are present. At first, the function of most organs is minimal; however, by the end of 9 months the fetus is prepared structurally, functionally, and metabolically for extrauterine existence. The most critical time for the fetus is in the first 8 weeks;

this is called the *organogenesis period*. In addition, each organ has a critical period when insults, such as teratogenic agents, can easily cause physical and functional defects to the central nervous system. However, the potential for harm caused by maternal malnutrition, chronic and acute diseases, and drugs continues until the infant is born.

References

Dickason, E. Z., Schultz, M. O., & Silverman, B. L. (1990). *Maternal-Infant Nursing Care.* St. Louis: C. V. Mosby.

Jones, K. L. (1988). *Smith's Recognizable Patterns of Human Malformations,* 4th ed. Philadelphia: W. B. Saunders Company.

Ladewig, P. W., London, M. L., & Olds, S. B. (1990). *Essentials of Maternal-Newborn Nursing,* 2nd ed. Redwood City, CA, Addison-Wesley Nursing.

Mattison, D. R., Kozolsski, K., Quirk, J. G., & Jelovsek, R. R. (1989). Effect of drugs and chemicals on the fetus. *Contemporary OB/GYN* 33:163–176.

Moore, K. L. (1989). *Before We Are Born: Basic Embryology and Birth Defects,* 3rd ed. Philadelphia: W. B. Saunders Company.

SUGGESTED ACTIVITIES

1. Review, in simple terms, how fertilization, sex determination, and implantation occur.
2. Explain the organogenesis period of embryonic development.
3. Prepare a diagram showing the differences between fetal circulation and adult circulation.
4. Make a list of circulatory changes that occur after birth.

REVIEW QUESTIONS

A. Select the best answer to each multiple-choice question.

1. Each body cell contains within its nucleus
   A. Chromosomes
   B. Genes
   C. Long chains of molecules
   D. A, B, C

2. During the process of *meiosis*, the number of chromosomes of the human ovum and sperm are reduced to
   A. 23
   B. 26
   C. 44
   D. 46

3. The union of the sperm and ovum normally occurs in the
   A. Abdominal cavity
   B. Ovary
   C. Fallopian tube
   D. Uterus

4. The sex chromosome(s) carried by the male sperm is (are)
   A. X chromosome
   B. Y chromosome
   C. XY chromosomes
   D. XX chromosomes

5. The fluid that surrounds the fetus is called
   A. Chorionic
   B. Amniotic
   C. Placental
   D. Umbilical

6. The structure that supplies oxygen and nutrients to the fetus and removes wastes products from the fetus is the
   A. Amniotic fluid
   B. Placenta
   C. Chorion
   D. Body stalk

7. The umbilical cord linking the fetus to the placenta contains
   A. One vein and one artery
   B. One vein and two arteries
   C. Two veins and one artery
   D. Two veins and two arteries

8. The amount of fetal nutrients necessary for growth, such as glucose, normally
   A. Increases steadily throughout pregnancy
   B. Remains the same throughout pregnancy
   C. Decreases throughout pregnancy
   D. Is unknown

9. During organogenesis, the main reason for adverse drug effects on the embryo is
   A. The cells are dividing rapidly into different functions
   B. The placental barrier is well defined but immature
   C. The yolk sac is still present
   D. None of the above

10. The product of conception, until the 8th week of gestation, is referred to as the
    A. Fetus
    B. Embryo
    C. Zygote
    D. Infant

11. The functions of the amniotic fluid include all of the following EXCEPT
    A. Preventing adherence of the amnion membrane to the fetus
    B. Allowing the fetus to move freely
    C. Maintaining a constant temperature for the fetus
    D. Restricting the movement of the fetus

12. The fetal membranes consist of two layers. The membrane layer that is next to the developing fetus is the
    A. Decidua capsularis
    B. Villi
    C. Amnion
    D. Chorion

13. The oxygen content is the highest in which of the following fetal structures?
    A. Umbilical artery
    B. Umbilical vein
    C. Ductus venosus
    D. Foramen ovale

B. Choose from column II the phrase that most accurately defines the term in column I.

I

1. Gene _____
2. Amnion _____
3. Placenta _____
4. Amniotic fluid _____
5. Umbilical cord _____
6. Ectoderm _____

II

A. Embryonic germ layer
B. Filters substances from maternal blood
C. Structure connecting placenta and fetus
D. Inner membrane of amniotic sac
E. Responsible for specific hereditary trait
F. Fluid that surrounds the fetus

C. Match the description in column II with the correct structure in column I.

I

1. Ductus arteriosus _____
2. Ductus venosus _____
3. Foramen ovale _____
4. Umbilical vein _____

II

A. Opening between right and left atria
B. Carries oxygenated blood from placenta to fetus
C. Fetal blood vessel that allows blood to bypass the liver
D. Fetal blood vessel connecting the pulmonary artery to the aorta

UNIT III

THE EXPECTANT MOTHER

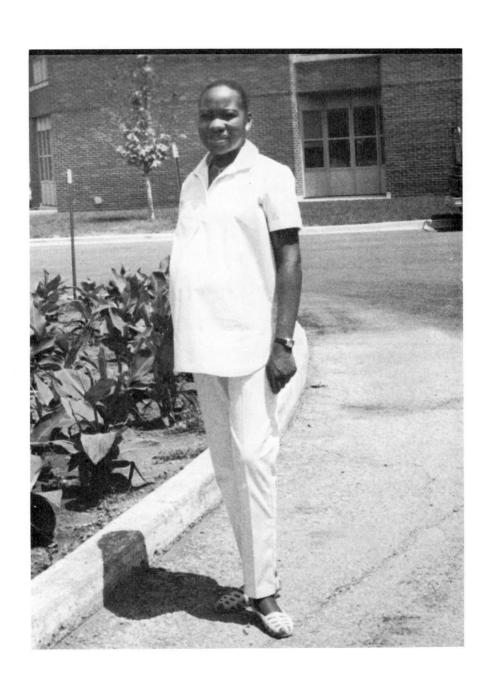

CHAPTER 5

Chapter Outline

Terminology
    Systematic method to indicate a woman's obstetrical history
Duration of Pregnancy
Signs and Symptoms
    Presumptive signs: Changes that suggest pregnancy
    Probable signs: Changes that strongly indicate pregnancy
    Positive signs: Changes that clearly establish pregnancy
Maternal Body Changes
    Changes in the endocrine system
    Changes in the reproductive system
    Changes in the musculoskeletal system
    Changes in the cardiovascular system
    Changes in the respiratory system
    Changes in the gastrointestinal system
    Changes in the renal (urinary) system
Psychological Changes During Pregnancy
    Body image
    Developmental tasks

Learning Objectives

Upon completion of Chapter 5, the student should be able to

- Define the terminology used in discussing pregnancy.
- Determine the duration of pregnancy by days, calendar months, lunar months, and trimesters.
- Explain Nägele's rule in determining the duration of pregnancy.
- Define the terms *gravida, para, embryo,* and *fetus.*
- Name four signs and symptoms of pregnancy that suggest, but do not clearly establish, pregnancy.
- Name three positive signs of pregnancy.
- Describe the changes that occur in the ovaries during pregnancy.
- Explain the changes in the uterus and vagina that are necessary for birth.
- Explain how pregnancy affects blood volume and blood plasma.
- Identify factors that influence posture during pregnancy.
- Explain the cause of the supine hypotension syndrome during pregnancy.
- Explain why frequency of urination occurs early and late in pregnancy.
- List the pigmentation changes of the skin during pregnancy.
- Recall how the hormones estrogen and progesterone influence pregnancy.
- Identify the psychological changes that occur during pregnancy.
- Define the developmental tasks of pregnancy.

PHYSICAL AND PSYCHOLOGICAL CHANGES IN PREGNANCY

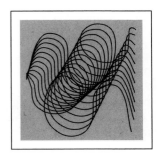

If the promotion of health and prevention of complications are to take place during pregnancy, the nurse and other caregivers need to understand the physical and psychological changes that occur during pregnancy. In addition, the nurse should be acquainted with appropriate medical and nursing interventions for the uneventful (normal) pregnancy. With this knowledge, the nurse can develop adequate nursing care plans that include nursing diagnoses, nursing interventions related to body changes, and appropriate outcomes. Patient self-care should be a part of the care plan.

Terminology

The following are definitions of some terms applied to pregnancy:

- *ante*—before.
- *antepartum*—the time before delivery.
- *prenatal*—the time before birth.
- *gravida*—the number of pregnancies a woman has had, regardless of the outcome. It includes the present pregnancy.
- *para*—the number of pregnancies a woman has had that have continued to the period of fetal viability.
- *primigravida*—a woman pregnant for the first time.
- *multigravida*—a woman who has been pregnant more than once.
- *nulligravida*—a woman who has never been pregnant.
- *primipara*—a woman who has given birth to a fetus (dead or alive) that has reached the stage of viability.

- *multipara*—a woman who has given birth or is in labor for at least the second time.
- *viability*—the capability of the fetus to live outside the uterus. The age of viability previously was 28 weeks, but many states now accept 20 weeks or more, or a fetus weighing 500 g or more.

SYSTEMATIC METHOD TO INDICATE A WOMAN'S OBSTETRICAL HISTORY

One quick method used to indicate not only the number of pregnancies the woman has had but also the outcomes involves five digits separated by dashes. The first digit refers to the total number of pregnancies, including the present one; the second is the number of full-term births; the third is the number of premature births; the fourth indicates the number of abortions; and the fifth is the number of children currently living. Using this system, a pregnant woman who has four living children, all single births, and who has had no preterm births and no abortions would be a gravida 5–4–0–0–4.

First digit:	Number of times pregnant.
Second digit:	Number of full-term births.
Third digit:	Number of premature births.
Fourth digit:	Number of abortions.
Fifth digit:	Number of living children.

A two-digit system provides less information about the woman's history but is simpler and is still used in some institutions. This system uses *gravida*, which indicates the number of pregnancies including the present pregnancy, and *para*, which indicates the number of previous pregnancies that terminated after the infant was *viable*, whether born alive or stillborn. With this system a woman who is pregnant for the first time (primigravida) and has not carried a pregnancy to viability is gravida 1 para 0. During subsequent pregnancies she is a gravida 2, a gravida 3, and so forth. After the woman has given birth to her first child, if she becomes pregnant again she is a gravida 2 para 1.

Duration of Pregnancy

The duration of pregnancy is usually estimated by counting from the first day of the last normal menstrual period (LMP). Using Nägele's rule, the expected date of delivery or expected date of confinement (EDC) is determined by adding 7 days to the first day of the LMP and subtracting 3 months (first day of LMP + 7 days − 3 months = EDC). For example, if the woman's LMP began on July 10, the EDC would be April 17. Remember that this is an *estimated* date and the birth may not occur on this date. Only a small number of births occur on the estimated date; most occur before or after it.

1st day of LMP	November	18
Add 7 days	+ 7 days =	25
Minus 3 months	= August	25

When the LMP is January through March, it may be easier to add 9 months rather than subtracting 3 months. For example, if the LMP is January 17, by adding 9 months and 7 days the EDC would be October 24.

McDonald's rule is used in some institutions to attempt to add precision to the measurement of fundal height during the second and third trimesters. Calculation is as follows:

Height of fundus (cm) × 2/7 (or = 3.5)
= Duration of pregnancy in lunar months
Height of fundus (cm) × 8/7
= Duration of pregnancy in weeks

The average duration of pregnancy is approximately 280 days. This period of time is calculated in 28-day months called *lunar months*. There are 10 lunar months (40 weeks, 280 days) in a full-term pregnancy. This is approximately the same as 9 calendar months. For convenience, the 9 months of pregnancy are divided into three *trimesters*, each representing a 3-month period.

Not all pregnancies continue to term. A pregnancy that terminates before the fetus is viable is called an *abortion* (laypersons use the term *miscarriage*). A pregnancy that terminates after the age of viability but before full term is called a *preterm* (premature) *birth*. A pregnancy that terminates 2 weeks after the EDC (42 weeks' gestation) is called a *postterm birth*.

Signs and Symptoms

It is important to establish the diagnosis of pregnancy or confirm that the woman is pregnant. Many signs characteristic of pregnancy assist in confirmation. Signs and symptoms of pregnancy are divided into three categories: (a) presumptive signs, which suggest pregnancy; (b) probable signs, which indicate that the woman is likely pregnant; and (c) positive signs, which give definite evidence that the woman is pregnant. The three positive signs are the only signs that clearly establish a diagnosis of pregnancy. It is important to remember that many of the signs and symptoms that are present in pregnancy may also be present in other conditions.

PRESUMPTIVE SIGNS: CHANGES THAT SUGGEST PREGNANCY

Amenorrhea is frequently the first sign that alerts the woman to a possible pregnancy. It is a valuable clue in the woman who menstruates regularly; however, amenorrhea, or cessation of menses, also may result from other conditions such as emotional stress, chronic disease, environmental changes, and the beginning of menopause. In addition, oral contraceptives cause cessation of menses.

Nausea with or without vomiting occurs in about one-half of pregnancies. Because it most often occurs in the morning, it is referred to as "morning sickness." Usually the nausea disappears in a few hours, although it may persist throughout the day. It appears early in pregnancy but usually does not persist after 16 weeks. Frequently, the woman can obtain relief by eating carbohydrates such as dry crackers before rising in the morning. This will dilute the concentration of hormones accumulated in her body during the night.

Breast changes may be noted early in pregnancy. Heaviness, tingling, tenderness, and heightened sensitivity may be noted early in pregnancy. The pigmentation of the nipple and areola darkens, and by the second month the breasts begin to increase in size. These changes are due to higher levels of certain hormones during pregnancy.

Urinary frequency occurs from pressure exerted on the bladder by the enlarging uterus. However, other conditions, such as infection, can cause the same sign.

Quickening is the term used to describe the mother's first recognition of the baby's movements. Because these movements are slight and fluttery, they can be mistaken for active gas movements within the bowel. This presumptive sign is helpful in estimating the duration of pregnancy when the obstetric history is vague. Quickening is often noticed by the mother between 18 and 20 weeks of pregnancy.

PROBABLE SIGNS: CHANGES THAT STRONGLY INDICATE PREGNANCY

Uterine enlargement, enlargement of the abdomen, is due to the growth of the baby, uterus, and the placenta. This enlargement can also occur when a tumor is present. In pregnancy, the enlargement of the uterus is judged over time, with a progressive enlargement being significant.

Hegar's sign is present when there is a softening of the lower uterine segment. It becomes soft by about 6 weeks of pregnancy. This softening can be felt by the examiner as he or she compresses the uterus manually.

Goodell's sign is a softening of the cervix at 8 weeks of pregnancy. Normally, the cervix is quite firm.

Chadwick's sign is the bluish or purplish discoloration of the vagina and vulva. This sign is caused by greater vascularity or pelvic congestion due mainly to an increase in the hormone estrogen. There are other conditions that can cause pelvic congestion.

Ballottement is a rebounding of the fetus against the examiner's fingers after the fetus is pushed upward through the vagina or the abdomen. Ballottement can be felt during the fourth or fifth month when the fetus is small in comparison with the amount of amniotic fluid present.

Braxton Hicks contractions are painless uterine contractions that begin early in pregnancy. They are present through the pregnancy, becoming noticeable as pregnancy advances. They may be felt by the woman as a tightening across her abdomen. Near the end of pregnancy, these contractions become stronger and may be mistaken for labor contractions.

Pregnancy tests, when done properly, are accurate 90% to 98% of the time. Most pregnancy tests are based on the presence of human chorionic gonadotropin (hCG), a hormone produced by the chorionic villi of the placenta. This hormone appears in the urine or blood 10 to 12 days after conception. Tests may be done by immunological assay. If urine is used, it should be the woman's first voided specimen of the day, in which hCG concentration is highest.

One of the most sensitive and accurate tests for pregnancy is the *radioimmunoassay* test. This test is capable of detecting hCG in the maternal serum about 8 days after fertilization. Because no pregnancy test is 100% accurate, all of the tests fall in the probable category of signs of pregnancy.

POSITIVE SIGNS: CHANGES THAT CLEARLY ESTABLISH PREGNANCY

Fetal heartbeat can be heard as early as 10 to 12 weeks of pregnancy with a Doppler amplifier device (Figs. 5–1 and 5–2). The standard fetoscope detects fetal heart tones (FHT) by about 18 to 20 weeks (Fig. 5–3). The fetal heart rate is rapid, ranging from 120 to 160 beats per minute, or about twice the maternal pulse rate. To avoid error, the mother's radial pulse should be felt at the same time the FHT are auscultated. A fetoscope or Doppler amplifier device is used in outpatient clinics and on low-risk patients.

Other sounds that may be heard while listening to the fetal heartbeat are the funic souffle and the uterine souffle. The *funic souffle* is a soft, swishing sound heard from the blood as it passes through

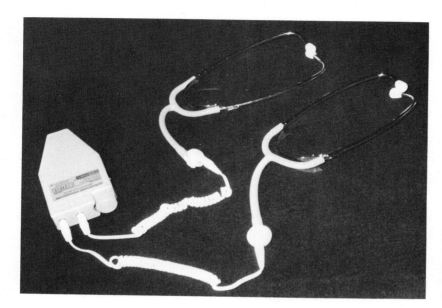

▲ FIGURE 5–1

The Doppler fetal pulse detector picks up fetal heart tones as early as the third month of pregnancy, reassuring the expectant mother.

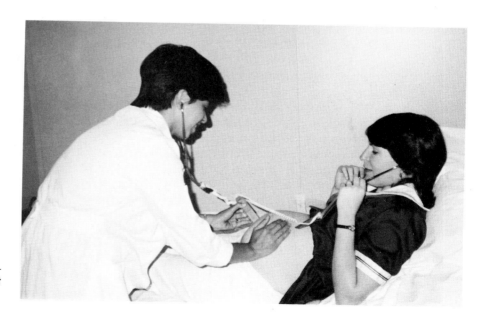

▲ FIGURE 5–2

Mother listening to fetal heart tones with second headset.

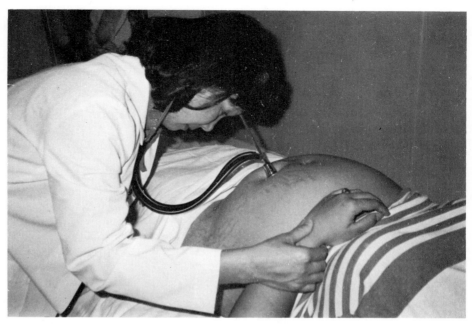

▲ **FIGURE 5–3**

Counting the fetal heart rate with a fetoscope. Note striae gravidarum on abdomen.

the umbilical cord vessels. The *uterine souffle* is a soft, swishing sound made by maternal blood as it rushes through the large vessels of the uterus. The mother's pulse rate is the same as the rate of the uterine souffle.

The presence of *active fetal movements,* as palpated by the examiner, is diagnostic of pregnancy. Because to the mother bowel activity can appear similar to fetal movements, the movements must be felt by the examiner. Fetal activity is noticeable by 18 to 20 weeks' gestation. Ultrasonography can detect fetal movements much earlier.

Ultrasonography can detect the gestational sac by 4 weeks' gestation. In addition, fetal heart pulsation can be seen at this time. By the third month of gestation, ultrasound scanning is very accurate in diagnosing pregnancy.

SIGNS AND SYMPTOMS OF PREGNANCY

Presumptive Signs: Changes That Suggest Pregnancy

- Amenorrhea
- Nausea with or without vomiting
- Breast changes
- Urinary frequency
- Quickening

Probable Signs: Changes That Strongly Indicate Pregnancy

- Uterine enlargement
- Hegar's sign
- Goodell's sign
- Chadwick's sign
- Ballottement
- Braxton Hicks contractions
- Pregnancy tests

Positive Signs: Changes That Clearly Establish Pregnancy

- Fetal heartbeat
- Fetal movements felt by examiner
- Detection of embryo or fetus by ultrasonography

Maternal Body Changes

Many physiological changes occur during pregnancy. Because of these changes, a number of minor symptoms or discomforts result. Most of these complaints do not require medical therapy. However, they do require explanation and reassurance, because most women cannot assess the seriousness of a particular symptom. Also, a number of complaints during pregnancy can be alleviated by relatively simple nursing (including patient self-care instruction) and medical measures.

The two major sources of the physiological changes during pregnancy are changes in the endocrine system and physical changes in the body.

CHANGES IN THE ENDOCRINE SYSTEM

Several hormones are necessary to maintain pregnancy. Most of these are produced initially by the corpus luteum and later by the placenta. The increased production of hormones affects all the major systems in the body.

Human Chorionic Gonadotropin

Human chorionic gonadotropin (hCG) is produced early in pregnancy. By day 14, it is secreted by the trophoblastic tissue. It stimulates progesterone and estrogen production by the corpus luteum to maintain the pregnancy until the placenta is developed sufficiently to assume the function.

The presence of hCG is used in pregnancy tests to determine if a woman is pregnant.

Human Placental Lactogen

Human placental lactogen (hPL) affects both glucose and protein metabolism. It allows more protein to be available for fetal and maternal growth needs. HPL has a diabetogenic effect in the mother (allowing increased glucose to stimulate the pancreas to produce more insulin). This can cause a "burnout" effect, resulting in maternal gestational diabetes.

Melanocyte-Stimulating Hormone

Melanocyte-stimulating hormone (MSH) causes darkening in the pigmentation of the skin in localized areas of the woman's body. It works in concert with estrogen. It produces darkening of the nipples and areola. A brown line called the *linea nigra* appears in the middle of the woman's abdomen (Fig. 5–4). Brownish patches called *chloasma* appear in the face, and freckles and moles become darker. These changes occur in the middle of pregnancy and usually fade after birth of the baby.

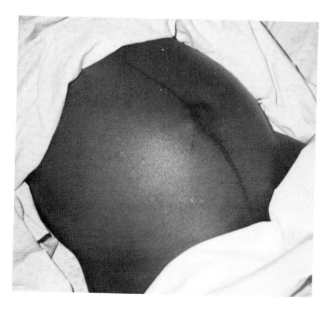

▲ FIGURE 5–4

Pregnant woman's abdomen showing linea nigra.

Aldosterone

Aldosterone is an adrenal hormone that increases by about week 15 of pregnancy. It stimulates the kidney tubules to reabsorb sodium and water. The increases in aldosterone and progesterone counterbalance each other during pregnancy. Elevated progesterone levels result in sodium loss by the renal tubules. When aldosterone and progesterone are out of balance, hypertension is likely to occur.

Estrogen

Estrogen has profound effects on the woman's body during pregnancy. Its principal source is the placenta. Estrogen stimulates uterine development to provide a suitable environment for the fetus. It also helps to develop the breasts' ductal system in preparation for lactation. Estrogen has an indirect effect on the dermal elastic tissue. Its elevation causes a rise in adrenal function. An increase in adrenal steroid concentration results in a weakening of the dermal elastic tissue. Therefore, this hormone plays a role in the development of *striae gravidarum* (stretch marks) on the abdomen, thighs, and breasts (see Fig. 6–3).

The increased estrogen level causes flushing and erythema of the skin, and the woman's body becomes more vascular, increasing the flow of blood to the fetus. Pregnant women are more likely to have nosebleeds (epistaxis) because of increased estrogen.

ESTROGEN (Effects During Pregnancy)

- Causes enlargement of uterus, breasts, and genitals.
- Plays a role in development of striae gravidarum.
- Causes vascular changes.
- Promotes nutrient availability.
- Stimulates MSH, which is responsible for increased pigmentation.

Progesterone

Progesterone also has profound effects on the maternal systems during pregnancy. Its principal source is the placenta. It maintains the endometrium and inhibits uterine contractions, thus preventing abortions. Progesterone also helps develop the breasts for lactation. It causes the body to lose sodium and increases the sensitivity of the respiratory center.

Progesterone provides a regulatory mechanism by helping the woman to eliminate carbon dioxide. It maintains the basal metabolic rate, which causes the woman to feel warm when others are comfortable. It reduces smooth muscle tone, which reduces gastric motility and relaxes sphincters. This action causes many minor complaints during pregnancy, such as constipation, heartburn, and varicosities.

PROGESTERONE (Effects During Pregnancy)

- Promotes development of the lining of uterus.
- Assists implantation.
- Decreases contractility of uterus.
- Promotes development of secretory ducts of breast (for lactation).
- Stimulates sodium excretion (natriuresis).
- Reduces smooth muscle tone (causing discomforts such as constipation, heartburn, and varicosities).
- Helps woman eliminate waste products of fetus.

CHANGES IN THE REPRODUCTIVE SYSTEM

Uterus

The uterus changes dramatically during pregnancy. Before pregnancy, the uterus is a small, semisolid, pear-shaped organ weighing about 2 oz (60 g). At the end of pregnancy, it is a thin-walled, muscular container housing the fetus, placenta, and amniotic fluid with a capacity of 2 lb (1000 g).

This enlargement is primarily the result of an increase in size (hypertrophy) of preexisting muscle cells. The ease with which the fetus can be palpated through the abdominal wall indicates its thin structure (Table 5–1).

The circulatory requirements of the uterus greatly increase as the uterus enlarges and the

TABLE 5–1. CHANGES IN THE REPRODUCTIVE SYSTEM DURING PREGNANCY

PHYSIOLOGICAL CHANGE	CLINICAL SIGNIFICANCE
UTERUS	
Growth: Increases from 2 oz to 2 lb (60 g to 1000 g)	Estrogen and progesterone stimulate uterine enlargement to accommodate fetus
Position: Lifts into pelvis at 12 wks	Uterus os is palpable:
	3 mos (12 wks) at symphysis
	5 mos (20 wks) at umbilicus
	9 mos (40 wks) at xiphoid process
Circulation: By term, 1/6 of maternal blood volume is within uterus	Increased vascularity meets oxygen needs of growing uterus and fetus
Cervix: Increase in vascularity, softness, hypertrophy of cervical glands	Estrogen is responsible for cervical changes
	Mucus plug forms in cervical canal that protects fetus from infection
Contractions: Begin early in pregnancy; later called Braxton Hicks contractions	Oxytocin causes myometrial cells to contract
	Irregular, nonrhythmic contractions assist movement of blood to fetus; later cause effacement and slight dilatation of cervix
BREASTS	
Increase in size and sensitivity; nipples enlarge, darken, and become erect	Primarily under stimulation of estrogen and progesterone, breast changes occur in preparation for lactation
	Sensations of tingling, tenderness, and fullness are felt
Secretion of colostrum begins early in pregnancy	Prelactation secretion; lactation occurs after delivery

fetus and placenta develop. By the end of pregnancy, one-sixth of total maternal blood volume is contained within the uterus. The growth of the uterus is stimulated by hormones and by pressure of the growing fetus against the uterine wall.

Early in pregnancy, irregular, painless uterine contractions occur. As pregnancy progresses, these contractions are palpable and easily detected. These contractions help move the blood through the placenta to the fetus.

Cervix

The cervix of the uterus becomes shorter and softer during pregnancy. These adjustments prepare the cervix for the thinning (*effacement*) and the enlargement (*dilatation*) of the opening of the cervix. This is necessary to permit the baby to pass from the uterus at birth.

The softening of the cervix is due to (a) a hormonal influence that causes an increased blood supply and (b) an increase in secretions from the cervical glands. The secretions from the cervical glands form a mucus plug in the cervical canal that acts as a barrier to prevent organisms from entering the uterus. The mucus plug is expelled from the vagina during labor.

Ovaries

During pregnancy, follicles in the ovaries cease to develop to maturity. Ovulation does not occur. The corpus luteum persists and produces hormones until about 10 weeks of pregnancy to maintain the pregnancy until the placenta takes over.

Vagina

The changes that occur in the vagina prepare it for the tremendous stretching necessary for the birth of the baby. The proliferation of cells and hyperemia of the vaginal connective tissue cause the vaginal walls to become thickened, pliable, and distendable.

Breasts

Several hormones, including estrogen, progesterone, prolactin, and hPL, interact during pregnancy to prepare the breasts for *lactation* (milk production). Estrogen and progesterone seem to be the most important. The breasts rapidly enlarge in the first 8 weeks, owing mostly to vascular engorgement. Thereafter, the breasts enlarge progressively throughout pregnancy as a result of ductal growth stimulated by estrogen and alveolar hypertrophy stimulated by progesterone. Little if any of the increase in breast size is attributable to the deposition of fat.

The breast changes during pregnancy can be summarized as follows: Size increases, beginning the sixth to eighth weeks of pregnancy; breasts become full and tender; the pigmentation of the areolar and nipple darkens; Montgomery's glands become more prominent and promote elasticity and lubrication of the nipple in preparation for breastfeeding; colostrum is excreted from breasts as early as the tenth week of gestation and continues until about the third postpartum day, when it is replaced by milk; and lactation is initiated by the profound drop in estrogen and progesterone levels after delivery of the placenta, allowing an increase in prolactin production (Table 5–1).

CHANGES IN THE MUSCULOSKELETAL SYSTEM

The principal musculoskeletal changes during pregnancy are the hormonal relaxation of the joints and the adjustments in posture caused by the growth of the uterus. The relaxation of the pelvic joints is primarily due to the hormone relaxin. This increases preparation for a vaginal delivery and causes a "waddling gait." As the uterus enlarges, lordosis shifts the center of gravity over the woman's legs; otherwise, the center of gravity would shift forward and make it difficult for the woman to stand or walk. Both the change in posture and the mobility of the joints contribute to backache during pregnancy (Table 5–2).

Enlargement of the uterus stretches the round ligaments that support the uterus, and this can cause a quick, sharp pain when the woman moves quickly, such as getting up from a chair. In addition, as the abdominal muscles are gradually stretched during pregnancy, the rectus muscles may separate, a condition called *diastasis recti abdominis*. The muscles return to their normal position sometime after delivery. This process is facilitated by exercise.

During pregnancy, weight gain and edema can produce a compression of the medial nerve, particularly around the wrist. This is referred to as carpal tunnel syndrome. Commonly this syndrome consists of pain, numbness, or tingling in the hand and wrist. In severe cases, weakness and decreased motor function occur. Supportive therapy is usually adequate, and the symptoms sub-

TABLE 5–2. CHANGES IN MUSCULOSKELETAL SYSTEM DURING PREGNANCY

PHYSIOLOGICAL CHANGE	CLINICAL SIGNIFICANCE
PELVIC JOINTS RELAX UNDER INFLUENCE OF HORMONE RELAXIN	Ligaments of the pubic symphysis and sacroiliac joints become more pliable, causing backache
POSTURE CHANGES OCCUR	Center of gravity shifts anteriorly
Lordosis occurs	Protuberant abdomen and lordosis lead to an unsteady gait and backache
UTERINE WEIGHT INCREASES	Round ligament pain may occur, especially with quick movements
DIASTASIS RECTI MAY OCCUR	Abdominal recti muscles may separate
CARPAL TUNNEL SYNDROME MAY OCCUR	Muscle numbness, weakness, and tenderness may be experienced in the wrist and thumb

side in the postpartum period as the total body fluid volume returns to normal. Sometimes splints are placed on the dorsum side of the hand to keep the wrist in a neutral position (Table 5–2).

CHANGES IN THE CARDIOVASCULAR SYSTEM

The cardiovascular system exhibits profound changes during pregnancy. These changes are essential to deliver oxygen and nutrients to the growing fetus and the enlarging uterus. Blood must be delivered into uterine vessels at pressures sufficient to meet the requirements of the placental circulation, which is necessary for an adequate exchange of oxygen between mother and fetus.

Anatomical Changes

Enlargement of the heart (myocardial hypertrophy) begins to occur early in pregnancy. This change is attributed mainly to the increase in *stroke volume,* the amount of blood ejected per heartbeat. Most likely, in addition to the extra work the heart must do because of the increased stroke volume, the elevation in hormone levels plays a role in cardiac enlargement (Fig. 5–5).

Position of the Heart

Change in the position of the heart is attributed to an elevation of the diaphragm, which is noticeable in the second half of pregnancy. The heart rotates forward and to the left; this position change may cause electrocardiogram changes. In addition, heart sounds are often louder and more forceful. Women may notice slight palpitations and may need reassurance that during pregnancy these are common. Benign arrhythmias can occur, and systolic murmurs are not uncommon. Diastolic murmurs, however, are considered pathologic.

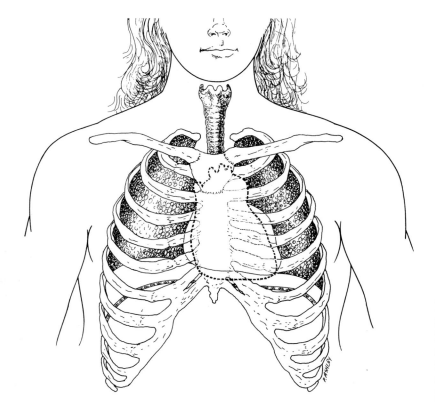

▲ FIGURE 5–5

Changes in the position of the heart, lungs, and thoracic cage during pregnancy. The broken line indicates the nonpregnant position; the solid line indicates changes that occur during pregnancy.

Cardiac Output

Cardiac output—blood volume injected into the system—is increased 30% to 50% over normal. This greater output is noticeable as early as 10 weeks. The increased cardiac output is necessary to meet the demands of the enlarging uterus and growing fetus. In addition, the increased cardiac output acts as a reserve in case of blood loss at birth. The cardiac output also increases in response to the elevation in metabolic needs (Table 5–3).

Blood flow is greater in some areas than in others; for example, the blood flow to the skin can increase as much as 70% by the thirty-sixth week of pregnancy. This can cause the woman to experience a feeling of warmth, clammy or moist skin, sweating, and nasal congestion.

During pregnancy, there is a greater renal blood flow, facilitating adequate maternal kidney function. Urinary output increases to remove the waste products for both mother and fetus. Increased cardiac output allows adequate blood flow to the uteroplacental unit to meet the demands of the fetus.

Pulse Rate and Stroke Volume

As a result of the increase in blood volume, the pulse rate increases approximately 10 beats per minute. Also, the stroke volume (the amount of blood ejected per heartbeat) is elevated. Hence, not only is the heart beating faster, but also with each beat the heart has to pump out more blood. This means that the relaxation period (diastolic period) in the cardiac cycle is shortened. These adjustments are well tolerated by most women. However, if a woman has a history of previous heart problems, she should be carefully monitored during pregnancy.

Blood Volume

Blood volume begins to increase during the first trimester or as early as the tenth week of gestation. The increase is most rapid during the second trimester, appears to peak at approximately 30 to 34 weeks, and then seems to plateau. The average increase in blood volume is about 33% (range = 30% to 50%). This increase in blood volume involves a greater increase in fluid content than in cellular content, allowing increased fluid to the maternal and fetal tissues.

Plasma Volume and Red Blood Cell Count

Both plasma volume and red blood cell (RBC) count increase during pregnancy. Increased plasma volume (the fluid component of blood) is necessary to dissipate fetal heat production, and an elevated RBC count (the cellular component) is necessary for fetal oxygen needs. The increases in plasma and RBCs are disproportionate; there is a greater increase in the plasma volume than in the number of RBCs. This results in a hemodilution or "physiological anemia." It is generally accepted that the hemoglobin should not be less than 11 g/dL, and the hematocrit value should not be less than 35%. If these values are below the arbitrary lower limits of normal, the woman is considered to have anemia secondary to some other condition, generally iron deficiency anemia. Oral supplementation of elemental iron (60 to 80 mg/day) is routine during pregnancy. A therapeutic amount is 120 to 240 mg/day.

White Blood Cell Count

The white blood cell count increases to 15,000 on the average (normal range = 5000 to 10,000). This increase in WBCs protects against infection. If the WBC count is above 15,000 the woman should be evaluated for infection.

Blood Clotting Factors

Blood clotting factors increase during pregnancy. In fact, pregnancy places a woman in a "hypercoagulable state" with an increase in fibrinogen and other blood clotting factors. Hence, there is a faster response in stopping the bleeding at the placental site after delivery. At the same time, there is a greater potential for the development of an embolism during the postpartum period. For this reason, women are asked to ambulate quickly and frequently during the postpartum period.

TABLE 5–3. CHANGES IN THE CARDIOVASCULAR SYSTEM DURING PREGNANCY

PHYSIOLOGICAL CHANGE	CLINICAL SIGNIFICANCE
HEART DISPLACED BY ELEVATION OF DIAPHRAGM	Palpitations, benign arrhythmias, and systolic murmurs are result of change in position of heart
CARDIAC OUTPUT INCREASES	Cardiac output or volume of blood injected into system is increased 30–50% to meet demands of enlarging uterus and fetal oxygenation
Blood flow increases in skin	Feelings of warmth, moist skin, and nasal congestion are experienced
Blood flow increases to kidneys	Improves removal of waste products for mother and fetus
PULSE RATE AND STROKE VOLUME INCREASE	Pulse rate increases approximately 10 beats/minute, and stroke volume increases
BLOOD VOLUME INCREASES 30–50%	Blood volume increases early in pregnancy; begins at about 10 wks; peaks at 34 wks
	Blood volume increase hydrates maternal and fetal tissues
PLASMA AND RED BLOOD VOLUME INCREASE	Plasma volume increases more than red cell mass, causing hemoglobin and hematocrit to fall; oral supplementation of 60–80 mg/day of elemental iron is routine
	If hemoglobin drops below 11 g/dL or hematocrit below 35%, woman should be evaluated for anemia
WHITE BLOOD CELL COUNT INCREASES (average >15,000)	A protective mechanism against infection
BLOOD CLOTTING FACTORS INCREASE	Provides rapid blood clotting mechanism at placental site when expelled, increasing risk of postpartum embolism; therefore, women are asked to ambulate frequently after delivery
FEMORAL VENOUS PRESSURE INCREASES	Enlarged uterus places pressure on veins of lower extremities, and stagnation of blood in lower extremities may occur
SUPINE HYPOTENSIVE COMPRESSION MAY OCCUR	Compression of the inferior vena cava in third trimester by gravid uterus can decrease cardiac output; women are instructed to lie on left side
ORTHOSTATIC HYPOTENSION MAY OCCUR	Decrease in cardiac output may occur when a woman moves from a recumbent to an upright position
BLOOD PRESSURE DOES NOT INCREASE	An arbitrary upper limit of normal is 140/90 mm Hg; an increase of 30 mm Hg or more systolic or 15 mm Hg or more diastolic is indicative of a potential hypertensive disorder

Femoral Venous Pressure

As the enlarged uterus places pressure on the veins of the lower extremities, femoral venous pressure increases. For this reason, pregnant women should be instructed to avoid sitting or standing for long periods of time. Also, they should be instructed not to sit with their legs crossed, because this decreases venous blood flow. Lying on the left side increases venous blood return; the woman should be encouraged to lie on her left side whenever she is in a recumbent position.

Supine Hypotension Syndrome

The vena cava is compressed to some degree when pregnant women lie on their backs during the last half of pregnancy. This is referred to as *supine hypotension syndrome* (Fig. 5–6). When pressure from the pregnant uterus places pressure on the inferior vena cava, the venous blood return is reduced, which in turn reduces the cardiac output. If pressure on the veins is prolonged, the woman may experience shock symptoms including dizziness, faintness, fast pulse, moist skin, nausea and vomiting, and decreased blood pressure. These conditions can compromise the fetus. If the woman lies on her left side (the inferior vena cava

is on the right side), the venous blood return will revert back to adequate circulation.

Orthostatic Hypotension

A decrease in cardiac output may occur whenever a woman moves from a recumbent position to a standing position; this is referred to as *orthostatic hypotension.* A decrease in venous return is the cause of orthostatic hypotension.

Varicose Veins

Obstructed venous return by the gravid (enlarged) uterus and relaxation of the smooth muscle owing to progesterone are causes for varicose veins in the vulva and anal area (hemorrhoids). Varicose veins usually diminish in size after the birth of the baby.

Blood Pressure

Blood pressure should be the same during pregnancy as it is in the nonpregnant state. An elevation of blood pressure during pregnancy indicates a potential hypertensive disorder. An arbitrary upper limit of normal blood pressure is 140/90,

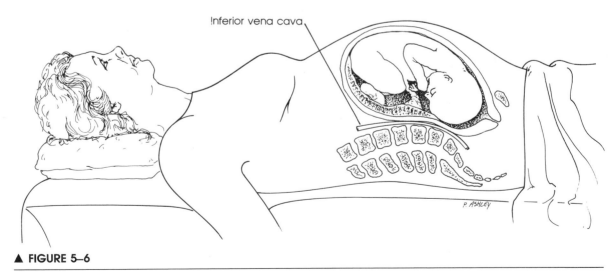

Inferior vena cava

P. ASHLEY

▲ FIGURE 5–6

Supine hypotensive syndrome. Gravid uterus compresses vena cava when the woman is in a supine position. The blood flow returning to the heart is decreased, and maternal hypotension may result.

but more important is a 30-mm Hg or more increase in the systolic pressure and a 15-mm Hg or more increase in the diastolic pressure above the nonpregnant state. Pregnant women who demonstrate these levels of blood pressure need further medical attention (Table 5–3).

CHANGES IN THE RESPIRATORY SYSTEM

Thoracic circumference increases during pregnancy because of the relaxation of the ligaments (primarily owing to progesterone) and a flaring of the lower ribs. Therefore, despite the elevation of the diaphragm (as much as 4 cm) in the later part of pregnancy, the lung capacity remains the same.

Inspiration increases during pregnancy, allowing greater intake of oxygen. Increased expiration facilitates carbon dioxide removal. In other words, the exchange of carbon dioxide and oxygen that takes place at the alveolar cell level is improved. The pregnant woman breathes more deeply and more frequently to maintain oxygen for herself and her fetus.

Dyspnea

Shortness of breath—dyspnea—is a common complaint of pregnancy. The sensation of dyspnea appears to be related to a greater sensitivity of the respiratory system caused by increased progesterone. Dyspnea is also related to pressure of the gravid uterus on the diaphragm.

Epistaxis

Nosebleeds and nasal ''stuffiness'' are common during pregnancy. These discomforts are thought to be due to the increased vascularity that results from increased estrogen. Another change that can occur is a change in the woman's voice. A pregnant woman's voice may become deeper because of an increase in the size of the vocal cords that is caused by increased progesterone (Table 5–4).

CHANGES IN THE GASTROINTESTINAL SYSTEM

Changes in the mouth frequently occur during pregnancy. Some pregnant women complain that their gums bleed easily when they brush their teeth. The bleeding is due to a softening of the gums because of the increased amount of estrogen present during pregnancy. Women should be instructed to use a soft toothbrush and practice good oral hygiene. An increase in appetite and thirst is common and facilitates growth of the fetus and uterus. Saliva production (ptyalism) is often increased; the etiology is unknown. Nausea with or without vomiting is common during the first part of pregnancy and is thought to be due to the rising level of estrogen in the blood (Table 5–5).

During pregnancy, the peristaltic action of the gastrointestinal tract decreases. This is mainly due to the increase in progesterone. With the relaxation of the cardiac sphincter, gastric contents can reach the esophagus and cause heartburn, a common discomfort of pregnancy. Pregnant women should be urged to sit up for 30 minutes after eating, rather than immediately lie down, to lessen heartburn (Fig. 5–7).

With the loss in muscle tone, there is a delayed emptying time of the intestines, which allows more water to be absorbed from the bowel. This change causes constipation, another common complaint.

Metabolic changes occur during pregnancy. Carbohydrate metabolism alters, allowing the fetus to have a source of high energy, in the form of glycogen. Fat metabolism also alters, which facilitates fetal growth and provides maternal stores for lactation.

CHANGES IN THE RENAL (URINARY) SYSTEM

Early in pregnancy the growing uterus puts pressure on the bladder, causing frequent urination. Later in pregnancy, as the fetus settles down in the pelvic cavity, the woman again experiences pressure on the bladder, and frequency of urination returns (Fig. 5–8).

Because renal blood flow is increased, the substances in the blood are cleared more efficiently.

TABLE 5–4. CHANGES IN RESPIRATORY SYSTEM DURING PREGNANCY

PHYSIOLOGICAL CHANGE	CLINICAL SIGNIFICANCE
LOWER RIBS FLARE	Lower ribs attached to relaxed ligaments flare, increasing the thoracic circumference and movement and allowing improved gaseous exchange to occur
	Inspiration and oxygen intake increase; greater expiration facilitates carbon dioxide removal
DIAPHRAGM RISES 4 CM (THIRD TRIMESTER)	Despite the elevation of the diaphragm, the lung capacity remains the same
DYSPNEA OFTEN OCCURS	Dyspnea occurs as result of greater sensitivity of respiratory center and mechanical pressure

TABLE 5–5. CHANGES IN GASTROINTESTINAL SYSTEM DURING PREGNANCY

PHYSIOLOGICAL CHANGE	CLINICAL SIGNIFICANCE
ORAL CHANGES OCCUR	Gums become more vascular and bleed easily; saliva production (ptyalism) is increased
APPETITE AND THIRST INCREASE	Appetite and thirst increase, which facilitates growth of fetus and uterus; an alteration in taste buds may occur
NAUSEA AND VOMITING ARE COMMON	Nausea and vomiting are a common complaint early in pregnancy; usually disappear by week 16
MUSCLE TONE AND MOTILITY DECREASE	Constipation, esophageal reflux (heartburn), and nausea may occur; water absorption within colon causes constipation
METABOLIC CHANGES OCCUR	Carbohydrate metabolism is altered, which allows the fetus to have a source of high energy; fat metabolism is altered, which facilitates fetal growth and maternal stores for lactation

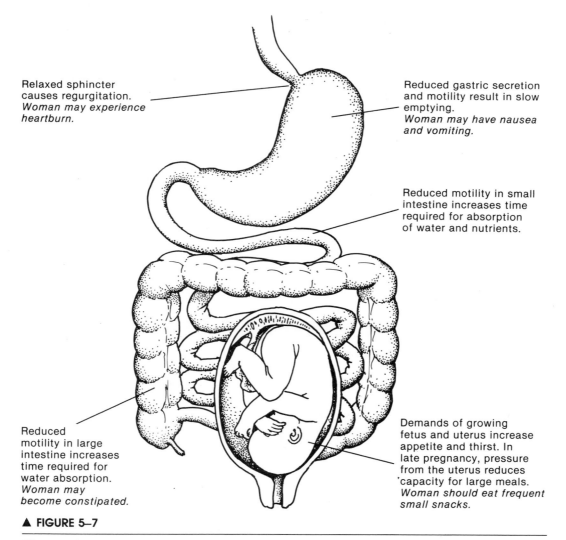

Relaxed sphincter causes regurgitation. *Woman may experience heartburn.*

Reduced gastric secretion and motility result in slow emptying. *Woman may have nausea and vomiting.*

Reduced motility in small intestine increases time required for absorption of water and nutrients.

Reduced motility in large intestine increases time required for water absorption. *Woman may become constipated.*

Demands of growing fetus and uterus increase appetite and thirst. In late pregnancy, pressure from the uterus reduces capacity for large meals. *Woman should eat frequent small snacks.*

▲ **FIGURE 5–7**

Changes in the gastrointestinal system related to pregnancy.

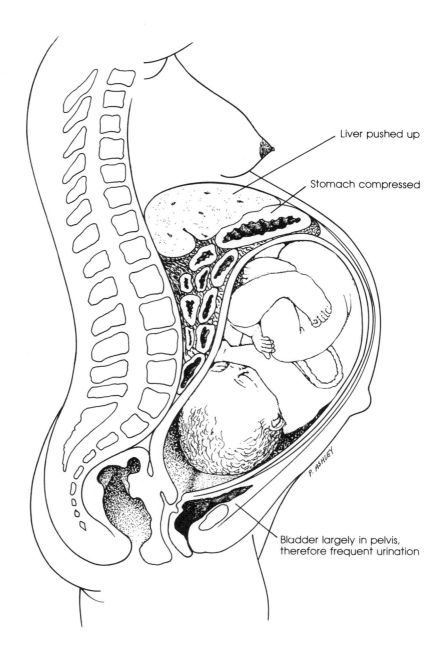

Liver pushed up

Stomach compressed

Bladder largely in pelvis, therefore frequent urination

▲ **FIGURE 5–8**

Crowding of abdominal contents late in pregnancy causes urinary frequency.

With a decrease in the smooth muscle function, the peristaltic action necessary to propel the urine from the kidneys to the bladder decreases. This places the woman at risk for urinary infection. Because of this, pregnant women are instructed to drink eight 8-oz glasses of fluid every day (Table 5–6).

Psychological Changes During Pregnancy

Pregnancy is a profound event in the life of a woman and her family. It is a time when she and her significant others are faced with the challenges of redefining their present roles, working through previous conflicts, and taking on the parent role. The emotional and physical adjustments of pregnancy plus those required to become parents cause varying levels of stress and anxiety.

Some specific factors that contribute to either a positive or a negative psychological response of a woman to her pregnancy include body image changes, emotional security, cultural expectations, support from significant others, whether the pregnancy is unexpected, and financial situation. A major factor that influences the psychological impact of pregnancy is a woman's level of maturity and readiness for childbearing.

BODY IMAGE

Body image is a person's perception of his or her own body. Body image can be grouped into four main categories: appearance, function, sensation, and mobility.

Appearance

As some women enter later adulthood, greater emphasis is placed on their inner selves and less emphasis is placed on physical appearances. However, during pregnancy, changes in their body's shape and functions are so noticeable that they may become threatening. The speed with which the changes occur makes it difficult for women to integrate them into their self-perception (Fig. 5–9).

The change in body shape alone can cause women to feel negative about their pregnancy. They may feel ugly and fat and as if they are a "big bulge." These women need reassurance and physical closeness. Women must recognize that their feelings are normal and understandable. The expression of physical love is a good way to lessen their negative feelings about their pregnancies.

Other women feel beautiful during their pregnancies and will say things like "I feel good when I am pregnant."

Function

The pregnant woman often experiences a decline in body control. Her physical discomforts frequently cause her great anxiety. For example, if she experiences urinary incontinence, she may feel out of control of her body, and this feeling will reinforce negative feelings about her pregnancy. If the body adjustments that she will likely

---

TABLE 5–6. CHANGES IN RENAL SYSTEM DURING PREGNANCY

PHYSIOLOGICAL CHANGE	CLINICAL SIGNIFICANCE
URINARY FREQUENCY OCCURS	Early and late in pregnancy, the uterus exerts pressure on the bladder, causing frequent urination
RENAL BLOOD FLOW INCREASES	Improves renal function; substances are cleared from blood more efficiently
TONE AND MOTILITY DECREASE	Decrease in smooth muscle function puts woman at risk for urinary stasis and infection; increased fluid intake decreases risk

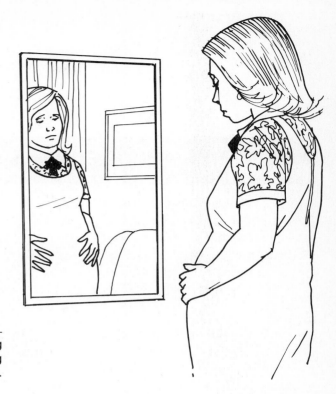

▲ FIGURE 5–9

Body image. A woman's appearance changes during pregnancy; some women have difficulty integrating these changes with previous perceptions of themselves.

experience are explained to her and if she is reassured that these changes are normal, she will be able to accept them with less difficulty.

Sensation

During pregnancy, the physical senses may become more acute. Pregnant women may be more sensitive to touch. The change in sexuality varies, and the libido may be increased or decreased from the nonpregnant state. The apparent physiological basis of heightened sexuality is the greater vasocongestion in the pelvic area during pregnancy.

Mobility

The pregnant woman often feels restricted in physical activities that were part of her usual routine before pregnancy. She should be encouraged to participate in the same activities (including many sports) that she participated in before she became pregnant, as long as participation creates

no problem with her pregnancy. Moderation is the key instruction to physical activities during pregnancy.

DEVELOPMENTAL TASKS

Pregnant women are known to go through certain developmental tasks. Tasks relate to the sequence of trimesters and are more apparent in some women than in others.

Task 1: Pregnancy Validation

In the first trimester (first 3 months), the pregnancy is confirmed, and frequently introversion occurs and may continue during the first part of pregnancy. The behavior is an acceptable coping mechanism for this period of time. Introversion is encouraged by weight gain, wearing of maternity clothes, and other outward signs of pregnancy. At this time, the woman may question her identity as a woman and as a mother.

NURSING CARE PLAN 5–1

EFFECT OF PHYSICAL AND PSYCHOLOGICAL CHANGES DURING PREGNANCY

Potential Problems and Nursing Diagnoses	Nursing Interventions
1. Anxiety related to the unknown (if woman is/is not pregnant).	Explain the suggestive signs and positive signs of pregnancy.
2. Ineffective coping related to being pregnant.	Acknowledge the woman's feelings about the changes in family structure and economic status caused by the addition of a new member to the family.
3. Knowledge deficit related to changes that occur in the various body systems.	Discuss what physical changes will occur in her body during pregnancy and why.
4. Knowledge deficit related to changes in pigmentation of the skin.	Explain that an increase in hormones causes some areas of the skin to darken.
5. Sleep pattern disturbance related to frequent voiding.	Explain how the gravid uterus places pressure on the bladder.
6. Body image disturbance related to physical appearance.	Encourage the woman to express her feelings about changes in her appearance during pregnancy.

Expected Outcomes

1. Patient communicates an understanding of the suggestive and positive signs of pregnancy.
2. Patient expresses relief that health care provider is willing to listen to her feelings.
3. Patient demonstrates understanding of the various body changes that occur during pregnancy.
4. Patient recognizes that pigmentation changes occur during pregnancy but usually will lighten or disappear after the baby is born.
5. Patient verbalizes an understanding of why frequent voiding occurs during pregnancy.
6. Patient expresses confidence in her ability to accept changes in her body image (weight gain, pigmentation changes, etc.).

Task 2: Fetal Embodiment

During the second trimester (second 3 months), the woman usually attempts to incorporate the fetus into her body image as an integral part of self. She begins to readjust to her life roles and often reviews her conflicts with others. At this time, repressed thoughts can be dealt with, and it can be a time of maturation. She may experience greater inner strength to take on her new role.

Task 3: Fetal Distinction

When the woman feels quickening or fetal movements, the fetus begins to become distinct and apart from herself. At this time, she starts to form concepts of what type of mother she should be. The woman frequently daydreams about what her baby will be like. She begins to envision a perfect, beautiful baby and speaks of the baby as a certain sex. Her dreams may become unrealistic ("He is going to be a professional football player.").

Task 4: Role Transition

During the last trimester (third 3 months), the pregnant woman usually psychologically separates the fetus from herself and makes concrete plans for the baby. For example, she often purchases a crib and layette. At this time, she may show greater irritability, complain about her physical discomforts, and want the pregnancy to end. Her normal coping mechanisms frequently do not work quite as well for her, and she may need additional emotional support and anticipatory guidance.

In summary, mood swing, introversion, and passivity are common and normal during pregnancy. Women frequently experience emotional lability, heightened sensitivity, increased need for affection, greater irritability, fear, and anxiety. The expectant mother needs to receive rather than to give emotional support. She demonstrates an increased need for affection and caring so that she can later nurture her baby. Pregnancy can be a maturing experience for a woman in that she accepts the role of a woman and a mother. Guidance and instruction are an important part of nursing care (see Nursing Care Plan 5–1). They can help make pregnancy a more positive and enjoyable experience.

References

Auvenshine, M. A., & Enriquez, M. G. (1990). *Comprehensive Maternity Nursing: Perinatal and Women's Health*, 2nd ed. Boston: Jones and Bartlett.

Danforth, N. D., & Scott, J. R. (1986). *Obstetrics and Gynecology*, 5th ed. Philadelphia: J. B. Lippincott.

Ladewig, P. W., London, M. L., & Olds, S. B. (1990). *Essentials of Maternal-Newborn Nursing*, 2nd ed. Redwood City, CA: Addison-Wesley Nursing.

Lederer, J. R., Marculescu, G. L., Mocnik, B., & Seaby, N. (1990). *Care Planning Pocket Guide: A Nursing Diagnosis Approach*. Redwood City, CA: Addison-Wesley Nursing.

Lederman, R. (1984). *Psychological Adaptation in Pregnancy*. Beverly Hills, CA: Sage.

Parmley, T., & O'Brien, T. (1990). Skin changes during pregnancy. *Clinical Obstetrics and Gynecology* 33:713–717.

Sherwen, L. N. (1987). *Psychological Dimensions of the Pregnant Family*. New York: Springer.

SUGGESTED ACTIVITIES

1. Explain the physical adjustments that occur during pregnancy.
2. Describe the developmental tasks of pregnancy.
3. List the common discomforts of pregnancy and the appropriate nursing actions to relieve them.
4. List the positive signs of pregnancy.

REVIEW QUESTIONS

A. Select the best answer to each multiple-choice question.

1. Ms. Johnson's initial history reveals that she is gravida 3 para 2. Which of the following best explains this statement?

   A. She is pregnant for the first time

   B. She has delivered her third child

   C. She is pregnant for the third time and has had two other viable pregnancies

   D. She is pregnant for the third time and has had two abortions

2. If Ms. Johnson, 7 months pregnant, complains of nasal congestion and epistaxis, the nurse could advise her that these symptoms are related to
   A. Increase in prolactin
   B. Increase in estrogen
   C. Increase in human placental lactogen
   D. Increase in aldosterone

3. If Ms. Johnson, 8 months pregnant, complains of backache, the nurse should explain to her that a relaxation of the pelvic joints causing backache is primarily due to the hormone
   A. Estrogen
   B. Prolactin
   C. Relaxin
   D. Aldosterone

4. Plasma and blood volume change during pregnancy. The changes include
   A. Increase in plasma and in red blood cells
   B. Decrease in plasma and in red blood cells
   C. Increase in plasma, but decrease in red blood cells
   D. Decrease in plasma, but increase in red blood cells

5. Ms. Johnson should be instructed that breast changes that occur during pregnancy are mainly due to an increase in hormones. These changes will include
   A. Enlargement of the breasts
   B. Secretion of colostrum
   C. Sensation of tingling and tenderness
   D. All of the above

6. Respiratory changes that occur during pregnancy include all of the following EXCEPT
   A. Increased inspiration
   B. Increased expiration
   C. Flaring of the lower ribs
   D. Decreased carbon dioxide removal

7. Gastrointestinal changes that occur during pregnancy include all of the following EXCEPT
   A. Increase in appetite and thirst
   B. Decrease in water absorption from the colon
   C. Relaxation of the cardiac sphincter
   D. Increase in saliva production

8. The complaints of nausea and vomiting and amenorrhea are
   A. Presumptive signs of pregnancy
   B. Positive signs of pregnancy
   C. Probable signs of pregnancy
   D. Signs of labor

9. The following is a positive sign of pregnancy:
   A. Positive pregnancy test result
   B. Fetal heart tones
   C. Uterine enlargement
   D. Amenorrhea

10. The duration of a full-term pregnancy in weeks is
    A. 36
    B. 40
    C. 42
    D. 280

11. Using Nägele's rule, if a woman had her last normal menstrual period on May 10, her expected date of confinement would be
    A. January 10
    B. February 10
    C. February 17
    D. March 17

12. The pregnant woman's circulatory system adjustments include all of the following EXCEPT
    A. Increased blood volume
    B. Decreased pulse rate
    C. Increased blood flow to the kidney
    D. Increased white cell count

13. During the last trimester, the pregnant woman may experience dizziness, faintness, and a decreased blood pressure when she lies on her back. This is referred to as
    A. Lightening
    B. Supine hypotension syndrome
    C. Circulatory insufficiency
    D. None of the above

14. The arbitrary upper limits of "normal" blood pressure during pregnancy are
    A. 135/80
    B. 120/88
    C. 138/86
    D. 140/90

15. During pregnancy, the renal system changes include all of the following EXCEPT
    A. Increased renal blood flow
    B. Occasional trace of glucose in urine
    C. Additional risk for urinary infection
    D. Decrease in kidney function

16. Fetal movements felt by the woman are referred to as
    A. Quickening
    B. Lightening
    C. Ballottement
    D. Engagement

B. **Choose from column II the phrase that most accurately defines the term in column I.**

I	*II*
1. Human chorionic gonadotropin _____	A. Sodium-retaining hormone
2. Aldosterone _____	B. Causes vascular change
3. Estrogen _____	C. Critical to maintain corpus luteum in early pregnancy
4. Progesterone _____	D. Relaxes smooth muscle

C. **Choose from column II the phrase that most accurately defines the term in column I.**

I	*II*
1. Physiological anemia _____	A. Spillage of glucose in urine.
2. Heartburn _____	B. Water absorbed from bowel
3. Dyspnea _____	C. Greater increase of plasma volume than red cell volume
4. Constipation _____	D. Relaxation of cardiac sphincter
5. Glucosuria _____	E. Increased sensitivity of respiratory center
6. Backache _____	F. Pressure on bladder by gravid uterus
7. Body image _____	G. Change in posture
8. Urinary frequency _____	H. Person's perception of own body

D. **Match the developmental task during pregnancy in column II with its definition in column I.**

I	*II*
1. Pregnancy validation _____	A. Woman separates fetus from self
2. Role transition _____	B. Fetal movements increase thoughts about mothering role
3. Fetal distinction _____	C. Introversion occurs as pregnancy is confirmed

CHAPTER 6 _____

Chapter Outline

Significance of Prenatal Care
Promotion of Health
Prenatal Visits
    Initial history
    Subsequent visits
Nutrition
    Importance of nutrition
    The basic nutrients
    Nutritional risk factors during pregnancy
    Guidelines for nutritional assessment and intervention
Common Discomforts: Nursing Interventions and Self-Care
    Nausea with or without vomiting
    Heartburn
    Constipation
    Urinary frequency and urgency
    Flatulence
    Backache
    Varicose veins
    Dyspnea
    Faintness and dizziness
    Leg cramps
    Swelling of feet and ankles
    Carpal tunnel syndrome
    Round ligament pain
Education for Self-Care
    Bathing
    Physical activity
    Sexual activity
    Douching
    Dressing
    Breast and nipple care
    Dental care
    Travel and work
    Medications
    Danger signs
Substance Abuse
    Cocaine
    Caffeine
    Alcohol
    Cigarette smoking
    Drug dependency: Assessment and management
Nursing Diagnoses to Consider During Pregnancy

Learning Objectives

Upon completion of Chapter 6, the student should be able to

- Explain the significance of prenatal care.
- Describe the importance of promotion of health.
- Describe the care given during the first prenatal visit.
- Explain what is done on subsequent prenatal visits and how the visits are scheduled.
- Name the laboratory tests to be performed at each prenatal visit.
- Identify the components of an adequate prenatal diet.
- Name three minerals and three vitamins whose intake should be increased during pregnancy and identify the need for and sources of each.
- List five nutritional risk factors during pregnancy.
- Identify five common discomforts of pregnancy and the nursing interventions for each.
- Describe nipple care during pregnancy.
- Outline the instructions of self-care for the woman's personal hygiene.
- Describe how the use of nicotine, alcohol, or cocaine can harm the fetus.
- Relate the dangers that are associated with the use of caffeine during pregnancy.
- List four health disorders commonly found in women who are chemically dependent.

Health care during pregnancy

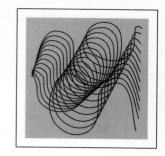

Significance of Prenatal Care

Improved prenatal care has dramatically reduced infant and maternal mortality. Detecting potential problems early leads to prompt assessment and treatment, which greatly improves the pregnancy's outcome. Because so much of the wellness of pregnancy depends on the woman's and family's assuming responsibility for the health of the woman and her fetus, preventive measures such as adequate nutrition, proper exercise, assessment of pregnancy, and a planned regimen of care are essential. Clearly, prenatal care is the greatest "insurance policy" a woman can invest in during her pregnancy.

Promotion of Health

When a woman suspects she is pregnant, she should consult medical and nursing assistance as early as possible. The course of pregnancy depends on a number of factors: the woman's pre-pregnancy health, the present status of her health, her emotional status, and past health care. All of these factors are assessed and evaluated during prenatal visits. Appropriate medical and nursing interventions are then suggested. Without doubt, the woman who obtains the earliest prenatal care possible, continues to obtain adequate care, and practices good health habits has fewer risks and discomforts during pregnancy.

THE GOALS OF PRENATAL CARE
SHOULD BE AS FOLLOWS:

- A pregnancy with minimum physical and emotional discomfort and maximum gratification

- Establishment of good health habits for the benefit of mother and baby
- A birth under the most desirable circumstances
- A normal, healthy baby
- Preparation for early motherhood
- Establishment of positive relationships between the infant and mother and significant others

Prenatal Visits

The first prenatal visit is often stressful to the woman. Establishing a comfortable environment in the first as well as subsequent visits is very important.

INITIAL HISTORY

A health history summary, including a thorough medical and obstetric history, is taken during the first examination to determine the present status of the woman's health. First, personal information is obtained, including age, marital status, education, and occupation. Second, the patient's and her family's medical history is taken. The family history is important to identify certain health problems, such as heart disease and genetic disorders, that could affect the outcome of pregnancy. The woman's personal history is important to assess her present and past health. Third, information about the woman's obstetric history is obtained. It includes the number of previous pregnancies (if this is not her first pregnancy); birth weight of previous infants; length of previous labor; and what, if any, problems arose during previous pregnancy, labor, birth, and puerperium. This information can give clues of what to expect during the present pregnancy (Figs. 6–1 and 6–2).

87

Health History Summary

Date: mo / day / yr

HOLLISTER® maternal/newborn RECORD SYSTEM

PATIENT IDENTIFICATION

Patient's name _____

Home address _____

STREET

CITY   STATE   ZIP

Age _____ Date of birth mo/ day / yr   Race or ethnicity _____ Religion _____   Marital status _____   Years married _____ Education _____

Social Security number _____   Occupation _____   Work Tel. no. _____   Home Tel. no _____

Alternate contact _____   Relation to patient _____   Work Tel. no. _____   Home Tel. no. _____

Referring physician _____   Attending physician _____   OPTIONAL FOR INSURANCE. ETC.

Medical History

Patient / Family

Check and detail positive findings including date and place of treatment. Precede findings by reference number.

1. Congenital anomalies
2. Genetic diseases
3. Multiple births
4. Diabetes mellitus
5. Malignancies
6. Hypertension
7. Heart disease
8. Rheumatic fever
9. Pulmonary disease
10. GI problems
11. Renal disease
12. Genitourinary tract problems
13. Abnormal uterine bleeding
14. Infertility
15. Venereal disease
16. Phlebitis, varicosities
17. Neurologic disorders
18. Metabol./endocrine disorders
19. Anemia/hemoglobinopathy
20. Blood disorders
21. Drug abuse
22. Smoking/alcohol use
23. Infectious diseases
24. Operations/accidents
25. Allergies/meds sensitivity
26. Blood transfusions
27. Other hospitalizations
28. _____
29. _____
30. **No known disease/problems**

Preexisting Risk Guide

Indicates pregnancy/outcome at risk

31. ☐ Age < 15 or > 35
32. ☐ < 8th grade education
33. ☐ Cardiac disease (class I or II)
34. ☐ Tuberculosis, active
35. ☐ Chronic pulmonary disease
36. ☐ Thrombophlebitis
37. ☐ Endocrinopathy
38. ☐ Epilepsy (on medication)
39. ☐ Infertility (treated)
40. ☐ 2 abortions (spontaneous/induced)
41. ☐ ≥ 7 deliveries
42. ☐ Previous preterm or SGA infants
43. ☐ Infants ≥ 4,000 gms
44. ☐ Isoimmunization (ABO, etc.)
45. ☐ Hemorrhage during previous preg.
46. ☐ Previous preeclampsia
47. ☐ Surgically scarred uterus
48. ☐ Preg. without familial support
49. ☐ Second pregnancy in 12 months
50. ☐ Smoking (≥ 1 pack per day)
51. ☐ _____
52. ☐ _____
53. ☐ _____

Indicates pregnancy/outcome at high risk

54. ☐ Age ≥ 40
55. ☐ Diabetes mellitus
56. ☐ Hypertension
57. ☐ Cardiac disease (class III or IV)
58. ☐ Chronic renal disease
59. ☐ Congenital/chromosomal anomalies
60. ☐ Hemoglobinopathies
61. ☐ Isoimmunization (Rh)
62. ☐ Alcohol or drug abuse
63. ☐ Habitual abortions
64. ☐ Incompetent cervix
65. ☐ Prior fetal or neonatal death
66. ☐ Prior neurologically damaged infant
67. ☐ Significant social problems
68. ☐ _____
69. ☐ _____
70. ☐ _____

Historical Risk Status

71. ☐ No risk factors noted
72. ☐ At risk
73. ☐ At high risk

Signature

Menstrual History	Onset age	Cycle q.	days	Length	days	Amount		L M P	mo/day/yr	quality

Pregnancy History		Grav	Term	Pret	Abort	Live		E D C	mo/day/yr	

No.	Month/ year	Sex	Weight at birth	Wks. gest.	Hrs. in labor	Type of delivery	Details of delivery: Include anesthesia and maternal or newborn complications. Use Risk Guide numbers where applicable.
1							
2							
3							
4							
5							
6							
7							
8							

Hollister™

HOLLISTER INCORPORATED. 2000 HOLLISTER DR. LIBERTYVILLE. IL 60048
*TRADEMARK OF HOLLISTER INCORPORATED

HEALTH HISTORY SUMMARY

5870-4/86

MOTHER'S PHYSICIAN COPY

▲ **FIGURE 6–1**

Health history summary. (Permission to reproduce this copyrighted material has been granted by the owner, Hollister Incorporated.)

Prenatal Flow Record

HOLLISTER®
maternal/newborn
RECORD SYSTEM

PATIENT IDENTIFICATION

Patient's name _____

Historical Risk Factors and Assessment

_____

☐ Has no known risk
☐ Is "at risk"
☐ Is at high risk

Continuing Risk Assessment Guide (revise RISK STATUS)

Date	At risk factors	Date	High risk factors
/	Uterine/cervical malformation	/	Diabetes mellitus
/	Suspect pelvis	/	Hypertension
/	Rh negative (nonsensitized)	/	Thrombophlebitis
/	Anemia (Hct <30%:Hgb <10%)	/	Herpes (type 2)
/	Venereal disease	/	Rh sensitization
/	Acute pyelonephritis	/	Uterine bleeding
/	Failure to gain weight	/	Hydramnios
/	Abnormal presentation	/	Severe preeclampsia
/	Postterm pregnancy	/	Fetal growth retardation
/	Alcohol use	/	Premature rupt. membranes
/		/	Multiple pregnancy (preterm)
/		/	Alcohol and drug abuse
/		/	

Medication Sensitivity ☐ None known or: _____

Initial Prenatal Screen / Additional Lab Findings

Date : mo/day /yr	Test	Date	Result	Date	Result
Hct/Hgb	Hct/Hgb	/		/	
Patient's Blood type and Rh	Blood sugar	/		/	
Antibody	Antibody	/		/	
Serology		/		/	
Rubella titer	Bacteriuria	/		/	
Urinalysis micro		/		/	
Pap test		/		/	
Cervical culture		/		/	
		/		/	

LMP mo/day /yr   EDC mo/day /yr   Quickening date mo/day /yr

☐ Initial prenatal instructions   **Amniocentesis**
☐ Attends prenatal classes   Explained on __mo / day__
☐ Do herpes culture   ☐ Accepted ☐ Rejected by patient
☐ Do antenatal RhoGam   **VBAC or C-Section**
☐ For sterilization   ☐ OR records reviewed
☐ Circumcision   Explained on __mo / day__
☐ Needs rubella vaccine   ☐ Candidate for VBAC
☐ Breast ☐ Bottle feeding   ☐ For Cesarean section

Baby's physician _____

G	T	Pt	A	L	Age	Visit date 19 ___	Weight this visit	Pre-gravid	Blood pressure	Base line	Urine protein	Urine Sugar	Est. weeks gestation	(dates/size)	Fundal height	Fetal heart rate/quadrant	Edema	RISK STATUS (0, 1, 2)		Return visit	Sig
						/			/			/		+							
						/			/			/		+							
						/			/			/		+							
						/			/			/		+							
						/			/			/		+							
						/			/			/		+							
						/			/			/		+							
						/			/			/		+							
						/			/			/		+							
						/			/			/		+							
						/			/			/		+							
						/			/			/		+							

Physician's signature

✖ Hollister™
HOLLISTER INCORPORATED. 2000 HOLLISTER DR. LIBERTYVILLE. IL 60048
*TRADEMARK OF HOLLISTER INCORPORATED

PRENATAL FLOW RECORD   MATERNAL RECORD COPY   5872-4/86

▲ **FIGURE 6–2**

Prenatal flow record. (Permission to reproduce this copyrighted material has been granted by the owner, Hollister Incorporated.)

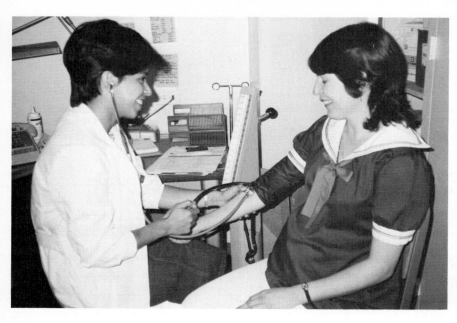

▲ **FIGURE 6–3**

Measurement of blood pressure during prenatal visit.

In the physical examination, the physician or midwife examines all body systems. This includes a head-to-toe examination. The patient's weight and blood pressure are recorded and a microscopic urine examination is done in the first visit. Obtaining the baseline weight and blood pressure is important because a sudden change in either could be significant; a sudden elevation in blood pressure or sudden excessive weight gain is a symptom of pregnancy-induced hypertension, a serious complication (see Chapter 21).

A pelvic examination is performed to determine the status of the reproductive organs and the birth canal. Pelvic measurements are taken to determine whether the pelvis will allow the passage of a fetus at delivery. A manual pelvic measurement, the *diagonal conjugate* (see Fig. 2–7), extends from the inferior margin of the symphysis bladder pubis to the sacral promontory. To measure the diagonal conjugate, the examiner inserts the fingers into the vagina to see if the fingertips reach the sacral promontory (to assess adequacy of the pelvis). Before the pelvic examination is conducted, the nurse should instruct the woman to empty her bladder and to take deep breaths during the examination to lessen her discomfort.

The following laboratory values are obtained during the first visit: hemoglobin concentration, hematocrit value, blood type, and Rh factor. In addition, a Papanicolaou (Pap) smear is done to screen for cervical precancerous cells, a plasma reagin (RPR) serologic test or Venereal Disease Research Laboratories (VDRL) test is used to detect untreated syphilis, and a rubella antibody titer may be measured. The tuberculin skin test (tine test) may be given to screen for tuberculosis in high-risk individuals.

SUBSEQUENT VISITS

Prenatal visits are scheduled every month for 7 months, every 2 weeks during the eighth month, then every week during the last month, if the pregnancy is uneventful (normal).

The woman's weight and blood pressure are recorded (Fig. 6–3), and the urine is checked for protein and glucose. These three assessments are for early detection of hypertension and diabetes. In addition, the physician or midwife measures the height of the uterus to see if the pregnancy is progressing at the expected rate (Figs. 6–4 and 6–5). The woman's abdomen is palpated using Leopold's maneuvers to assess the presentation and position of the fetus (Fig. 6–6). There are four basic maneuvers: (a) Determining what is in the

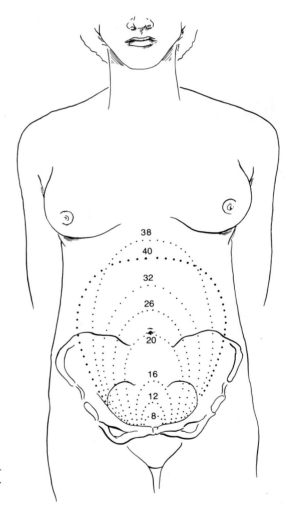

▲ FIGURE 6–4

The relative position of the uterus in different weeks of pregnancy.

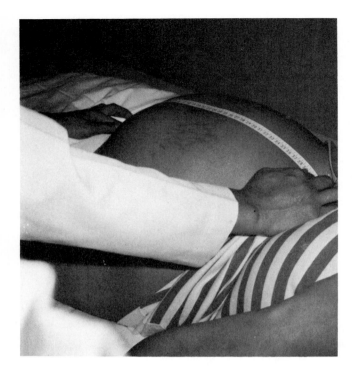

▲ **FIGURE 6–5**

Measuring fundal height.

fundus, either breech or head (the head is firm and round, whereas the breech feels softer); (b) Determining the position of the fetal back (opposite from the extremities); (c) Noting what part of the fetus is above the symphysis pubis, either head or breech; and (d) Noting the position of the cephalic prominence. Having determined the presentation and position of the fetus, the nurse should listen to the fetal heart rate. The fetal heart rate can be counted with a Doppler device or with a fetal stethoscope (see Chapter 5). Assessment for tenderness over the woman's kidney area (costovertebral angle, or CVA) or tenderness in the calf of her legs (Homans' sign) is done because during pregnancy a woman is at greater risk for renal infection and thrombophlebitis.

The woman is asked if she has any discomforts that trouble her. Sometimes vague symptoms or subtle clues are the first indication of an impending complication. If the woman has complaints, medical or nursing measures are suggested to relieve them. Routinely, women are given vitamins and iron supplements. During each visit the woman should be asked if she is taking them, and if not, why. Early in the subsequent visits, the

type of delivery anticipated and how she intends to feed her baby should be discussed. Reassurance of the woman's capacity to be a good mother is important in her decision making during her pregnancy. It is also important that she develop a feeling of trust in caregivers; if she trusts her health care providers, she will be more likely to comply with health care requirements.

Nutrition

IMPORTANCE OF NUTRITION

A woman's nutritional status before, during, and after pregnancy contributes to the well-being of both the woman and her infant. Despite what we know about the relationship between nutrition and health, the medical community in general does not emphasize the need for good nutrition. Referrals to dieticians are often initiated by nurses.

Mothers who are underweight or who have small weight gain during pregnancy place their infants at a higher risk for low birth weight,

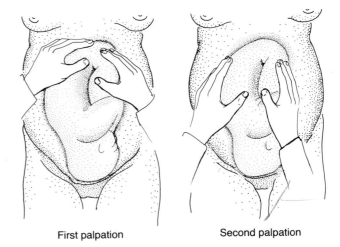

First palpation   Second palpation

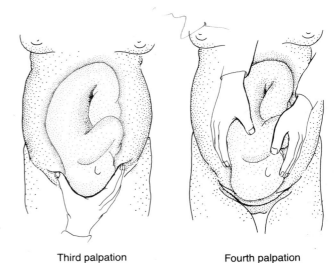

Third palpation   Fourth palpation

▲ **FIGURE 6–6**

Abdominal palpations (Leopold's maneuvers) to determine presentation, lie, and position of the fetus.

prematurity, low Apgar scores, and morbidity. The accepted weight gain in pregnancy, for a healthy outcome, is 25 to 30 lb (Fig. 6–7). During the first trimester, the expected weight gain is 3 to 4 lb, and after the first trimester 1 lb a week. The weight gain during the first trimester is almost entirely growth of maternal tissues. In the second trimester, growth is primarily maternal tissue with some fetal tissue. Growth is mainly fetal in the third trimester. From the third month until term, the fetal weight increases nearly 500-fold. Although obese women face greater risk of certain medical complications, it is not advisable to have them limit their diet during pregnancy. Dietary restriction might reduce not only calories but important nutrients in the woman's diet, which can be harmful to the fetus.

The dietary allowances recommended by the Food and Nutrition Board of the National Research Council, National Academy of Sciences, Washington, DC, provide a margin of safety for health (Table 6–1). The actual requirements for an indi-

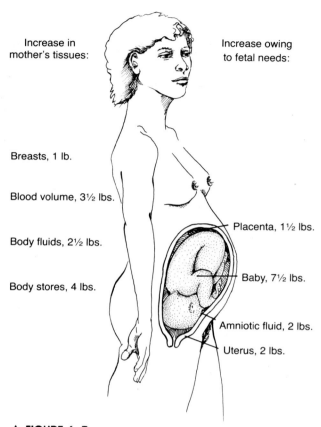

Increase in
mother's tissues:

Increase owing
to fetal needs:

Breasts, 1 lb.

Blood volume, 3½ lbs.

Body fluids, 2½ lbs.

Body stores, 4 lbs.

Placenta, 1½ lbs.

Baby, 7½ lbs.

Amniotic fluid, 2 lbs.

Uterus, 2 lbs.

▲ FIGURE 6–7

Weight gain in an average pregnancy.

vidual differ according to body size, age, activity level, and state of health. The recommended increases over usual caloric intake suggested by the Food and Nutrition Board are an increase of 300 calories per day during pregnancy and an increase of 500 calories per day during breastfeeding. These calories should be in foods that provide additional protein, vitamins, and minerals needed during pregnancy.

An ideal diet for pregnancy consists of the daily intake of 1 quart of milk; two or more servings of meat, poultry, fish, eggs, or cheese; three or more servings of vegetables and fruits; and four or more servings of cereals or bread. In addition to these basic food groups, the expectant mother should drink approximately eight glasses of fluids daily. For women who do not like to drink milk, it should be suggested that milk be used in cooking

or combined with cereals. Fortified skim milk may be used instead of whole milk when there is a need to reduce the fat intake.

Breads and cereals should be those made with enriched flour or whole grains. This will add vitamins and minerals to the diet.

Vegetables should be dark green, leafy, or yellow, and yellow fruits should be purchased. This will increase the amount of vitamin A ingested. Citrus fruits, tomatoes, and other fruits will increase the vitamin C content of the diet.

THE BASIC FOUR FOOD GROUPS

- THE MILK OR DAIRY GROUP: 1 quart of milk daily (four 8-oz glasses)
- THE MEAT GROUP (two servings daily): May include chicken, beef, lamb, pork, veal, fish, eggs
- THE VEGETABLE AND FRUIT GROUP: Dark green or deep yellow vegetables (two servings daily), other vegetables (one daily), and fruit (one or more servings of fruit daily)
- THE BASIC BREAD AND CEREAL GROUP (four servings daily)

THE BASIC NUTRIENTS

Protein

Protein is a building material necessary to the development of new cells for the woman's body and for the growth of the fetus. Protein is required to increase the maternal circulatory blood volume. The expectant mother should have a daily protein intake of 60 g. Protein may be derived from both animal and vegetable sources. Meats and milk are good sources, though relatively expensive. Legumes, such as beans and peas, are less expensive but do not contain all eight amino acids. Thus, animal protein should be included. One quart of milk contains 32 g of protein.

Minerals

Pregnant women need to increase their intake of calcium, phosphorus, and iron. Calcium and

TABLE 6–1. NUTRIENT REQUIREMENTS FOR PREGNANCY

NUTRIENT	NONPREGNANT NEEDS	PREGNANT NEEDS	RATIONALE	NUTRIENT SOURCES
Calories Pregnant Lactating	2200	+ 300 + 500	Growth of fetus, placenta, and maternal tissues. To spare protein for tissue synthesis. Needed as a buffer against food deprivation and prevents catabolism of the mother's tissues. Steady but slow rise in basal metabolism, while decreased activity depresses caloric requirement. Increase in body fat represents storage of sufficient energy to subsidize labor and lactation.	Breads Cereals Milk Fruits Vegetables Fat Margarine
Protein Pregnant Lactating	50 g	60 g* 60 g 65 g	To meet the needs for growth of fetal and maternal tissue and increase in maternal circulatory blood volume. Influences birth size of fetus within limits determined by heredity. Low-birth-weight infants are more susceptible to problems and have lessened chance of survival. Restriction during fetal life is associated with a decline in the number of cells in tissues at time of birth. This decline is particularly serious in the brain.	Milk Cheese Fish Poultry Eggs Legumes Nuts Grains
Calcium	800 mg	1200 mg	Essential element for the construction and maintenance of bones and teeth. Important constituent of the blood clotting mechanism. To deposit approximately 23 g of calcium in the body of the infant. Used in normal muscle action. There should be a storage rather than a depletion of calcium in the mother's tissues during pregnancy to help anticipate demands during lactation. The infant will draw from mother's maternal reserves to fulfill needs of its own development.	Milk Cheese Ice cream Enriched cereals Green leafy vegetables Current recommended daily allowance is contained in 1 L of milk

Table continued on following page

TABLE 6–1. NUTRIENT REQUIREMENTS FOR PREGNANCY *Continued*

NUTRIENT	NONPREGNANT NEEDS	PREGNANT NEEDS	RATIONALE	NUTRIENT SOURCES
Iron	15 mg	30 mg	Mother must transfer about 300 mg of iron to fetus during gestation. Fetus needs to store a 5–6 month supply of iron in its liver. Placenta needs 70 mg of iron. Hemoglobin formation need is 500 mg, which is the result of the increase in red blood cell mass associated with the increase in blood volume. Supplemental iron (30–60 mg) (150–300 mg of ferrous sulfate) recommended because iron is poorly absorbed.	Eggs Beans Beef Clams Lima beans Heart Beef kidney Beets Greens Lentils Liver Shrimp Oysters Dandelion greens Soybeans
Folic acid	400 μg	400 μg	Promotes normal fetal growth. Prevents macrocytic anemia of pregnancy. Evidence of marked decrease in dietary folate absorption and increase in urinary excretion, which may contribute to the depletion of maternal reserves. Key substance in cell growth and reproduction. Aids in formation of hemoglobin and nucleoproteins.	Liver (organ meats) Green, leafy vegetables Asparagus Bananas Oranges
Vitamin C (ascorbic acid)	60 mg	70 mg	Necessary for fetal and placental storage. Low maternal intake of ascorbic acid is associated with premature rupture of fetal membranes and higher neonatal death rates. Needed for formation of intercellular cement substance in developing connective tissue and vascular system. Resistance to infection. Improves absorption of iron. No cases of fetal hypervitaminosis C are known; however, possibility exists that fetal metabolism could be adversely affected by high levels of an oxidizing agent such as vitamin C. Caution against use of excessive supplementation.	Tomato juice Orange juice Cucumbers Grapefruit Berries Melons Cabbage Green, leafy vegetables

TABLE 6–1. NUTRIENT REQUIREMENTS FOR PREGNANCY *Continued*

NUTRIENT	NONPREGNANT NEEDS	PREGNANT NEEDS	RATIONALE	NUTRIENT SOURCES
Vitamin D	8 μg	10 μg	To promote the body's absorption and use of calcium and phosphorus, which are essential in bone formation. No need exists for additional source if 1 qt of milk fortified with 400 IU is consumed per day	Butter Fortified milk Fortified margarine Egg yolk
Vitamin B$_{12}$	2 μg	2.2 μg	Controls pernicious anemia. Is an extrinsic factor that combines with intrinsic factor (microprotein enzyme of gastric secretion) to be absorbed and used in the body. May activate folic acid.	Liver Lean meat Eggs Cheese Milk Fish, shellfish
Iodine	150 μg	175 μg	To prevent goiter during pregnancy, especially in adolescents. To replace increased losses of iodine in urine during pregnancy. To prevent cretinism (severe form of iodine deficiency). In infants, incidence of cretinism rises 1% when incidence of goiter among mothers reaches 55%. When mother has goiter, the chances of the child's having goiter are increased 10-fold. Restriction of salt intake may deprive a woman of her only reliable source of iodine.	Eggplant Seafood Iodized salt
Vitamin A	800 μg	800 μg	Essential factor in cell development, in maintenance of the integrity of epithelial tissue, in tooth formation, and in normal bone. Deficiency during early stages of fetal development (in animals) has been implicated in cleft palate, skeletal, and eye defects. Resistance to infections owing to healthy epithelial tissue.	Beef Butter Dark green and yellow vegetables Egg yolk Fortified margarine Canteloupe Watermelon Peaches

*Dietary requirements vary according to body size, height, and age.

Adapted from *Recommended Dietary Allowances*, rev. ed., Food and Nutrition Board (National Academy of Sciences, National Research Council, Washington, D.C.) 1989.

phosphorus are essential elements of bone and teeth. The fetus acquires most of its calcium during the last trimester, when the skeletal growth is greatest and the teeth are being formed. Calcium is also necessary for the clotting of blood, contractibility of muscles, and maintenance of the heartbeat. The mother's calcium, which is stored in the long bones, may be used to supply the needs of the fetus if her intake is insufficient. Milk is the best source of calcium.

Phosphorus is found in most foods rich in calcium, such as milk. Other good sources of phosphorus are cheese, ice cream, and green leafy vegetables.

Iron is essential for the production of hemoglobin, which functions in the delivery of oxygen to the maternal and fetal tissues. Because iron is poorly absorbed, a woman's intake of iron is usually supplemented by 60 to 80 mg of ferrous sulfate per day (120 to 240 mg/day for women with low hemoglobin values). The following foods are rich in iron: eggs; dark green, leafy vegetables; dried fruit; red meat; organ meat (for example, liver); shellfish; legumes; and enriched whole grain breads and cereals.

Vitamins

Vitamins should be increased in the pregnant woman's diet. Higher levels of vitamins A, C, and D are needed especially. Vitamin C (ascorbic acid) is necessary for the formation of connective and vascular tissues and reduces susceptibility to infection. It is found in citrus fruits, tomatoes, cantaloupes, strawberries, green peppers, broccoli, cabbage, cucumbers, and potatoes.

Vitamin D is essential for the absorption of iron and the body's use of calcium and phosphorus in bone formation. Sources of vitamin D include fortified milk, fish liver oil, butter, cheese, and green vegetables. Vitamin D is also produced when the body is exposed to sunlight.

Vitamin A is essential to cell development, tooth formation, and bone development. Vitamin A is important for fetal growth. However, ingestion of excessive amounts of vitamin A can be harmful to the fetus. Excessive intake of fat-soluble vitamins—A and D—can be toxic to the fetus because excess amounts are not excreted in the urine.

Studies have shown that excessive amounts of vitamin A can cause fetal malformations (eye or ear damage, cleft palate, and central nervous system damage). Overdoses of vitamin A should be avoided.

Sources of vitamin A are butter; cheese; beef; liver; cod-liver oil; dark green, leafy vegetables; yellow vegetables; and yellow fruits. If the woman is accustomed to taking mineral oil for constipation, she should be instructed *not* to take it during pregnancy because it reduces the absorption of fat-soluble vitamins such as vitamin A. Instead, she should be instructed to increase fluid intake and increase the amount of bulk foods in her diet.

NUTRITIONAL RISK FACTORS DURING PREGNANCY

The following factors place a pregnant woman at risk of poor nutrition:

- Adolescence (demands of growth spurt and pregnancy)
- Short interval between pregnancies, because depleted nutrient stores are not replenished
- Bizarre eating patterns (such as pica, the eating of laundry starch or red clay)
- Vegetarian diets with incomplete intake of the eight essential amino acids
- Previous anemia
- Inadequate nutritional intake
- Low income
- Inadequate weight gain
- Sudden weight gain
- Weight loss
- Smoking, alcohol use, or other drug addiction
- Medical conditions such as diabetes, kidney dysfunction

GUIDELINES FOR NUTRITIONAL ASSESSMENT AND INTERVENTION

In counseling the pregnant woman on nutrition, the nurse should be aware of the woman's food habits, attitudes, cultural preference, and economic status. A dietary 24-hour recall of her food intake is helpful in the analysis of the intake of nutrients. A dietary recall is a good way to see if a woman who is a vegetarian is ingesting all the essential proteins (Table 6–2). Some vegetarians include vegetables, fruit, legumes, and grains in their diet, but no dairy products or eggs. Their diet needs to be carefully planned to obtain all essential amino acids. If milk and cheese can be added to the diet, the protein requirement will be complete. Through the dietary 24-hour recall, the health care provider can also note an excessive intake of foods with a high sodium content (Table 6–3). Although the pregnant woman should not be placed on a low-sodium diet, she should not consume too much sodium. The assistance of a dietician is helpful in women with a poor income as well as a poor diet. Dieticians know how a woman may obtain assistance from government programs. One form of assistance is the Federal Food Stamps Program for Women, Infants, and Children (WIC). WIC is available for low-income women and provides highly nutritional foods.

Common Discomforts: Nursing Interventions and Self-Care

During the 9 months of pregnancy, women experience various types of discomfort. Many of the discomforts are a result of physical changes that take place during pregnancy (discussed in Chapter 5). Nurses and other health professionals often refer to these discomforts as minor, but they are not considered minor by the pregnant woman. If they are not expected, they can make her feel anxious and worried (Table 6–4). These discomforts usually can be relieved or prevented by simple measures. Self-care instruction is important.

NAUSEA WITH OR WITHOUT VOMITING

One of the first discomforts experienced by pregnant women is nausea (with or without vomiting). It is a common discomfort of early pregnancy and usually does not last beyond 16 weeks. Many women experience nausea on arising in the morning, and others experience nausea throughout the day. Nausea with or without vomiting

TABLE 6–2. VEGETARIAN DIETS	
BASIC TYPES	**FOOD SOURCES**
Lacto-ovovegetarian	Vegetable diet is supplemented with milk, eggs, and cheese. No problems with obtaining complete proteins.
Lacto-vegetarian	Vegetable diet is supplemented with milk and cheese. Milk products add to complete protein.
Pure vegetarian	All-vegetable diet includes vegetables, fruits, legumes, nuts, and grains. Not supplemented with any animal foods (dairy products or eggs). Careful planning is necessary for including essential amino acids. Vitamin B_{12} deficiency is potential problem.

appears to be caused by the elevation in hormone levels, decrease in gastric motility, fatigue, and emotional factors.

Women can prevent or lessen nausea and vomiting by avoiding an empty or full stomach, offending odors, and foods high in fat content. Eating dry crackers about ½ to 1 hour before getting up often makes the nausea subside. Another measure is drinking hot tea or fruit juice. Women are instructed to eat more frequently and a smaller amount, and to avoid fried, odorous, spicy, greasy, or gas-forming foods. If the vomiting persists and becomes severe, the woman should see her physician: A more serious condition called *hyperemesis gravidarum* may exist.

HEARTBURN

Heartburn is the regurgitation (backward flow) of gastric contents into the esophagus. It causes a burning sensation felt behind the sternum or in the lower chest. It is often accompanied by burping (gas) and by a little sour taste in the mouth.

TABLE 6-3. PRODUCTS HIGH IN SODIUM CONTENT			
COMMERCIAL ITEMS	**CURED, SALTED, OR CANNED MEAT**	**SEASONINGS**	**MISCELLANEOUS ITEMS**
Canned soups	Ham	Seasoned salts	Cheese
Dry soup mixes	Bacon	Garlic salt	Buttermilk
Bouillon cubes	Sausage	Onion salt	Pickles
Gravy	Corned beef	Celery salt	Sauerkraut
Catsup	Dried beef	Meat tenderizers	Pretzels
Prepared mustard	Hot dogs		Potato chips
Barbecue sauce	Luncheon meats		Corn chips
Soy sauce	Canned salmon		Salted crackers
Steak sauce	and tuna		Salted nuts
Worchestershire sauce			Salted popcorn
Chili sauce			Peanut butter
Horseradish			
Salad dressing			
Frozen TV dinners and pot pies			
Canned dinners			

Although this discomfort is called heartburn, it does not involve the heart. It appears to be caused by the relaxation of the smooth muscle, including the esophageal sphincter, and the displacement of the stomach by the enlarging uterus. The woman should be instructed to sit up for about 30 minutes after eating a medium or large meal, in order to soothe the irritation of the esophagus. Also, she should avoid gas-forming or greasy foods. With the physician's approval, antacids, such as Maalox or Gelusil, may be used, especially at bedtime. Sodium bicarbonate (baking soda) and Alka-Seltzer should not be taken because their high sodium content causes a retention of fluids.

CONSTIPATION

Constipation is a common problem during pregnancy because of the decreased peristalsis of the intestine and hence the increased water absorption of stool content. Decreased smooth muscle tone of the intestinal tract is due in large part to progesterone. In addition, pressure is placed on the enlarging uterus as pregnancy advances. Changes in eating habits and a reduction in exercise also encourage constipation. To lessen this discomfort,

the woman should drink lots of fluids, increase roughage in the diet (cereals, fresh fruits, and vegetables), and have a regular schedule for bowel movements. The woman should be instructed not to take stool softeners, laxatives, or enemas without consulting the physician.

URINARY FREQUENCY AND URGENCY

The pressure of the enlarging uterus on the bladder causes urinary frequency and urgency (see Fig. 5–7). This problem occurs early in pregnancy and again late in pregnancy when the fetus descends (drops) downward in the pelvis, pressing against the bladder.

Because progesterone relaxes the smooth muscle of the urinary system, the chance of urinary infection is higher. Tenderness over the kidney area or a burning sensation on urination should be reported to the physician. The woman should be encouraged to increase her daily fluid intake to avoid urinary infection.

FLATULENCE

Flatulence is attributed to the relaxation of the gastrointestinal tract during pregnancy. If this

TABLE 6–4. PRENATAL TEACHING GUIDE

Weeks 1–12

Woman more concerned with herself; her physical changes with pregnancy, and her feelings about the pregnancy.

Changes that are normal for pregnancy:
  Breast fullness
  Urinary frequency
  Nausea and vomiting
  Fatigue
Estimated date of conception:
  Calculate and explain
  Compare with uterine size
Expectation for care:
  Initial visit
  Subsequent visits
Clinic appointments
Need for iron and vitamins
Resources available:
  Education
  Dental evaluation
  Medical service
  Social service
  Emergency room
Danger signs:
  Drugs, self-medication
  Spotting, bleeding
  Cramping, pain

Weeks 12–24

Woman has usually resolved the issue of the pregnancy and becomes more aware of the fetus as a person.

Growth of fetus:
  Movement
  FHR (fetal heart rate)
Personal hygiene:
  Comfortable clothing
  Breast care and supportive brassiere
  Recreation, travel
  Vaginal discharge
Employment or school plans
Method of feeding baby:
  Breast or bottle
  Give literature about methods
Avoidance or alleviation of the following:
  Backache
  Constipation
  Hemorrhoids
  Leg ache, varicosities, edema, cramping
  Round ligament pain
Nutritional guidance
Weight gain
Balanced diet
Special nutritional needs

Weeks 24–32

Woman becomes more interested in baby's needs as a corollary to her own needs now and after birth.

Fetal growth and status:
  Presentation and position
  Well-being–FHR
Personal hygiene:
  Comfortable clothing
  Body mechanics and posture
  Positions of comfort
Physical and emotional changes
Sexual needs and changes; intercourse
Alleviation of the following:
  Backache
  Braxton Hicks contractions
  Dyspnea
  Round ligament pain
  Leg ache or edema
Confirm infant feeding plans:
  Prepare for breast or bottle feeding
  Nipple preparation
  Massage and expression of breast
Preparation for baby:
  Supplies
  Household assistance
Danger signs:
  Preeclampsia
  Headache, excessive swelling, blurred vision
Tubal ligation (papers prepared ahead)

Weeks 32–36

Woman anticipates approaching labor and caring for baby after birth.

Fetal growth and status
Personal hygiene:
  Positions of comfort
  Rest and activity
  Vaginal discharge
Alleviation of discomfort:
  Backache
  Round ligament pain
  Constipation or hemorrhoids
  Leg ache or edema
  Dyspnea
Recognition of "false labor" contractions
  Braxton Hicks contractions
  How to cope and "practice" with these
Nature of "true labor":
  Signs
  Difference between "bloody show" and bleeding
What happens during labor:
  Labor contractions and progress
  What she will experience

Table continued on following page

TABLE 6–4. PRENATAL TEACHING GUIDE *Continued*

Weeks 32–36 *Continued*
Relaxation techniques
Breathing techniques:
  Abdominal
  Accelerated pattern
  Panting and pushing
Involvement of father or significant other
Provision for needs of other children:
  Anticipation of baby
  Care for children at home while mother is in
    hospital
 	
Week 36 to term
Woman should feel "ready" for labor and for the
  assumption of care-taking responsibilities for baby,
  even though she may feel anxious about both of
  these as well.
Review signs of labor (or teach)
Review or continue instruction concerning
  relaxation and breathing techniques
Finalize home preparations
	Week 36 to term *Continued*
	Anticipation of hospitalization:
	  Admission (emergency room and labor admitting
	    room)
	  Examination, shave, possible enema, intravenous
	    solutions
	  Care in labor
	  Medication and anesthesia available
	  Postnatal care
	  Supplies needed: bra, personal items, money
	  May have 2 visitors
	  Tour of maternity unit
	Confirm plans to get to hospital (when to go and
	  where)
	Consider family planning needs
	Emergency arrangements:
	  Precipitate delivery
	  Premature rupture of BOW (bag of waters) with or
	    without contractions
	  Care away from home
	  Vaginal bleeding

Adapted from Roberts, J. E. (1976). Priorities in prenatal education, *Journal of Obstetric, Gynecologic, and Neonatal Nursing* 5:17–20.

problem occurs, the woman should be instructed to eat small meals, omit foods from her diet that are likely to form gas, and try to be regular in her elimination.

BACKACHE

Backache is a common complaint. The enlarging uterus alters a woman's center of gravity. To compensate for the alteration, the woman often walks with her head and shoulders thrust backward. Lordosis results, producing strain on the lower back muscles and causing backache. Excessive weight gain also puts strain on the back muscles. In addition, the pelvic joints and ligaments are relaxed by the hormone relaxin (see Chapter 9).

The woman should be instructed to use good body mechanics and practice good posture. Pelvic rocking exercises will strengthen muscle tone and provide muscle tension relief. She should avoid bending at the waist to pick up objects but rather should bend at the knees. She should place her feet about 12 to 18 inches apart to maintain body balance. Local application of heat to the back will increase the blood flow and temporarily decrease the discomfort. Adequate rest will also help relieve backache.

VARICOSE VEINS

Varicosities, or varicose veins, are caused by relaxation of the smooth muscle wall of the vessel. In addition, pressure of the enlarging uterus on the inferior vena cava and pelvic blood vessels impairs circulation to the vulva, rectum, and legs.

The woman should be instructed to sit with her legs elevated whenever possible, take rest periods lying down, and avoid wearing constricting clothes, such as tight knee-high or thigh-high stockings. Local applications of witch hazel compresses or analgesic ointments (Nupercainal) or special suppositories may be necessary to lessen discomfort of hemorrhoids (varicosities of the rectum). Sitz baths or soaking in a warm tub of water may be helpful.

DYSPNEA

Shortness of breath—dyspnea—is a complaint that occurs late in pregnancy. Dyspnea occurs as the uterus rises into the abdomen and gets more pronounced in the last trimester as the uterus presses directly on the diaphragm. The discomfort may disturb the woman's sleep. She should be instructed to sleep with several pillows under her head. Deep chest breathing may help just before she goes to sleep. Sometimes lying on her back with her arms extended above her head will give temporary relief. This position stretches the thoracic cavity maximally and allows the fullest possible expansion of the lungs.

FAINTNESS AND DIZZINESS

When the pregnant woman is in a warm, crowded areas, faintness and dizziness may occur. Faintness can be caused by changes in the blood volume and pooling of blood in the lower extremities. Sudden change of position or standing for prolonged periods can cause her to feel faint. The woman should be instructed to change her position frequently and, if she feels faint, to sit down and lower her head between her legs. She should be assisted to an area where she can lie down.

Faintness may occur when a pregnant woman lies on her back. In this position the enlarging uterus presses on the large blood vessel (inferior vena cava), causing a decrease in venous return to the heart, cardiac output, and blood pressure (hypotension), referred to as "supine hypotensive syndrome" (see Chapter 5). The woman should be instructed to lie on her side, preferably the left, and avoid lying on her back. Sometimes faintness is due to hypoglycemia (low blood glucose levels). In this case, she should have a snack containing carbohydrates.

LEG CRAMPS

Leg cramps are common during pregnancy. They are caused by pressure of the gravid uterus on the blood vessels, which impairs circulation to the legs, and by muscle strain and fatigue. The effect of imbalance in the calcium/phos-

phorus ratio as a cause of leg cramps remains unclear.

Leg cramps can be lessened by having the woman elevate her legs as often as possible. Oral intake of calcium by tablet may be prescribed. Also, the woman should be instructed to dorsiflex her foot while straightening her leg by exerting downward pressure on her knee or to stand up with her feet flat on the floor when leg cramps occur (Fig. 6–8).

SWELLING OF FEET AND ANKLES

Edema is a common complaint during the latter part of pregnancy. Many pregnant women have some edema in the feet and ankles by the end of the day. This swelling is due to the increased difficulty of venous blood return from the lower extremities. The swelling should lessen after a night's rest. The woman should be advised to increase rest periods, lie on her left side, and elevate her legs when sitting. If it persists or gets worse, it may be a sign of pregnancy-induced hypertension (PIH), and the physician should be notified.

CARPAL TUNNEL SYNDROME

Compression of the median nerve around the thumb and second and third fingers causes carpal tunnel syndrome. This syndrome manifests as tenderness, numbness, and tingling, particularly of the thumb. Reassurance that this usually disappears when her pregnancy ends will relieve the woman's anxiety.

ROUND LIGAMENT PAIN

Round ligament pain is a common discomfort. Sudden or jerky movement of the torso pulls the ligaments, causing pain in the lower part of the abdomen, where the ligaments are stretched by the enlarged uterus. The woman should be instructed to have pillow support for her abdomen and use good body mechanics, avoiding jerky or quick movements.

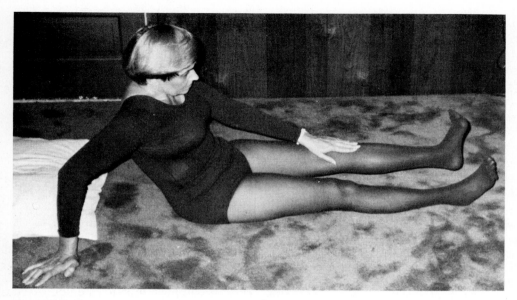

▲ **FIGURE 6–8**

Relieving a leg cramp in pregnancy. Pressing down on the knee and forcing toes upward relieves most cramps.

Education for Self-Care

The nurse should make sure that the woman and her family have an opportunity to ask questions about her care (and the care of the baby, discussed in Chapter 19). Teaching the woman how to carry out self-care and report changes that may indicate health problems is an important part of the nursing care plan. The nurse should provide anticipatory guidance of changes to expect during pregnancy, labor, and birth and after childbirth. Some of the common pregnancy concerns that women have are discussed below.

BATHING

A woman is likely to perspire profusely during pregnancy. Frequent baths, in either the tub or shower, are needed. Bathing in the tub may become a problem later in pregnancy because of awkwardness; caution should be advised. Studies have shown that the bath water does not enter the vagina, so there is no need to fear infection.

PHYSICAL ACTIVITY

Pregnant women should be encouraged to continue some kind of physical activity. Women may benefit both psychologically and physically by retaining some portion of their prepregnancy fitness. Women should be encouraged to do low-intensity and non-weight-bearing exercises (e.g., walking and stationary bicycling). Health care providers' major concern is the possibility that vigorous exercises may compromise the fetal oxygen supply by diverting blood from the placenta to the mother's working muscles. Some of the findings from animal research demonstrate fetal risk. Although the risk of human fetal risk is small, the American College of Obstetricians and Gynecologists (ACOG) prefers to err on the conservative side (see ACOG Exercise Guidelines in Chapter 9).

The goal of exercising should be muscle strengthening that minimizes the risk of joint and ligament injuries (with increased connective tissue laxity and resulting joint instability) and correcting postural changes that cause lower back pain. Fatigue should be avoided, and exercise periods should be interspersed with rest and relaxation.

Strenuous exercises (in recreational sports) should not exceed 15 minutes' duration, and the maternal heart rate should not exceed 140 beats/minute. In addition, women should pay particular attention to avoid dehydration and hyperthermia during exercise (see ACOG Exercise Guidelines).

A distinction should be made between childbirth preparatory programs and recreational and sports activities. Childbirth preparatory education emphasizes the learning of relaxation techniques that aid coping with the discomfort/pain of labor and birth. Recreational and sport activities vary from low- to high-intensity exercises. The key word to remember concerning physical exercise during pregnancy is MODERATION.

SEXUAL ACTIVITY

Instructions regarding sexual intercourse during pregnancy are more liberal than in the past. Most physicians allow couples to have sexual intercourse until the woman reaches full term. In fact, many women experience heightened sexual tension during pregnancy. This is partly due to greater blood congestion of the vulva. Sexual intercourse should not be engaged in after the "bag of waters" (the membranes containing the amniotic fluid that surrounds the fetus) ruptures or after labor begins.

Some women experience discomfort because of their shape, and the couple may want to try different positions while having sexual intercourse. Some health professionals believe that orgasm may initiate preterm labor. If the woman has a history of abortion or preterm labor, she will likely be advised to discontinue or limit sexual relations.

DOUCHING

Although normal vaginal secretions are intensified during pregnancy, the pregnant woman should NOT douche unless douching is prescribed for a vaginal infection. Douching changes the vaginal pH and alters the normal vaginal flora that has a protective effect against pathogenic organisms. If a douche is ordered by a physician, specific instructions should be given to keep the douche

bag no more than 6 inches above the level of the vagina while douching, so the water pressure is kept low.

DRESSING

Clothing should be adjustable, loose fitting, washable, and lightweight. For greatest comfort, maternity dresses should hang from the shoulders and allow for the expansion of the uterus.

The woman should avoid wearing such articles as knee-high or thigh-high stockings, tight garters, or panty girdles because they can interfere with the blood circulation of the legs. When constriction of the blood vessels in the legs occurs, edema and varicose veins are encouraged.

Maternity girdles, specially designed for pregnancy, may be worn. They should be loose fitting in front. It is important that the pregnant woman wear a good support brassiere to prevent the breakdown of elastic tissue. During pregnancy, the breasts increase one to two cup sizes. If the woman plans to breastfeed her baby, she should buy nursing brassieres.

As pregnancy progresses, the woman's center of gravity moves forward, and she will have a greater tendency to fall. Thus, it is best for her not to wear high-heeled shoes.

BREAST AND NIPPLE CARE

Whether the woman plans to breastfeed or bottle-feed her infant, proper support of the breasts is important to promote comfort. If she plans to nurse her baby she can prepare her nipples for breastfeeding. There is some question about the merits of "nipple preparation," however. Some health care providers may ask the woman to dry her nipples with a turkish towel after bathing (starting about seventh month of pregnancy). Very limited soap should be applied to the breasts because soap removes the natural oils provided by Montgomery's glands. The woman may be further instructed to grasp the nipple firmly between the thumb and index finger, pull the nipple out slightly, then twirl it back and forth several times, as a daily exercise. Women who have had preterm births are discouraged from nipple rolling because of the possibility of stimulating uterine contractions.

Women should be informed that their breasts will secrete a substance called *colostrum,* a yellow fluid, before or during the last trimester. It is important for the woman to know that the size of her breasts has nothing to do with the production of sufficient milk for the baby.

DENTAL CARE

Pregnant women can have routine dental care. It is advisable to have cavities filled and infected teeth treated. The nurse can encourage the woman to use a soft toothbrush to lessen bleeding from the gums, which increase in vascularity during pregnancy.

TRAVEL AND WORK

Most women employed outside the home can continue working as long as they are comfortable. By midpregnancy, rest periods should be a daily routine, and they are allowed in most places of work. Pregnant women should not work in any setting where radiation is present.

MEDICATIONS

It is important that the woman be told to not take any drugs during pregnancy unless they are prescribed by the physician. This means that she should not take either over-the-counter drugs or illicit drugs. These precautions are necessary to protect the embryo and fetus against the harmful effects of drugs (see Appendix B). The woman should be informed about the effects of substance abuse on the baby.

DANGER SIGNS

The woman should be instructed about danger signs that must be reported to the physician or necessitate a trip to the clinic. Each woman should receive a booklet listing the important signs.

DANGER SIGNS TO REPORT TO THE PHYSICIAN

- Bleeding from the vagina
- Leakage of water from the vagina
- Severe or continuous headache
- Disturbance in vision
- Chills and fever
- Swelling of face or hands
- Pain in the abdomen or chest
- Persistent vomiting
- Scant or bloody urine
- Temperature above 101° F and chills
- Painful urination
- Absence of fetal movement

Substance Abuse

The greatest potential for gross abnormalities in the fetus occurs during the 1st trimester of pregnancy; however, drugs can be damaging to the fetus throughout the pregnancy. Several drugs are known to have teratogenic effects on the fetus and are capable of disrupting fetal growth and producing malformations. Some of the substances commonly used are cocaine, caffeine, alcohol, and tobacco.

COCAINE

Pregnant women who use cocaine place their infant at risk. Cocaine use during pregnancy is a major problem with users in all economic levels in our society. The number of childbearing women who take cocaine is unknown, but studies demonstrate that it involves a large number in both the adolescent and adult pregnant populations, and the number is increasing.

Cocaine is derived from the leaves of the *Erythroxylon coca* plant. Its use has been dated as far back as 600 A.D. Recently its price decreased and its purity increased, making it available and affordable to numerous people. This has led to widespread abuse. In 1987 a New York hospital reported that 10% of all newborns born there had a positive urine test for cocaine. The magnitude of maternal cocaine abuse is just beginning to surface.

Cocaine is a central nervous system stimulant

that produces mood-altering effects such as euphoria, hyperactivity, excitement, and hallucinations. Cocaine stimulates the peripheral nervous system and prevents the reuptake of norepinephrine, leading to a high level of norepinephrine in the baby's circulation. At this level, the cardiovascular system experiences peripheral vasoconstriction, leading to an increased heart rate and blood pressure. These may lead to arrhythmias, myocardial infarction, stroke, pulmonary edema, and often sudden death.

Pregnancy Complications

Numerous complications occur in pregnancies during which cocaine is used. During the 1st trimester, women who use cocaine are at risk for a spontaneous abortion related to the vasoconstriction of vessels in the placenta that cocaine use causes. Hypertension resulting from cocaine use increases the incidence of premature separation of the placenta (abruptio placentae). This may occur within 1 hour after use. Sudden onset of uterine contractions, premature labor, and precipitous labor can all be induced by cocaine use.

Effects During Labor and Delivery

Cocaine use can cause a sudden onset of strong uterine contractions and a precipitous labor. These signs should alert the health care provider to have the urine examined; cocaine can be detected as long as 24 hours after its use, and blood sampling can indicate the quantity of the drug in circulation.

If the woman shows a positive test for the drug, the goal of treatment is to stabilize the mother and fetus. The fetus often shows tachycardia (fast heart beat) and is excessively active, and its oxygenation may be impaired owing to the strong contractions. Oxygen is administered by face mask to improve fetal oxygenation. The nurse should continually assess the neurological condition of the pregnant woman. Headache, abdominal pain, and excessive vaginal bleeding (signs of separation of placenta) are complications of cocaine use.

Effects on the Newborn

Cocaine is transferred to the fetus through the placenta. The newborn's signs and symptoms are increased irritability, tremors ranging from mild to moderate, and muscular rigidity. Other common findings include poor feeding, associated with a poor sucking reflex, and an irregular sleeping pattern. Elevated heart rate and respiratory movements have also been linked to cocaine exposure. More infants must be evaluated before specific congenital malformations can be said to be clearly caused by cocaine.

Infants born to cocaine-using mothers are at increased risk for sudden infant death syndrome (SIDS). Intrauterine growth retardation (IUGR) is seen in these infants. They display poor motor responses. Thus, infant–parent interactions such as eye contact and grasping (components of the bonding process) are reduced. Because studies have shown that malattachment is linked to child abuse, these mothers need to be continually assessed for coping with their infants.

In conclusion, the use of cocaine is becoming a grave problem, and health care providers need to instruct expectant parents about the seriousness of taking the drug, not only for themselves but for their infants. Additional attempts should be made to try to get the pregnant woman into counseling and/or a community program.

SUMMARY OF ADVERSE COCAINE EFFECTS

Maternal
- Hypertension
- Abruptio placentae
- Tachycardia
- Cardiac failure
- Convulsions
- Respiratory failure
- Death

Neonatal/Fetal
- Small for gestational age
- Preterm birth
- Behavioral problems
- Congenital malformations
- Fetal distress
- Stillbirth

CAFFEINE

There is reason to believe that caffeine, especially in large quantities, can affect the infant. The

TABLE 6-5. COMMON SOURCES AND AMOUNTS OF CAFFEINE

BEVERAGES	CAFFEINE (mg/oz)
Brewed coffee	17
Instant coffee	12
Coca-Cola	5.4
Dr. Pepper	5.0
Brewed black tea	10
Cocoa	4.6
Mountain Dew	4.5
Diet Dr. Pepper	4.5
Brewed green tea	6.0
Instant tea	6.0
Tab	3.3
Pepsi-Cola	3.5
RC Cola	2.8
Chocolate milk	3.0
Decaffeinated coffee	0.6

Food and Drug Administration (FDA) issued a caution to pregnant women to limit their caffeine intake (Table 6–5). Recently, caffeine has been linked to potential fetal anomalies, although the studies have been scant (Fig. 6–9). Caffeine may act as a mutagen because its chemical structure is that of a purine, one of the constituents of deoxyribonucleic acid (DNA). Caffeine demonstrates the ability to alter genes and break down chromosomes. In animal studies, caffeine has shown vasoconstrictive properties that can alter both uterine and placental blood flow. There is evidence from studies that caffeine can cause congenital abnormalities such as cleft palate and heart anomalies. By studying past histories of pregnant women, researchers have shown that an excessive caffeine intake—600 mg or more a day—is associated with a high incidence of abortions, stillbirths, and premature births. Side effects of caffeine are restlessness, insomnia, increased heart rate, heart palpitations, stomach irritation, and diarrhea.

Infants can accumulate caffeine. If a breastfeeding mother drinks six to eight cups of caffeine-containing beverages (coffee, tea, and colas) per day, her infant is likely to show hyperactivity and wakefulness. Nurses should know the common sources of caffeine (Table 6–4).

During prenatal instruction, the woman's caffeine intake should be assessed. She should be told which beverages have a high caffeine content, and alternative fluids should be suggested.

ALCOHOL

According to some studies, there is no safe threshold for alcohol consumption during pregnancy (Fig. 6–10). Any ingestion of alcoholic beverages, such as beer, wine, and liquor, during pregnancy should be discontinued. Mothers who

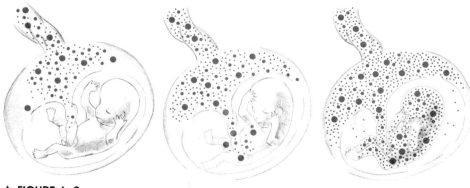

▲ FIGURE 6–9

Most chemical agents, including alcohol, the by-products of tobacco smoking, caffeine, and medications, readily cross the placenta into all of the fetus' tissues. The chemical agent is shown as dots in this illustration. (From Smith, D. W. (1979). *Mothering Your Unborn Baby*. Philadelphia, W. B. Saunders Company.)

It is estimated that as many as 1 to 2 per 100 liveborn infants have a variety of psychosocial, behavioral, and neurological disorders, such as hyperactivity, as a result of maternal alcohol consumption. Also, many pregnancies in which al-

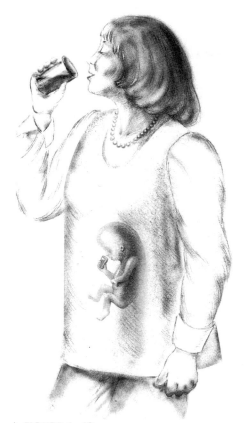

▲ **FIGURE 6–10**

When the mother takes an alcoholic drink, the baby takes an alcoholic drink. (From Smith, D. W. (1979). *Mothering Your Unborn Baby*. Philadelphia, W. B. Saunders Company.)

consume alcohol during their pregnancy place their infant at risk for *fetal alcohol syndrome* (FAS).

Infants born with FAS exhibit an altered pattern of growth in height and weight. Special facial anomalies are present: short palpebral fissures, short upturned noses, and hypoplastic upper lips, all of which give the distinctive flattened facial appearance of FAS.

The greater the degree of facial disorders, the more likely the infant is to have psychosocial, behavioral, and neurological disorders. The severity of the disorders appears to be related to both the amount of alcohol consumed and the time of pregnancy it was consumed (Fig. 6–11). Although not all women who drink heavily throughout their pregnancy give birth to infants with FAS, studies have shown that at least 40% do.

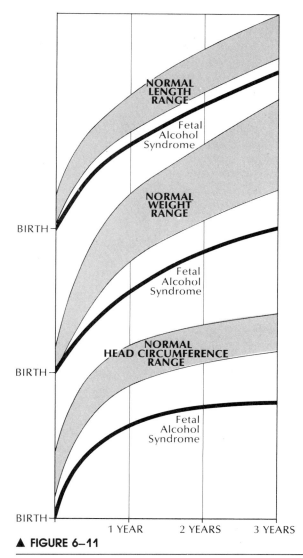

▲ **FIGURE 6–11**

The reduced growth of children (length, weight, and head circumference) with fetal alcohol syndrome (indicated by dark curves). They tend to be underweight for their height. The most worrisome feature is growth deficiency of the brain. (From Smith, D. W. (1979). *Mothering Your Unborn Baby*. Philadelphia, W. B. Saunders Company.)

cohol was consumed end in abortion or stillbirth. In the United States, alcohol may be the number one fetal teratogen.

It is recommended that pregnant women abstain from drinking from conception throughout pregnancy. Although fetal damage may have already occurred by the time the woman seeks prenatal care, abstinence even as late as the 3rd trimester may limit the extent of damage.

CIGARETTE SMOKING

The suspicion that exposure to tobacco and to cigarette smoke is hazardous to both reproductive function and fetal development has been expressed for many years (Fig. 6–12). It has been documented that three compounds found in tobacco smoke—nicotine, carbon monoxide, and benzo(a)pyrene—have harmful effects on the fetus. All of these substances, relative to the number of cigarettes smoked by the mother, can readily cross the placental barrier and build up levels in the fetus.

Carbon monoxide readily crosses the placenta and binds to sites available on the hemoglobin, preempting the binding of oxygen to these sites. Increasing concentrations of fetal carboxyhemoglobin cause fetal hypoxia because fetal tissues do not receive an adequate oxygen supply. Hypoxia puts the fetus at risk for asphyxia and impaired fetal growth.

It cannot be overemphasized that nicotine has a number of effects that may impair maternal nutrients. Among these is the sympathetic stimulation of epinephrine release from the adrenal medulla and the subsequent increase in basal metabolic rate. A breakdown in fat in the tissues (lipolysis) results. Many smokers find nicotine addiction so intense that they continue smoking despite the dangers of this drug.

Nicotine contained in cigarette smoke depletes vitamin C (ascorbic acid) levels. Vitamin C is needed to produce collagen to help preserve capillary health, assist tissue healing, and reduce risk of infection. Also, vitamin C enhances the absorption of iron needed during pregnancy.

The metabolism of calcium appears to be impaired by smoking. Therefore, smoking may jeopardize the woman's as well as the fetus's calcium stores. An adequate maternal serum calcium level also is necessary for blood clotting, maintaining muscle tone, and preventing irritability. Many women who smoke do not drink as much milk because they are accustomed to caffeine-containing beverages. This finding is significant to the changes in diet needed during pregnancy.

Benzo(a)pyrene also readily crosses the placental barrier. It stimulates the production of enzymes that compete for the same pathways as the enzymes of cells that process nutrients and provide oxygen to the developing fetus. Thus benzo-(a)pyrene is one of the substances that can cause harm to the fetus.

The majority of women who smoke have low-birth-weight infants. Many have premature infants. Both conditions place the infants at greater risk for respiratory distress. The impairment of oxygen delivery to the fetus appears to affect

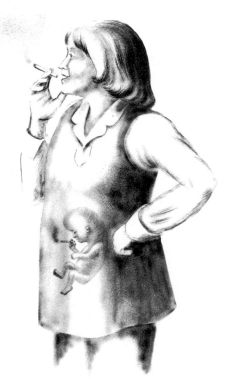

▲ FIGURE 6–12

When the mother smokes a cigarette, the unborn baby smokes a cigarette. (From Smith, D. W. (1979). *Mothering Your Unborn Baby.* Philadelphia, W. B. Saunders Company.)

central nervous system development (Fig. 6–13). It has been reported that children of mothers who smoke have lower intelligence quota (IQ) scores and a higher incidence of minimal brain dysfunction than children of nonsmoking mothers.

Cigarette smoking should be stopped or reduced to a minimum during pregnancy. To help the pregnant woman stop smoking, the nurse may inform her of the risks to maternal and fetal life and recommend the following: destroying the cigarette after a few puffs, keeping a record of each cigarette smoked, smoking low-tar and low-nicotine cigarettes, not inhaling smoke, and calling on a nonsmoking friend for support. Group discussions as well as individual counseling are often helpful to the woman who is trying to stop smoking during pregnancy.

Women who want to nurse their infants should be counseled to discontinue or reduce smoking. Nicotine is secreted into human breast milk and can be detected as long as 7 to 8 hours after smoking. The concentration of nicotine in breast milk varies according to the number of cigarettes smoked. In large doses, nicotine inhibits lactation. Also, it has been noted that smokers tend to be

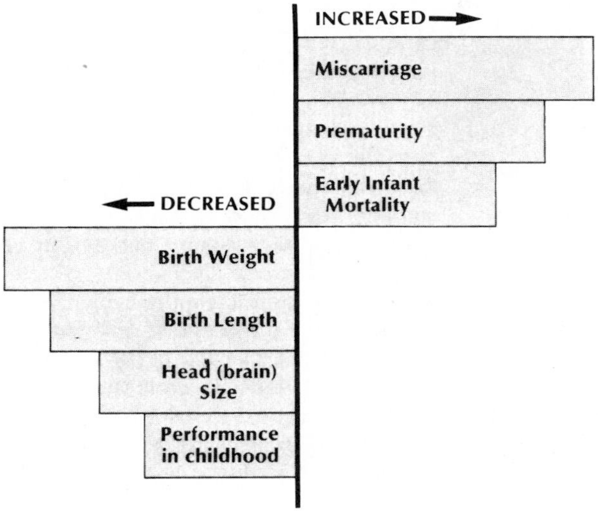

more anxious than nonsmokers, and anxiety could be a factor responsible for poor lactation.

There is overwhelming evidence that smoking during pregnancy is associated with a greater incidence of low-birth-weight infants. Studies also report fetal risk when the mother is exposed to passive smoking, such as being in a smoked-filled room. Considering that infants with low birth weight have higher morbidity rates, the effects of the mother's smoking on the infant are obvious. In contrast to infants whose low birth weight is the result of malnutrition, who tend to exhibit rapid catch-up growth, infants who are prenatally exposed to cigarette smoke tend to remain below average in height and weight. In other words, the effects of in utero exposure to tobacco smoke may be long-lasting.

DRUG DEPENDENCY: ASSESSMENT AND MANAGEMENT

Many women who have a chemical dependence will not admit to their problem. A number of symptoms aid in the diagnosis of maternal drug addiction and withdrawal: fatigue, headache, nausea and vomiting, and hot sweats or flashes. Fetal and infant withdrawal symptoms include agitation, convulsions, high shrill crying, poor sucking reflex, and even intrauterine death.

Antepartum Management

The drug-dependent woman needs special attention and support throughout her pregnancy. A complete medical and drug history is important. Medical problems commonly found among drug addicts who are pregnant include anemia, sexually transmitted diseases, urinary tract infections, tuberculosis, abscesses, and edema. A positive history of hepatitis is common. Often, drug-dependent women have poor diets and need instruction to eat properly and take prenatal vitamins and iron supplements.

Fetal Assessment

It is important to understand that detoxification during pregnancy, if too rapid, may provoke un-

▲ **FIGURE 6–13**

Effects of heavy smoking on the unborn baby. (From Smith, D. W. (1979). *Mothering Your Unborn Baby.* Philadelphia, W. B. Saunders Company.)

NURSING CARE PLAN 6–1

HEALTH CARE DURING PREGNANCY

Potential Problems and Nursing Diagnoses	Nursing Interventions
1. Anxiety related to the initial physical examination, including a pelvic examination.	Explain how the pelvic examination is performed and why it is necessary ("to assess the adequacy of the pelvis") Instruct patient to empty her bladder before the examination Encourage patient to take deep breaths just before and during the examination
2. Altered nutrition: less than body requirements.	Explain to patient that her weight gain is too small; this could place her infant at risk Review foods in the basic four food groups. Explain why protein, minerals, and vitamins are essential for an uneventful pregnancy and a healthy baby Review the nutritional intake by a 24-hour dietary recall Refer patient to the dietician for further counseling and assistance from the federal WIC program
3. Constipation related to gastrointestinal system changes during pregnancy.	Explain cause: because of the decrease in peristalsis in the gastrointestinal system, there is increased water absorption in the stool content Instruct patient to increase intake of fluids and roughage
4. Altered health maintenance.	Encourage patient to increase her physical activity by walking for 5 to 15 minutes/day Instruct patient to take rest periods twice a day Explain the importance of keeping prenatal clinic appointments to ensure a good pregnancy outcome
5. Fatigue related to physical discomforts.	Instruct relaxation techniques agreeable to patient Encourage rest periods to decrease fatigue
6. Fluid volume excess, causing edema of the lower extremities.	Explain cause: the gravid uterus puts pressure on veins in the lower extremities, causing edema (swelling) of the feet and ankles Encourage patient to elevate her legs whenever possible
7. Sexual dysfunction related to discomfort.	Encourage patient to discuss, with her partner, the use of different positions during intercourse. Explain that it is common for a woman to feel uncomfortable because of the change in body shape (uterine/abdominal enlargement)

NURSING CARE PLAN 6–1 *Continued*

HEALTH CARE DURING PREGNANCY

Potential Problems and Nursing Diagnoses	Nursing Interventions
8. Knowledge deficit related to sensations of dizziness or faintness.	Explain that she may feel dizzy or faint when making a sudden position change, standing in the same position for a long time, or lying supine.
	Instruct patient to immediately sit down and lower her head between her legs when she feels faint and is in an upright position
9. Knowledge deficit related to self-care.	Explain self-care during pregnancy, such as bathing, appropriate clothing, travel, and work
	Emphasize the importance of not taking medications, unless prescribed by the physician, because of potential danger to fetus
10. Potential for injury related to substance abuse.	Explain that caffeine, smoking, alcohol, and drugs such as cocaine can be damaging to the baby

Expected Outcomes

1. Patient expresses less anxiety about the pelvic examination. She plans to take deep breaths before and during the pelvic examination.
2. Patient verbalizes an understanding of foods necessary for good nutrition during pregnancy. She communicates the desire to have a healthy baby.
3. Patient demonstrates understanding that an increased intake of fluids and roughage in her diet will likely decrease constipation.
4. Patient decides to walk for 5 to 15 minutes every day.
5. Patient verbalizes an understanding of why rest periods are necessary to reduce fatigue and how relaxation techniques can promote rest.
6. Patient recognizes the need to elevate her legs whenever she sits down.
7. Patient expresses relief to know that a position change in intercourse may be more comfortable.
8. Patient recognizes why dizziness and faintness occur during pregnancy. She will avoid standing or sitting for long periods of time and will lie on her side rather than assuming a supine position.
9. Patient verbalizes an understanding in self-care during pregnancy.
10. Patient expresses confidence in her ability to reduce intake of caffeine. She also states she will avoid the intake of alcohol and stop smoking.

desirable fetal side effects. The sequence of events observed with rapid detoxification of the fetus are hyperactivity, intrauterine convulsions, passage of meconium, and possible death. The fetus needs to be monitored for well-being.

Rehabilitation

The pregnant woman addicted to drugs may need to use medical, psychological, social, vocational, or legal services. However, the health care provider should be aware that there will be a percentage of women who will not respond to these services. Drug abuse in a pregnant woman is often complicated by intense feelings of guilt, fear, and shame of the harm that she has imposed on her baby.

Nursing Diagnoses to Consider During Pregnancy

Nursing interventions and self-care instructions that apply to common discomforts of pregnancy and substance abuse have been discussed. It is worthwhile to list nursing diagnoses applicable to the content of this chapter. The suggested nursing diagnosis may apply to the woman who has a healthy pregnancy. Because the nurse may see an individual woman only once a month during the first 7 months of pregnancy, developing a written care plan that incorporates knowledge-based information, nursing diagnoses, and expected goals is clearly important for continuity of patient care (see Nursing Care Plan 6–1). After the initial plan, the nurse should anticipate making changes in the care plan according to additional information received about the woman's needs and the physical and psychological changes that have resulted in various discomforts and concerns.

NURSING DIAGNOSES APPLICABLE TO PREGNANCY

- Activity intolerance
- Altered nutrition: less than body requirements
- Altered health maintenance

- Anxiety
- Body image disturbance
- Constipation
- Fatigue
- Fear
- Fluid volume excess
- Fluid volume deficit
- Health-seeking behaviors
- Impaired physical mobility
- Ineffective breathing pattern
- Noncompliance
- Potential for injury
- Sexual dysfunction
- Ineffective individual coping
- Knowledge deficit
- Self-care deficit
- Sleep pattern disturbance

References

Aaronson, L. S., & Macnee, C. L. (1989). Tobacco, alcohol and caffeine use during pregnancy. *Journal of Obstetric, Gynecologic, and Neonatal Nursing* 18:279–285.

Auvenshine, M. A., & Enriquez, M. G. (1990). *Comprehensive Maternity Nursing: Perinatal and Women's Health*, 2nd ed. Boston: Jones and Bartlett.

Barbour, B. G. (1989). Is fetal alcohol syndrome completely irreversible? *American Journal of Maternal-Child Nursing* 14:44–46.

Bernhardt, J. H. (1990). Potential workplace hazards to reproductive health: Information for primary prevention. *Journal of Obstetric, Gynecologic, and Neonatal Nursing* 19:53–62.

Dibrubbo, N. E. (1987). Condom barrier. *American Journal of Nursing* 87:1306–1309.

Dombrowski, M. P., & Sokol, R. J. (1990). Cocaine and abruption. *Contemporary OB/GYN* 35(4):13–19.

Food and Nutrition Board, Commission on Life Sciences, and National Research Council, National Academy of Sciences (1989). *Recommended Dietary Allowances*, 10th ed. Washington, DC: National Academy Press.

Hammond, T., Mickens-Powers, B., Strickland, K., & Hankins, G. (1990). The use of automobile safety restraint systems during pregnancy. *Journal of Obstetric, Gynecologic, and Neonatal Nursing* 19:339–343.

Helton, A. S. (1990). A buddy system to improve prenatal care. *American Journal of Maternal-Child Nursing* 15:234–237.

House, M. A. (1990). Cocaine. *American Journal of Nursing* 90:41–45.

Jaffee, M. S., & Melson, K. A. (1989). *Maternal-Infant Health Care Plans*. Philadelphia, Springhouse.

Ladewig, P. W., London, M. L., & Olds, S. B. (1990). *Essentials of Maternal-Newborn Nursing*, 2nd ed. Redwood City, CA: Addison-Wesley Nursing.

Lynch, M., & McKeon, V. A. (1990). Cocaine use during pregnancy. *Journal of Obstetric, Gynecologic, and Neonatal Nursing* 19:285–291.

Mattison, D. R., Kozlowski, K., Quirk, J. G., & Jelovsek, F. R. (1989). Effects of drugs and chemicals on the fetus. *Contemporary OB/GYN* 33(3):163–176.

McMahon, A., & Maibusch, R. M. (1988). How to send quit-smoking signals. *American Journal of Nursing* 88:1498–1499.

National Academy of Sciences, Institute of Medicine (1990).

Nutrition during Pregnancy: Weight Gain and Nutrient Supplements. Washington, DC: National Academy Press.

Roberts, J. E. (1976). Priorities in prenatal education. *Journal of Obstetric, Gynecologic, and Neonatal Nursing* 5:17–20.

Tiedje, L., & Collins, B. (1989). Combining employment and motherhood. *American Journal of Maternal-Child Nursing* 14:29.

Worthington-Roberts, B. S., & Willimans, S. R. (1989). *Nutrition in Pregnancy and Lactation*, 4th ed. St. Louis: Times Mirror/Mosby.

SUGGESTED ACTIVITIES

1. Describe the pregnant woman's health care in the initial prenatal visit, including the diagnostic laboratory tests.
2. Reveiw the important nutrients necesary during pregnancy. List food sources for each nutrient.
3. Explain reasons why use of cocaine, cigarettes, alcohol, and caffeine should be reduced during pregnancy.
4. Explain the woman's common concerns and discomforts during pregnancy. Include appropriate nursing interventions for each discomfort.

REVIEW QUESTIONS

Select the best answer to each multiple-choice question.

Clinical Situation: Ms. Jackson is married, age 20 years, and 2 months pregnant and has come to a prenatal clinic to receive care. Her history reveals that her only complaint is nausea, usually without vomiting, during the morning. She states that she smokes 1 package of cigarettes a day and drinks 5 to 6 cups of coffee most days. She denies taking nonprescription drugs.

1. The care given to Ms. Jackson during pregnancy is called
   A. Antepartum care
   B. Intrapartum care
   C. Postpartum care
   D. Neonatal care

2. Ms. Jackson should receive medical supervision
   A. Monthly until the eighth month
   B. Twice a month during the eighth month
   C. Every week during the ninth month
   D. All of the above

3. Ms. Jackson's complaint of nausea, usually without vomiting, is considered a normal symptom of pregnancy of the
   A. first trimester
   B. second trimester
   C. third trimester
   D. first through third trimester

4. A complete history should be obtained from Ms. Jackson. This would include
   A. The family history of diabetes
   B. Personal history of communicable diseases
   C. Personal history of past illness
   D. All of the above

5. Ms. Jackson asks the nurse how much weight she can expect to gain during pregnancy. The nurse should reply
   A. 10 to 12 lb
   B. 12 to 15 lb
   C. 18 to 20 lb
   D. 24 to 30 lb

6. Ms. Jackson asks the nurse if she should increase her protein intake since she does not eat meat. The nurse should tell her to eat
   A. Green vegetables, eggs, and fruit
   B. Milk, vegetables, and pudding
   C. Eggs, green vegetables, and cheese
   D. Milk, cheese, and eggs

7. Ms. Jackson is instructed to bring a urine specimen each time she comes to the clinic. The urine will be tested for
   A. Protein and glucose
   B. Glucose and acetone
   C. Protein and acetone
   D. Bacteria

8. Ms. Jackson is instructed to increase her calcium intake. The best source of calcium is
   A. Poultry
   B. Milk
   C. Fresh fruit
   D. Green leafy vegetables

9. Ms. Jackson is instructed to include additional iron in her diet during pregnancy, because iron is necessary for all of the following EXCEPT
   A. Hemoglobin formation
   B. Increased number of red blood cells to carry oxygen
   C. Demand on mother by fetus for iron
   D. Prevention of goiter during pregnancy

10. Ms. Jackson's daily intake of calcium should be increased because calcium is
    A. An important element in blood clotting
    B. Used in muscle action
    C. Used in maintenance of bone and teeth
    D. All of the above

11. Mineral that Ms. Jackson does NOT have to increase is
    A. Phosphorus
    B. Calcium
    C. Iron
    D. Sodium

12. Vitamin C, ascorbic acid, is necessary during Ms. Jackson's pregnancy for all of the following reasons EXCEPT
    A. Increasing resistance to infection
    B. Improving absorption of iron
    C. Improving formation of connective tissue
    D. Decreasing hemoglobin formation

13. Ms. Jackson should be instructed that the best sources of iron are
    A. Soybeans, eggs, and tomato juice
    B. Eggs, liver, and milk
    C. Soybeans, eggs, and liver
    D. Seafood, milk, and butter

14. Ms. Jackson is instructed to discontinue or reduce cigarette smoking during pregnancy because smoking
    A. Contains nicotine that depletes vitamin C levels
    B. Contains carbon monoxide that can decrease oxygen to tissues
    C. Impairs the metabolism of calcium
    D. All of the above

15. Ms. Jackson is instructed to reduce her caffeine intake because caffeine
    A. Is a potential cause of fetal anomalies
    B. Stimulates heart rate
    C. Increases insomnia
    D. All of the above

16. Ms. Jackson says she is planning to breastfeed her baby and asks if there is any special breast care during pregnancy. She should be instructed to do all of the following EXCEPT
    A. Limit the amount of soap applied to her breasts because it can remove the natural oils
    B. Limit exposure of breasts to air
    C. Dry breasts well after bathing
    D. Wear a supportive brassiere

17. Ms. Jackson receives a list of danger signs to report. They include the following EXCEPT
    A. Bleeding from the vagina
    B. Severe or continuous headache
    C. Swelling of face or hands
    D. Fatigue

Clinical Situation: Debbie Brown is a clinic patient who is 6 months pregnant. She is interested in anticipatory guidance and wants to be informed of the common discomforts of pregnancy. Also, she asks what she can do to alleviate the discomforts and assist the baby to have a healthy environment. The nurse develops a teaching care plan.

18. To promote the best fetal perfusion during pregnancy, the teaching plan instructs Debbie to
    A. Avoid venal caval compression
    B. Modify her exercise
    C. Assume the left-side position when lying down
    D. All of the above

19. To decrease edema of the extremities, the teaching plan instructs Debbie to do all of the following EXCEPT
    A. Change position frequently and not stand for long periods of time
    B. Wear whatever type of stockings she feels is helpful
    C. Elevate her legs when she sits down
    D. Lie on her side when resting

20. The teaching plan encourages Debbie to stop smoking because of the potential effects on the baby, such as
    A. Decrease in birth weight
    B. Decrease in head (brain) size
    C. Increase in prematurity
    D. All of the above

21. The teaching plan encourages Debbie to omit alcohol during pregnancy because of the potential effects on the baby, such as
    A. Facial disorders
    B. Neurological disorders
    C. Psychological disorders
    D. All of the above

22. The woman who uses cocaine during pregnancy should be instructed that she is placing her infant at risk for
    A. Growth retardation
    B. Sudden death syndrome
    C. Postbirth withdrawal symptoms
    D. All of the above

CHAPTER 7 _____

Chapter Outline

General Information about Sexually Transmitted
   Diseases
      Key Points in Education
Bacterial Sexually Transmitted Diseases
     Syphilis
     Gonorrhea
Viral Sexual Infections
     Chlamydia
     Herpes simplex virus
     Cytomegalovirus
     Hepatitis B
     Human immunodeficiency virus and acquired
        immune deficiency syndrome

Learning Objectives

Upon completion of Chapter 7, the student should be
able to
- Describe the methods of transmission, treatment, and
  prevention of syphilis.
- Explain how gonorrhea is transmitted and treated.
- Explain the potential effect on the infant of delivery
  through a gonorrhea-infected birth canal.
- Identify chlamydia infection relative to childbirth.
- List the potential risk of herpes simplex to the new-
  born infant.
- List the secretions that may be reservoirs for cyto-
  megalovirus.
- Identify the populations at high risk for hepatitis B
  infection.
- Describe the populations at high risk for infection
  with human immunodeficiency (HIV) virus and ac-
  quired immune deficiency syndrome.
- List the behaviors that risk HIV infection.
- Describe the early symptoms of HIV infection.
- Identify the two most common forms of infections
  that occur as the HIV-positive infection progresses.
- Outline the universal precautions suggested by the
  Centers for Disease Control to reduce sexually trans-
  mitted infections.
- List methods to prevent transmission of infections
  acquired through blood and body fluids.

SEXUALLY TRANSMITTED DISEASES

Sexually transmitted diseases (STDs) are specific infections that are transmitted primarily during sexual contact. The term *STDs* has replaced the term *venereal diseases*. The shift in terminology recognizes an expanded awareness of infectious diseases transmitted through sexual contact as well as an expanded array of diseases. These sexually transmissible infections have become a major health priority. They may be caused by bacteria, viruses, protozoa, or fungal agents. A wide variety of STDs have been associated with serious complications during pregnancy. The infections may affect the mother or the infant. Complications include spontaneous abortion, preterm birth, intrauterine growth retardation, prematurity, neonatal death, congenital infection, and postpartum uterine infection. The STDs constitute a major, largely preventable health threat to women and infants. Care has been directed to education, disease detection, partner tracing, and improved treatment. Some of the STDs are more difficult to identify then others. Frequently, complications can occur even if no symptoms are present. The effects of STDs present a challenge to medical and nursing management in this country and the world.

General Information about Sexually Transmitted Diseases

Populations with high rates of STDs are an obvious focus for prevention, screening, and education efforts (Table 7–1). In addition, individuals in certain groups are more likely to have one or more STDs because their sexual partners are usu-ally in the same high-risk group and practice the same sexual behaviors.

High-risk groups for STDs include people under age 25, racial/ethnic minorities, homosexual males, both males and females with more than one sexual partner, and drug-addicted individuals who share intravenous needles. Two-thirds of reported cases of gonorrhea occur in persons 24 years of age or younger. Rates of syphilis, gonorrhea, and hospitalization for pelvic inflammatory disease (PID) are the highest in adolescents and decline with increasing age.

In many STDs, women suffer more severe long-term consequences, including PID, ectopic pregnancy, chronic pelvic pain, infertility, and cervical cancer. In addition, women are apparently more likely than men to acquire a sexually transmitted infection from any single sexual encounter; for example, the risk of acquiring gonorrhea from a single coital event (in which one partner is infectious) is approximately 25% for men and 50% for women.

Counseling individuals about STDs is important and should include discussions of prevention, the prevention of new infections, compliance with treatment and follow-up, and provision of comfort measures, and it should include an offer to discuss the infection, treatment, and consequences with the partner.

Bacterial Sexually Transmitted Diseases

SYPHILIS

Syphilis is now at its highest prevalence in the past 40 years. Recent syphilis outbreaks have been

KEY POINTS IN EDUCATION: SEXUALLY TRANSMITTED DISEASES

- Make sure the patient understands what disease he or she has, how it is transmitted, why it must be treated, and when and how to take prescribed medications (for example, taking tetracycline on an empty stomach may cause nausea.)
- Impress upon the patient the need to take medications as prescribed, even though the symptoms of the disease may have disappeared. Discontinuing antibiotics before the infection is completely gone not only leads to recurrent infection, but also increases the likelihood that hard-to-cure strains of pathogen may flourish.
- Prevent reinfection by treating the sexual partner.

- Advise patients to avoid sexual intercourse while completing the full course of therapy. After the infection is cured, urge the patient to continue to use condoms to prevent repeated infections.
- Recognize that good health habits require regular assessment of one's body, including the genital self-examination (for the sexually active person).
- Mention that the American Social Health Association maintains a hotline for people to call for recent information about STDs.

TABLE 7–1. PRINCIPLES TO REDUCE THE RISK OF ACQUIRING STDs

BASIC INFORMATION	HEALTH PROTECTION
Know that sexual activity provides potential contact with STDs and that precautions reduce risk.	Abstinence or restriction to one partner. Increased number of partners increases risk.
Practice sexual activities that do not cause exchange of bodily fluids with unknown partners.	STD organisms are transmitted by direct contact with mucous surfaces or open skin.
Understand that use of barrier forms of contraception reduces risk.	Properly used, condoms along with spermicides (contraceptive foam or jelly) reduce risk of many STDs. If an individual's infectious lesions or secretions are exposed, the contraceptive devices will not be helpful.
Avoid unsafe sex practices.	Avoid practices that may cause skin or mucous membrane injury. Avoid anal contact, e.g., anal intercourse. Avoid sexual activities that cause bleeding.
Recognize importance of periodic screening for STDs.	Individuals at high risk should be screened or tested frequently, especially those with more than one sex partner.
Recognize individuals at high risk for AIDS.	Recognize those who share intravenous needles; engage in anal sex, oral–genital sex, or vaginal intercourse without a condom; who have sex with someone who has or who themselves have multiple partners; also individuals who received blood products between 1977 and 1985.
Ask for partner's cooperation.	Recognize that individuals with STDs may or may not have symptoms (e.g., chlamydia, gonorrhea, or HIV infections).

associated with the exchange of sex for drugs. Congenital syphilis occurs in about 1 in 10,000 pregnancies.

Syphilis is caused by an organism called *Treponema pallidum,* a thin, mobile spirochete (bacteria). The spirochete is capable of penetrating intact skin or mucous membranes and is transmitted by direct contact with skin lesions or blood, primarily during sexual intimacy, including kissing. Infective lesions develop by 3 weeks after exposure; however, lesions have been known to appear as late as 1 year after exposure. Once contracted, the disease progresses slowly, taking anywhere from a couple of weeks to several months before it makes itself known. The earliest sign of *primary syphilis* is an infectious lesion on the skin called a *chancre.* This lesion is usually painless and may appear on the genitals or lips. At this stage syphilis may be transmitted by kissing, sexual intercourse, and oral-genital relations.

Maternal Issues

If a mother is untreated for syphilis, she can transmit the infection to the fetus in utero; this is called *congenital syphilis.* Untreated, syphilis is responsible for many stillbirths, spontaneous abortions, and live-born infants with congenital syphilis.

In the *primary stage* of syphilis, the chancre is located at the site of exposure. Although the chancre heals within about a month, the infection has not ended. The infection can then spread by the bloodstream throughout the body. During this *second stage,* or about 6 weeks to 6 months later, symptoms can include aching, rash, fever, large genital warts, and joint pains. Even without treatment, these second-stage syphilitic symptoms may disappear. During the *third,* or *latent, stage* of syphilis, the heart muscle and the central nervous system are targets for the spirochete. Cardiovascular (thoracic aortic aneurism and aortic insufficiency) and neurological (general paresis, tabes dorsalis, and focal neurological signs) effects are sequelae of both congenital and late syphilis. For this reason, transmission of syphilis to the fetus is of grave concern.

All women should be tested early in pregnancy for syphilis. Laboratory tests that have a definitive diagnosis for syphilis include dark-field microscopy and fluorescent antibody techniques. An antibody technique used is the rapid plasma reagin (RPR). The RPR is used to screen for syphilis and to follow the response of the therapy.

The treatment of syphilis depends on whether is it primary or secondary and whether early syphilis is less than 1 year's duration.

Treatment for Syphilis

This text presents the standard treatment of syphilis.

Primary, secondary, or syphilis of less than 1 year's duration is treated with benzathine penicillin G, 2.4 million units intramuscularly. Syphilis of indeterminate length or more than 1 year's duration is treated with benzathine penicillin G, 7.2 million units (2.4 million units weekly, for 3 successive weeks) intramuscularly. Patients who are allergic to penicillin are treated with doxycycline, 100 mg taken orally twice a day. If the duration of the disease is less than 1 year, treatment lasts for 15 days; otherwise, 30 days. For penicillin-allergic pregnant women or for doxycycline-intolerant patients, treatment is erythromycin 500 mg orally, four times a day for 2 weeks.

Newborn Issues

All infants born to women with a reactive syphilis screening test who were not treated before 20 weeks' gestation need to be evaluated. The most common characteristics of the syphilitic infant is the presence of nasal discharge associated with a "sniffling" sound on respiration, blistering and peeling of the palms of the hands and soles of the feet, and open fissures around the lips or anus. Also, the liver and spleen are often enlarged. Signs appearing later, indicating presence of congenital syphilis, are notched teeth (Hutchinson's teeth) and "saddle nose." Treatment for newborns infected with congenital syphilis is penicillin.

GONORRHEA

Gonorrhea is a common STD, occurring most frequently among adolescents and young adults.

It is caused by the organism *Neisseria gonorrhoeae*. This disease is extremely communicable as long as the organism is present. Because the organism thrives in wet, mucus-lined body areas such as the vagina, rectum, and genitourinary tract, several forms of sexual relations are an ideal way for transmission.

The signs of gonorrhea in men are usually obvious within 2 or 3 days after exposure. There is a burning sensation during urination (dysuria) and a cloudy or purulent discharge from the penis. In a some instances, mild symptoms are present and overlooked by men; in fact, infected men can be asymptomatic.

In most women the early symptoms of gonorrhea are urinary burning and vaginal discharge. Some women are asymptomatic and are not aware that they have been infected by their male partner.

Maternal Issues

Gonorrhea is a common cause of PID in women. This can produce a narrowing of the fallopian tubes and can later cause a tubal pregnancy or even sterility. Infections during pregnancy are usually mild; however, infection of the amniotic fluid can occur, as well as can an increased risk of postpartum uterine infection (endometritis). Risk for a premature labor or a prolonged labor is high. Treatment for gonorrhea during pregnancy is penicillin. Penicillin-resistant gonococci should be treated with spectinomycin.

If the woman has a past history of gonorrhea, there is a strong possibility that it may recur during pregnancy. Partners should be treated, because reinfection after treatment is common.

About one-fourth of men and women with gonococcal infections have coexistent chlamydial infection. For this reason, the treatment of choice is dual therapy consisting of a single dose of ceftriaxone (or penicillin), 250 mg intramuscularly, and doxycycline, 100 mg orally, two times a day for 7 days.

Newborn Issues

For the infant delivered through an infected birth canal, a gonococcal eye infection known as *ophthalmia neonatorum* is possible. In the past, a silver nitrate 1% solution placed in the infant's eyes soon after birth was the treatment of choice. Today erythromycin is preferred because it is effective against both gonorrhea and chlamydia pathogens. *Neisseria gonorrhoeae* has been isolated in the newborn infant's gastric aspirate as well as the eyes. Because of the maternal and infant risks, testing for gonorrhea is important during pregnancy.

Viral Sexual Infections

CHLAMYDIA

The organism *Chlamydia trachomatis* is responsible for a widespread STD infection. Because about 50% of affected persons have a concomitant infection, the actual incidence of chlamydia infection is difficult to determine. A high-risk group is adolescent single mothers from the lower economic population.

Maternal Issues

Genital chlamydia infections are very common bacterial infections in the United States. The infection usually is asymptomatic; however, it may involve the cervix, tubes, urethra, and lining of the uterus. Women may experience chronic pelvic pain. During pregnancy, cervical chlamydia infection increases the risk of tubal pregnancy, premature labor, premature rupture of membranes, and preterm birth. If the membranes have ruptured prematurely or an internal fetal scalp monitor is used, the risk of infection from the birth canal to the infant is increased.

Doxycycline, 100 mg taken orally twice a day for 7 to 10 days, is usually the antibiotic of choice for all sites of chlamydia infection.

Newborn Issues

Chlamydia conjunctivitis appears as a watery discharge from the eyes that progresses to a thick and purulent discharge. It is most common during the first month of life. This infection can be eliminated by using erythromycin ointment rather than silver nitrate drops as prophylaxis against gonococcal ophthalmia. Erythromycin is effective against gonococcus infection as well as chlamydia and is less irritating to the eye than silver nitrate drops.

HERPES SIMPLEX VIRUS

Herpes is the name of a family of viruses. The specific virus that causes lesions is the herpes simplex virus (HSV). This virus can cause lesions on the lips and in the mouth and also cause genital lesions. When HSV lesions appear in the mouth area, they are commonly called cold sores. More than a decade ago, the HSV virus apparently became more active and more contagious. Very likely a viral mutation occurred and a new strain appeared. The HSV virus began to appear increasingly in the genital area.

A primary infection with HSV has been proved to place the newborn infant at risk. The clinical signs in the mother include burning, tingling, or itching at the site of the lesion. Within 1 to 2 days, a fluid-filled blister appears on the area. During the next 1 to 2 weeks the blister breaks and a scab forms or the lesion crusts over. These lesions, referred to as HSV-1 (nongenital herpes), commonly occur on the mouth, eyes, or other parts of the face. Lesions referred to as HSV-2 (genital herpes) occur on the vagina, vulva, cervix, or penis. Recurrent infections of herpes infection are thought to be related to heat, cold, stress, and sunshine.

Nursing care is generally supportive for pregnant women with HSV. Primary nursing responsibilities include education about direct transmission of HSV through lesion-skin contact. The implementation of universal precautions as a hospital policy makes protection easier (Table 7–2). This includes the barrier method of protection—using gowns, gloves, and masks to minimize transmission by direct contact with viral lesions and secretions.

No cure for HSV has been found; however, the antiviral drug acyclovir has helped reduce or suppress the symptoms. The safety of systemic acyclovir in pregnant women has not been established.

Maternal Issues

HSV infection during pregnancy may cause spontaneous abortion, prematurity, or even congenital anomalies. Women with HSV should be monitored during pregnancy. Sexual contact should be discouraged during the last months of pregnancy.

Maternal infection with HSV has serious implications for the infant. If transmission occurs, the infant mortality is approximately 60%. Newborn infants are at risk for seizures, blindness, and mental retardation. One way to screen women for HSV is through Papanicolaou (Pap) smears, which pick up about 75%; however, viral cultures are more accurate. Because HSV infections have been associated with cervical cancer, annual Pap smears are recommended.

The infant can be delivered vaginally if the woman has been virus free for at least 1 week before delivery. Otherwise, a cesarean birth is recommended to prevent infection of the newborn when traveling through the mother's birth canal.

Assessment of the status of fetal membranes at the time of labor is important. Internal fetal monitoring is discouraged because an open fetal scalp lesion would provide entrance for the virus.

Newborn Issues

If the newborn infant is infected with HSV, generalized systemic infection can result, involving the central nervous system, liver, and other organs. Local infection may be seen in the skin, eyes, and mouth. Infants may have respiratory distress, sepsis, and seizures. These infants should be isolated from infection-free infants in the newborn nursery. HSV-infected infants are at risk for low birth weight and prematurity.

If the mother has an active lesion at the time of labor, a cesarean section is performed. The infant should be carefully observed for 7 to 10 days after birth. The American Academy of Pediatrics recommends that nursery and other personnel who have active HSV infections such as cold sores

TABLE 7–2. UNIVERSAL PRECAUTIONS TO REDUCE THE RISK OF STDs, INCLUDING RISK OF HIV INFECTION

Body fluids of high risk (all universal precautions apply):

Blood, semen, vaginal secretions, amniotic fluid, tears, saliva, cerebrospinal fluid

Breast milk is source of perinatal transmission; health care worker may wish to wear gloves if exposed

Body fluids of low risk (all universal precautions may not apply):

Feces, nasal secretions, sweat, urine, and vomitus

Precautions

1. Use appropriate barrier precautions to prevent skin and mucous membrane contact with bodily fluids.
2. When caring for all patients, gloves should be worn for:
   - Contact with blood (venipuncture; finger stick; changing perineal pads, chux, or linen)
   - Contact with bodily fluids (changing any saturated pad, chux, or linen; saturation after rupture of membranes)
   - Contact with mucous membranes (vagina, etc.)
   - Contact with nonintact skin
   - Handling things soiled with blood or bodily fluids (soiled pads, chux, bedding, or clothing)
3. Gloves should be changed after contact with patient and between patient contacts.
4. Medical gloves (vinyl or latex sterile or nonsterile) should not be washed and reused.

5. Masks, protective eyewear, or face protection should be worn during procedures that cause splashes of blood or bodily fluids on mucous membranes of eyes, nose, or mouth, e.g.:
   - Vaginal or cesarean birth
   - Cutting of umbilical cord
   - Rupture of membranes under pressure
6. Fluid-resistant gowns or aprons should be worn during procedures likely to cause splashes of bodily fluids:
   - Vaginal or cesarean birth
   - Artificial rupture of membranes
7. Gowns and gloves should be worn by health care workers handling placenta or infant until blood and amniotic fluid have been removed from infant's skin. Gloves should be worn for care of umbilical cord after delivery.
8. Removal of infant nasopharyngeal secretion at birth should not be done by mouth but by mechanical suction. Resuscitation should be done by ventilation equipment.
9. Gloves torn or punctured by needle stick or other injury should be removed and replaced promptly.
10. Precautions should be taken to prevent injury from needles and surgical instruments:
    - Needles should not be recapped, bent, or removed from disposable syringes by hand.
    - After use, needles and other sharp items should be placed in puncture-resistant containers for disposal.
    - Surgical instruments should be carefully cleaned to avoid injury.
11. Health care workers who have frequent exposure to breast milk may wear gloves.

Adapted from Centers for Disease Control (1988): *Universal precautions for prevention of transmission of human immunodeficiency virus, hepatitis B virus and other blood-borne pathogens in health care settings.* Atlanta, GA.

should have limited contact with the mother and newborn infant. Proper instruction of the barrier method of infection control are important. Gloves should be worn by caregivers with hand infections. Personnel should wear gowns and gloves when they have contact with these infants until the exposed lesions are healed.

CYTOMEGALOVIRUS

The organism cytomegalovirus (CMV) is a member of the herpes family and is one of the common STD infections. It has been defined as a sexually transmitted disease because viral shedding is observed more in young persons who have multiple sexual partners than those with single partners. Infected secretions, including breast milk, cervical mucus, semen, saliva, and urine, are the reservoirs of this disease. CMV can also be contacted through blood transfusions. In general, men are at less risk for CMV than women. The underprivileged population is at a greater risk for CMV, most likely because of crowding, poor hygiene, and lower economic status.

Maternal Issues

CMV can present symptoms similar to those of infectious mononucleosis—fatigue, fever, and possible liver involvement. The virus can be transmitted to the fetus through the maternal blood by way of the placenta. If the mother has a cervical infection, the newborn may acquire the CMV virus perinatally. CMV-infected breast milk can also transmit the virus to the newborn.

Good personal hygiene is important during pregnancy. This includes frequent handwashing, particularly when there are frequent contacts with other infants and toddlers.

The treatment is supportive and symptomatic. The acquired illness is usually self-limiting in immunocompetent individuals.

Newborn Issues

Infants may be infected with CMV before birth. These infants may have intrauterine growth retardation, jaundice, deafness, and blindness.

Treatment is not very clear for this infection. Good handwashing and appropriate barrier methods of infection control are important for protection from body fluids. A small percentage of newborn infants may excrete the CMV virus. Thus, it is especially important to protect the preterm infants, whose immune system may be compromised. New tests for specific CMV antibodies are being developed.

HEPATITIS B

Hepatitis B (HBV) infection can be transmitted through blood or body secretions. Certain blood products can be contaminated with HBV and transmit the virus. The virus produces systemic illness, with weakness, jaundice, and nausea. It is one of the most common causes of hepatitis. An HBV vaccine is a recommended prophylaxis for the high-risk population.

Maternal Issues

Women with HBV are at risk for transmitting the organism to their offspring transplacentally. Women who have been identified to be at greatest risk are those of Asian, Pacific island, or Alaskan Eskimo descent. Women may be asymptomatic for liver disease. They can develop a subclinical infection and be in a chronic carrier state. The sharing of bodily secretions during sexual intercourse can result in transmission of the disease. HBV has a long period of incubation, 50 to 190 days after exposure, before the potential onset of symptoms such as jaundice. Serological testing for HBV antigen is useful. It is recommended that pregnant women in the high-risk group or who have sexual partners with HBV be screened and follow-up provided. Mothers should be taught to carefully wash their hands before handling the infant and to avoid placing the infant in contact with lochia or soiled linen.

Supportive and symptomatic care should be provided. Clinical follow-up care is important to assess the symptoms and the results of liver function tests.

Universal precautions (see Table 7–2) in hospital infection control should be strictly adhered to. Health workers should assume that all blood and other body fluids, including urine, saliva, feces, and wound drainage, are potentially infectious, and therefore use barrier protection. Vaccination is recommended after pregnancy for individuals who are most at risk to contract HBV. These persons include intravenous drug users, those with many sexual partners, and health care workers.

Newborn Issues

Infants born to mothers who are HBV positive should receive immunization. All infants should have pediatric follow-up care. Nurses should use universal infection control precautions when handling these newborns, including wearing gowns and gloves while holding these infants before the first bath.

HUMAN IMMUNODEFICIENCY VIRUS AND ACQUIRED IMMUNE DEFICIENCY SYNDROME

New information has increased our understanding of the human immunodeficiency virus (HIV) and acquired immune deficiency syndrome (AIDS). It is now known that infection with HIV has a variety of manifestations, with AIDS considered the most extreme end of the HIV spectrum. The broad continuum of effects in HIV-infected persons ranges from acute infection to an asymptomatic state to full-blown AIDS. HIV infection and AIDS have become among the greatest health problems the world has ever known. In 1981, the first cases of AIDS were identified in the United States, although earlier cases have now been found to have occurred. It is estimated that 1 million or more Americans are already infected with HIV. It is believed that most of these people feel well, are not under medical care, and may not be protecting sexual partners or needle-sharing partners from HIV. There is evidence that the AIDS rate is higher in big cities such as New York and San Francisco. Also, the incidence of AIDS is high in parts of Africa and some of the Caribbean countries. Because of the nature of the disease and ongoing research, health care providers are encouraged to be familiar with up-to-date information.

Etiology

AIDS is caused by the HIV. The AIDS virus attacks lymphocytes—white blood cells that play a major role in defending the body against disease. HIV causes a defect in the body's immune system by invading and multiplying within certain white blood cells (T-4 lymphocytes). Once released from the infected cells, the virus attacks more cells. Ultimately the body is left without any effective immune system, and the person with AIDS becomes helpless against opportunistic diseases.

Cultural Changes

Social and cultural changes have contributed to sexual experimentation and freedom. These changes include a weakening of traditional values; an increase in number of sexual partners; an openness about homosexuality; and increased use of air transportation, which allows greater intermingling.

Transmission of HIV

Transmission of HIV can occur by contact of various body fluids: blood, semen, saliva, urine, feces, amniotic fluid, breast milk, and vaginal secretions. HIV can be transmitted by sexual contact between men, between men and women, and between women. Also, HIV transmission occurs from seropositive mothers to their infants.

Clinical Course of HIV

The initial HIV infection may be accompanied by a mononucleosis-like illness with symptoms including fatigue, fever, and enlargement of the lymph glands. A rash may or may not develop. Servoconversion occurs in the beginning stage of HIV infection. Asymptomatic infection may be the next stage of HIV infection. In this stage the infection may remain silent, yet transmissible, for 2 to 10 years before progressive symptoms of immune deficiency develop.

The patient may experience many opportunistic infections, including herpes simplex, toxoplasmosis, candidiasis, histoplasmosis, CMV, tuberculosis, and pneumocystis carinii.

Prognosis and Treatment

The two most common forms of the HIV infection that later overwhelm the body (cause death) are pneumonia caused by *Pneumocystis carinii* and a form of cancer called *Kaposi's sarcoma*, both ordinarily rare diseases.

HIV infections and AIDS are currently incurable. However, extensive research is being done to find adequate treatment. The discovery of effective treatments has been hindered by the biology of the virus and the nature of the infection. HIV has the ability to invade a variety of cell types rather than a specific type cell. Azidothymidine (AZT) has shown promise in prolonging the lives of some individuals. It is hoped that sometime in the future, a vaccine will be developed, but at this time a breakthrough has not been found.

An approach to the treatment of individuals with HIV is as follows:

- Therapy aimed at combating HIV itself or preventing reactivation or progression
- Strengthening of the individual's immune system
- Therapy aimed at treatment of the opportunistic coexistent infections

Risk Behaviors

Studies have identified several groups of individuals who are at highest risk for HIV infection. This information is very important in educational programs aimed at decreasing the spread of HIV infection. The following are risk behaviors that may communicate AIDS:

- Intravenous drug use
- Sharing of needles among intravenous drug users
- Vaginal intercourse without a condom
- Oral–genital sexual relations
- Anal intercourse without a condom
- Sharing objects (such as a vibrator) that are inserted into the anus or vagina
- Intercourse with someone who has had multiple partners, who presently has multiple partners, who has a history of high-risk behaviors, or whose sexual history is not known
- Homosexuality and male bisexuality
- The receipt of blood products between 1977 and 1985

Counseling

In the absence of adequate treatment, the most effective means to decrease the incidence of the disease is to provide education and screening in an attempt to prevent the spread of the infection. Screening involves careful history taking of risk behaviors as well as of the signs and symptoms of illness. Physical examination and serological testing is also a way to identify individuals who are HIV positive. Individuals should be advised about high-risk behaviors and the benefits of antibody testing, procedure of testing, the meaning of the possible results, the confidentiality of results, and the psychological and social impacts of a positive test.

Maternal Issues

It is estimated that women compose 7% of the patients with AIDS in the United States today. Approximately 80% of these women are of childbearing age, or between 15 and 49 years of age. Many of these women are latino or black, and there is a higher incidence in large urban cities.

Recent studies have shown that AIDS-infected pregnant women maintain their pregnancies and give birth to their infants. It is important to remember that most people infected with AIDS may be asymptomatic and that the onset of symptoms may be delayed for 5 to 10 years. Women in the high-risk group should be encouraged to find out their antibody status. Pregnant women who test positive early in pregnancy should be followed carefully. Those whose initial antibody testing is negative but whose behaviors currently are or previously were high risk should be tested again later in pregnancy.

Newborn Issues

Maternal transmission of HIV to unborn infants is estimated to be 40% to 60%. Infants are believed to become infected transplacentally (from the mother's blood through the placenta to the infant). Infants can also be exposed to the HIV virus in the birth canal. Cases have been reported of infants' becoming infected from the breast milk of women who were HIV positive. Because of the poor prognosis of the disease when contracted, breastfeeding is discouraged if women are known to be HIV positive.

Infants born to HIV-positive mothers need to be screened at birth and followed for indications of the infection. Infected infants demonstrate repeated viral and bacterial infections and often die before they are 2 years old. Infants at birth may not show symptoms initially but then may suffer symptoms such as failure to gain weight, fever, enlarged lymph nodes, diarrhea, yeast infections such as thrush, enlarged liver or spleen, and pneumonia.

In summary, the number of individuals in the United States and in the world who are HIV seropositive (with or without full-blown AIDS) has increased greatly during the past decade. In addition, it appears that a cure for HIV infections and AIDS will not be available for some time. This means that health care providers should take all the necessary precautions to avoid coming in contact with the disease. The public should continue to be informed about precautions to prevent the possibility of becoming HIV seropositive.

Health care providers have a great challenge in caring for HIV-infected persons. It is important to be truthful about the progressive and ultimately fatal nature of HIV infection. At the same time, it is important to be hopeful with them about future improvements in treatment, which may make HIV a manageable illness.

References

Barrick, B. (1990). Light at the end of a decade. *American Journal of Nursing* 90:37–40.

Centers for Disease Control (1990). *HIV/AIDS. Surveillance Report.* Atlanta, GA: Centers for Disease Control.

Centers for Disease Control (1988). AIDS due to HIV-2 infection in New Jersey. *Morbidity and Mortality Weekly Report* 37:33–35.

Davies, K. (1990). Genital herpes: An overview. *Journal of Obstetric, Gynecologic, and Neonatal Nursing* 19:401–406.

Dickason, E. J., Schult, M. O., & Silverman, B. L. (1990). *Maternal-Infant Nursing Care.* St. Louis: C. V. Mosby.

Durham, J. D., & Cohen, F. (1991). *The Person with AIDS: Nursing Perspectives,* 2nd ed. New York: Springer.

Flaskerud, J. H. (1989). *AIDS/HIV Infection: A Reference Guide for Nursing Professionals.* Philadelphia: W. B. Saunders Company.

Friedland, G., Kahl, R., & Saltzman, B. (1990). Additional evidence for lack of transmission of HIV infection by close interpersonal (casual) contact. *AIDS* 4:639–614.

Gershon, R. R., Valahov, D., & Nelson, K. E. (1990). The risk of transmission of HIV-1 through non-percutaneous, non-sexual modes: A review. *AIDS* 4:645–650.

Hatcher, R. A., Stewart, F., Trussell, J., Kowal, D., Guest, F., Stewart, G. K., & Cates, W. (1990). Sexually transmitted diseases. In *Contraceptive Technology,* 15th ed. New York: Irvington.

Holmes, K. (1990). *Sexually Transmitted Diseases,* 2nd ed. New York: McGraw-Hill Information Services.

Minkoff, H. L. (ed.) (1990). AIDS/HIV Diseases in pregnancy. *Obstetrics and Gynecology Clinics of North America* 17(3).

National Academy of Sciences (1990). Substance use and abuse during pregnancy. In *Nutrition during Pregnancy* (pp. 390–405). Washington, DC: National Academy Press.

Nattina, S. L. (1990). Syphilis: A new look at an old killer. *American Journal of Nursing* 90:68–70.

Prince, N. A., Beard, B. J., Ivey, S. L., & Lester, L. (1989). Perinatal nurses' knowledge and attitudes about AIDS. *Journal of Obstetric, Gynecologic, and Neonatal Nursing* 18:363–369.

Scherer, P. (1990). How HIV attacks the peripheral nervous system. *American Journal of Nursing* 90:67–70.

Taber, J. (1989). Nutrition in HIV infection. *American Journal of Nursing* 89:1446–1451.

Talashek, M., Tichy, A., & Salmon, M. (1989). The AIDS pandemic: A nursing model. *Public Health Nursing* 6(4):182–188.

Tinkle, M. B. (1990). Genital human papillomavirus infection: A growing risk. *Journal of Obstetric, Gynecologic, and Neonatal Nursing* 19:501–507.

Wendel, G. D., & Gilstrap, L. C. (1990). Syphilis rise calls for accurate diagnosis. *Contemporary OB/GYN* 35(6):37–46.

Wiley, K., & Grohar, J. (1988). Human immunodeficiency virus and precautions for obstetric, gynecologic, and neonatal nurses. *Journal of Obstetric, Gynecologic, and Neonatal Nursing* 17:165–168.

SUGGESTED ACTIVITIES

1. List four precautions that health care providers should take when coming in contact with body fluids such as blood from a patient with a potential or known STD.
2. List four factors that increase the risk of obtaining an STD.
3. List the stages of syphilis and summarize the symptoms and treatment.
4. Describe the symptoms of HIV infection and AIDS.

REVIEW QUESTIONS

A. Select the best answer to each multiple-choice question.

1. All of the following statements are true EXCEPT
   A. Primary syphilis presents itself with a painless lesion called a chancre
   B. A chancre is not infectious
   C. The second stage includes a rash, fever, and joint pains and is infectious
   D. The latent stage can cause heart and central nervous system damage; during this stage the disease can be spread, if untreated

2. Gonorrhea is a sexually transmitted disease that can cause
   A. Dysuria
   B. Pelvic inflammatory disease of the woman
   C. Female tubal obstruction
   D. All of the above

3. Chlamydia is a common sexually transmitted disease. All of the following statements are true EXCEPT
   A. Often the infection is asymptomatic
   B. Chlamydia increases the risk of tubal pregnancy
   C. The infection increases the risk of premature rupture of membranes
   D. Chlamydia does not affect the newborn

4. Herpes simplex virus is a sexually transmitted disease. If a lesion is present, which management of labor and birth is used?
   A. Nursing care is supportive
   B. Barrier method of protection is used
   C. Vaginal birth is the mode of delivery
   D. Cesarean birth is performed

5. The incidence of immunodeficiency virus (HIV) infection is increasing in the population of pregnant women. The history of the woman is important because of known risk factors, which are
   A. Intravenous drug use
   B. Sexual intercourse with multiple partners
   C. Vaginal intercourse without use of a condom
   D. All of the above

6. The health care provider should take the following precautions to avoid contacting HIV infection:
   A. Wearing gloves, masks, and protective eyewear during procedures that cause splashes of blood or bodily fluids on face and hands
   B. Wearing gown and gloves when handling the placenta
   C. Wearing gown and gloves when giving initial care to the newborn infant
   D. Using precautions to prevent injury from needles (needles should not be recapped or removed from disposable syringes)
   E. All of the above

B. Choose from Column II the phrase that most accurately defines the term in Column I.

I	II
1. Syphilis _____	A. Virus that produces potential liver involvement
2. Hepatitis B _____	B. May cause mouth or genital lesions
3. Chlamydia _____	C. Symptoms similar to those of infectious mononucleosis
4. Herpes simplex _____	D. Latent, untreated stage can cause a congenital newborn infection
5. Cytomegalovirus _____	E. Responsible for newborn conjunctivitis

CHAPTER 8 _____

Chapter Outline

Identification of a Fetus at Risk
Fetal Assessment During Pregnancy
    Ultrasonography
    Amniocentesis
    Maternal estriol levels
    Chorionic villus sampling
    Fetoscopy
    Maternal assessment of fetal activity
    Intermittent monitoring of fetal heart rate by auscultation
    Breast self-stimulation
    Electronic fetal heart rate monitoring
        Electronic monitoring of fetal heart rate during pregnancy
        Electronic monitoring of fetal heart rate during labor

Learning Objectives

Upon completion of Chapter 8, the student should be able to
- Describe the fetus's status in terms of well-being and maturity.
- List five factors that place the fetus at risk.
- Name four methods for assessing the fetal condition during the antepartum period.
- Explain the uses of ultrasonography during pregnancy.
- State the use of amniocentesis as a diagnostic tool.
- Identify the most important indicator of fetal maturity that can be determined by amniocentesis.
- Describe chorionic villus sampling.
- Compare chorionic villus sampling with amniocentesis.
- Explain the technique of fetoscopy.
- Explain maternal assessment of fetal activity.
- Describe the purpose of the nonstress test.
- List the advantages that the nonstress test has over the contraction stress test.
- Explain the purpose of the oxytocin challenge test (OCT).
- Describe the procedure of the OCT.
- Describe the breast self-stimulation test.
- List three factors that could affect the fetal heart rate during labor.
- Compare the advantages and disadvantages of external electronic fetal monitoring during labor.
- Describe internal electronic fetal monitoring during labor. List its advantages and disadvantages.
- Define terms used in electronic fetal monitoring.
- Identify interventions used when fetal heart rate patterns suggest fetal distress.
- Describe fetal blood sampling and explain why it is done.
- Describe the mother's psychological reactions to electronic fetal monitoring.

ASSESSMENT OF FETAL HEALTH

Diagnostic tests of fetal health give health care providers and the expectant mother information about the health of the fetus. Fetal health is determined by fetal well-being and fetal maturity. *Fetal well-being* is a term used to describe appropriateness of growth for gestation, normality of body structures, and adequacy of oxygenation from the placenta. *Fetal maturity* refers to the maturity of the body systems, with an emphasis on the pulmonary system. Diagnostic tests can predict both placental insufficiency and the fetus's ability to survive outside the uterus. Although the fetus usually matures best in the intrauterine environment, the proper timing of the delivery depends on placental adequacy (oxygenation) as well as the fetus's ability to tolerate the outside world.

Nurses should be careful to not let the highly technical nature of today's methods of fetal assessment and screening distance them from their patients. Machines should not replace hands-on clinical skills such as listening and touching.

Identification of a Fetus at Risk

Many women have pregnancies that proceed normally and require only basic assessment to ensure their own health and that of the fetus. However, a certain percentage of women are known to be at risk for intrapartum complications because of preexisting conditions. Others may encounter unanticipated problems during pregnancy. The basic factors used to assess the fetus's health are estimating the number of gestational weeks by calculations from the woman's last menstrual period, observing fundal height (see Figs. 6–4 and 6–5), and hearing fetal heart tones (see Figs. 5–2 and 5–3). If the woman's history is vague or the fundal height appears low, further assessment usually is carried out.

The woman's history is important to determine potential risks to the infant's health. For example, a medical condition such as essential hypertension can cause damage to maternal vascular organs which can contribute to placental insufficiency and thereby compromise the infant's health. Maternal smoking is related to low birth weight in infants. Women in lower socioeconomic groups frequently have poor nutrition and inadequate prenatal care. These factors can also place the infant at risk. In addition, studies have shown that older women (over 35 years of age) are more likely to give birth to infants with congenital defects or chromosomal abnormalities. Finally, the woman's work environment, such as one in which she is exposed to irradiation or cigarette smoke, can injure the fetus.

RISK FACTORS BY HISTORY

- Uterine fundal height relative to estimated date of confinement
- Maternal medical conditions that may contribute to vascular organ damage and placental insufficiency
- Maternal smoking
- Poor nutrition
- Older age of woman (over 35)
- Adolescence or young age
- Prior poor obstetrical history
- Woman's work environment (for example, exposure to irradiation)

131

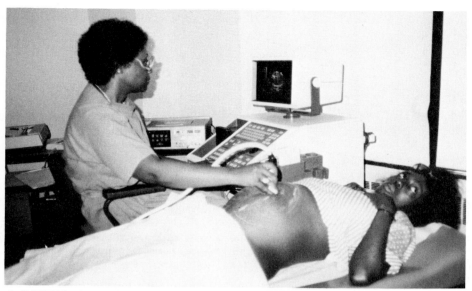

▲ FIGURE 8–1

Ultrasonography is a noninvasive, painless method of scanning a pregnant woman's abdomen with high-frequency waves to determine fetal growth and development.

Fetal Assessment During Pregnancy

Methods used to assess the condition of the fetus during pregnancy include ultrasonography, amniocentesis, chorionic villus sampling, fetoscopy, determination of estriol levels, the nonstress test, and the contraction test (oxytocin challenge test).

The nurse or other health professional has an opportunity to inform the woman about the test to be administered and provide support. The woman should be instructed about what to expect during the procedure, and her concerns regarding the specific test should be listened to. Usually, receiving knowledge about the procedure decreases the woman's anxiety (see Nursing Care Plan 8–1, pp. 147–148).

ULTRASONOGRAPHY

Valuable information about the fetus can be obtained by ultrasonography. This technique involves the rebounding of high-frequency waves, which are reflected off tissues of different densi-

ties. When an ultrasound transducer is passed over the skin of the abdomen, the sound waves are changed to electrical, visible signals that produce a picture. With sophisticated equipment, visible signals can be photographed for a permanent record.

The procedure is simple, noninvasive, and painless (Fig. 8–1). However, ultrasonography needs to be investigated further before it can be used liberally as a screening device or be performed without a good reason. To date, no harmful effects have been identified for either the woman or fetus. Ultrasound is used in most instances to identify fetal problems, because x-ray (rarely used) is known to have harmful effects on the fetus.

It is important for the nurse to explain the ultrasound procedure to the expectant mother to lessen her anxiety. Because a full bladder displaces the uterus upward, making the fetal head more accessible for measurement, the woman should not empty her bladder until the procedure is completed. The woman is placed in supine position (on her back), and her abdomen is exposed. A lubricant is applied to her abdomen to reduce friction and increase conductivity. Ultrasound scanning usually takes about 20 minutes.

The most common use of ultrasonography is to detect retardation of fetal growth and to determine gestational age. Measurement of the biparietal (widest) diameter of the fetal head provides valuable information about continued growth. Other measurements for monitoring fetal growth are crown-to-rump length and femur length. Ultrasonography can confirm a diagnosis of pregnancy as early as 6 to 8 weeks' gestation. At this time, the gestational sac can be seen, and the pulsating heart can be detected (Fig. 8–2). Other clinical uses of ultrasonography are identification of multiple fetuses (Fig. 8–3); detection of fetal anomalies, such as hydrocephaly; detection of hydramnios and hydatidiform mole; detection of fetal malposition; determination of placental location

for amniocentesis; and determination of placenta previa.

USES OF ULTRASONOGRAPHY IN THE FIRST TRIMESTER

- Early confirmation of pregnancy
- Diagnosis of pregnancy outside the uterus
- Assessment of placenta location (placenta previa)
- Diagnosis of hydatidiform mole
- Diagnosis of multiple gestation

USES OF ULTRASONOGRAPHY IN THE SECOND AND THIRD TRIMESTERS

- Assessment of fetal growth
- Assessment of fetal abnormalities

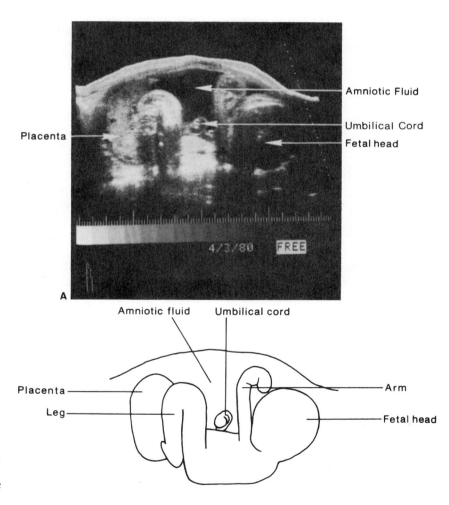

Placenta
Amniotic Fluid
Umbilical Cord
Fetal head

4/3/80   FREE

A

Amniotic fluid   Umbilical cord
Placenta
Leg
Arm
Fetal head

B

▲ **FIGURE 8–2**

A. Fetus as seen ultrasonographically at 32 weeks' gestation. (Ultrasound and photography by Dr. Lewis Nelson.) **B.** Outline of fetus as seen ultrasonographically in **A.** (From Moore, M. L. (1983). *Realities in Childbearing*, 2nd ed. Philadelphia, W. B. Saunders Company.)

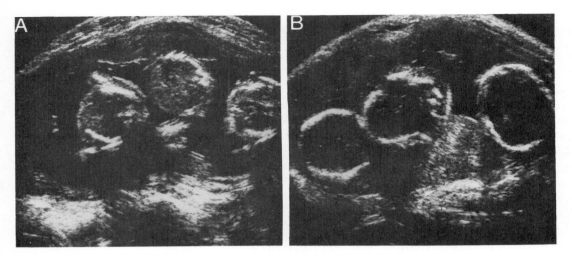

▲ FIGURE 8–3

Ultrasonograms of triplets at 18 weeks' gestation, showing trunk areas (A) and cross sections of the three heads (B). (From Creasy, R. K., & Resnik, R. (1984). *Maternal–Fetal Medicine*. Philadelphia, W. B. Saunders Company.)

- Assessment of fetal position and presentation
- Assessment of fetal viability (living or dead)

AMNIOCENTESIS

Amniocentesis is the withdrawal of some of the amniotic fluid surrounding the fetus. The fluid is analyzed for fetal maturity and well-being. The procedure can be done as early as 14 weeks, at which time the amniotic fluid volume has increased enough to make the procedure safe for the fetus. Amniocentesis is a fairly simple procedure and can be done on an outpatient basis. Risks are greatly reduced if ultrasonography is used to locate the placenta and the position of the fetus just before the amniocentesis is performed. This reduces the incidence of direct fetal injury and fetomaternal hemorrhage with possible resultant isoimmunization. The complications (1% chance) include possible spontaneous abortion, fetal trauma, fetal infection, and Rh sensitization of an Rh− mother as a result of fetal bleeding (from an Rh+ fetus). Although complications are rare, many health care facilities require a woman to sign a consent form before the procedure is done.

Indications

The main indications for doing an amniocentesis are to detect birth defects, genetic defects, and fetal maturity and evaluate the progress of a pregnancy in which isoimmunization has occurred. In addition, Down's syndrome (trisomy 21), Tay-Sachs disease, sickle cell disease, and hemophilia can be detected by this method. Testing for neural tube defects (indicated by the presence of α-feto-protein) such as spina bifida, anencephaly, or meningomyelocele is also possible. Although the sex of the fetus can also be determined, because of the potential risks this is not a justifiable reason for performing the procedure.

To detect the presence of a genetic disorder, amniocentesis is performed between the fourteenth and sixteenth weeks of gestation. It takes 3 to 5 weeks for the growth of the cultured cells that would indicate the presence of a genetic disorder.

If there is uncertainty regarding the maturity of the fetus, the maternal status, or both, amniocentesis should be done at 34 to 36 weeks' gestation.

Amniotic Fluid Analyses

The fetal organs that can be assessed by amniocentesis are the lungs, liver, kidneys, and skin.

Specific diagnostic tests using the amniotic fluid to determine fetal maturity are the lecithin/sphingomyelin (L/S) ratio (for lung maturity) and the following, less reliable, tests: creatinine values (for kidney function), bilirubin levels (for liver function), and fetal skin cells. One important organ that cannot be assessed by amniocentesis is the heart.

Lecithin/Sphingomyelin Ratio. Lung maturity is the most important indicator of fetal maturity that can be determined by amniocentesis. Lecithin and sphingomyelin phospholipids (fat-like substances) are produced in the fetal alveoli (air sacs) of the lung. The concentration of lecithin correlates highly with the degree of fetal lung maturity. Lecithin increases markedly at approximately 35 weeks' gestation. It is associated with a greater production of surfactant by the alveolar cells. Surfactant is necessary for the expansion of the lungs at birth and for the maintenance of the end-expiratory expansion after birth. Without enough surfactant, the infant's lungs would be unable to take over the task of gas exchange; when the infant began to breathe on his or her own, many of the alveoli would not stay expanded and would collapse. The amount of lecithin is compared with the amount of sphingomyelin in the amniotic fluid to give the L/S ratio. When the L/S ratio is greater than 2/1, the lungs are considered mature enough for infant survival, and there is a decreased potential that the infant will develop respiratory distress syndrome.

Amniotic Fluid Bilirubin. It is possible to measure the amount of bilirubin and other breakdown products of hemoglobin in the amniotic fluid. Presumably because the fetal liver is able to conjugate bilirubin, the concentration peaks at midpregnancy and decreases to zero at term. The amount of bilirubin in the amniotic fluid has been found to be helpful in determining if the fetus of an Rh-sensitized mother is in jeopardy.

Amniotic Fluid Creatinine. The creatinine level in the amniotic fluid seems to have some correlation with fetal renal maturity. Creatinine is excreted by the fetal kidneys as growth occurs.

Fetal Skin Cells. Examination of samples of fetal squamous cells from the amniotic fluid can detect some genetic abnormalities. However, it takes an average of 3 weeks before the cells in the tissue culture grow sufficiently to make chromosomal assessments significant.

Procedure

The woman is requested to empty her bladder before the amniocentesis so that the bladder is not entered instead of the amniotic sac within the uterus. The procedure should be fully explained to the woman. Discomfort is caused mainly by the injection of the local anesthetic. The woman, or couple, should be instructed about the need for ultrasonography to determine the fetal and placental locations before amniocentesis. The possible risks should be stated along with the indications. Usually, the need for doing the procedure outweighs the potential risks.

An initial ultrasound scan is performed to confirm fetal position and location of the placenta. A site for needle insertion is chosen where there is a pocket of amniotic fluid. Using aseptic technique, the physician inserts a sterile needle through the abdominal wall and uterine wall into the amniotic sac. The first few drops of fluid are discarded because they many contain maternal cells. Then, approximately 10 to 30 mL of amniotic fluid is withdrawn and the needle is removed (Fig. 8–4). The site of injection is covered with an adhesive bandage. Fetal heart tones are checked after the procedure is completed.

MATERNAL ESTRIOL LEVELS

The estriol level in samples of maternal blood or urine (urine collected over a 24-hour period) is an indicator of fetoplacental well-being. Both the fetus and the placenta must be intact to produce estriol. If either the fetus or the placenta is compromised, decreased production of the hormone will occur. Using a blood sample is more convenient than using a urine sample, and the findings are not affected by maternal renal function. Serial estriol determinations provide more information about the stability of the fetoplacental unit than does a single test. Instead of assessing absolute values, the physician looks for a pattern of values. A progressive or dramatic fall in estriol values may signify danger to the fetus. Placental insufficiency can occur in diabetes, hypertension, and suspected postmaturity and can compromise the fetus.

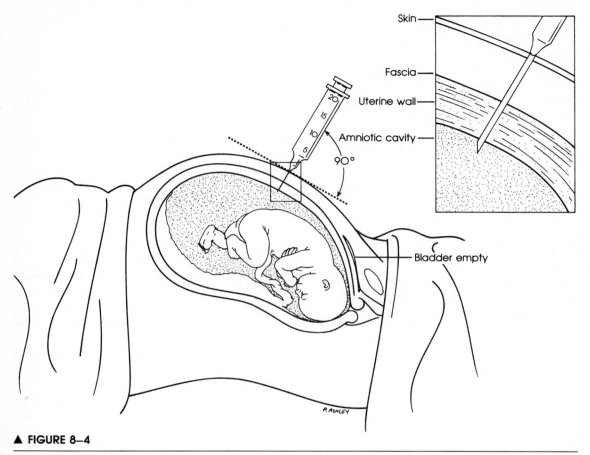

Skin

Fascia

Uterine wall

Amniotic cavity

90°

Bladder empty

P. ASHLEY

▲ **FIGURE 8–4**

Amniocentesis. The woman is scanned to locate the placenta and to determine the position of the fetus. A needle is inserted through the skin, fascia, and uterine wall. When the needle is within the uterine cavity, amniotic fluid is withdrawn.

CHORIONIC VILLUS SAMPLING

Chorionic villus sampling (CVS) is a relatively new diagnostic method. CVS can be done as early as 8 to 12 weeks' gestation for early identification of genetic problems. Two techniques have been developed to obtain small fragments of the chorionic villi from the developing placenta: transcervical sampling and transabdominal sampling. The advantage of CVS over amniocentesis is that CVS can be done earlier (that is, at 8 to 12 weeks); this technique can be performed during the 1st trimester, which allows for the termination of early gestation with greater safety and less psychological trauma. CVS has the potential for diagnosing the same disorders that are detected by the amniocentesis. Women at risk as a result of older age or a previous delivery of a child with a genetic defect are candidates for this procedure.

Using ultrasound, a transcervical catheter is introduced and chorionic villi are aspirated into a syringe (Fig. 8–5). The cells are then prepared for diagnostic assessment. Transabdominal sampling of chorionic villi can also be performed.

Complications of CVS are similar to those of amniocentesis. They include amniotic fluid leakage, infections, Rh isoimmunization, and fetal death. The risk increases if the catheter has to be passed more than one time.

FETOSCOPY

Fetoscopy is a new technique of fetal assessment and currently is performed at only selected medi-

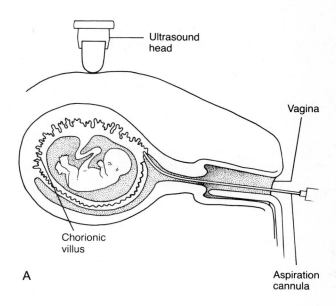

Vaginal sampling

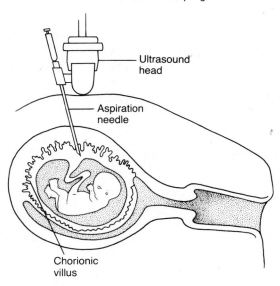

Abdominal sampling

▲ FIGURE 8–5

Chorionic villus sampling (CVS). Chorionic villi may be obtained either vaginally (**A**) or transabdominally (**B**) by an aspirating needle guided by ultrasonography. The test can be done at 8 to 10 weeks' gestation, and the results can be available within 48 hours.

cal centers. It requires specialized equipment and experience. Fetoscopy is used to diagnose problems such as sickle cell anemia and hemophilia and treat the fetus in the uterus. The diagnostic benefit must outweigh potential fetal risks. Pregnancy wastage can be as high as 12%. The procedure begins with ultrasound to locate the placenta and umbilical cord and assess the fetus. Direct visualization of the fetus is possible through the insertion of a fiberoptic telescope transabdominally into the uterine cavity under ultrasound guidance. Blood or a sample of fetal skin is obtained for diagnosis of fetal genetic disorders (Fig. 8–6). Treatment can then be given; for example, the fetus who is severely anemic can receive an intrauterine blood transfusion. After the procedure, the fetal heart rate (FHR) is monitored for possible fetal distress.

MATERNAL ASSESSMENT OF FETAL ACTIVITY

The expectant woman may be asked to count fetal movements during the third trimester as a screening device, if she states she notices less fetal activity. The woman's perceptions of fetal movements and her accuracy of documenting them influence the reliability of her information. Two or more fetal movements per hour are reassuring; however, the fetus has rest–sleep periods during which minimal or no movement may occur. If there are fewer than two fetal movements for an extended period of time it should be reported to the physician for evaluation with a nonstress test.

INTERMITTENT MONITORING OF FETAL HEART RATE BY AUSCULTATION

In low-risk pregnancies the FHR may be obtained by intermittent FHR monitoring using a *fetal stethoscope* or a *Doppler* device (see Chapter 5). However, monitoring of FHR by intermittent auscultation has several limitations: (a) The evaluation of FHR is restricted to the interval between uterine contractions; (b) the FHR cannot be heard during contractions, when assessment is crucial; (c) changes in FHR cannot be detected early; and (d) errors in counting FHR are made. Because during

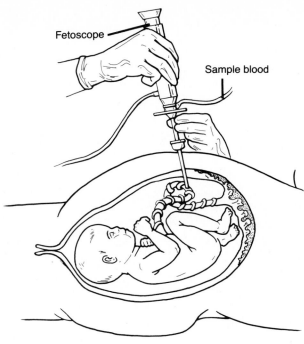

▲ **FIGURE 8–6**

Fetoscopy and fetal blood sampling. A fine fiberoptic telescope may be passed into the amniotic sac under ultrasound control.

labor it is necessary to frequently count and record the FHR to know the fetal status, continuous monitoring is preferred.

BREAST SELF-STIMULATION TEST

The breast self-stimulation test (BSST) is carried out by applying warm washcloths and/or manually rolling one nipple at a time to stimulate contractions. When the contractions are sufficient to interpret the results, the nipple stimulation is stopped. Breast stimulation is discontinued if late decelerations occur.

ELECTRONIC FETAL HEART RATE MONITORING (Table 8–1)

Maternal indications for electronic FHR monitoring during pregnancy are as follows:

TABLE 8–1. TERMS USED IN ELECTRONIC FETAL MONITORING

TERM	DEFINITION	CHARACTERISTIC	CAUSE	INTERVENTION
Baseline FHR[a]	FHR between contractions	Normal rate 120–160 bpm	—	—
Baseline variability	Irregularity (change) of baseline FHR Fluctations of FHR	Variability of >6 bpm Flat (smooth) baseline of <6 bpm	— CNS[b] depressants Uteroplacental insufficiency (UPI)	— Change maternal position to side (left side, if possible) Oxygen; notify physician
Bradycardia	Abnormally slow heart rate (<120 bpm)	FHR of <120 bpm	Drugs Heart block	Discontinue drugs (if cause)
Tachycardia	Abnormally fast FHR	FHR of 160 bpm	Maternal fever Fetal hypoxia Fetal infection	Change maternal position to side Check maternal temperature Assess emotional status (anxiety) Oxygen; notify physician
Early deceleration	Slowing of FHR when contraction begins FHR returns to normal at end of contraction	Mirrors contraction; FHR returns to baseline at end of contraction FHR usually stays within range of 120–160 bpm	Compression of head Uterine contraction Vaginal examination Fundal pressure	Change maternal position to side
Late deceleration	Slowing of FHR as contraction begins Recovery to normal is delayed	FHR does not return to normal baseline until well after uterine contraction	UPI Inadequate fetal oxygen	Change maternal position to side Oxygen Correct hypotension if present Elevate legs Discontinue oxytocin infusion Notify physician
Variable deceleration	Slowing of FHR	Abrupt, transitory decrease in FHR that is variable in duration, intensity, and timing relative to contraction	Compression of cord Short cord Compression of head Pushing during second stage Vaginal exam	Change maternal position Oxygen, if FHR does not respond Correct hypotension, if present Notify physician, if above measures do not correct FHR
Acceleration	Short-term increase in FHR above baseline	Usually during contraction; occurs in breech presentation		Change maternal position to side

[a]Fetal heart rate.
[b]Central nervous system.

- Maternal complications (for example, hypertension, diabetes, renal disease)
- History of previous stillbirth
- Rh sensitization
- Abnormal estriol excretion pattern
- Postterm pregnancy
- Premature rupture of membranes
- Maternal age over 35

Fetal indications for electronic FHR monitoring are as follows:

- Intrauterine growth retardation
- Multiple gestation
- Assessment of fetus after amniocentesis
- Decreased fetal movement
- Placental perfusion problems

Electronic Monitoring of Fetal Heart Rate During Pregnancy

NONSTRESS TEST

The nonstress test (NST) is used clinically to evaluate FHR acceleration in response to fetal movement. An acceleration in FHR is expected with fetal activity and indicates a *reactive fetus* (Fig. 8–7). Observation of baseline variability and accel-

eration of the FHR indicates that central nervous and autonomic nervous systems are intact and are not being affected by hypoxia. Lack of fetal movement during a 20-minute test may indicate fetal sleep. Attempts to arouse the fetus may be made by rubbing the woman's abdomen or giving her fruit juice or even a light meal.

If the fetus does not show movement during the 20-minute period, the period may be extended to approximately 40 minutes. If there is no movement by this time, the fetus is referred to as *nonreactive*. A nonreactive NST is taken as an indication for further evaluation of the fetus by a contraction stress test (CST), such as the oxytocin challenge test (OCT). If the fetus is at the period of viability, the CST may be done the same day.

ADVANTAGES OF THE NST

- Quick to perform
- Noninvasive and inexpensive
- Can be done in the clinic or office
- No side effects

DISADVANTAGES OF THE NST

- Fetus may remain inactive despite stimulation

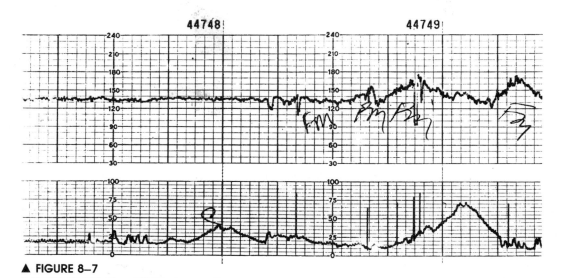

▲ FIGURE 8–7

The reactive nonstress test tracing the onset of fetal activity with increased fetal heart rate. (From Creasy, R. K., & Resnik, R. (1984). *Maternal–Fetal Medicine.* Philadelphia, W. B. Saunders Company.)

• May be difficult to obtain a good tracing

During an NST, an electronic fetal monitor is used to obtain a tracing of FHR and fetal movement. Two belts are placed on the woman's abdomen. One belt contains a device that detects fetal movement and uterine activity, and the other belt holds a device that detects FHR. As the fetal movement occurs, it is documented so the associated or simultaneous FHR changes can be evaluated.

ACOUSTIC STIMULATION TEST

A new method, the *acoustic stimulation test*, which uses sound to stimulate the fetus, is being evaluated. The fetus has been demonstrated to respond to vibroacoustic stimulation as early as 26 weeks' gestation. This technique begins with the NST. If after 5 to 10 minutes spontaneous accelerations do not occur, an artificial larynx box that produces both vibratory and acoustic frequencies is applied to the maternal abdomen over the fetal head. It is then activated with a 2- to 3-minute stimulus that has shown to provoke a response from a healthy fetus. Use of the Artificial Larynx Stimulator (Corometrics, Wallingford, CT, Model 146) has reduced the number of nonreactive NSTs reported as well the time required for the NST.

CONTRACTION STRESS TEST (OXYTOCIN CHALLENGE TEST)

The CST is helpful in assessing the circulatory–respiratory function (oxygen and carbon dioxide exchange). The CST is conducted after the 28th week of gestation if the physician suspects placental insufficiency. It is not done earlier because it could stimulate the woman to go into labor before the fetus is likely to survive.

During contractions, the intrauterine pressure increases, and blood flow to the fetus (via intervillous spaces in the placenta) momentarily decreases. This reduces the oxygen received by the fetus. A healthy fetus usually tolerates this reduction; however, if the placental reserve is insufficient, the fetus can be compromised.

Indications for a CST are those conditions in which uteroplacental insufficiency may occur, including chronic hypertension, pregnancy-induced hypertension, diabetes, intrauterine growth retardation, suspected postmaturity (more than 42 weeks' gestation), Rh sensitization, heart disease, renal disease, history of previous stillbirths, and nonreactive NST.

Procedure. A necessary component of the CST is the presence of uterine contractions. The contractions usually are induced with intravenous administration of oxytocin (Pitocin). This method is known as the OCT. Alternatively, some clinics are using the BSST. This method is based on the knowledge that the woman's body produces oxytocin when the nipples of the breasts are stimulated.

The woman is placed on her left side or in semi-Fowler's position. An electronic monitor is used, with an ultrasonic transducer to evaluate FHR, and a pressure transducer called a *tocodynamometer* is placed on the woman's abdomen, over the uterine fundus, to record uterine contractions. The ultrasonic transducer and the tocodynamometer are secured in place with belts. A continuous recording with tracing is done with the electronic fetal monitor. The woman's blood pressure and pulse rate are assessed during the recording. After a 15-minute baseline reading of uterine activity and FHR is obtained, the tracing is assessed for spontaneous contractions. If no contractions have occurred, oxytocin is administered intravenously to produce contractions of good quality, that is, three or four contractions that last longer than 30 seconds each within a 10-minute period. The OCT is discontinued if late decelerations occur.

ASSESSMENT OF CST (OCT)

• CST is negative if no change in FHR occurs during three uterine contractions lasting more than 30 seconds each within a 10-minute period.
• CST is positive if repetitive late FHR decelerations occur, demonstrating the stress of uterine contractions on FHR.
• Hyperstimulation occurs when contractions occur more frequently than every 2 minutes or last more than 90 seconds each.
• The CST is termed *suspicious* when there are inconsistent but definite late decelerations in FHR.

ADVANTAGES OF THE CST

- CST provides information about how the fetus tolerates or reacts to the stress of uterine contractions.
- CST can demonstrate that the fetal environment is deteriorating.

DISADVANTAGES OF THE CST

- CST needs to be administered in hospital setting.
- OCT is an invasive procedure using an intravenous line.
- CST may initiate uterine contractions and start labor.

Electronic Monitoring of Fetal Heart Rate During Labor

Because labor is a period of stress for the fetus, *continuous assessment of fetal health by electronic FHR monitoring is almost always instituted.* The FHR provides important information about the fetal status, especially as it relates to uterine contractions. The normal range of the FHR is 120 to 160 beats per minute. A sudden rise or fall in the FHR, prolonged periods above or below the normal range, decreased variability (decrease in fluctuations) in the FHR, or marked slowing of the number of beats per minute indicates fetal distress.

Factors that affect FHR during labor contractions include compression of the fetal head, compression of umbilical cord, and compression of vessels (uteroplacental insufficiency).

CONTINUOUS EXTERNAL FETAL ELECTRONIC MONITORING DURING LABOR

In external monitoring of the fetus, two separate transducers are used to record the FHR and uterine contractions. The FHR ultrasound transducer picks up the sound waves from the fetal heart and valves, and a tocotransducer (a pressure-sensing device) picks up the abdominal tension of contractions. The separate transducers are held in place by Velcro-like straps that are placed around the woman's abdomen (Fig. 8–8). The FHR transducer should be placed where the FHR is heard most clearly; the electronic signals are recorded on a graph and displayed on a screen. Conductive gel is applied to the crystals to promote conduction of the FHR. The tocotransducer is placed over the fundus of the uterus, where contractions are felt most strongly. The tocotransducer can measure the frequency and duration, but not the intensity, of the contractions.

External electronic monitoring is easily applied by the nurse, but the transducers need to be repositioned if the mother or fetus changes position. The pressure-sensitive dial on the tocotransducer usually has to be adjusted periodically for tracing of the uterine contractions. Also, the FHR transducer has to be readjusted frequently for FHR tracing.

ADVANTAGES OF EXTERNAL ELECTRONIC FETAL MONITORING DURING LABOR

- Because it is noninvasive, it reduces the chance of infection.
- It can be conducted at any time (before membranes have ruptured and before cervix is dilated).
- Placement of transducers can be done by the nurse.
- Tracing gives a permanent record.

DISADVANTAGES OF EXTERNAL ELECTRONIC FETAL MONITORING DURING LABOR

- Uterine contraction intensity is not calibrated.
- FHR variability is not accurate; it is subject to maternal and fetal movement.
- Movement of woman requires frequent repositioning of transducers.
- Obesity and fetal position affect quality of recording.
- If the woman is kept in supine position, maternal hypotension may result.

CONTINUOUS INTERNAL FETAL ELECTRONIC MONITORING DURING LABOR

Internal fetal monitoring requires the use of a fetal electrode and an intrauterine pressure cath-

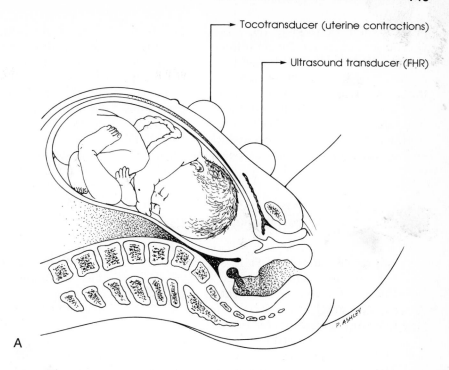

Tocotransducer (uterine contractions)

Ultrasound transducer (FHR)

A

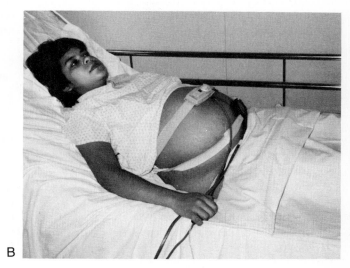

B

▲ **FIGURE 8–8**

Diagrammatic representation of external fetal monitoring (**A**). Placement of external transducers: tocotransducer is placed above the umbilicus, and ultrasound transducer is placed below the umbilicus (**B**).

eter that is inserted into the cervix and passed inside the uterine cavity above the presenting part (usually the fetal head). Before insertion of the catheter, the cervix must be dilated at least 2 cm, the fetal presenting part must be specified and felt by vaginal examination, and the amniotic sac must have ruptured (spontaneously or artificially).

After the perineum is cleansed, the physician, midwife, or specially trained registered nurse inserts a sterile internal electrode through the vagina into the uterine cavity, where it is placed against the presenting part. The electrode is rotated clockwise until it is attached to the fetal head. Wires that extend from the electrode are attached to a leg plate (which is secured to the woman's thigh by Velcro-like straps or adhesive tape) and the plate is then attached to the monitor (Fig. 8–9). Uterine contractions are monitored by placing a sterile catheter, filled with sterile water, inside the uterine cavity. It is connected to a strain gauge that is attached to the monitor. This allows uterine contractions to be evaluated by the intrauterine pressure that is present both during and between contractions. Also, the relationship between FHR and uterine contractions can be more accurately evaluated.

ADVANTAGES OF INTERNAL ELECTRONIC MONITORING DURING LABOR

- Abnormal patterns of FHR, suggestive of fetal distress, can be detected early.
- Intensity of uterine contractions is recorded with accuracy.
- Obesity and fetal/maternal movement do not affect the recording.
- FHR variability can be assessed.
- The woman is allowed greater freedom of movement in bed without compromising the monitor tracing.

DISADVANTAGES OF INTERNAL ELECTRONIC MONITORING DURING LABOR

- Membranes must be ruptured and cervix somewhat dilated.
- There is potential risk to the fetus if fetal electrode is not correctly applied.
- Potential risk of infection in fetus and woman exists.
- Procedure must be done by physician, midwife, or specially trained registered nurse.

INTERPRETATION OF FHR DURING LABOR

To interpret the FHR during labor, the nurse must know (a) the baseline FHR, (b) whether the rate is above or below the normal 120 to 160 beats per minute, and (c) whether the variability of FHR is adequate. Emphasis is placed on the fetus's receiving adequate oxygen because hypoxia (lack of oxygen) can compromise the fetus (Fig. 8–10).

Baseline variability refers to beat-to-beat varia-tions (that is, fluctuations) in FHR. Fluctuations of the FHR baseline indicate normal neurological control of the heart rate and a measure of fetal reserve. In contrast, if each interval between heartbeats was the same, the baseline would be flat, indicating central nervous system depression associated with hypoxia.

Variability is further described as short- or long-term. *Short-term variability* is a change in FHR from one beat to the next. *Long-term variability* is the rhythmic fluctuation, or waves, generally 3 to 5 cycles per minute. Accurate short- and long-term variability evaluation is possible with the internal mode of monitoring using the spiral fetal electrode.

FHR fluctuations correlate with normal acid–base status and fetal health. Variability decreases with fetal sleep, certain drugs, and lack of oxygen. Average baseline variability is 6 to 10 beats per minute. Minimal baseline variability (3 to 5 beats per minute) indicates potential fetal distress. Absence of variability (0 to 2 beats per minute) is referred to as a smooth or *flat* baseline and is considered an important warning for fetal jeopardy.

Tachycardia is a baseline FHR of more than 160 bpm. This problem may be due to maternal fever, certain drugs, or, if persistent, fetal distress.

Bradycardia is a baseline FHR of less than 120 bpm. Persistent bradycardia, especially when it follows the uterine contraction, indicates fetal distress. Although rare, bradycardia can signal fetal heart abnormality. Other causes of bradycardia are severe contractions due to oxytocin, supine maternal position (maternal hypotension), paracervical block or regional anesthetics, and maternal "bearing down" (when woman exerts pressure by contracting her abdominal muscles).

RELATIONSHIP OF FHR TO UTERINE CONTRACTIONS DURING LABOR

It is important that the nurse understand the relationship between the FHR and uterine contractions during labor.

Accelerations are transient increases in FHR above the baseline. They usually occur in response to uterine contractions and fetal movements caused by the pressure of the contractions. Accel-

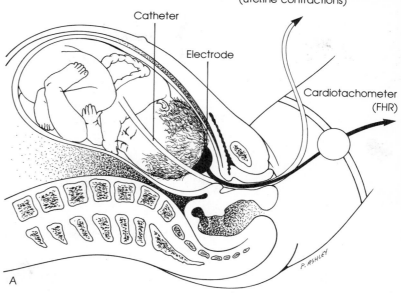

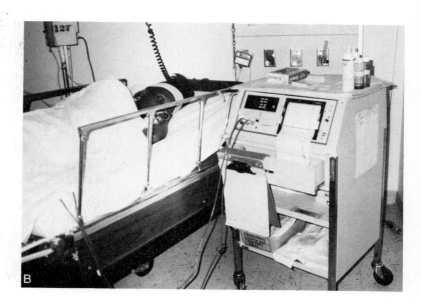

▲ FIGURE 8–9

Diagrammatic representation of internal fetal monitoring with intrauterine catheter and spiral fetal electrode in place (**A**). Electronic fetal heart rate monitor with internal mode of monitoring (**B**).

erations of this type are considered a sign of well-being.

Decelerations are temporary decreases in FHR from the baseline that are classified into types—early, late, and variable—according to the time of their occurrence during the contraction (Fig. 8–10).

Early decelerations are usually due to head compression during the contraction. The deceleration starts with the contraction and ends with it. The uniform wave shape reflects the shape of the contraction (mirrors the contraction) and is considered benign. No intervention is necessary.

Variable deceleration is a transient drop in the FHR before, during, or after the uterine contraction. There is no uniformity of the FHR pattern. It may be related to a brief compression of the umbilical cord. If encountered, it usually can be

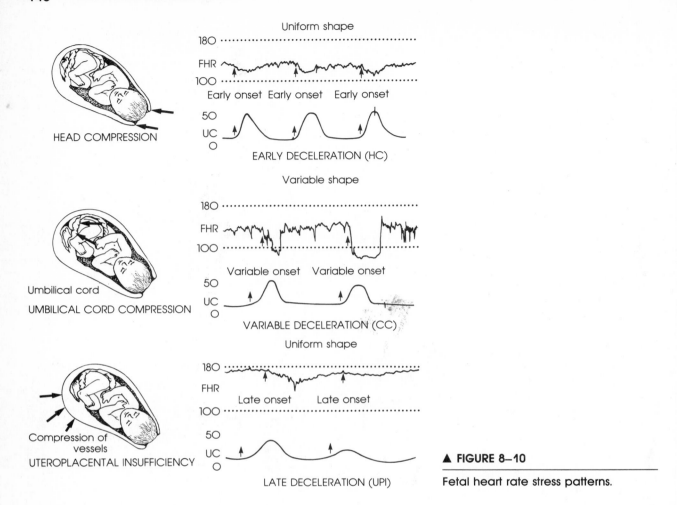

Uniform shape

EARLY DECELERATION (HC)

HEAD COMPRESSION

Variable shape

VARIABLE DECELERATION (CC)

Umbilical cord
UMBILICAL CORD COMPRESSION

Uniform shape

LATE DECELERATION (UPI)

Compression of vessels
UTEROPLACENTAL INSUFFICIENCY

▲ FIGURE 8–10

Fetal heart rate stress patterns.

eliminated by having the mother change position. In the second stage of labor, it may result from cord compression during fetal descent. If variable deceleration is severe or prolonged, it may indicate a tight cord around the baby's neck, which may require an emergency cesarean birth.

Late decelerations are decelerations that begin *after* the contraction has been established and continue after the contraction ends (Fig. 8–11). They are usually caused by uteroplacental insufficiency. The depth and the time to return to baseline are significant. Persistence or frequent recurrence of late decelerations usually indicates hypoxia or lack of oxygen to the fetus. A late deceleration can be caused by maternal hypotension, excessive uterine activity (for example, during induction of labor), and deficient placental perfusion. Any drop of 30 bpm or baseline variability (less than 3 to 5 bpm) is a significant indicator of fetal distress.

Fetal blood sampling is obtained from the fetal scalp when fetal distress is suspected. This procedure is often done after variable or late fetal heart decelerations are observed. Analysis of the fetal blood for pH reveals whether the fetus is acidotic. The blood sample is obtained from the fetal scalp transcervically. The amniotic membranes must be ruptured and the cervix dilated before this procedure is possible. Prompt delivery of the infant is necessary if the pH is below 7.20. If acidosis is uncorrected, the fetus would soon be in jeopardy.

NURSING INTERVENTIONS TO CONSIDER IN ELECTRONIC FETAL MONITORING DURING LABOR

- Interpret various FHR patterns
- Report significant changes in FHR

NURSING CARE PLAN 8–1

ASSESSMENT OF FETAL HEALTH

Potential Problems and Nursing Diagnoses	Nursing Intervention
1. Knowledge deficit related to the ultrasound procedure.	Explain that the ultrasound procedure is noninvasive and painless. Explain that it gives valuable information about fetal growth, placental location, and whether there is more than one fetus. Encourage verbalization about the procedure. Try to decrease the anxiety and make patient feel more positive about having an ultrasound.
2. Anxiety related to having an amniocentesis.	Listen to patient's concerns about having an amniocentesis. Explain that the procedure can determine if the baby's lungs are mature. Reassure patient that amniocentesis is a common procedure.
3. Knowledge deficit related to maternal assessment of fetal activity.	Instruct woman to count each time the baby moves for a 2-hour period on two or three occasions. Explain that babies demonstrate little movement during their sleep periods, which can last 20 to 30 minutes. Tell patient that counting the number of times the baby moves for a 2-hour time period is a screening technique, and thus the accuracy of reporting is important.
4. Knowledge deficit related to internal electronic fetal monitoring during labor.	Explain the electronic monitoring equipment to patient. Reassure patient that someone will be with her at all times. Explain that the electronic fetal monitoring procedure is commonly used. It is a way to safeguard the baby's health. Encourage patient to ask questions about the procedure. Ask patient to remain on her left side as much as possible. Attempt to keep patient comfortable.
5. Noncompliance related to position assumed during labor.	Provide an opportunity for patient to state reasons for assuming the supine position rather than the side-lying position during electronic fetal monitoring.
6. Powerlessness related to health care environment; health-related regimen.	Create an environment to facilitate patient's participation in her basic care (brushing her teeth, etc.).

Nursing Care Plan continued on following page

NURSING CARE PLAN 8–1 *Continued*

ASSESSMENT OF FETAL HEALTH

Expected Outcomes

1. Patient verbalizes understanding of the ultrasound procedure. She recognizes that it will provide information about the baby's growth.
2. Patient communicates a more positive feeling about the amniocentesis procedure. She recognizes it is to assess the baby's health.
3. Patient verbalizes understanding of the importance of accuracy in counting the baby's movements and plans to keep a record of movements.
4. Patient verbalizes an understanding of why the internal electronic fetal monitoring procedures is performed.
5. Patient verbalizes her misconception that there is no difference between the supine position and the side position during internal electronic fetal monitoring.
6. Patient identifies the reason why powerlessness is felt.

(tachycardia, loss of baseline variability, or decelerations)
- Change the woman's position, preferably so that she is lying on her left side (assess the woman's comfort, offer bedpan, etc.)
- Evaluate excessive uterine contractions
- Decrease uterine activity by discontinuing oxytocin infusion
- Administer oxygen to the woman, usually by mask

- Correct hypotension by repositioning woman to side
- Report status to physician

MEDICAL AND NURSING GOALS IN ELECTRONIC FETAL MONITORING DURING LABOR

The primary goal is to have optimal maternal and fetal outcome. Nurses as well as physicians

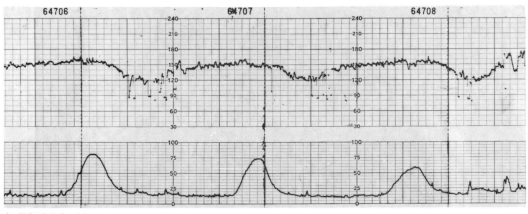

▲ **FIGURE 8–11**

Internal fetal monitor tracing showing late decelerations. Note the late onset and late recovery of fetal heart rate. (From Creasy, R. K., & Resnik, R. (1989). *Maternal–Fetal Medicine: Principles and Practice*, 2nd ed. Philadelphia, W. B. Saunders Company.)

in the labor care settings should be able to recognize FHR patterns, beat-to-beat variability, and intensity of uterine activity. In addition, the nurse should remember that the monitor cannot replace hands-on assessment. Sometimes, the mother states that her contractions are stronger than those seen on the monitor. It could be the perception of the woman, or it is possible the equipment is not recording correctly. If the labor pattern does not correlate with the tracing, the physician or midwife should be notified. In addition, the woman should be instructed about the procedure, because good FHR patterns can be reassuring to the woman that her baby is tolerating the contractions well and that the labor can continue its course.

References

Chez, B. F., Skurnick, J., Chex, R., Verklan, M., Biggs, S., & Hage, M. (1990). Interpretations of nonstress tests by obstetric nurses. *Journal of Obstetric, Gynecologic, and Neonatal Nursing* 19:227–231.

Cooper, R. L., & Goldberg, R. L. (1990). Catecholamine secretion in fetal adaptation to stress. *Journal of Obstetric, Gynecologic, and Neonatal Nursing* 19:223–226.

Creasy, R. K., & Resnik, R. (1989). *Maternal-Fetal Medicine: Principles and Practice,* 2nd ed. Philadelphia: W. B. Saunders Company.

Cundiff, J. L., Haubrich, K. L., & Hinzman, N. C. (1990). Umbilical artery Doppler flow studies during pregnancy. *Journal of Obstetric, Gynecologic, and Neonatal Nursing* 19:475–481.

Dickason, E. J., Schult, M. O., & Silverman, B. L. (1990). *Maternal-Infant Nursing Care.* St. Louis: C. V. Mosby.

Fetal Heart Rate Auscultation. (1990). *OGN Nursing Practice Resource.* Washington, DC: Organization for Obstetric, Gynecologic, and Neonatal Nurses.

Gaffney, S., Salinger, L., & Vintzileos, A. (1990). The biophysical profile for fetal surveillance. *American Journal of Maternal-Child Nursing* 15:356–360.

Galvan, B. J., Van Mullem, C., & Broekhuizen, F. F. (1989). Using amnioinfusion for the relief of repetitive variable decelerations during labor. *Journal of Obstetric, Gynecologic, and Neonatal Nursing* 18:222–229.

Koehl, L., & Wheeler, D. (1989). Monitoring uterine activity at home. *American Journal of Nursing* 89:200–203.

Ladewig, P. W., London, M. L., & Olds, S. B. (1990). *Essentials of Maternal-Newborn Nursing,* 2nd ed. Redwood City, CA: Addison-Wesley Nursing.

Morrison, J. C. (1990). Antepartal fetal surveillance. *Obstetrics and Gynecology Clinics of North America* 17:1–266.

Organization for Obstetric, Gynecologic, and Neonatal Nurses (1988). *Nursing Responsibilities in Implementing Intrapartum Fetal Heart Rate Monitoring.* Washington, DC: Author.

Parer, J. T. (1983). *Handbook of Fetal Heart Rate Monitoring.* Philadelphia: W. B. Saunders Company.

Sleutel, M. R. (1990). Vibroacoustic stimulation and fetal heart rate in nonstress tests. *Journal of Obstetric, Gynecologic, and Neonatal Nursing* 19:199–294.

SUGGESTED ACTIVITIES

1. Describe various methods of evaluating fetal well-being and maturity. List nursing actions for each method.
2. Explain the nonstress test (NST) and the contraction test (OCT). List two nursing interventions for each.
3. Describe two methods of continuous electronic fetal heart rate (FHR) monitoring.
4. Explain why the three common FHR patterns occur in continuous (FHR) monitoring. List two nursing interventions when each pattern arises.

REVIEW QUESTIONS

A. Select the best answer for each multiple-choice question.

Clinical Situation: Ms. Barber is pregnant for the first time. Her history reveals that she has chronic hypertension, is unsure of the date of her last normal menstrual period, and has edema of her face and hands. The physician has ordered an ultrasound test and an amniocentesis to be done to obtain information about fetal gestational age and fetal maturity.

1. When explaining the ultrasound scanning procedure to Ms. Barber, the nurse could say
   A. The procedure is painless
   B. The procedure will take approximately 20 minutes
   C. The procedure is a means of determining fetal gestational age
   D. All of the above

2. When explaining the procedure for an amniocentesis to Ms. Barber, the nurse can say all of the following EXCEPT
   A. A needle prick, with local anesthetic, will be injected through the skin
   B. A needle will be inserted through the abdomen into the amniotic sac to withdraw fluid
   C. The procedure will cause no painful sensation
   D. The fetal condition will be observed before and after the procedure

3. Amniocentesis is done most often to test a fetus for the following EXCEPT
   A. Chromosomal abnormalities
   B. Neural tube defect
   C. Fetal maturity
   D. Fetal size

4. Diagnostic tests of the amniotic fluid done to determine fetal maturity include all of the following EXCEPT
   A. Lecithin/sphingomyelin ratio (L/S ratio)
   B. Creatinine levels
   C. Bilirubin levels
   D. Heart formation maturity

5. The fetus is unlikely to develop respiratory distress if the L/S ratio is at least
   A. 1/8
   B. 1/2
   C. 2/1
   D. 1/10

6. Maternal blood estriol levels are ordered to determine the functioning of
   A. The maternal–fetoplacental unit
   B. The fetal kidneys
   C. The placenta
   D. The maternal kidneys

7. Ultrasonography is a useful tool in all of the following EXCEPT
   A. Detecting fetal heart beat
   B. Determining if multiple fetuses are present
   C. Locating the placenta
   D. Determining the duration of labor

8. The nonstress test (NST) is used clinically to evaluate the fetus
   A. Who responds to movement with a decreased heart rate
   B. Whose heart rate increases with fetal movement
   C. With anoxia
   D. Who is large for gestational age

9. The oxytocin challenge test (OCT) is done for which of the following reasons?
   A. To determine the fetus's capability to withstand the stress of labor
   B. To assess the maturity of the fetus
   C. To assess for fetal genetic defects
   D. None of the above

10. There are known maternal risk factors that can be detrimental to the fetus. These factors include
    A. Maternal age, uterine fundal height, weight gain beyond 15 lb
    B. Maternal age, poor nutrition, smoking, weight gain beyond 15 lb
    C. Poor nutrition, poor work environment, smoking
    D. Poor work environment, uterine fundal height, uneventful obstetric history

11. The advantages of external electronic fetal monitoring include
    A. It is noninvasive and convenient
    B. Minimal training is required to apply the external monitor
    C. It can be conducted at any time, regardless of whether or not the cervix is dilated
    D. All of the above

12. The disadvantages of external electronic fetal monitoring include all of the following EXCEPT
    A. The fetal heart rate (FHR) may be lost if the mother changes position
    B. The heart rate tracing does not give accurate information about FHR variability
    C. Maternal complications impede its use
    D. Obesity and fetal position affect the quality of recording

13. The advantages of internal electronic fetal monitoring include
    A. FHR variability can be assessed
    B. Internal monitoring reveals accurate measurement of the intensity of the contraction
    C. Obesity and maternal movement do not affect the recording
    D. All of the above

14. Uterine contractions affect the FHR by three primary mechanisms. The three mechanisms are
    A. Compression of the fetal head
    B. Compression of the uterine myometrial vessels
    C. Compression of the umbilical cord
    D. A and C
    E. A, B, and C

15. Which of the following recordings would indicate no fetal distress?
    A. Early decelerations, no variability
    B. Early decelerations, good variability
    C. Late decelerations, good variability
    D. Variable decelerations, no variability

B. Choose from Column II the words that most accurately refer to the terms in Column I.

I

1. Oxytocin challenge test _____
2. Amniotic fluid analysis _____
3. Nonstress test _____
4. Ultrasonography _____
5. Baseline FHR _____
6. Baseline variability _____
7. Bradycardia _____
8. Tachycardia _____
9. Early deceleration _____
10. Late deceleration _____
11. Variable deceleration _____

II

A. Genetic defect
B. Biparietal diameter of fetal head
C. Heart rate increase in response to fetal movement
D. Assessment of fetus's ability to withstand mild contractions
E. Abnormally fast FHR
F. Nonuniform slowing of FHR, which bears no relationship to uterine contractions
G. Slowing of FHR when contraction begins that returns to normal when contraction ends
H. FHR between contractions
I. Beat-to-beat fluctuations of FHR
J. Slowing of FHR that begins at, or soon after, the peak of the contraction and does not return to baseline until well after the contraction ends
K. A baseline FHR below 120 beats per minute

CHAPTER 9 _____

Chapter Outline

Learning Objectives

Upon the completion of Chapter 9, the student should be able to

- Identify the basic philosophy in preparation for child-birth.
- Compare two methods of preparation for childbirth.
- Explain the use of the coach during the labor period.
- Describe the use of breathing techniques to reduce discomfort during labor.
- Describe four exercises to strengthen and stretch muscles in preparation for childbirth.
- Explain how the endorphin system decreases discomfort during labor.
- Identify the role of the nurse as health teacher in preparation for labor and birth.

PREPARATION FOR CHILDBIRTH

For an expectant couple, the 9 months of pregnancy can serve as a period of time to learn together. They can use this time to become informed about the changes that occur during pregnancy, the process of childbirth, the postpartum period, the care of the newborn infant, and parenthood in general.

An increasing number of hospitals, private groups, public health clinics, and Red Cross chapters offer classes to meet varied needs of expectant and new parents (Fig. 9–1). Nurses usually conduct the classes, although an obstetrician and a pediatrician may also participate.

The content of the courses is usually similar, although some courses are designed with emphasis on preparation for the birth itself than on preparation for parenthood. Almost every community has both day and evening classes, and the couple can select the time that best suits their schedule. The classes are usually repeated every 5 or 6 weeks. Thus, if a class is missed it can be made up in the next series.

Classes early in pregnancy focus on pregnancy and the physical and emotional changes that occur during pregnancy. In midpregnancy classes the attention is often centered on the baby; therefore, information about the growing fetus is emphasized. Also, the physical changes, appearance, and other concerns of pregnancy are discussed. Appropriate clothing, physical activities, proper body mechanics, and employment safety are mentioned. Because the couples usually have questions specific to their activities, an informal discussion is conducted to address the needs of the couples in that particular class.

Later in pregnancy, expectant parents' attention is focused on preparation for the birth and for care of the infant after birth. Class discussions about the birth usually include information about relevant maternal anatomy and physiology as well as specific ways to better cope with the birth. Classes later in pregnancy are directed toward helping the couple (woman and significant other) to approach the birth experience with confidence in their ability to help themselves in the normal process of labor. The goals are to help the woman remain in control of herself and actively participate in the birth of her child. The father or significant other can also participate in the birth of the infant.

Many clinics are beginning to offer classes for pregnant adolescents. When such classes are held separately from the adult classes, the adolescents feel more comfortable and ask questions more freely. In addition, the information given to them can be adjusted to their level of interest and understanding.

Other areas covered are parent preparation for cesarean birth, sibling preparation, and grandparent preparation. Grandparents are a vital link between the parents and infant. If they live close by, they can be of assistance to the mother after birth, while the mother becomes more secure in the care of her infant. Many expectant parents are concerned about the older child's response to the birth of a new sister or brother. Discussion of ways to help prepare children at different ages is beneficial to the couple.

TOPICS OFTEN COVERED IN PRENATAL CLASSES

- Anatomy and physiology of the reproductive organs
- Physical and emotional changes that occur during pregnancy
- Growth and development of the fetus

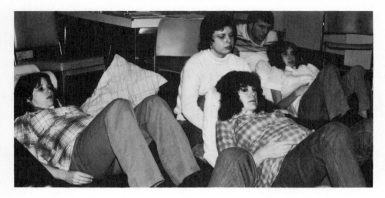

▲ FIGURE 9–1

Classes in preparation for childbirth involve active participation by the woman, the coach, and the nurse. The coach may be the husband, the boyfriend, or anyone the mother chooses to be with her during labor. (From Moore, M. L. (1983). *Realities in Childbearing*, 2nd ed. Philadelphia, W. B. Saunders Company.)

- Nutritional needs of the mother and fetus
- Prenatal care
- The birth process (including muscle strengthening and relaxation exercises)
- Care of the newborn infant
- Cesarean birth
- Sibling preparation

Preparation Methods

Classes on preparation for childbirth often emphasize a particular method that has become known by the name of the founder of the method. The three most common methods are the Dick-Read, Lamaze, and Bradley. Despite theoretical differences, the three methods have similarities: information about the labor process, some type of physical preparation, and belief in continuous and informed support during labor. They all teach that the woman, not the obstetrician, is the "star performer" in the birth process.

DICK-READ METHOD

Dr. Grantly Dick-Read, in the 1930s, recognized that two factors—fear and tension—intensified pain during labor. He called this phenomenon the *fear–tension–pain syndrome.* Dick-Read contended that the fear–tension–pain cycle needed to be broken. His book *Childbirth Without Fear* changed ideas that had been held for centuries.

Dick-Read taught that pain during childbirth increased when the woman was terrified because she did not know what was happening to her body. As an example, people often feel tense and perspire when they go the dentist until they hear that they have no cavities to be filled or the dentist explains what is to be done.

The Dick-Read method includes education about the physiology of childbirth, exercises for the abdominal and perineal muscles, and relaxation techniques. Dick-Read advocated the learning of relaxation by concentration on each part of the body separately, from the toes to the head, contracting and then relaxing the muscles. He believed that it was important for the woman in labor never to be left alone, because being alone generated fear. Although his philosophy included the use of analgesics when necessary, he emphasized the avoidance of "unnatural aids," which made the Dick-Read method the foundation for organized programs of childbirth preparation.

BRADLEY METHOD

The Bradley method is named after Dr. Robert Bradley of Denver, Colorado. Like Dick-Read, Bradley stressed that labor is a normal process. His method focuses on environmental variables such as darkness and quiet to make childbirth a more natural experience. In the Bradley method the husband's support is of foremost importance. The American Academy of Husband-Coached Childbirth was founded to prepare instructors, so the Bradley method could be more accessible to expectant parents.

In early labor the woman is encouraged to be

up and about or to engage in diversionary activities such as playing cards with her husband. When not ambulating, the woman is encouraged to assume the tailor sitting position (Fig. 9–2). The Sims position is recommended when the woman is lying down. To simulate sleep during each contraction, the woman is encouraged to close her eyes and let each muscle in her body relax. Slow, deep abdominal breaths (in through her nose and out through her mouth) are encouraged throughout the contractions. During each contraction the husband is supportive. He is encouraged to touch his wife and to place his hand on her abdomen during labor contractions. The Bradley method is referred to as husband-coached childbirth.

LAMAZE METHOD

The Lamaze method of childbirth was named after Dr. Fernand Lamaze of Paris. He attended a conference in Russia where he became convinced that psychoprophylaxis (mental prevention of pain) is a method that could be used in childbirth. The woman could be taught to substitute responses to pain, fear, and loss of control with more positive behavior. The Lamaze method is based on the Pavlov conditioned-reflex theory. The Lamaze method of preparation for childbirth currently is the most popular method.

Controlled muscular relaxation and breathing techniques are combined in the Lamaze method. The woman is taught to contract specific muscle groups while she relaxes other muscles. She is also taught to practice focusing on some small object that will be used as a focal point during labor (see Fig. 9–2). During labor, the object is placed where it can be seen easily by the woman. Specific exercises (how to breathe) are explained thoroughly in the classes before labor. The Lamaze method includes the husband (or significant other) and encourages the woman to be an active participant in her labor and delivery.

The Lamaze classes are usually taught in small groups and frequently begin about the twelfth or thirteenth week of pregnancy. A support person (husband or significant other) is encouraged to attend the classes along with the pregnant woman. The physiology of labor and birth is discussed. Practice sessions include types of breathing at various stages of labor, methods for relaxing certain muscle groups, and measures to use during labor to increase comfort.

Typically, when labor is established, the woman is positioned on her side (unless she is ambulating), with two pillows under her head and one pillow between her knees. When contraction starts, she takes a deep, cleansing breath, focuses her attention on a selected object, and takes slow, deep breaths using her chest. At the end of the

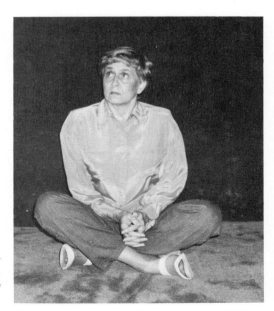

▲ FIGURE 9–2

Mother practices focusing, relaxing, and breathing techniques. She is focusing with her eyes opened and her body relaxed. (Note tailor sitting position.)

contraction, she again takes a deep, cleansing breath. The cleansing breaths in the beginning and at the end of the contraction give the woman a chance to pull herself together and rest. As labor intensifies, the slow chest breathing usually becomes less effective. She is then encouraged to start with slow chest breathing, modify her breathing to more shallow breathing as the contraction reaches its peak, and then return to slow chest breathing. Continued rapid breathing can cause hyperventilation, a state in which the carbon dioxide level in the blood is decreased. This is undesirable because it can compromise the infant. Actually, variations are used in the breathing patterns. Some women find their own pattern of breathing that is comfortable for them. The partner plays an active role in counting or relaying to the woman, at 15-second intervals, the length of time of the contraction. Throughout labor, the husband or significant other is asked to remind the woman in labor to relax.

Gate Control Theory

The gate control theory has been used to explain the effectiveness of techniques to reduce pain during childbirth. The theory proposes that there is a gate-like mechanism involved in the transmission of pain (discomfort) impulses to the brain (cerebral cortex). It is believed that the intensity of labor pain can be decreased if the gate can be closed. Some caregivers think that this mechanism can be used effectively during labor. If something can close the gate, messages will not travel up the spinal cord to the brain. Cutaneous stimuli, such as touching, rubbing, or fingertip massage (*effleurage*), can close the gate. For example, if we hit our finger we can suck on it and lessen the discomfort; if we have a backache we can have someone stroke our back and lessen the discomfort. The same suggestions to close the gate are included in the Lamaze method of childbirth preparation, namely, distraction or active focusing of attention; continuous stimulation; knowledge about the labor process; and relaxation and breathing exercises.

Endorphin System

The discovery of the *endorphin system* increased our understanding of how and why certain pain-prevention techniques (including acupressure) work. A chemical substance was found to be released from the brainstem and the pituitary gland. This opiate-like substance is referred to as *endorphin*, which is pharmacologically similar in makeup to morphine. They both block transmission of pain impulses. Endorphin can make a person feel relaxed and drowsy. In 1984, Dr. Newnham found endorphin blood levels at delivery to be much higher than in nonpregnant women. The discovery of endorphin and its action is consistent with methods used in preparation for childbirth.

The method of preparation for childbirth is most effective if the couple feels comfortable with that method. Frequently, a combination of different methods is used; however, most emphasize aspects of the Lamaze method.

Breathing Patterns and Relaxation

Breathing techniques are used to help the woman to relax and override the pain of the uterine contractions. Paced breathing is a method whereby the woman "paces" herself in breathing rhythmically and by self-regulation is able to conserve energy. The breathing patterns commonly used during labor are a slow paced breathing or a modified paced breathing. The breathing techniques may be referred to as slow chest breathing, shallow chest breathing, a combination of the two, and a cleansing breath. A cleansing breath should be as effortless and as deep as is comfortable. It helps the woman to relax and, indeed, may play a role in enhancing oxygenation.

Relaxation is the foundation for all breathing patterns. The breathing rate should be comfortable for the woman. If the woman chooses to inspire through her mouth, instead of her nose, she should be taught ways to protect the mucous membranes from drying, such as by taking crushed ice or clear liquids. Also, she can be instructed to place her tongue gently against the roof of her mouth during breathing to trap moisture and lessen dryness of the mouth. The overall goals of teaching breathing techniques (or paced breathing) are to (a) maintain adequate oxygenation of the mother and fetus, (b) increase physical and psychological relaxation and possibly decrease discomfort and anxiety, and (c) provide a means of attention focusing.

There is no "right" breathing technique to teach to prepare the woman for childbirth. The woman should be allowed to do what is most comfortable for her (Fig. 9–3).

Certain breathing patterns and nursing interventions are commonly used. They are directed toward the patient's comfort and relaxation during labor.

BREATHING PATTERNS AND NURSING INTERVENTIONS BY STAGE OF LABOR

Early (Latent) Labor. In the latent phase, the woman uses slow chest breathing. At beginning and end of contraction she takes a cleansing breath. If woman is not ambulating, lying on her side is best. Back massage given by support person is helpful.

Early (Active) Labor. In the active phase, the woman uses shallow chest breathing. At the beginning and end of each contraction she takes a cleansing breath. Gentle stroking (by nurse or significant other) of mother's abdomen with both hands in circular movement (called *effleurage*) is often helpful.

Transition Labor. Pant–blow breathing during the contraction helps override the contraction. Counterpressure on sacrococcygeal area and effleurage are usually helpful.

Expulsion Labor. The woman uses modified pant–blow breathing. The nurse positions the woman with her head and shoulders bent forward, leaning on diaphragm, to encourage the "pushing sensation." Also, the woman can assume a 45-degree recumbent position. The woman or the support person can hold her legs under or on top of the knees, bringing the legs as close to the shoulders as possible (Fig. 9–4).

KEY POINTS IN EDUCATION: BREATHING TECHNIQUES

- Breathing techniques are used only during the contraction.
- Inspiration and expiration should be equal.
- Hyperventilation (a decrease in carbon dioxide) can occur as a result of rapid or deep breathing. Carbon dioxide depletion can cause tingling of finger, hands, and mouth. Dizziness may also occur. If hyperventilation occurs, the woman should be instructed to rebreathe some carbon dioxide from cupped hands or breathe normally while compressing one nostril with the index finger. If hyperventilation is allowed to continue, the infant can be deprived of oxygen.
- A cleansing breath, or deep breath, before and after each contraction helps the woman to relax. If the woman inhales through her nose (rather than her mouth) she will lessen dryness of her mouth.
- Shallow costal breathing is like breathing with an imaginary butterfly on the chest. This type of breathing prevents "blowing off" too much carbon dioxide.
- A combination of any two methods can be used.
- "Pant–blow" breathing is rapid, shallow, or light chest breathing used later in labor.
- Expulsive breathing is modified pant–blow breathing. The woman can set a pattern of five to seven panting breaths for each blowing breath. Blowing breaths are important to avoid hyperventilation.

FIRST STAGE OF LABOR

Phase I: Early (Also known as latent, entertainment, or preliminary phase.)

Slow Chest Pattern

Contractions:

Respiration

Characteristics—Mild intensity, reaching a peak and diminishing gradually

Interval—5–20 min
Length—30–60 sec

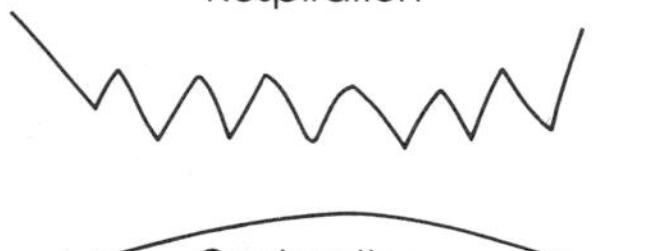

Contraction

Complete Effacement
Dilatation 0–3 cm

Phase II: Active

Accelerated-Decelerated Pattern
(4/4, Yankee Doodle)

Contractions:

Respiration

Characteristics—greater intensity; harder to manage, yet manageable; reach a peak and diminish gradually

Interval—3–5 min
Length—45–60 sec

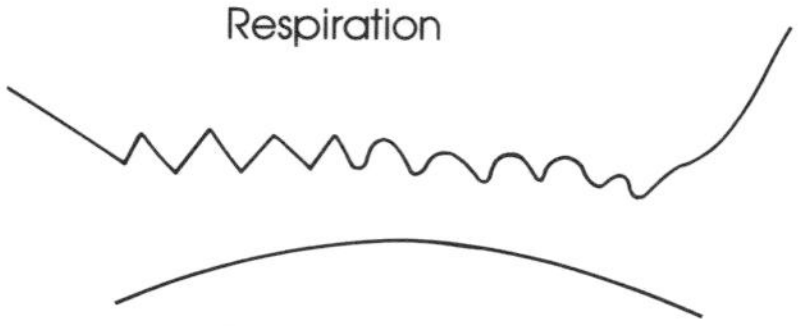

Contraction

Dilatation 3–7 or 8 cm

Phase III: Transition

4-6-8 Pant Blow Pattern
Respiration

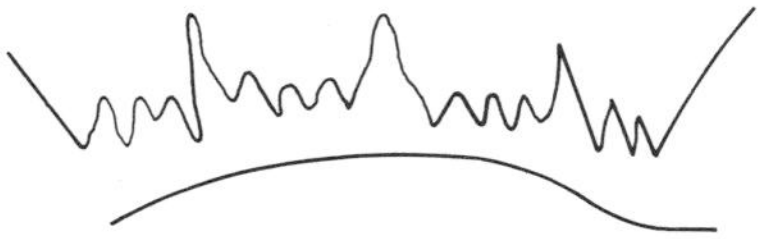

Contractions:

Characteristics—Reaching a peak within 2–3 sec of onset; multipeaked, quite overwhelming if not prepared

Interval—90–120 sec
Length—60–90 sec

Contraction

Dilatation Complete
8–10 cm

SECOND STAGE OF LABOR

Expulsion of Baby

Respiration
catch breath

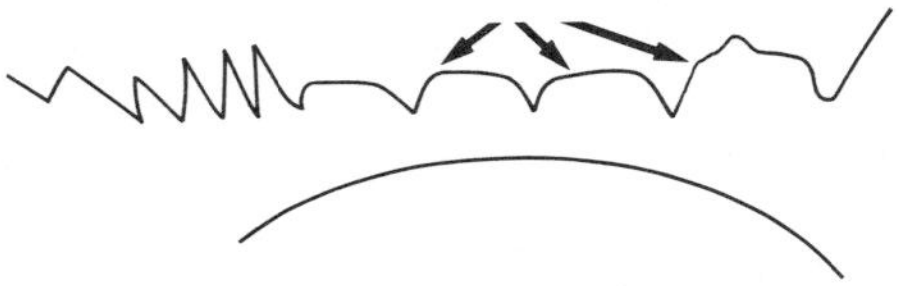

Contractions:

Characteristics—Decreased intensity as compared with transitional contractions, once again reaching a peak and diminishing gradually

Interval—2–4min
Length—60 sec

Contraction

Breathing techniques are used according to need. Phase does not dictate which technique should be used.

▲ **FIGURE 9–3**

Stages of labor, their characteristics, and Lamaze breathing techniques that may be applied. Breathing techniques are used according to need. Phase of labor does not dictate which technique should be used. (Redrawn from Huprich, P. A. (1977). Assisting the couple through a Lamaze labor and delivery. Copyright 1977 American Journal of Nursing Company. Reprinted from American Journal of Maternal–Child Nursing, 1977, vol 2. Used with permission. All rights reserved.)

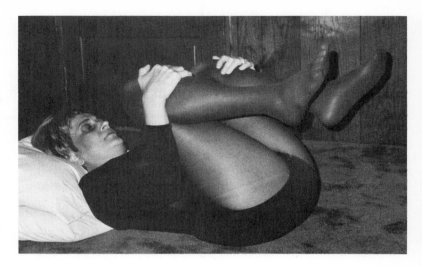

▲ FIGURE 9–4

Assuming a C-shaped position facilitates the forward movement of the baby through the pelvis.

Exercises for Childbirth

The safety of the mother and infant is the primary concern in any exercise program suggested during pregnancy. The potential for maternal and fetal injury is important because of the musculoskeletal and cardiovascular changes during pregnancy. Although the risk of fetal injury is probably small, exercise recommendations must err on the conservative side. To date, information gained about exercising during pregnancy is primarily on aerobic exercises and/or exercises that are intense in nature. Because pregnant women may be involved in swimming, bicycling, and other recreational sports activities, the American College of Obstetrics and Gynecology (ACOG) developed *Guidelines for Exercise During Pregnancy and the Postpartum Period.* The guidelines offer restrictions on and modifications to sports activities that ACOG believes are necessary because of the physiological changes of pregnancy (Table 9–1).

The ideal exercise program offers women a variety of options, including walking, swimming, stationary cycling, and modified forms of dancing. No single exercise program can meet the needs of all women. Health care personnel should alert the pregnant woman about the potential hazards of exercise of certain recreational and sport activities. In addition, health care personnel should be aware

of the application of the ACOG guidelines to the exercises included in childbirth preparation classes.

Exercises for Childbirth Preparation Classes

The goal of childbirth exercise programs is to maintain physical fitness within the physiological limitation of pregnancy. Childbirth preparation classes should be directed toward strengthening muscles to minimize the risk of joint and ligament injuries and correcting postural changes that result in lower back pain (Fig. 9–5). Health care providers should note that strain and fatigue should be avoided, and exercise periods should be interspersed with rest and relaxation. In addition, the woman should not lie supine, twist, bounce, or make jerky movements during exercise. She should be alert to unusual pain.

The exercises generally emphasize the upper body, the abdomen, and the legs. Specific exercises include posture reeducation, pelvic tilt–back muscle strengthening, abdominal muscle strengthening, pelvic floor muscle toning, squatting, leg muscle conditioning (increasing venous return), and Kegel exercises to strengthen pelvic muscles. Exercising the muscles groups provides relaxation as well as strengthening muscles.

TABLE 9-1. ACOG EXERCISE GUIDELINES

During pregnancy only
1. Maternal heart rate should not exceed 140 beat/minute.
2. Strenuous activities should not exceed 15 minutes' duration.
3. No exercise should be performed in the supine position after the fourth month of gestation is completed.
4. Exercises that employ the Valsalva maneuver should be avoided.
5. Caloric intake should be adequate to meet the extra energy needs not only of pregnancy but also of the exercises performed.
6. Maternal core temperature should not exceed 38.5° C.

During pregnancy and the postpartum period
1. Regular exercise (at least 3 times per week) is preferable to intermittent activity. Competitive activities should be discouraged.
2. Vigorous exercise should not be performed in hot, humid weather or during a period of febrile illness.
3. Ballistic movements (jerky, bouncy motions) should be avoided. Exercise should be done on a wooden floor or a tightly carpeted surface to reduce shock and provide a sure footing.
4. Deep flexion or extension of joints should be avoided because of connective tissue laxity. Activities that require jumping, jarring motions, or rapid changes in direction should be avoided because of joint instability.
5. Vigorous exercise should be preceded by a 5-minute period of muscle warm-up. This can be accomplished by slow walking or stationary cycling with low resistance.
6. Vigorous exercise should be followed by a period of gradually declining activity that includes gentle stationary stretching. Because connective tissue laxity increases the risk of joint injury, stretches should not be taken to the point of maximum resistance.
7. Heart rate should be measured at times of peak activity. Target heart rates and limits established in consultation with the physician should not be exceeded.
8. Care should be taken to rise gradually from the floor to avoid orthostatic hypotension. Some form of activity involving the legs should be continued for a brief period.
9. Liquids should be taken liberally before and after exercise to prevent dehydration. If necessary, activity should be interrupted to replenish fluids.
10. Women who have led sedentary life-styles should begin with physical activity of very low intensity and advance activity levels very gradually.
11. Activity should be stopped and the physician consulted if unusual symptoms appear.

Adapted from American College of Obstetricians and Gynecologists (1985). *Exercises during Pregnancy and the Postnatal Period: Home Exercise Programs Educational Bulletin.* Washington, DC.

- PELVIC TILT: Seated with knees bent and arms in back for support, the woman arches lower back in (inhaling) and out (exhaling). This exercise strengthens back and abdominal muscles (Fig. 9–6).
- STRAIGHT-LEG LIFT: In a sitting position with one knee bent and one leg extended with the foot flexed, the woman lifts the extended leg up a comfortable distance from floor (inhaling), then lowers the leg slowly to the floor (exhaling); this is repeated with the other leg. This exercise promotes venous return (Fig. 9–7).
- FOOT ROTATION: Seated with legs straight, the woman rotates first one foot, then the other. Movements promote venous return.
- KEGEL EXERCISES (perineal muscles tightening): The woman contracts the anal sphincter, vagina, and urethra. This exercise strengthens pelvis muscles.
- RELAXATION: The woman relaxes body muscle groups starting from head to toe. She relaxes all of the body, including face and hands.

Many traditional back-strengthening exercises

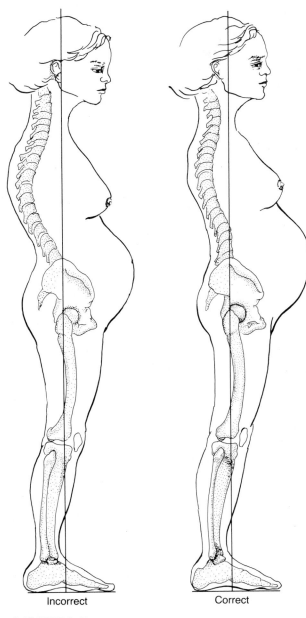

Incorrect   Correct

▲ **FIGURE 9–5**

Correct postural changes to decrease lordosis and lower back discomfort during pregnancy.

EXERCISES FOR MUSCLE STRENGTHENING AND RELAXATION

- TAILOR SITTING: The woman sits cross-legged on the floor to strengthen thigh and pelvic muscles (see Fig. 9–2).

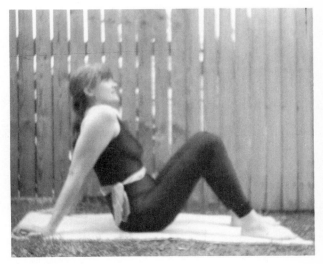

▲ **FIGURE 9–6**

Pelvic tilt: Seated with knees bent and arms in back for support, the woman arches her lower back in (inhaling) and then out (exhaling). This exercise strengthens back and abdominal muscles.

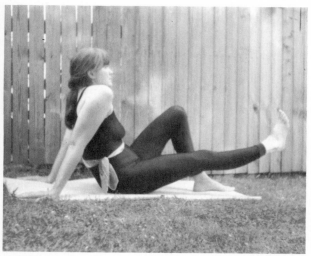

▲ FIGURE 9–7

Straight-leg lift. While in sitting position, the woman has one leg flexed. She lifts the extended leg up a short distance from the floor (inhaling), then lowers leg to the floor (exhaling). This exercise promotes venous return.

are no longer recommended during pregnancy because they required the supine position or the Valsalva maneuver. Also, some of these exercises include bounces and fast swings that should be avoided because jerky movements can stress lax joints and muscle attachments.

Differences in childbirth preparation may be found from community to community. Major considerations are to be flexible, avoiding rigidity. The learners (the couple) should be comfortable in what they are doing. Also, it is very important that the woman and significant other receive support from the health care personnel during the actual labor. The couple should not be made to feel guilty if what they learned and practiced before labor is not satisfying to them. In addition, they should not feel uncomfortable if they decide to discontinue the method at any time they so choose.

Principles of Teaching and Learning

The first basic principle of teaching and learning is that learning must be active. The couple must be involved in the learning process. The second basic principle is that learning must be meaningful. For example, if the nurse tries to instruct the expectant mother about the care of her infant when she wants to know what is happening to her body (early pregnancy), very little learning will likely take place. A third principle of learning is that the learner (the woman) must be motivated. Most couples are motivated to learn about pregnancy because they want the pregnancy to result in a healthy baby and be a positive experience for them. Finally, the nurse (the teacher) should attempt to make the couple comfortable. This can be accomplished by providing a relaxed environment.

References

American College of Obstetricians and Gynecologists. (1985). *Exercises during Pregnancy and the Postnatal Period: Home Exercise Programs Educational Bulletin.* Washington, DC.

Artal, R., & Wiswell, R. (1986). *Exercise in Pregnancy.* Baltimore: Williams & Wilkins.

De Grez, S. A. (1988). Bend and stretch. *American Journal of Maternal-Child Nursing* 13:357–359.

Dickason, E. J., Schult, M. O., & Silverman, B. L. (1990). *Maternal-Infant Nursing Care.* St. Louis: C. V. Mosby.

Dick-Read, G. (1959). *Childbirth Without Fear,* 2nd ed. New York: Harper & Row.

Fishbein, E. G., & Phillips, M. (1990). How safe is exercise during pregnancy? *Journal of Obstetric, Gynecologic, and Neonatal Nursing* 19:45–49.

Nichols, F. H., & Humenick, S. S. (1988). *Childbirth Education: Practice, Research, and Theory.* Philadelphia: W. B. Saunders Company.

Mittelmark, R. A., Wiswell, R. A., & Drinkwater, B. L. (1991). *Exercise in Pregnancy,* 2nd ed. Baltimore: Williams & Wilkins.

SUGGESTED ACTIVITIES

1. Describe the basic components of a woman's preparation for childbirth.
2. Practice the exercises described in this chapter so that you can show them to the woman and her significant other.
3. List three different methods of administering anesthesia to the woman in labor.
4. Name two nursing measures that should be carried out when a woman receives an epidural block.

REVIEW QUESTIONS

A. Select the best answer to each multiple-choice question.

1. The basic components of childbirth preparation include
   A. Muscle strengthening
   B. Relaxation and breathing
   C. Knowledge about the labor process
   D. All of the above

2. The gate control theory of pain proposes all of the following EXCEPT
   A. Distraction
   B. Cutaneous stimulation
   C. Relaxation and breathing exercises
   D. Rapid breathing during contractions

3. Opiate-like substances that occur naturally in the body are called
   A. Endorphins
   B. Ectrophins
   C. Morphines
   D. Catecholamines

4. The major goals of nonpharmacological pain relief measures are
   A. Promoting relaxation
   B. Reducing anxiety
   C. Decreasing painful impulses
   D. All of the above

5. The woman should be encouraged to use the breathing pattern that is comfortable for her. However, she should be reminded to avoid fast deep breathing because the resultant hyperventilation may cause the following EXCEPT
   A. An imbalance of oxygen and carbon dioxide
   B. A decrease in carbon dioxide in the blood
   C. Fetal compromise with potential anoxia, if hyperventilation is allowed to continue
   D. An increase in carbon dioxide in the blood

6. There are potential risks of strenuous exercise during pregnancy; therefore, the American College of Obstetricians and Gynecologists developed guidelines that include all of the following EXCEPT
   A. Maternal heart should not exceed 140 beats per minute
   B. Jerky, bouncy movements should be avoided
   C. Care should be taken to rise gradually from the floor to avoid orthostatic hypotension
   D. Exercise can be performed in supine position

7. Exercises for childbirth preparation are directed toward
   A. Maintaining physical fitness within the physiological limitations
   B. Posture reeducation
   C. Muscle strengthening
   D. All of the above

B. Choose from Column II the phrase that most accurately defines the term in Column I.

I
1. Kegel exercises _____
2. Pelvic rocking _____
3. Cleansing breath _____
4. Hyperventilation _____
5. Effleurage _____
6. Tailor sitting _____

II
A. Carbon dioxide depletion
B. Sitting with knees spread apart with arms resting on knees
C. Gentle stroking of abdomen in a circular motion
D. Contraction of muscles of anal sphincter, vagina, and urethra
E. Arching back upward and then flattening the arch
F. Taking a deep breath in through mouth and exhaling out through the nose

UNIT IV

Labor and birth

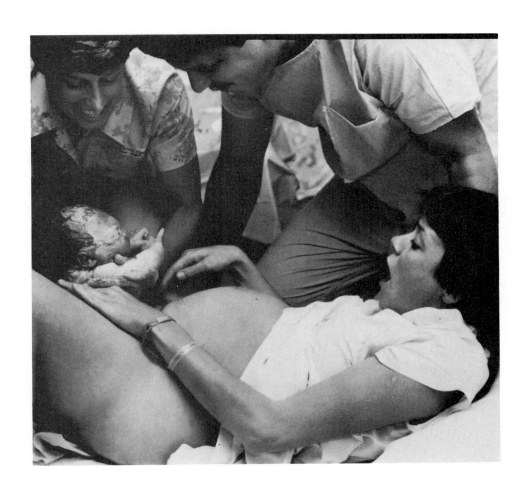

CHAPTER 10

Chapter Outline

Events Before the Onset of Labor
    Lightening
    Vaginal discharge (show)
    False labor
    Spontaneous rupture of membranes
    Cervical changes
Major Variables in the Birth Process
    Uterine contractions (powers)
    Passage and passenger: The fetopelvic relation-
      ship
The Four Stages of Labor
    Factors that influence the course of labor
Maternal Systemic Response to Labor
    Cardiovascular system
    Respiratory system
    Renal system
    Gastrointestinal system
    Fluid and electrolyte balance
Psychological and Sociological Factors That Affect
  Labor

Learning Objectives

Upon completion of Chapter 10, the student should be able to

- Define labor, lightening, vaginal show, effacement, and cervical dilatation.
- Identify spontaneous rupture of membranes.
- List the events that signal approaching labor.
- List the four main variables in the birth process.
- Explain the ability of the uterine muscles to contract and relax.
- Explain the importance of the period of uterine muscle relaxation between contractions.
- List three distinctive characteristics of labor contractions.
- Explain how frequency, duration, and intensity of contractions are monitored.
- Differentiate between false and true labor.
- Explain how the fetal head is able to withstand the pressure of labor.
- Describe fetal attitude, fetal lie, and fetal presentation.
- List the six positions the occiput of the fetal head may occupy in relation to the mother's pelvis.
- Describe the term *station* as it relates to the maternal pelvis.
- Describe the fetal positional changes that occur in the mechanisms of labor.
- List six factors that influence the course of labor.
- State what is accomplished in each of the four stages of labor.
- List the major body systems and identify the response of each to labor.
- State the psychological factors that influence labor.

Pʀocess of Normal Labor and Birth

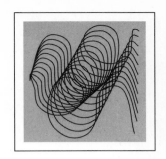

The time of labor and birth, though short in comparison with the length of pregnancy, is perhaps the most dramatic and significant period of pregnancy for the expectant mother, infant, and family. Many physiological and psychological changes occur during labor and birth that provide opportunities for nurses and other caregivers to use their skills.

The process by which the fetus is expelled from the uterus is called *labor*. Labor is accomplished by regular, rhythmic contractions of the uterine muscles. What actually causes labor to begin is not known, but several factors are believed to be involved. As pregnancy reaches term, there is a shift in hormone levels. Oxytocin is believed to increase and stimulate the uterus to contract. In addition, the uterus at term is greatly extended, and the stretching of the muscles appears to increase their irritability, causing them to contract.

Events Before the Onset of Labor

Any of the following signs noticed by the expectant woman indicates that labor usually is not far away: lightening, vaginal discharge (show), false labor, spontaneous rupture of membranes, and cervical changes.

LIGHTENING

About 2 weeks before labor, the fetal head settles deeper into the maternal pelvis. This is called *lightening*. At this time, the uterus actually shifts forward. In referring to lightening, some women say, "The baby has dropped down." The physical changes that occur because of lightening are easier breathing and more frequent urination. These signs indicate that there is more pressure because the baby is lower in the pelvis. Multigravidae may not experience lightening until labor begins (Fig. 10–1).

VAGINAL DISCHARGE (SHOW)

With cervical changes caused by increased pressure, a blood-tinged mucus plug becomes dislodged. The blood is from the rupture of superficial blood vessels.

FALSE LABOR

Later in pregnancy the expectant mother notices contractions that are painless but frequently can be felt as she places her hand on her abdomen. During the last 2 to 3 weeks of pregnancy, uterine activity increases, but the contractions remain uncoordinated. These contractions help to demarcate the uterus into the upper segment (the muscular, contractile portion) and the lower segment. Because of these contractions, the cervix prepares for changes.

Sometimes the contractions are quite noticeable, and the woman comes to the hospital. If the cervix has not dilated and the contractions stop, the condition is called *false labor*. False labor has no clinical significance except that it causes maternal anxiety and premature admission to the hospital. This experience may be disappointing and embarrassing to the woman and her family (Table 10–1).

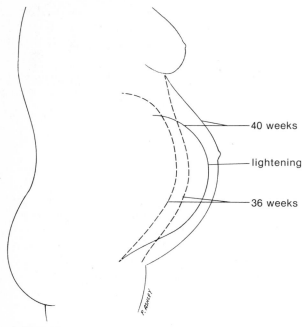

▲ **FIGURE 10–1**

Lightening. Fetal presenting part settles deeper into maternal pelvis. Breathing is easier; pressure on bladder increases, as does urinary frequency.

SPONTANEOUS RUPTURE OF MEMBRANES

Spontaneous rupture of the amniotic membranes (ROM) occasionally occurs before labor begins. ROM is what is meant when people say, "The bag of waters broke." At full term, it is not unusual for women to go into labor within 24 hours after ROM. If labor does not begin within a few hours, the risk of fetal and maternal infection increases. There is also danger of a prolapsed cord if the fetal head has not settled in the pelvis (the umbilical cord can be washed out along with the discharge of amniotic fluid). Initially there can be either a trickle or a rush of fluid. In order to differentiate ROM from urine or vaginal fluid, Nitrazine paper is used to test the pH. Amniotic fluid is slightly alkaline, whereas urine is generally acidic.

CERVICAL CHANGES

Cervical changes include cervical effacement and dilatation. Cervical effacement is the shortening and thinning out of the cervix. Normally, the cervix is 1 to 2 cm in length. When effacement is complete (100%), the cervix has almost disappeared (Fig. 10–2).

Cervical dilatation is the enlargement of the cervical opening (os) from 0 to 10 cm (complete dilatation). Both cervical effacement and dilatation are measured by vaginal examination. If the cervix is beginning to dilate or is thinned out, the onset of labor is near. Dilatation of 4 cm is significant

CHARACTERISTIC	TRUE LABOR	FALSE LABOR
"Show" (pinkish mucus)	Usually present; increases as the cervix changes	None present
Contractions	Regular with increases in intensity and duration	Irregular; frequency and intensity do not change
Discomfort	Frequently begins in lumbar region and then felt in abdomen	Often located in abdomen
Activity	Activity (walking) may intensify contractions	Often contractions lessened by walking
Cervical changes[a]	Cervix becomes effaced and dilates progressively	No cervical changes

TABLE 10–1. COMPARISON OF TRUE LABOR AND FALSE LABOR

[a]The most distinguishing characteristics between true and false labor are the cervical changes in true labor.

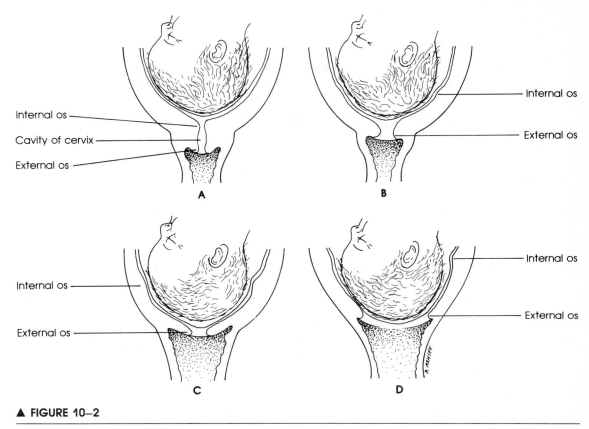

Internal os

Cavity of cervix

External os

A

Internal os

External os

B

Internal os

External os

C

Internal os

External os

D

▲ **FIGURE 10–2**

Cervical effacement and dilatation. **A.** Before labor. **B.** Beginning effacement. **C.** Complete effacement (100%). **D.** Complete dilatation (10 cm).

because at this point the woman's active labor usually progresses to completion (Fig. 10–3).

Major Variables in the Birth Process

Four factors are significant in the process of labor: *Passage* (size of pelvis), *Passenger* (baby), *Powers* (effectiveness of contractions), and *Psyche* (preparation, previous experience). These are known as the "Four P's." An ideal labor is one in which the bony pelvis is adequate, the infant is of average size, and the strength of the uterine contractions increases sufficiently to cause the cervix to fully efface and dilate. The woman's psyche—her ability to relax and concentrate on muscle groups, as well as maintain a low level of anxiety—

also plays a role in the normal progress of her labor. Each of the Four P's is discussed in this chapter.

UTERINE CONTRACTIONS (POWERS)

The anatomy of the uterus and pelvis is discussed in Chapter 2. However, in order to understand labor, it is important to understand the dramatic and unique physiology of the uterus. The uterine muscle (myometrium) is a smooth muscle that possesses the same properties as other smooth muscles in the body. Each muscle can contract and relax in a coordinated manner. Uterine contractions occur when uterine cells are stimulated to contract, and the stimulation spreads throughout the uterus. During pregnancy, contractions are present but are of low intensity and

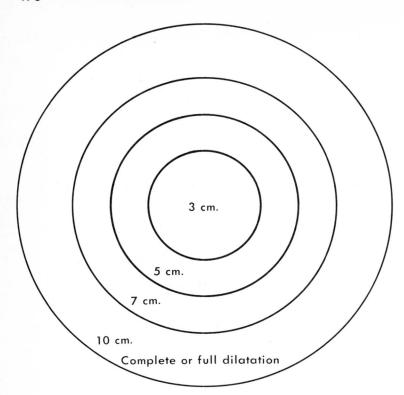

3 cm.

5 cm.

7 cm.

10 cm.

Complete or full dilatation

▲ **FIGURE 10–3**

Measurement of cervical dilatation.

remain in a small localized area of the uterus. During labor, the contractions begin in the top of uterus (fundus) and spread throughout the uterus in approximately 15 seconds. Because each contraction starts at the top, in the assessment of contractions, the nurse is able to ascertain the beginning of the contraction by placing her/his hands on the fundus.

A unique property of the uterine muscle is its ability to retain some of the shortening achieved during the contraction. This ability is called retraction or "brachystasis." When the myometrium cells contract, the fibers of both the fundus and the body of the uterus shorten. When the contraction ends and the muscles relax, the fibers do not return to their original size but remain shorter than before the contraction. This continued shortening of the muscle fibers in the upper portion of the uterus results in a progressive decrease in the size of the uterine cavity and a thickening of the muscle tissue of the upper portion. These changes supply the force needed to advance the fetus. With less room at the top of the uterus, the fetus is forced to descend.

Uterine contractions are referred to as the "source of power" that brings about the birth of the baby. Because these contractions cause discomfort, they are frequently called "labor pains." The amount of discomfort produced by the contractions varies with the intensity of the contraction and with the woman's tolerance of discomfort (her psyche). During labor, the woman may first perceive the contractions as back discomfort. The discomfort then radiates to the front of the abdomen.

Labor contractions have the following distinctive characteristics:

1. They are involuntary.
2. They are intermittent but recur in a regular pattern of frequency.
3. They occur in a bell-shaped curve in three phases: *increment* (period of building intensity), *acme* (peak or maximum intensity), and *decrement* (period of decreasing intensity).

Significant Facts About Labor Contractions

Each contraction is followed by a period of *relaxation;* thus relaxation is the interval between contractions. This period is significant to the mother and her fetus. During the contraction, there is decreased blood flow through the uterine arteries and intervillous spaces. This decline in blood flow lowers the fetal heart rate. If the mother is being observed by means of fetal electronic monitor, the decrease in fetal heart rate during contractions is carefully assessed (see Chapter 8). If the contractions become more frequent and prolonged, the decrease in blood flow can be cumulative and compromise the infant. In other words, the infant receives a *decreased oxygen supply* and experiences "fetal stress" during contractions. For this reason, it is important that the caregiver report to the physician when labor contractions are so close that there are no relaxation periods between them or if the intervals are progressively shortened so as to cause significant patterns of bradycardia.

Labor contractions are affected by *maternal position.* When a woman lies on her back, the contractions are likely to be more frequent but of lower intensity. When she lies on her side, the contractions are likely to be less frequent but of greater intensity; therefore, side lying improves progress of labor. In addition, side lying improves oxygenation to the fetus (see Chapter 8).

When the cervix is fully dilated (second stage of labor), the woman is often asked to use her abdominal muscles to superimpose intra-abdominal pressure on the contraction pressure. The *bearing-down* effort using the abdominal muscles is consciously controlled and is of great assistance in the final expulsion of the baby. It is important that someone (the nurse or significant other) coach the woman in her bearing-down effort during labor contractions.

Assessment of Labor Contractions

Uterine contractions are the important source of power that (a) produces cervical effacement and dilation, (b) causes the fetus to engage and rotate, (c) causes the fetus to be delivered, and (d) detaches and expels the placenta (afterbirth). Therefore, to assess the progress of labor, it is important to know the type of contractions the woman is experiencing. The characteristics of labor contrac-

tions include the frequency, duration, and intensity (Fig. 10–4).

The *frequency* of contractions is determined by the amount of time between the beginning of one contraction and the beginning of the next. The frequency of contractions increases as labor progresses. The contractions often start every 20 minutes at the beginning of labor and are as frequent as 2 to 3 minutes at the end of labor.

The *duration* of a contraction is the time from the onset of the contraction to its end. Contractions may last only 15 seconds at the beginning of labor but last longer as labor advances. Toward the end of labor, the contractions usually last at least 45 seconds, and during transition, the last phase of Stage 1, contractions last 60 to 90 seconds.

The *intensity* of a contraction is the strength of the contraction. A rough estimation is made by palpation of the fundus to determine the firmness of the uterus during a contraction; however, direct measurement may be obtained with an intrauterine catheter (see Chapter 8). Intensity of the contraction is described as mild, moderate, or strong. During a contraction, if there is little firmness of the uterus and it can be easily indented with the fingertips, the contraction is a mild one. In a moderate contraction, the fundus of the uterus is firmer, but it is possible to indent it. In a strong contraction, the fundus of the uterus is very firm, and indentation is difficult. The measurement of intensity is more accurate if the woman is observed using an internal electronic monitor that measures the strength of the contraction by recording the amniotic fluid pressure. The woman usually begins to feel some discomfort with the contraction, although the contraction appears mild on palpation, when the tracing shows a pressure of 25 mm Hg (Fig. 10–5). Electronic fetal monitoring is discussed in Chapter 8.

The contraction pattern of frequency, duration, and intensity should be recorded by the nurse at least every hour during the beginning of labor and more frequently as labor progresses. This information is valuable in evaluating the normal progress of labor.

PASSAGE AND PASSENGER: THE FETOPELVIC RELATIONSHIP

The accommodation between the passenger (baby) and the maternal passage (pelvis and soft

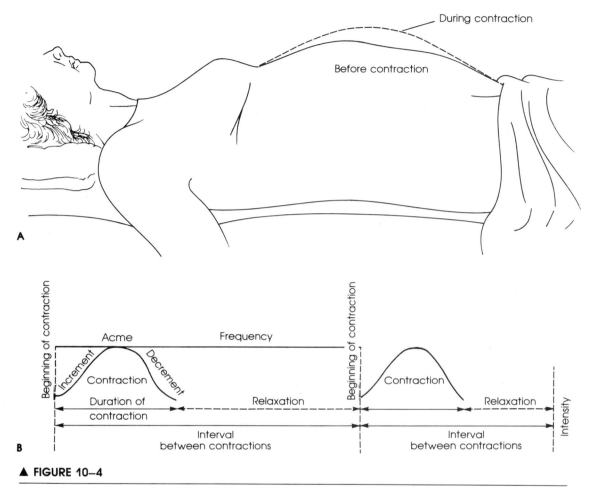

▲ **FIGURE 10–4**

A. Changes in abdominal contour before and during uterine contraction. **B.** Assessment of frequency, duration, and intensity of uterine contractions during labor.

structures) is referred to as the *fetopelvic relationship*. The relationship of the fetus to the maternal passageway is of great importance to the progress of labor. The relationship between passenger and passage affects the length of labor, potential types of complications encountered, and status of the infant when born.

Maternal Passage

The anatomy of the pelvis and uterus is discussed in Chapter 2. Estimation of the adequacy of the pelvis is important and is part of the prenatal physical examination. The angles of the birth canal are downward, forward, and upward, somewhat similar to the angles of a stovepipe. This pelvic curve must be negotiated by the fetus during the birth process. If the pelvic anterior–posterior diameter is shortened by the sacral promontory, by narrowing of the transverse diameter as a result of protrusion of the ischial spines, or by the presence of a narrow pubic arch, the fetus will have added difficulty in coming through the birth canal.

Passenger

Fetal Head. The fetal head is engineered to withstand the pressure of uterine contractions and descent through the birth canal. Great pressure is

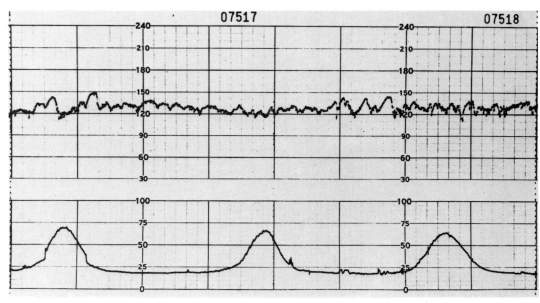

▲ **FIGURE 10–5**

Normal fetal heart rate (FHR) pattern with normal rate (about 130 beats/minute) and FHR variability (range = 15 beats/minute). This pattern represents a normally oxygenated fetus. Uterine contractions are 2 to 3 minutes apart and about 60 mm Hg in intensity. (From Creasy, R. K., & Resnick, R. (1989). *Maternal–Fetal Medicine*, 2nd ed. Philadelphia, W. B. Saunders Company.)

exerted on the fetal head during labor, and even stronger pressure is applied to the head after the rupture of membranes.

Bony Skull. The bones in the fetal skull are thin and poorly ossified. The skull is made up of small, slightly curved little bones, connected by very flexible elastic membranous tissues (sutures). This construction allows for an overlap and reduction of the fetal head circumference necessary to squeeze through the narrow birth canal. Frequently, the fetal head elongates in the anterior–posterior diameter. The bones of the head may overlap at the suture lines as the head passes through the birth canal; this overlapping is called *molding*. A few days after birth, the head returns to its normal shape (Fig. 10–6).

Fetopelvic Relationship: Terminology

Some common terms are used in a special way to describe the fetopelvic relationship. It is impor-

tant to know each term in order to understand the course of labor and birth.

Fetal attitude is the relation of the fetal parts to one another. The normal attitude of the fetus is one of flexion. The fetus is flexed with head on chest, arms and legs folded, and legs drawn up onto the abdomen. Changes in fetal attitude, particularly in flexion or extension of head, cause the fetus to present larger or smaller diameters of the fetal head to the maternal pelvis. Extension of the fetal head, especially full extension in which chin or face presents, makes vaginal birth difficult and sometimes impossible.

Fetal lie is the relationship of the *longitudinal axis* of the fetus to the longitudinal axis of the mother. The ideal is a parallel relationship where the long axes of the fetus and mother are the same. In rare instances, the fetus lies crosswise in the uterus (transverse lie), which necessitates a cesarean birth.

Fetal presentation is determined by the body part of the fetus that is lowest in the mother's pelvis (Fig. 10–7). A cephalic, breech, or shoulder pres-

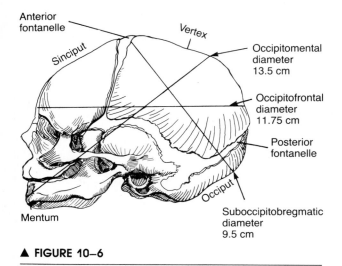

Anterior fontanelle

Sinciput

Vertex

Occipitomental diameter 13.5 cm

Occipitofrontal diameter 11.75 cm

Posterior fontanelle

Occiput

Mentum

Suboccipitobregmatic diameter 9.5 cm

▲ **FIGURE 10–6**

The fetal head. Note the lengths of the diameters.

entation may occur. Cephalic (head first) presentation is the most common, occurring in about 95% of all births. If the head is flexed it is referred to as a vertex presentation. Breech presentation occurs in approximately 4% of all births. In the breech presentation, the presenting parts may be either the buttocks (frank breech) or one or both feet (footling breech). The rarest (approximately 1% of births) type of presentation is the transverse, described above.

Fetal position, a more specific indication of the fetopelvic relationship, is the relationship of some designated point on the presenting part to the four quadrants of the maternal pelvis: anterior, posterior, left side, and right side. If the reference point is directed toward the transverse diameter of the maternal pelvis, it is referred to as a transverse position.

Three aspects of the fetal position are noted:

- Side of maternal pelvis: right (R) or left (L).
- Designated point of fetal presenting part: occiput (O), sacrum (S), mentum/chin (M), brow/forehead (Fr), or shoulder/acromion process (A).
- Location of the designated point to the left or right of the maternal pelvis, anterior or posterior to the maternal pelvis, or to the transverse diameter of the maternal pelvis: (anterior, A), (posterior, P), or (transverse, T).

The abbreviations help the caregivers in communicating fetal position. If the back of the head (occiput) is directed to the left and anteriorly, it is described as LOA (left occiput anterior). When the head is directed to the back (posterior to the pelvis), the labor is often longer and the woman experiences more backache (see Fig. 10–8 for various positions). The left occiput anterior and right occiput anterior positions are the most common:

SIX POSSIBLE OCCIPUT POSITIONS

- Left occiput anterior (LOA)
- Left occiput posterior (LOP)
- Left occiput transverse (LOT)
- Right occiput anterior (ROA)
- Right occiput posterior (ROP)
- Right occiput transverse (ROT)

Station is the relationship of the presenting part of the fetus to an imaginary line drawn between the ischial spines of the maternal pelvis (Fig. 10–8). To put it simply, station is how far the fetal presenting part has descended into the mother's pelvis. Station defines the progression of (usually) the fetal head down toward the pelvic floor. It is measured in centimeters above or below the ischial spines. When the presenting part is above the ischial spines, it is at −1 or −2 station. When the presenting part is 1 to 2 cm below the spines, it is at +1 or +2 station. When the presenting part is level with the spines, it is said to be 0 station, in which case the head is referred to as *engaged*. This is significant because the widest biparietal diameter of the baby's head has entered the inlet (middle of pelvis). Before the head becomes engaged, it is said to be *floating*. When the station is +2 or +3, the mother's perineum begins to *bulge*. *Crowning* takes place when the fetal head is forced against the pelvic floor and can be seen during contractions.

Mechanisms of Labor

The mechanisms of labor are a series of movements that reflect changes in the posture of the fetus as the fetus conforms itself to the birth canal. Most of the changes in posture take place during the second stage of labor; however, descent and some flexion take place earlier.

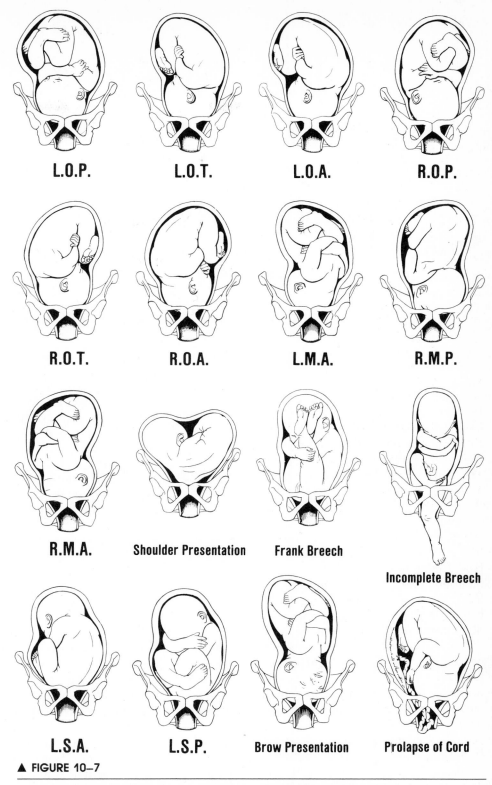

▲ FIGURE 10–7

Various presentations. (From Ross Laboratories (1980). *Clinical Education Aid No. 18, G174.* Columbus, Ross Laboratories. Reprinted with permission of Ross Laboratories, Columbus, OH 43216.)

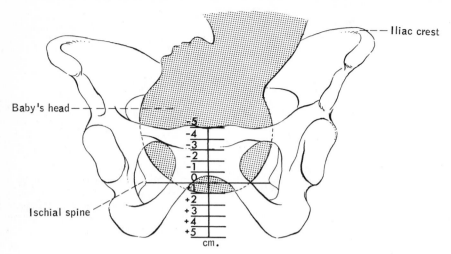

Baby's head

Iliac crest

Ischial spine

-5
-4
-3
-2
-1
0
+1
+2
+3
+4
+5
cm.

Perineum

▲ **FIGURE 10–8**

Stations of presenting part (degree of engagement). In this diagram, the presenting part has reached a +1 station.

The posture changes (mechanisms of labor) are dictated by the pelvic diameters, maternal soft tissues, the size of the baby, and the strength of contractions. The fetus must turn and twist to locate the easiest path to be expelled. In essence, labor proceeds along the path of least resistance through adaptation of the smallest achievable fetal dimensions to the contour of the maternal pelvis. The series of adaptive movements of the fetal head and shoulders are (a) engagement and descent, (b) flexion, (c) internal rotation, (d) extension, (e) external rotation, and (f) expulsion (Fig. 10–9).

Descent cannot be isolated from the other adaptive movements. As the head moves toward the pelvic inlet, it is described as floating. Once the biparietal diameter of the head passes through the inlet, the head becomes engaged. This may occur before or after labor begins and is due to pressure of contractions and of amniotic fluid.

Flexion occurs as the fetal head descends. The head flexes so that the chin rests on the chest. Flexion reduces the presenting fetal diameter. It normally occurs when the fetal head meets resistance from the pelvis and soft tissues of the pelvic floor.

Internal rotation occurs as the fetal head rotates from the transverse position to the anteroposterior position, aligning itself with the anteroposterior diameter of the maternal pelvis. Pressure from the pelvic floor encourages the fetal head to rotate anteriorly.

Extension occurs as the fetal head reaches the pelvic floor, at which point it pivots under the symphysis pubis and advances upward. This occurs as a result of a combination of pressure from the uterine contractions, abdominal pressure exerted by the mother's pushing, and resistance from the pelvic floor. As extension occurs, first the occiput appears, then the forehead, nose, mouth, and chin.

External rotation occurs after the head is delivered. It immediately rotates back to the transverse position, as the shoulders align themselves to the anterior–posterior diameter of the pelvic outlet.

Expulsion usually proceeds as follows: First the anterior shoulder rotates forward and is delivered, followed by delivery of the posterior shoulder, followed by delivery of the rest of the infant's body.

Placental expulsion or expulsion of the afterbirth is NOT one of the mechanisms of labor but normally occurs between 5 and 30 minutes after the delivery of the infant. The uterus begins to contract, reducing its size, immediately after birth of the baby and is sheared off from the endometrium. Signs of placental separation are (a) lengthening of the cord, (b) change in the shape of the uterus, and (c) a trickle or gush of vaginal blood. If the dull (maternal) side appears first, it is referred to as *Duncan's mechanism;* if the shiny (fetal) side of the placenta appears first, it is referred to as *Schultz's mechanism.* Periodic studies have not shown any significant differences between the Schultz and Duncan mechanisms.

The Four Stages of Labor

Traditionally, labor was divided into three stages in which specific developments occur. In recent years, however, a fourth stage has been identified as crucial in the birth process. This text discusses four stages. Each stage is divided from the next, and the first stage has three distinct phases. All stages are carefully observed to assess the progress of normal labor. The average lengths of the first and second stages differ between primigravidae and multigravidae. However, the average lengths of the third and fourth stages are similar for both (Table 10–2).

FACTORS THAT INFLUENCE THE COURSE OF LABOR

Several factors influence the course of labor. These factors should be considered in the assessment of the course of a woman's labor. The factors are as follows:

1. Parity—First labor is longer.
2. Uterine contractions—Effective contractions are necessary for labor to progress.
3. Presentation—The fetal head is a more effective mechanical dilating wedge than the buttocks.
4. Position—When the baby is in a posterior position, the labor tends to be longer and more painful.
5. Status of membranes—Cervical dilatation can be enhanced by the rupture of membranes. This action brings the firm fetal head in contact with the cervix.
6. Fetopelvic diameters—Flexion of the head is a significant factor in duration of labor.
7. Muscles—Strength and relaxation of pelvic floor muscles are important in aiding the expulsion of the infant's head.
8. Psyche—Childbirth preparation and a positive attitude toward labor appear to shorten the duration of labor.

FIRST STAGE

The first stage of labor is the longest and most variable stage. The first stage begins with the onset of regular contractions; cervical changes have already begun. It is complete when the cervix is fully dilated and effaced. The first stage is referred to as the "stage of dilatation." The contractions bring about two important changes in the cervix:

- Complete effacement of the cervical canal (100%)
- Complete dilatation of the cervix (10 cm)

As already stated, effacement of the cervix is the shortening and thinning of the cervix during the first stage of labor. The cervix goes from being about 2 to 3 cm in length and about 1 cm thick to being nearly obliterated or "taken up" by a shortening of the uterine muscle cells. When effacement is complete (100%), only a thin edge of the cervix can be palpated.

Dilatation of the cervix is the widening of the opening of the cervix (cervical os) from 0 cm to 10 cm to allow delivery of the term infant. When the cervix is fully dilated, it can no longer be palpated by vaginal examination. As dilatation of the cervix progresses, there is an increased amount of bloody show.

The Three Phases of the First Stage

The first stage of labor is divided into the latent, active, and transition phases, each characterized by certain physical and psychological changes.

Latent Phase. The *latent phase* is the early, slow part of labor, which begins with the onset of regular contractions and lasts until the cervix is dilated 4 cm. During this phase the contractions become stabilized and are usually mild. They occur about every 10 to 15 minutes and last about 15 to 20 seconds. The woman feels that she is able to cope with the discomfort. She is often talkative and smiling and is relieved that labor has finally started. She is usually up and about, watching TV or talking with her partner. This is a good time to ask the woman if she has any questions about what to expect and, if she is anxious, teach her some of the relaxation techniques. At this time, she is able to focus clearly on what is being taught.

Text continued on page 182

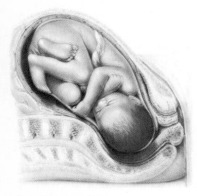
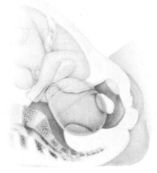
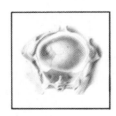

▲ **FIGURE 10–9**

MECHANISM OF NORMAL LABOR IN A LEFT OCCIPITOANTERIOR POSITION.
A. *Engagement and descent* occur as the head moves toward the pelvic inlet; descent continues. *Flexion* reduces the diameter of the fetal head to adjust to the pelvic measurements. (From Ross Laboratories (1964). *Nursing Education Aid No. 13.* Columbus, Ross Laboratories. © Ross Laboratories, Columbus, OH 43216.)

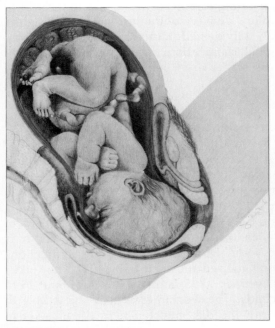
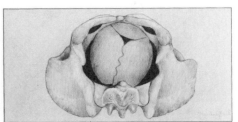
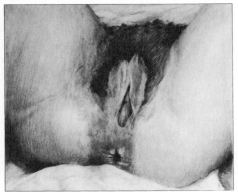

▲ **FIGURE 10–9** *Continued*

B. *Internal rotation* occurs as the fetal head rotates, bringing it into anteroposterior alignment with the anteroposterior diameter of the maternal pelvis. This position facilitates birth. (© 1984 Childbirth Graphics, Rochester, NY)

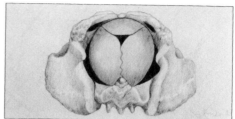

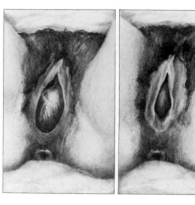

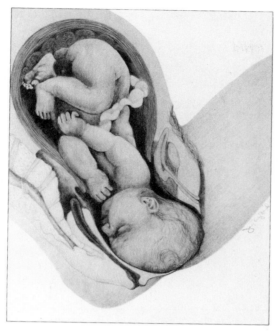

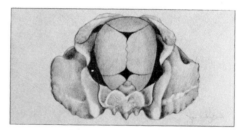

▲ **FIGURE 10–9** *Continued*

C. *Extension begins* when the fetal head reaches the pelvic floor. The distention of the perineum becomes apparent. The fetal head advances with uterine contractions and bearing-down efforts of the woman. (© 1984 Childbirth Graphics, Rochester, NY)

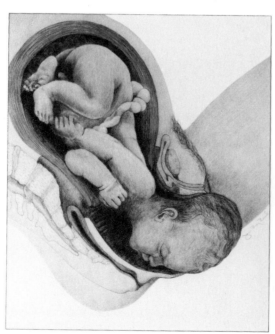

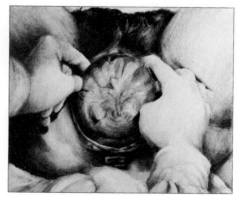

▲ **FIGURE 10–9** *Continued*

D. *Crowning* occurs when the head distends the perineum and is visible. (© 1984 Childbirth Graphics, Rochester, NY)

Illustration continued on following page

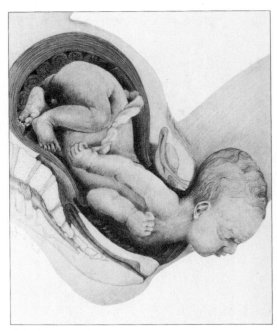
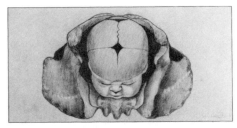
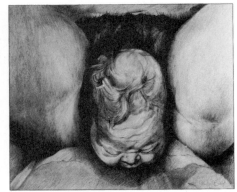

▲ **FIGURE 10–9** *Continued*

E. *Extension is complete* as the fetal head pivots the symphysis pubis and pressure is exerted on the neck, which forces the baby's head upward. This is accomplished by the continued force of contractions and bearing-down efforts. (© 1984 Childbirth Graphics, Rochester, NY)

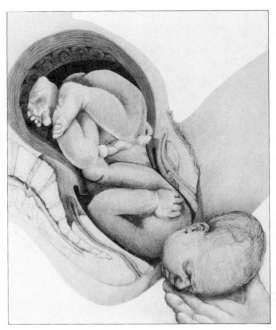
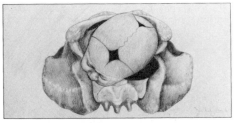
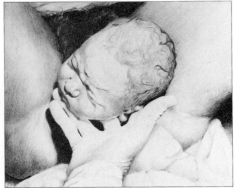

▲ **FIGURE 10–9** *Continued*

F. *External rotation* (shoulder rotation) *occurs* when the fetal head rotates back to the side or oblique position in which it entered the pelvis, thus realigning the head with the shoulders. (© 1984 Childbirth Graphics, Rochester, NY)

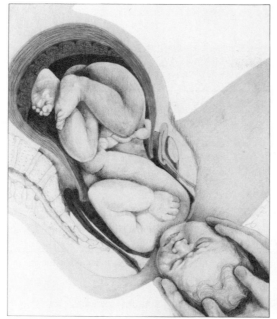
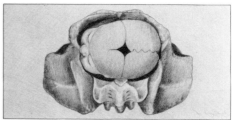
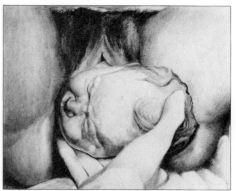

▲ **FIGURE 10–9** *Continued*

G. *External rotation continues* as the shoulders rotate from the transverse to the anterior–posterior position for delivery. The anterior shoulder is often delivered first, followed quickly by the posterior shoulder. (© 1984 Childbirth Graphics, Rochester, NY)

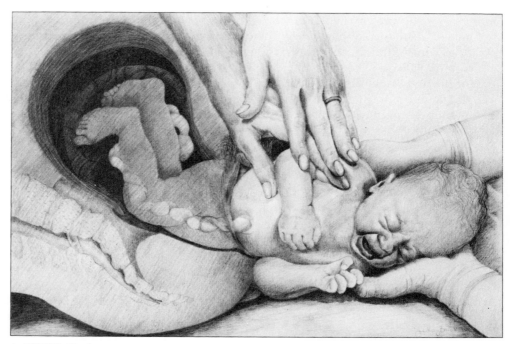

▲ **FIGURE 10–9** *Continued*

H. *Expulsion* occurs as the rest of the body is born. (© 1984 Childbirth Graphics, Rochester, NY)

TABLE 10–2. STAGES OF LABOR

| | FIRST STAGE | | | SECOND STAGE |
	Latent Phase	Active Phase	Transition Phase	
Primigravida	8–10 hr	6 hr	1–2 hr	1 hr
Multipara	5 hr	4 hr	30 min to 1 hr	15 min
Cervical dilatation	0–4 cm	4–8 cm	8–10 cm	
Contractions				
Frequency	10–15 min	2–3 min	1–2 min	2–3 min
Duration°	15–20 sec	30–45 sec	60–90 sec	60–90 sec
Intensity	Begin mild and become moderate	Begin moderate and become strong	Strong	Strong

°Duration of labor varies. Figures presented represent average length of labor at various times.

Active Phase. The *active phase* causes the woman different degrees of discomfort. The contractions are stronger and last longer, with the result that cervical dilation progresses from 4 cm to 8 cm. Fetal descent proceeds. The duration of contractions increases to 30 to 45 seconds. During this phase the woman can be assisted in her breathing techniques and relaxation. She may continue to ambulate until she is uncomfortable or until her membranes rupture. As her contractions increase, her anxiety increases. She may begin to doubt her ability to cope with the labor contractions.

Transition Phase. The *transition phase* is the last part of the first stage. Cervical dilatation continues at a slower rate (8 to 10 cm) but becomes complete. The contractions now become more frequent, longer (60 to 90 seconds), and stronger. During this phase, the woman may exhibit decreased ability to cope with her contractions and pain. Often, the woman becomes very restless, frequently changing positions and feeling as if she has been abandoned. It is crucial that the nurse stay with the woman at this time as a backup or relief for the support person. Often, the woman needs to be reminded of how to relax and focus or refocus with each contraction. She may become nauseated and even vomit. Also, she may become irritable and not want to be touched during her contractions.

The woman may feel a splitting sensation by the force of the contractions and pressure of the fetal head near the opening of the cervix. As the fetal head descends, she likely will feel the urge to push because of pressure of the fetal head on the sacral nerves. As she pushes, her abdominal muscles exert additional pressure, which helps the fetal head to descend. As the fetal head continues to descend the perineum begins to bulge and flatten, and soon the fetal head can be seen. Between contractions the fetal head appears to recede. With each contraction the fetal head descends further. When *crowning* occurs, the fetal head is seen in the external opening of the vagina and birth is imminent.

Medications are often administered during the active and transition phases to help the woman relax and get pain relief. However, the woman should not be given medications earlier than 1 to 2 hours before birth because the effect may depress the infant at birth. Demerol and phenergan are common drugs given (see appendix on drugs).

CHARACTERISTICS OF THE TRANSITION PHASE

- Restlessness
- Sense of bewilderment and sometimes anger
- Statements that she "cannot continue" or "can't take it"
- Difficulty in following directions; needs instruction with each contraction
- Requests medication to ease the pain
- Hyperventilation, caused by increased breathing rate
- Beads of perspiration appear on face
- Belching, hiccuping
- Nausea and vomiting

- Increasing rectal pressure; states she has to have a bowel movement
- May feel warm and throw off covers (exposure may embarrass partner)
- May be very irritable
- Contractions may be only 1 to 2 minutes apart and last up to 90 seconds

SECOND STAGE

The second stage of labor begins when the cervix is completely dilated (10 cm) and ends with the birth of the infant. At this time the woman usually feels the urge to bear down (as if she has to have a bowel movement). She may now use her abdominal muscles to assist the involuntary uterine contractions as a force to cause the descent of the baby. Generally, the second stage is considerably shorter than the first stage, lasting from a few minutes to 2 hours. Descent of the fetal head causes bulging of the perineum. *Crowning* occurs when the fetal head is seen in the external opening of the vagina. Between contractions, the fetal head appears to recede. With succeeding contractions and the woman pushing, the birth is imminent. The uterine contractions are forceful, but now (generally) are only every 2 to 3 minutes and last 60 to 90 seconds. There is an increase in bloody show.

As the fetal head reaches the perineal floor, it appears in the vaginal opening. To prevent laceration, the physician or midwife may make an *episiotomy*, a midline or mediolateral incision in the perineum. The episiotomy often shortens the second stage of labor. The physician or midwife supports the fetal head as it delivers and rotates, the mouth and nose of the baby are suctioned, and the shoulders and rest of the baby's body appear. Before the delivery of the baby, a quick check is made to make sure there is no umbilical cord around the baby's neck. After the birth of the baby, the woman usually is relieved.

Anesthesia used during delivery must be safe for the baby. General anesthesia is not given if the woman has been given food or fluids by mouth. Regional anesthesia (see Chapter 11) is usually given, because it is safer for the baby and the mother is at risk for aspiration.

THIRD STAGE

The third stage of labor is referred to as the *placental separation stage*. It extends from the birth of the baby to the delivery of the placenta (30 minutes or less). After the birth of the infant, the umbilical cord is clamped in two places and cut between the two clamps. The nose and mouth of the baby are suctioned again to clear them of mucus (see Chapter 12). An oxytocin drug (Pitocin) is often given to keep the uterus firm and lessen the maternal blood loss.

FOURTH STAGE

The fourth stage is the time from 1 to 4 hours after birth, during which major readjustments of the mother's body occur. Blood loss ranges from 250 to 500 mL. This can result in a drop in blood pressure and an increase in pulse rate. The uterine muscles continue to contract and relax as they compress the open blood vessels at the placental site. For the first hour after delivery, it is critical to observe the mother for excessive bleeding.

The mother may feel thirsty and hungry. She may experience a shaking chill. Nursing care is discussed in Chapter 12.

Maternal Systemic Response to Labor

Knowing the responses of the various systems to labor is important in nursing assessment of and intervention for a woman in labor. Aspects of physical care are based on the alterations that occur in the major systems during labor.

CARDIOVASCULAR SYSTEM

Contractions cause an increase in the woman's blood pressure during the first and second stages of labor, with a return to prelabor level during the third stage. Because the elevation in blood pressure is most noticeable during contractions, maternal blood pressure should be taken between contractions. Other factors that cause a rise in blood pressure are anxiety, apprehension, and pain. The heart rate is increased during the second stage by the woman's bearing-down efforts.

Approximately 10% to 15% of women demonstrate clinical symptoms of hypotension and increased pulse rate as a result of supine vena cava syndrome (see Chapter 5).

RESPIRATORY SYSTEM

The oxygen consumption during labor is equal to that of moderate to strenuous exercise. The increase in ventilation continues throughout labor as long as the respiratory center is not depressed by medication. The woman is more prone to changes in blood gas levels during disturbances in ventilation. She may quickly develop hypoxia or acidosis, which in turn can compromise the infant. A decrease from the normal amount of carbon dioxide in the blood may also develop as a result of hyperventilation.

RENAL SYSTEM

As a result of muscle breakdown during labor, a trace of protein may be found in the urine. More than a trace is suggestive of preeclampsia. A distended bladder can obstruct the descent of the baby; therefore, assessment for a distended bladder is important. Urinary stasis may also occur, increasing the risk of infection. Often the woman has less urge to void during labor and needs to be encouraged to do so. Decreased urinary flow is more marked when the woman is on her back because of the compression of the ureters by the distended uterus.

GASTROINTESTINAL SYSTEM

During labor, gastrointestinal peristalsis and absorption decrease. Hence, the rate of absorption of solid food is slowed. It can take as long as 12 hours to digest a meal. Many hospital staffs withhold solid food during labor because there is always the potential for obstetrical surgery. Eating would increase the risk of aspiration of vomitus.

Gastrointestinal absorption of liquid is not changed; ice chips are frequently given to women in labor.

FLUID AND ELECTROLYTE BALANCE

The muscle activity increases the body temperature, which in turn increases the sweating and fluid evaporation from the skin. Thus, perspiration is profuse during labor. An increase in the respiratory rate occurs as the woman responds to the work of labor involving the muscles. The woman is also prone to hyperventilation during labor, which alters the electrolyte balance. Adequate hydration is an important aspect of care. Many hospital staffs routinely start intravenous fluid administration on patient admission, to prevent dehydration.

Psychological and Sociological Factors That Affect Labor

The woman's cultural beliefs about childbearing may influence whether she views childbirth as a meaningful or stressful event. Her beliefs about her feminine role and her self-concept can also influence her behavior during labor. Some women do not like to be touched, some cry for assistance, and others become quite negative and unhappy. Also, if the woman has had a poor previous experience in childbearing, she will be more likely to feel negatively about the present childbirth experience.

References

Auvenshine, M. A., & Enriquez, M. G. (1990). *Comprehensive Maternity Nursing: Perinatal and Women's Health*, 2nd ed. Boston: Jones and Bartlett.

Dickason, E. J., Schult, M. O., & Silverman, B. L. (1990). *Maternal-Infant Nursing Care*. St. Louis: C. V. Mosby.

Ladewig, P. W., London, M. L., & Olds, S. B. (1990). *Essentials of Maternal-Newborn Nursing*, 2nd ed. Redwood City, CA: Addison-Wesley Nursing.

Malinowski, J. S., Pedigo, C. G., & Phillips, C. R. (1989). *Nursing Care During the Labor Process*, 3rd ed. Philadelphia: F. A. Davis.

Oxhorn, H., & Foote, W. F. (1975). *Human Labor and Birth*, 3rd ed. New York: Appleton-Century-Crofts.

SUGGESTED ACTIVITIES

1. Explain the differences among the four stages of labor and the three phases of the first stage.
2. Identify the beginning and the end of the first through fourth stages of labor.

REVIEW QUESTIONS

A. Select the best answer to each multiple-choice question.

Clinical Situation: Ms. Leib (gravida 3, para 2, age 24 years, 40 weeks' gestation) was awakened during the night as the result of a gush of fluid from her vagina. Within one hour labor contractions became noticeable every 10 minutes. Ms. Leib was accompanied to the hospital by her husband. She was immediately admitted to the labor suite.

1. Ms. Leib's sudden gush of fluid from the vagina is referred to as
   A. Bloody show
   B. Lightening
   C. Rupture of membranes
   D. Dilatation of cervix

2. Ms. Leib experienced a settling of her baby into her pelvis 1 week ago, which is called
   A. Effacement of the cervix
   B. False labor
   C. True labor
   D. Lightening

3. On admission, Ms. Leib's cervical dilatation revealed that she was in active labor. Her cervical dilatation in centimeters was
   A. 2–3
   B. 4–6
   C. 4–8
   D. 6–10

4. Ms. Leib's temperature, pulse, and respirations were recorded on admission. This is important because
   A. It is a hospital policy
   B. It is the physician's orders
   C. An elevated temperature is indicative of infection
   D. None of the above

5. A vaginal examination was performed on Ms. Leib on admission. It reveals
   A. Degree of cervical dilatation
   B. Degree of cervical effacement
   C. Degree of fetal descent into the maternal pelvis
   D. All of the above

6. The oxygen consumption while Ms. Leib is in labor
   A. Is equal to that of moderate or strenuous exercise
   B. Decreases during labor
   C. Remains the same
   D. None of the above

7. The presenting part of the fetus becomes engaged in the pelvis when it reaches the level of
   A. Ischial tuberosities
   B. Ischial spines
   C. True pelvis
   D. Perineum

8. The first mechanism of labor is
   A. Descent
   B. Flexion
   C. Effacement
   D. Dilatation

9. True labor is differentiated from false labor by
   A. Intensity of contractions
   B. Duration of contractions
   C. Dilatation of cervix
   D. Amount of vaginal bloody show

10. If the fetal head is directed downward in the lower part of the uterus, with the occiput on the left anterior side of the maternal pelvis, the position is termed
    A. LOA
    B. LOP
    C. ROA
    D. ROP

11. The portion of the infant's body that can be felt by the examiner's finger in the woman's cervix is called the
    A. Presenting part
    B. Primary part
    C. Cephalic part
    D. Breech part

12. The assessment of contractions includes all of the following EXCEPT
    A. Frequency
    B. Duration
    C. Intensity
    D. Dilatation

13. During the first stage of labor, the following occurs:
    A. Effacement and dilatation
    B. Birth of the baby
    C. Expulsion of placenta
    D. Recovery period

14. During the second stage of labor, the following occurs:
    A. Effacement and dilatation
    B. Birth of the baby
    C. Expulsion of placenta
    D. Recovery period

15. During the third stage of labor, the following occurs:
    A. Effacement and dilatation
    B. Birth of the baby
    C. Expulsion of placenta
    D. Recovery period

16. A woman is more likely to have a normal labor if her uterine contractions become more frequent, more intense, and last longer. With this change in the contraction pattern, all of the following will likely occur EXCEPT
    A. The cervix will efface and dilate
    B. The fetus will engage and rotate
    C. The blood pressure will decrease
    D. The placenta, postbirth, will separate

17. Paula Miller is a nurse caring for a patient in active labor. Paula knows that in assessing the frequency of contractions she records the time
    A. From the beginning of one contraction until it is completely over
    B. From the beginning of one contraction to the beginning of the next
    C. From the end of one contraction to the beginning of the next
    D. From the end of one contraction to the end of the next

18. Paula knows that if the woman experiences a gush of fluid with the contraction, she should
    A. Notify the physician immediately
    B. Implement measures such as placing a chux under the woman's buttocks
    C. Check the fetal heart rate
    D. Instruct the woman that the birth of the baby is near

19. Paula recognizes that she must follow the Centers for Disease Control universal precautions to minimize the risk of exposure to blood and body fluids. She will
    A. Always wear protective coverings such as gloves, gowns/aprons, masks, and eye/face shields when doing procedures that may contaminate her with splashing blood or fluids
    B. Wear gloves when inserting or discontinuing an intravenous catheter or needle
    C. NEVER recap, bend, or break needles after use
    D. All of the above

20. Paula understands that the mechanisms of labor consist of a series of sequential movements with a change in the posture of the fetus to conform to the birth canal. The following correctly describes the order of fetal positional changes:
    A. Flexion, descent, internal rotation, extension, external rotation
    B. Descent, flexion, internal rotation, extension, expulsion
    C. Descent, flexion, internal rotation, extension, external rotation
    D. Flexion, internal rotation, extension, expulsion

B. Choose from Column II the phrase that most accurately defines the term in Column I.

I

1. Fetal lie _____
2. Breech presentation _____
3. Station _____
4. Position _____
5. Second stage of labor _____
6. Fourth stage of labor _____

II

A. Specific relationship of fetus to relationship of presenting part to maternal pelvis
B. Relationship of longitudinal axis of fetus to longitudinal axis of mother
C. The buttocks and/or feet of fetus are in the lowest part of maternal pelvis
D. The relation of the fetal presenting part to the ischial spines of mother's pelvis
E. Stage of recovery
F. Stage of delivery

CHAPTER 11 _____

Chapter Outline

The Nature of Pain During Labor
    Major causes of pain during labor and birth
    Reactions to pain
    Benefits of pain control
Nonpharmacological Pain Control Strategies
    Support
    Information
    Stimuli
    Cognitive control
    Cutaneous stimulation
    Systemic relaxation
Pharmacological Pain Control
    Basic principles for choosing the drug given during
      labor
    Analgesics
    Anesthesia
Summary

Learning Objectives

Upon completion of Chapter 11, the student should be able to

- Explain the physical causes of discomfort during labor.
- State the importance of controlling pain during labor.
- Name the sources of endorphins within the body.
- List nonpharmacological pain control strategies.
- Describe three ways to reduce discomfort during labor without the use of drugs.
- List and describe three types of analgesics used during labor.
- Differentiate the injection sites of pudendal, paracervical, epidural, and spinal blocks.
- Describe the risks from medication in relationship to phases of labor.
- List maternal side effects of narcotics, sedatives, epidural block, and spinal block anesthesia.
- List the potential effect on the newborn of sedatives, narcotics, epidural block, and spinal anesthesia.
- Identify risks of general anesthesia to the woman and infant.

Pain relief during labor and birth

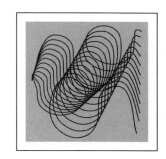

It is important to understand the woman's physiological and psychological reactions to pain and to be able to identify factors that affect the amount of pain she experiences during labor and birth. In addition, a nurse should be able to use nonpharmacological pain control strategies appropriate to the birth process. Drugs are used sparingly during labor because of their potentially harmful effects on the fetus.

The Nature of Pain During Labor

MAJOR CAUSES OF PAIN DURING LABOR AND BIRTH

First Stage

- Dilatation and stretching of cervix
- Uterine contractions
- Hypoxia (lack of oxygen) of uterine muscles
- Stress (feeling unprepared, anxious, and tense raises cortical and catecholamine levels)
- Low pain threshold (illness, fatigue, and lower endorphin levels)

Second Stage

- All First Stage factors
- Stretching of the perineal tissues and muscles, most pronounced during birth of baby
- Large baby
- Posterior position (especially with a large baby)
- Borderline or small pelvis (makes it difficult to deliver infant)

Third Stage

- Separation and expulsion of placenta
- Episiotomy and repair
- Laceration and repair
- Extreme exhaustion

REACTIONS TO PAIN

Because pain cannot be seen, but can only be reacted to, it is difficult to assess whether a person is having pain, to assess the amount of pain being experienced, and to assess the degree of the person's reaction to it. Pain is influenced by racial, cultural, and environmental factors. The differences among experiences of pain, discomfort, and unpleasantness are subjective.

The gate-control theory of pain has application to labor and childbirth. The gate mechanism in the spinal cord, cerebral cortex, and brain stem omits or decreases the sensation of pain by "closing the gate." It is now believed that many gates can be opened or closed by nursing interventions during labor and birth. Cutaneous stimulation such as effleurage may have a direct effect on closing the gate. What happens, physiologically, when a person experiences pain is the following: (a) The nerve cells carry the message of pain sensation to the spinal cord, (b) the gate opens, and (c) the transmittal cells send back the message of pain. The gate control theory, using descending and ascending pathways, helps to explain the effectiveness of various types of focusing strategies in prepared childbirth, such as breathing, listening to music, verbal coaching, and effleurage. Acupuncture, applying an external analgesic, and back massage provide relief because they help close the gate to the discomfort. The message of discomfort can accumulate to the point at which the sensation is felt as severe pain.

The endorphin system, recognized about 15 years ago, increased our understanding of why and how certain pain-prevention techniques work. It was found that endogenous (that is, originating within the body) chemicals that have a makeup similar to that of opiates (for example, morphine) are released from the brain stem and pituitary gland. These chemicals are natural pain inhibitors called *endorphins*. Endorphins seem to be able to make the woman drowsy and sleepy. It has been shown that the endorphin blood level in a woman in delivery is much higher than that of a nonpregnant woman. It now appears that women who have a positive attitude during labor have more natural protection by their bodies' ability to produce their own analgesia. This phenomenon can contribute to a more positive outcome of the woman's childbirth experience.

The pain of childbirth is unique because the woman in labor generally expects pain, knows why it happens, and knows how long it will last. In addition, the woman will receive a reward at the end—a baby.

Most labors are accompanied by some degree of pain or discomfort. The degree of discomfort varies according to (a) the individual, (b) the type of labor, (c) the size of the baby, and (d) the position of the baby. Generally, the pain initially occurs in the lower back, then circles through the torso to the abdomen. Sometimes the pain extends into the groin. In early labor, the pain is described as a deep aching sensation. As the fetus passes into the birth canal, the sensations change to feelings of pressure, tingling, burning, and so-called splitting. These sensations are more pronounced as the fetus presses on the perineum.

During labor, the woman's sense of time is altered, because most of her energy is directed inward. Her perceptions are also altered. The woman may be sensitive to voices out in the hall or at her bedside, yet she may respond only to specific instructions given in a one-to-one manner owing to her inward focus. The woman's behavior in response to the sensation of pain will vary. She may grimace, cry, moan, tense her muscles, or become hysterical. The fact that some women do not display reactions to pain does not necessarily mean they are not experiencing discomfort. The fear of pain is very obvious in some women and not so obvious in others.

BENEFITS OF PAIN CONTROL

Psychological Benefits

Controlling or decreasing pain helps the woman and significant other participate more actively in the birth of the baby. It promotes a positive relationship with the infant and increases the woman's self-esteem in achieving the tasks of delivering and caring for the infant. In addition, it has the potential to strengthen the bond between the infant and parents. Pain may elicit the fear response known as "flight-or-fight." This may be projected onto the infant and partner. Controlling pain lessens the chance that such projection will occur.

Physiological Benefits

The control or lessening of the sensation of pain decreases the fatigue of labor. Therefore, the woman has extra energy for increased cooperation and increased awareness of the environment. When less medication is required, the infant is more responsive at birth.

Nonpharmacological Pain Control Strategies

SUPPORT

Support can come from a husband, mother, friend, or the nurse. The woman can receive support from any person that she trusts. The nurse can also function as a support to the woman's support person.

INFORMATION

The woman in labor needs to continue to receive information on what to expect, when labor will start, how long it will last, what it will be like, and when it will be over. The nurse is in a key position to give this type of information in prenatal classes, during clinic visits, during the admitting procedures, and throughout labor and birth. If the woman or couple does not receive this type of communication during labor, what she or they have learned during prenatal classes may be of little benefit.

STIMULI

It is important to eliminate sources of noxious (unwholesome) stimuli whenever possible. The nurse can attempt to relieve thirst, sweating, heat, and tension by comfort measures. Repositioning the woman or adjusting tapes and monitoring belts may provide relief.

COGNITIVE CONTROL

Several cognitive methods of pain control may be tried. Dissociation may be used by helping the woman imagine more pleasant experiences (waves instead of contractions). Interference may work better than dissociation, however. The woman may be asked to look at a picture or TV or to talk to take her mind off the discomfort; this is called passive interference. In this instance the nurse is doing the distracting. Attention focusing—asking the woman to focus on something—may help her to block out painful sensations. For example, the woman can focus on breathing patterns or a spot on the wall. This behavior requires active participation by the woman in labor.

CUTANEOUS STIMULATION

Touching, rubbing, or massaging the back often decreases discomfort. Counterpressure with the palm or closed fist pressed at the point of back pain is often helpful. Hot and cold towels applied to the back may be effective for some women.

SYSTEMIC RELAXATION

Even if the woman has attended prenatal (for example, Lamaze) classes, she will need continued support in achieving relaxation of her voluntary muscles. The time for the most effective teaching is between contractions and the latent phase of the first stage of labor. Some women need to be shown the difference between relaxation and tension. The most effective strategy is the combination of the woman's "feedback" relaxation, in which the nurse or support person continually works with the woman to keep her relaxed, and have her attempt attention focusing.

After birth, the woman's assimilation of her labor and birth experience is significant. She will want to discuss how she behaved. She will seek confirmation of the events and of her acceptable behavior, namely, that she did what she had intended to do. Aftermath assimilation is the final stage of the pain experience. It is important that caregivers help the woman confirm that her behavior during labor and birth was acceptable.

Pharmacological Pain Control

The decision to prescribe and administer drugs during labor must be carefully weighed because of the effects on the infant. Dosage and time of administration must be calculated to avoid having the infant born depressed. This factor is extremely important. Because the fetus cannot metabolize the drugs as quickly as the mother, the fetal response may be intense and last much longer.

During the first stage of labor, administration of drugs may affect the progress of labor. If an analgesic is given too soon during the latent phase, it may slow down the labor. Usually, labor is well established, with a cervical dilatation of 4 cm (in active labor), before the woman receives medication.

BASIC PRINCIPLES IN CHOOSING THE DRUG GIVEN DURING LABOR

1. The drug should provide maximum relief to the woman, with minimal risk to the fetus.
2. The drug should have minimal side effects.
3. Labor should be well established.
4. If the drug affects uterine contractions, it should be given with the woman's knowledge.
5. Adequate fetal monitoring and emergency equipment should be available.
6. The drug must be one that will allow the uterus to contract during the postpartum period. Some general anesthetics relax the uterus and increase bleeding.
7. If the infant is preterm, risk is increased with drugs given during labor; therefore, they should not be given to reduce maternal discomfort during preterm delivery.
8. Preferably, drugs should not be given if less than 1 hour remains before delivery, because after birth the infant may have difficulty in metabolizing them and may experience respiratory depression.

ANALGESICS

Analgesics help a woman to cope with the stress and pain of labor by decreasing her perception of pain. Analgesics are categorized according to their actions and include sedatives, tranquilizers, amnesic narcotics, and narcotic antagonists. These medications are given to reduce the pain caused by uterine contractions, muscle stretching, and pressure on the nerves. The drugs commonly used during labor are presented in Table 11–1.

Sedatives

The sedatives, such as the barbiturates secobarbital (Seconal) and pentobarbital sodium (Nembutal) are not commonly used today because of their potential adverse effect on the infant. They may be used to allow rest and sleep for the anxious woman in very early labor when delivery is not anticipated for 12 to 24 hours. These drugs produce drowsiness and a feeling of well-being. Barbiturates may produce excitement and disorientation. Therefore, they should be used in conjunction with close observation. Barbiturates readily cross the placenta and can cause depression in the fetus. In addition, effects may persist for a prolonged time, as long as 2 to 10 days. Poor sucking behavior has been observed during the first 4 days of life in newborns whose mothers received secobarbital during labor.

Tranquilizers

Tranquilizers decrease anxiety and apprehension, thereby increasing the woman's ability to relax and cope with labor. The tranquilizers commonly given are promazine (Sparine), hydroxyzine (Vistaril), and promethazine (Phenergan). Vistaril should be given only in a deep intramuscular (IM) injection, using the Z tract method, because it can cause severe vessel irritation. Diazepam (Valium) is *not* used because it can severely affect the infant (the infant can be born with poor muscle tone and respiratory depression). Tranquilizers potentiate the action of barbiturates and narcotics so that smaller doses of both can be given. Tranquilizers can cause a decrease in beat-to-beat variability of the fetal heart rate.

Narcotics

Narcotics are frequently given in the active phase of labor. It is important that they not be

TABLE 11–1. DRUGS COMMONLY USED DURING LABOR

DRUG	DOSAGE (MG)	TIME OF ADMINISTRATION	ADVANTAGES TO WOMAN	DISADVANTAGES TO INFANT
Sedatives-Hypnotics				
Secobarbital sodium (Seconal)	50–100 PO or IM	Early labor latent phase	Provides rest Relieves tension	Fetal respiratory depression
Pentobarbital sodium (Nembutal)	50–100 PO or IM	Early labor latent phase	Provides rest Relieves tension	Same as secobarbital sodium
Narcotic analgesics				
Meperidine (Demerol)	50–100 IM or IV (onset: IM— 15 min, IV— 30 sec; duration; IM—2–3 hr IV—1½–2 hr)	After cervix is dilated 3–4 cm	Reduces pain Relaxes cervix	Mild respiratory depression; with excessive dose, severe respiratory depression CNS depression if delivery is <2 hr after administration
Alphaprodine (Nisentil)	15–40 IM or IV	After cervix is dilated 3–4 cm	Reduces pain	Same as meperidine
Butorphanol (Stadol)	2 mg IM, 1 mg IV (onset: IM—10 min IV—rapid)	After cervix is dilated 3–4 cm	Reduces pain	Respiratory distress (in woman, nausea and increased perspiration) 2 mg of Stadol depresses infant respirations equal to 75 mg of Demerol
Amnesic				
Scopolamine (rarely used today)	0.3–0.4 IM	Midlabor	Amnesia Produces drowsiness Lessens secretions (Woman is not responsible for her actions and *must not be left alone*)	Respiratory distress CNS depression
Tranquilizers				
Promethazine HCl (Phenergan)	20–50 IM	Early labor only (given with narcotic)	Decreases anxiety Potentiates effect of narcotic or CNS depression	May depress respirations of newborn
Hydroxyzine HCl (Vistaril)	20–50 IM			Decreases fetal beat-to-beat heart rate variability
Narcotic antagonist				
Naloxone (Narcan)	0.05–0.1 IM or IV (infant dose)	Administered to infant after birth to relieve narcotic side effects		Can precipitate withdrawal symptoms in infant of drug-dependent mother

administered to the mother within 1 to 2 hours before the birth. If the infant's central nervous system becomes depressed, a narcotic antagonist may be ordered. Naloxone (Narcan) may have to be given to correct the respiratory depression. Unfortunately, the narcotic antagonists do not alleviate the depressant effects of tranquilizers and barbiturates. Meperidine (Demerol) is a narcotic given during labor. Because it can have a depressant effect on the newborn, it should be used cautiously in women delivering preterm infants. The depressant effects of meperidine after intramuscular injection are manifested 1 to 4 hours after delivery. Intravenous administration is superior to intramuscular administration of narcotics because control of the analgesia is better, onset of action is quicker, and the duration of action is shorter. When 25 mg of meperidine is administered intravenously within 1 hour of delivery, the depressant effect is less pronounced. Side effects include nausea and vomiting and tachycardia.

Butorphanol (Stadol) is a relatively new synthetic narcotic that is used during labor. Use of 1 to 2 mg of butorphanol compares favorably with use of 40 to 80 mg of meperidine. The common dosage is 1 mg intravenously or 2 mg for an intramuscular injection. Nausea and vomiting occurs less with butorphanol than with other narcotics. Hence, use of butorphanol is increasing. Respiratory depression appears to be less with the low dosages required with butorphanol.

When analgesic drugs are administered to the woman in labor, the nurse should carefully monitor the woman's vital signs and the fetal heart rate. For patient safety, the bed's side rails should be up after medications have been administered.

Opiate Antagonist

Naloxone (Narcan) is used as an antagonist to the depressing effects of narcotic analgesics. It acts to combat central nervous system and respiratory system depression. There can be a return of depression as long as 6 to 8 hours later because naloxone is metabolized more rapidly than analgesics are.

ANESTHESIA

Anesthetics may provide local or regional numbness and loss of sensation of pain (Table 11–2). Anesthetics may also provide general loss of sensation and consciousness because of varying degrees of central nervous system depression. General anesthesia places the maternity patient at much more risk than regional anesthesia because of aspiration of stomach contents during induction and recovery. Every woman should be made aware of her choices of anesthesia before she signs a consent form.

Regional (Localized) Anesthesia

Regional anesthesia provides pain relief to a localized site while using small amounts of medication with minimal effects on the fetus. The physician, nurse anesthetist, or nurse midwife administers the regional anesthesia. However, the nurse must be able to explain the procedure to the woman and elicit her cooperation while it is being administered. The nurse should assist in monitoring both the maternal and the fetal status after administration. The common types of local anesthesia are local infiltration, pudendal block, paracervical block, epidural or caudal block, and spinal anesthesia. When specific nerves are injected, as in the pudendal and paracervical blocks, only the distribution area of those nerves is affected. In other words, the anesthetic is retained in a localized area (Fig. 11–1).

Local Anesthesia Infiltration. Local anesthesia infiltration in childbirth is an injection of an anesthetic drug (for example, lidocaine 1%) directly into the perineal area, where the episiotomy is made. This injection can be done just before or after the birth of the infant. This procedure is simple and free of complications.

Pudendal Block. A pudendal block is done when the woman is ready for delivery. It is a relatively simple and safe procedure that has no effect on the uterine contractions. The pudendal nerves supplying the perineum are injected with an anesthetic drug, such as lidocaine 1% (Xylocaine) (Fig. 11–2). Pudendal nerve block is performed 10 to 20 minutes before delivery. The most

TABLE 11-2. REGIONAL ANESTHESIA USED DURING LABOR AND BIRTH

TYPE OF BLOCK	PROCEDURE	AREA AFFECTED	WHEN GIVEN	EFFECT OF BLOCK	MAJOR DISADVANTAGES	NURSING INTERVENTIONS
Local infiltration	Local anesthetic injected	Perineum	At time of birth (just before birth of baby)	Causes perineal anesthesia before episiotomy and later for repair of episiotomy	May need large amount of local anesthetic	Instruct patient about method; provide support; assess for perineal edema and trauma
Pudendal	Local anesthetic injected transvaginally into space in front of pudendal nerve	Perineum, vulva, rectal area	Late second stage (just before birth of baby)	Causes perineal anesthesia for repair of episiotomy or lacerations	Broad ligament hematoma	Instruct patient about method; provide support; assess for hematoma
Paracervical	Local anesthetic injected transvaginally adjacent to the outer rim of cervix	Lower uterine segment and cervix and upper 1/3 of vagina	Active labor; lasts about 1 hr; may be repeated	Relieves pain of cervical dilation, does not anesthetize perineum; does not interfere with pushing	Fetal bradycardia; loss of FHR variability	Instruct patient about method; assess maternal BP and pulse; assess FHR; monitor FHR tracing; assess maternal bladder
Epidural	Local anesthetic injected into epidural space	Affects all nerves from the level of the umbilicus to the thighs	Active labor to relieve pain	Relieves discomfort of uterine contractions and fetal descent and anesthetizes perineum	Maternal hypotension; fetal bradycardia; loss of bearing-down reflex in second stage	Instruct patient about method; assess maternal BP and pulse every 15 min; assess FHR; assess maternal bladder at frequent intervals; do not let woman ambulate until all motor control had returned; assess for orthostatic hypotension
Spinal	Local anesthetic injected into spinal fluid	Affects all nerves from the level of the umbilicus to the feet	In late second stage or before cesarean birth; numbs body from waist to feet	Anesthesia given for vaginal birth; or used for cesarean birth	Maternal hypotension; fetal bradycardia; loss of bearing-down reflex in second stage; potential headache	Instruct patient about method; assess maternal signs frequently; assess uterine contractions; assess level of anesthesia; assess FHR tracing; provide safety and prevent injury when woman moves; recognize signs of potential impending birth; maintain bedrest for 6–12 hr after birth

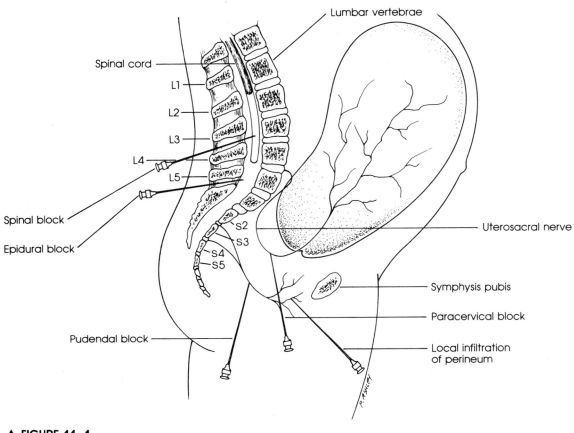

▲ **FIGURE 11–1**

Injection sites of regional anesthetics.

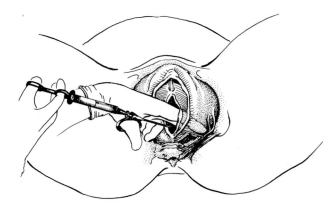

▲ **FIGURE 11–2**

Local infiltration of the pudendal nerve using the transvaginal technique.

common route is transvaginal insertion of a long (5 to 6 inches) needle in a guide into the pudendal nerve vicinity. The anesthetic is injected, on both sides, beneath the inferior tip of the ischial spine. This technique is particularly indicated for women who choose minimal analgesia and anesthesia but need an episiotomy (an incision of the perineum to substitute for a ragged laceration). Drugs such as lidocaine can produce relaxation of the perineum. In addition, the drug reduces pain before the episiotomy is done and often lasts through the repair of the episiotomy. The relaxation of the perineum can hasten the delivery, decreasing the time of the woman's discomfort.

Paracervical Block. In a paracervical block, nerve pathways from the uterus are blocked during labor. This measure relieves the pain of cervical dilation but does not anesthetize the lower vagina or perineum. It is given in the active stage of labor.

There are disadvantages to paracervical block. The perineum is not anesthetized, and another type of anesthesia must be added for delivery. More important, paracervical block has been found to cause *fetal bradycardia* (decreased fetal heart rate), decreased fetal viability, and fetal acidosis; therefore, it is rarely recommended for labor.

It is common for fetal bradycardia to occur after a paracervical block. It has been suggested that fetal bradycardia after this procedure is due to uterine artery spasm, causing decreased intervillous space blood flow and fetal hypoxia. It is mandatory that continuous electronic fetal heart rate monitoring be done and the woman's vital signs taken frequently. In most cases, a healthy fetus will tolerate the asphyxia that may accompany the paracervical block.

Epidural Block. Epidural block is also referred to as the *lumbar epidural block.* The anesthetic is injected into the epidural space, which is located inside the vertebral column surrounding the dural sac in the lumbar region of the spine. An epidural block provides regional anesthesia during the first and second stages of labor. A one-time medication injection may be done. A technique also used is continuous infusion of a dilute anesthetic with an infusion controller or pump. The infusion pump ensures a precise flow rate of the medication. The drug used in an epidural block, bupivacaine (Marcaine), is longer lasting than lidocaine or mepivacaine, and therefore should be used in a dilute dosage of 0.25% to 0.05% (lidocaine and mepivacaine are used in 1% dosage). The anesthetic reactions include central nervous system and cardiovascular components such as serious arrhythmias and marked cardiovascular depression. Because of the long-acting effect of bupivacaine, resuscitation of patients who experience undesirable cardiovascular effects is more difficult.

The administration of an epidural block requires special training and expertise by an obstetrician or anesthesiologist. The patient is positioned on her left side, with her legs partially flexed. The lumbar region is cleansed and draped. A needle or a catheter, if continuous, can be inserted in the epidural space in the lumbar region.

There are disadvantages to the epidural block. Because the catheter can go into the spinal column, the emergency cart should be readily available for cardiorespiratory resuscitation. In addition, epidural anesthesia can cause hypotension and a reduction in uteroplacental perfusion, which can cause fetal bradycardia. Finally, use of an epidural block increases the chances of a forceps delivery.

Nursing responsibilities include taking the vital signs every 5 minutes, observing the woman carefully to ensure that spinal anesthesia has not been given inadvertently, assessing the fetal electronic monitor tracing every 5 minutes, and immediately reporting to the physician any untoward cardiorespiratory signs.

Spinal Anesthesia. Spinal anesthesia (saddle block) is a type of anesthesia used primarily for delivery. It is given late in the second stage of labor. The anesthesia is injected into the dura of the spinal canal. The woman must sit still, with her head down and her lower back arched during the procedure (Fig. 11–3). She is asked to remain sitting (upright position) for 3 to 5 minutes to ensure that the anesthesia does not travel to the respiratory area. As with an epidural block, hypotension may result, followed by fetal bradycardia. Frequent monitoring of vital signs is important. Because the woman cannot feel her uterine contractions, she must be carefully observed so she does not deliver in bed without assistance.

After delivery, a temporary motor paralysis is present in the woman's legs. She usually remains in bed for about 6 hours after the block to prevent a headache caused by leakage of cerebrospinal fluid. The incidence of the postspinal headache

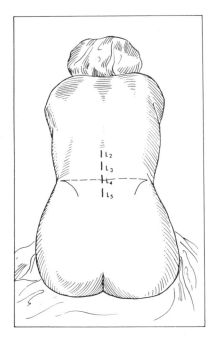

▲ FIGURE 11–3

Positioning for spinal anesthesia.

has decreased with the use of smaller-gauge needles. The woman may not have the sensation of urination and may need to be catheterized. The woman's vital signs should be observed until she is stable.

General Anesthesia

General anesthesia is often referred to as inhalation anesthesia. It is no longer an anesthesia of choice because of the danger it presents to the baby as well as the woman. It is most often used in emergency cesarean sections.

General anesthesia relieves pain through the loss of consciousness. The anesthetic drug may be administered by inhalation or intravenous infusion. This type of anesthesia provides immediate pain relief but crosses the placenta rapidly; therefore, the infant can be depressed. General anesthesia puts the woman at risk of regurgitation and aspiration of gastric contents. The physiological changes in the gastrointestinal tract during pregnancy include decreased gastric motility and delayed gastric emptying. The gastric contents are highly acidic and produce chemical pneumonitis if aspirated. Every woman in labor should be viewed as having a stomachful of hydrochloric acid. Because of this, prophylactic antacid therapy before administration of general anesthesia has become common practice.

Because of the risk of aspiration, the placement of an endotracheal tube is essential with the use of mask general anesthesia. Also, the woman should be preoxygenated. A continuous intravenous infusion is important so that access to the intravascular system is immediately possible.

Summary

Labor pains exist for only a short time. However, within that short time the discomfort progresses from a slightly unpleasant experience to intense sensations. To the woman in labor, the discomfort or pain may seem endless. She may wonder if she can tolerate it. To the nurse, the process of labor is a challenge. Armed with knowledge of the causes of pain in the various stages of labor and interventions for pain relief and comfort, the nurse designs a plan of care for the woman (see Nursing Care Plan 11–1). Working with the woman, family, and other health professionals,

NURSING CARE PLAN 11–1

PAIN RELIEF DURING LABOR

Potential Problems and Nursing Diagnoses	Nursing Interventions
1. Pain: Alteration in comfort related to labor and birth.	Discuss patient's/couple's knowledge regarding factors that influence pain during labor.
2. Knowledge deficit related to nonpharmacological comfort techniques during labor and birth.	Review nonpharmacological methods of coping with discomfort during labor and birth.
	Demonstrate and assist with breathing techniques appropriate for each stage of labor.
	Provide back massage, counterpressure, hot or cold compresses.
	Provide distraction (such as music)
3. Potential for (fetal) injury related to analgesics, sedatives, and narcotics.	Provide information about effect of drugs on baby, such as fetal distress.
	Support woman's/couple's decisions regarding choice of pain management.
	Administer ordered analgesic and monitor maternal and fetal response.
	Communicate with woman about expected sensations.
	Monitor maternal and fetal vital signs frequently.
	Record on fetal monitor strip and chart the type of drug given, the amount, and the route.
4. Altered tissue perfusion with decrease in fetal heart rate.	Recognize that some regional anesthetics can produce maternal hypotension and fetal bradycardia, such as paracervical and epidural blocks.
	Record time of administration on fetal monitor strip.
	Report changes to physician.

Expected Outcomes

1. Woman verbalizes factors that influence pain and discomfort during labor, such as cervical dilatation and uterine contractions.
2. Woman expresses relief obtained from breathing techniques, focusing, and cutaneous stimulation.
3. Woman expresses relief obtained from the pain medication given and exhibits appropriate coping behaviors, with use of medication and breathing techniques.
4. Fetal heart rate tracing is stable. Patient maintains stable blood pressure.

the nurse can meet the challenge of making each delivery a safe and a more pleasant birth experience.

References

Bucknell, S., & Sikorski, K. (1989). Putting patient-controlled analgesia to the test. *American Journal of Maternal-Child Nursing*, 14:37–40.

Dickason, E. J., Schult, M. O., & Silverman, B. L. (1990). *Maternal-Infant Nursing Care*. St. Louis: C. V. Mosby.

Henrikson, M. L., & Wild, L. R. (1988). A nursing process approach to epidural analgesia. *Journal of Obstetric, Gynecologic, and Neonatal Nursing*. 17:316–319.

Ladewig, P. W., London, M. L., & Olds, S. B. (1990). *Essentials of Maternal-Newborn Nursing*, 2nd ed. Redwood City, CA: Addison-Wesley Nursing.

SUGGESTED ACTIVITIES

1. Explain nonpharmacological ways to reduce discomfort during labor.
2. Identify different types of regional anesthesia given during labor. Discuss their effects on the infant.

REVIEW QUESTIONS

Select the best answer to each multiple-choice question.

1. During labor, the woman can be relieved of pain by nonpharmacological means, including
   A. Cutaneous stimulation
   B. Systemic relaxation
   C. Focusing of attention
   D. All of the above

2. Medications that relieve anxiety and apprehension are called
   A. Amnesic narcotics
   B. Tanquilizers
   C. Narcotic antagonists
   D. Barbiturates

3. The mother's blood pressure should be taken frequently to identify hypotension during
   A. Epidural anesthesia
   B. Local anesthesia
   C. Pudendal block
   D. Effleurage

4. The woman near time of delivery will continue to feel uterine contractions when administered all of the following EXCEPT
   A. Pudendal block
   B. Spinal anesthesia
   C. Paracervical block
   D. Local infiltration

5. The anesthesia used for repair of the perineum after an episiotomy is called
   A. Pudendal block
   B. Local infiltration
   C. Epidural block
   D. Paracervical block

6. The drug NOT given to the laboring woman to reduce anxiety because it can severely affect infant respiration and produce poor infant muscle tone is
   A. Hydroxyzine (Vistaril)
   B. Promethazine (Phenergan)
   C. Promazine (Sparine)
   D. Diazepam (Valium)

7. A natural pain inhibitor that originates in the body is
   A. An opiate
   B. An endorphin
   C. A tranquilizer
   D. An exogenous substance

8. Choose the block(s) that is (are) NOT associated with fetal bradycardia:
   A. Pudendal
   B. Paracervical
   C. Lumbar epidural
   D. None of the above

9. Disadvantages of an epidural block include
   A. The drug can go into the spinal column
   B. Maternal hypotension may result
   C. Fetal bradycardia can occur
   D. Chances of forceps delivery are increased
   E. All of the above

10. After the anesthesiologist injects the medications into an epidural catheter, the nurse must immediately check for
    A. Hypotension and fetal distress
    B. Change in the intensity of contractions
    C. Complaints of thirst and anxiety
    D. Signs of nausea

11. A narcotic antagonist that is used to counteract infant respiratory depression is
    A. Demerol
    B. Narcan
    C. Marcaine
    D. Pitocin

CHAPTER 12 _____

Chapter Outline

Nursing Assessments and Interventions During Admission
    to the Labor Suite
      Admission questions and decisions
      Admission procedures
Psychological Support During Labor and Birth
      Psychological/sociocultural assessment
Potential Nursing Diagnoses and Expected Outcomes
  During Labor
Physical Support, Assessment, and Interventions During
  Labor and Birth
Provision of Care During the Four Stages of Labor
      First stage (three phases)
      Second stage (birth of the baby)
      Third stage
      Fourth stage (immediate recovery)
Provision of Initial Care to the Newborn by the Nurse
Emergency Delivery by the Nurse (Without a Physician
  or Midwife)
Alternative Birth Settings
      In-hospital birthing rooms
      Out-of-hospital birthing centers
      Home birth

Learning Objectives

Upon completion of Chapter 12, the student should be
able to
- Describe the nurse's role in the woman's admission
  to the labor suite.
- State the importance of the admitting nurse's establishing rapport with the woman and family.
- List three admission questions and the rationale for
  each.
- List five procedures commonly performed when a
  woman is admitted in labor.
- Describe different procedures, such as the perineal
  prep.
- Explain why oral fluids and solid food intake may be
  withheld during labor.
- List three nursing assessments and interventions dur-
  ing each stage of labor.
- Explain the importance of not allowing bladder dis-
  tention during labor.
- State the significance of psychological support dur-
  ing labor.
- Name ways to protect the woman from infection.
- Describe signs characteristic of the transitional stage
  of labor.
- Identify principles of aseptic technique used in the
  delivery room.
- Describe the cleansing of the woman's perineum
  before delivery.
- List four items important to record about the birth
  itself.
- Name a common oxytocic drug given to reduce
  blood loss.
- Outline how maternal–infant bonding can be en-
  couraged after birth.
- Describe alternative birth settings.

Nursing Care During Labor and Birth

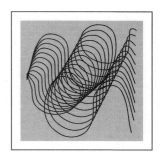

At no time in the childbearing cycle is the nurse's role more important than during labor and birth. Although the woman and her partner have waited long hours for the time when she would be in labor and give birth to the baby, this period can be overwhelming to them because of the many unfamiliar procedures and complicated technology facing them.

The nurse is in a position to be a support person and caregiver at one of the most exciting and important hours in the lives of the new family. How the nurse communicates to the expectant mother will make a difference in how the mother perceives being treated—as a person or as a "machine." The nurse can establish a positive relationship with the expectant mother by providing privacy, explaining each procedure before it is carried out, and caring for her in an unhurried manner.

Nursing Assessments and Interventions During Admission to the Labor Suite

Admission of a woman to the delivery suite entails standard nursing assessments and interventions. However, policies vary with different institutions. The woman should be given a preference when possible. For example, if a birthing room is an option, she should be able to choose that option over the traditional labor and delivery room.

Certain admission procedures are conducted as soon as the woman is admitted to the labor suite. They include

1. Placing an identification bracelet on the woman
2. Obtaining necessary information for the labor record
3. Taking vital signs: temperature, pulse, respirations, and blood pressure
4. Listening to the fetal heart rate
5. Taking care of the mother's clothing and other personal items
6. Assessing the progress of labor
7. Preparing the mother for labor and delivery

ADMISSION QUESTIONS AND DECISIONS

Immediately after admission, several questions are asked to obtain general information. These questions, and the rationale for each, are presented in Table 12–1. At this time, the nurse should orient the woman and her partner to the labor suite. Basic information such as how to adjust the bed position, how to summon assistance, and the location of the early-labor lounge area for ambulation should be given.

Some of the management decisions made at the time of admission depend on the physician's or midwife's routines. In some places, the woman is asked about her preference in some of the procedures. Decisions are made about the following:

1. Whether to give the woman an enema
2. Whether the woman is to have a perineal shave and, if so, what kind
3. Whether the woman can have fluids by mouth and, if so, precisely what is allowed
4. The frequency with which the woman's vital signs are checked
5. The frequency with which the fetal heart rate is checked and how this will be done

TABLE 12—1. ADMISSION QUESTIONS AND RATIONALES

QUESTIONS	RATIONALE
Name?	To immediately establish open communication.
When is baby due?	To determine if baby is full term or preterm.
What baby (first, second, etc.)?	To determine parity and length of labor.
Any medical problems during this pregnancy (bleeding, elevated blood pressure, etc.)?	To provide quick assessment of potential risks.
Any special tests during this pregnancy (ultrasonograph, blood tests)?	To provide information about potential risks to baby.
Any allergies (medications, food)?	To determine contraindications to medications or other substances.
Any problems with other pregnancies (bleeding, type of delivery, baby's health status)?	To determine if previous problems may be relevant to this birth.
When did labor start (frequency and duration contractions, bag of water rupture, bloody "show")?	To obtain basic information about progress of labor.
When was solid food last eaten?	To provide information if surgery is needed.

6. Identification of the woman's partner and his role

7. Whether the woman can ambulate

ADMISSION PROCEDURES

Physical Examination

Physical findings provide valuable information on which to base nursing care. Necessary information includes inspection (assessment), auscultation (listening), and palpation (feeling). These actions may be carried out by more than one person. A head-to-toe physical examination should be done. In addition, laboratory tests should be carried out. If a preadmission record is available, it will give information such as blood type and Rh factor determination.

Vital Signs

A maternal blood pressure of 140/90 or higher (or systolic increase of 30+ mm or diastolic in-

crease of 15+ mm) is of concern because of potential preeclampsia. Increased pulse and respiration rates may be indicative of stress, infection, or dehydration. A temperature elevation may indicate either infection or dehydration. Vital signs not within the normal range should be reported immediately to the physician or nurse midwife for modification of management.

Uterine Contractions

It is necessary to know the intensity, frequency, and duration of the woman's labor contractions. An assessment of labor contractions is described in Chapter 10. If the contractions are frequent and intense (strong) and if the woman has a previous history of short labor, the nurse will likely modify routine procedures accordingly.

Abdominal Palpation

By using abdominal palpation, the nurse can ascertain the position, presentation, and engagement of the fetus (see Chapter 6). Sometimes, abdominal palpation will reveal a multiple pregnancy at the time of admission. Also, because fetal heart tones are usually best heard through the fetus's back, determining the location of the back is helpful in finding them (Fig. 12–1).

Fetal Heart Rate

The fetal heart rate (FHR) provides important information about the fetal status. Normally, the FHR ranges between 120 and 160 beats per minute (bpm). Immediately upon admission, intermittent FHR monitoring is done (see Chapter 5). This is usually followed by continuous electronic fetal monitoring (see Chapter 8).

Vaginal Examination

Vaginal examinations are preferred over rectal examinations because they provide more accurate information. Cervical dilation and effacement, amniotic membrane status (ruptured or intact), position of the fetus, and station (degree of descent) can be determined by vaginal examination (Fig.

12–2). In other words, the progress of labor can be assessed. Aseptic technique should be conscientiously carried out when the procedure is done. Vaginal examinations must *not* be done when there is excessive bleeding, because if placenta previa or abruptio placentae exists, a fatal hemorrhage may result.

Perineal Shave

The perineal shave may be partial or full removal of hair. A full shave removes all of the hair from the perineum (hair on the mons pubis and from the vagina downward to the anus). A mini-preparation consists of shaving the hair between the lower border of the vagina downward to the anus. The mini-prep has replaced the complete shave. Sometimes, shaving of hair is omitted (no preparation is done). The purpose of shaving the hair is to provide a field for delivery that has a reduced bacteria-harboring potential. A preparation should be done with minimum discomfort and maximum privacy for the woman. Disposable shave kits are commonly used with Betadine or soapsuds. The important principle in doing the procedure is to stroke downward, from the clean to the unclean

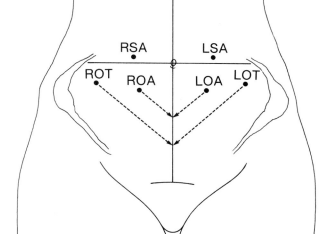

▲ **FIGURE 12–1**

Fetal heart tone locations on woman's abdomen, corresponding to fetal positions. RSA, right sacrum anterior; ROT, right occiput transverse; ROA, right occiput anterior; LSA, left sacrum anterior; LOT, left occiput transverse; LOA, left occiput anterior.

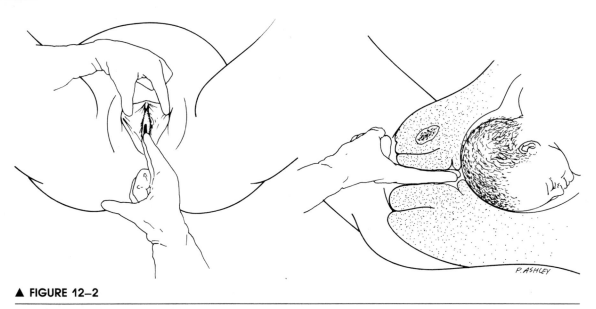

▲ **FIGURE 12–2**

Vaginal examination to determine dilation, effacement, and station.

areas. It is important *not* to contaminate the vagina or urinary meatus by passing over the rectum first.

Enema

Different types of enemas used during labor include a soapsuds enema, a tapwater enema, and a prepared enema (Fleet enema). The factors involved in deciding whether an enema should be given are the speed of the labor's progress, the amount of cervical dilatation, the status of lower bowel (presence of feces), the need for stimulation, and the woman's or physician's preference. An enema should not be given in cases of premature labor, unexplained vaginal bleeding, or breech presentation. Also, an enema is not given if the amniotic sac is ruptured.

When the nurse administers the enema, the woman should lie on her side while the solution is passed slowly into the rectum. Should a contraction occur while the enema is given, the flow of fluid should be stopped with the tubing left in place; after the contraction ends, the solution is begun again. The woman frequently is allowed to expel the enema in the bathroom, if her mem-

branes are intact (have not ruptured). If the woman's contractions are intense and frequent, or if she feels dizzy, the health care provider should stay nearby and assist the woman back to bed. The type of enema, the time it was given, and results should be noted on the woman's chart.

Psychological Support During Labor and Birth

Because the physical needs of the woman are the most apparent, it is easy to emphasize the physical aspect of care and neglect the psychological area of care. However, recognition of the importance of the psychological needs of the woman in labor has changed some hospital policies.

The goal of psychological care is to make labor a more pleasant and a satisfying experience and to allow more family participation. This can affect the course of labor, and the woman's attitude toward the father, the infant, and future pregnancies.

The nurse is in a key position to encourage the father or significant other to participate in the birth process. Nursing measures should be directed toward the promotion of self-confidence and reduction of fear. The mother must be reminded to rest between contractions. In addition, comfort measures (for example, wiping the woman's face with a cold, wet cloth) should be included in labor care. It is important that the nurse make every effort to keep the woman and her family informed about her labor progress.

PSYCHOLOGICAL/SOCIOCULTURAL ASSESSMENT

The following interventions are used to meet the psychological needs of the woman in labor:

1. Establish a therapeutic (caring) relationship with the woman and significant other.
2. Assess the degree of anxiety. If possible, prevent escalation of anxiety and fear to panic levels.
3. Assess the effectiveness of coping skills and behaviors.
   - Reinforce behaviors that facilitate positive feelings about labor's progress.
   - Modify less desirable behavior, such as loss of control.
4. Provide a PERSON-based support system.
   - Encourage participation of significant other.
   - Coach woman through labor.
5. Assess sensory stimulation:
   - Environmental stimuli: if not in a private room, encourage privacy by pulling drapes, etc.
   - Auditory stimuli: use a soothing voice when talking with woman: use music appropriately.
   - Visual stimuli: use eye-to-eye contact whenever possible to increase the sense of caring.
   - Touch: hold woman's hand, apply sacral pressure, or try rhythmic, soft rubbing of abdomen (effleurage).
6. Convey sincere concern and regard for well-being of mother and baby.

7. Recognize the woman's desire for independence in early labor and dependence in later labor (allow her to make decisions).
8. Facilitate maternal–infant attachment.
   - Allow mother to touch baby and see all fingers and toes immediately after birth (this will reassure mother infant is normal).
   - If the woman has decided to breastfeed her baby, encourage her to nurse the baby (get acquainted) right after birth.
9. Encourage the woman's labor experience to be integrated into a meaningful whole. Praise her cooperation.

Potential Nursing Diagnoses and Expected Outcomes During Labor

A number of problems may occur during labor. The nurse should determine the physical and psychological needs of the couple (the woman and her partner) and intervene to meet them. Nothing should be thought of as routine during the labor experience. The health of the mother and baby, the supportive role of the coach, and the mother's self-direction should be goals of nursing care. Nursing measures should support and facilitate the birth process and decrease the need for unnecessary medical interventions. Nursing measures that promote physical comfort should lessen anxiety and discomfort from medical procedures. Pertinent nursing diagnoses may be selected for each woman and her partner.

POTENTIAL NURSING DIAGNOSES DURING LABOR

- Impaired verbal communication related to inability to understand medical terminology or English
- Knowledge deficit related to the labor process
- Anxiety related to uncertain outcome of labor and birth
- Altered comfort related to pain during contractions

- Altered patterns of urinary elimination
- Ineffective coping related to age of mothers in young mothers and in those with prior negative experiences, with the stress of labor
- Altered nutrition: less than body requirements related to lack of nutrient intake
- Fluid volume deficit related to lack of fluid intake
- Altered uterine tissue perfusion related to strong uterine contractions
- Self-esteem disturbance related to body exposure
- Sleep pattern disturbance

EXPECTED OUTCOMES

- Verbalizes an understanding of the labor process
- Relates coping measures that can be used
- Understands the reason for the nursing interventions
- Verbalizes an understanding of medical interventions such as intravenous administration of fluids to keep from becoming dehydrated
- Verbalizes importance of the coach and appropriate support measures

Physical Support, Assessment, and Interventions During Labor and Birth

In addition to creating an environment of trust and security, meeting informational needs, promoting relaxation, and providing a support system, the nurse must address specific physical concerns throughout labor. All of these nursing assessments begin during the first stage and continue throughout the labor. The following nursing actions are important:

Monitor Maternal Vital Signs. It is important to know the baseline measurements and report significant changes. Monitoring vital signs includes taking the woman's blood pressure every 2 hours until active labor begins, then assessing blood pressure every 1 hour or 30 minutes. An elevation of blood pressure, especially the diastolic, is suggestive of preeclampsia. An elevated pulse rate may indicate hemorrhage or infection. Slowing of respirations may be due to an overload or toxicity of medication. This side effect can reduce the amount of oxygen the infant receives.

Monitor Fetal Status. The FHR should be assessed at least every 15 minutes if the woman is not being electronically monitored. An FHR outside the range of 120 to 160 bpm or a sudden change in FHR should be reported immediately. Also, FHR should be taken immediately after the rupture of membranes. The nurse should be familiar with normal FHR patterns when continuous electronic monitoring is done (see Chapter 8). If the woman is not electronically monitored, the FHR should be taken with a fetoscope between contractions.

Assess Status of Amniotic Fluid. It is important to know whether the membranes have ruptured or are intact. The time of rupture should be recorded because of the risk of infection to the mother and infant after rupture. At the time of rupture, the color of the fluid should be noted. Meconium stained fluid accompanied by cephalic (head first) presentation is indicative of fetal distress.

Monitor Uterine Contractions. One way to judge whether labor is progressing normally is to observe the pattern of uterine contractions. A summary of the frequency, duration, and intensity of contractions should be recorded on the woman's chart every hour. For example, one may observe and record that contractions occur every 2 or 3 minutes, with a duration of 35 to 40 seconds, and with strong intensity. The nurse should report when the contractions become weaker, shorter, and less frequent or when the contractions are almost continuous, with no relaxation between them.

Observe Eliminative Needs (Bladder Care). An important assessment in labor care is bladder distention. The woman should be encouraged to void at frequent intervals throughout labor, at least every 2 hours. A careful record should be kept of the amount and time of each voiding. A full bladder can prevent the descent of the baby and can predispose the woman to urinary stasis and infection. Also, it can cause an increased discomfort during labor. A full bladder can be palpated in the lower abdomen.

Give Enema if Appropriate. An enema may be

given to empty the lower bowel. In addition, it may stimulate peristalsis, causing the uterus to contract. A woman in advanced labor is not given an enema because she may only partly expel the enema before delivery, then contaminate the field by expelling feces at the time the baby is born.

Provide Protection from Dehydration. Ice chips or oral fluids should be given as tolerated and if allowed. In some hospitals, nothing is given by mouth (NPO) throughout labor. The NPO policy is designed to lessen the chance of aspiration (with possible later occurrence of pneumonia) if general anesthesia is given. Intravenous infusion of 5% dextrose and water is commonly ordered. It is important to maintain an open intravenous infusion to avoid dehydration and nutrient depletion.

Provide Protection from Aspiration. Vomiting is common during the active and transitional phases of labor. Positioning is important to facilitate drainage. The woman's head should be turned to one side during vomiting. The emesis basin should be readily available. Gastric contents may be present as long as 36 hours after an ingested meal. In addition ·to aspiration, the acidity of gastric contents creates a risk for the woman. Some women are given prophylactic antacid therapy to keep the gastric contents as neutral as possible.

Provide Protection from Infection. Strict asepsis in procedures involving skin penetration should be used. Perineal cleansing should be carried out after each voiding, defecation, and vaginal examination. Sterile technique should be carried out during artificial rupture of membranes, venipuncture, and internal electronic monitoring because all of these procedures provide potential sites for infection.

Because sexually transmitted diseases (STDs) involve blood, amniotic fluid, and other secretions, *health care providers should use the Centers for Disease Control (CDC) universal precautions* (see Chapter 7) to protect the woman as well as themselves.

Provide Protection from Injury. One of the most important nursing actions is to keep the bed's side rails up to avoid injury for all women who have been medicated with analgesics, tranquilizers, or anesthetics. Uncluttered passageway for the woman with bathroom capability and adequate lighting reduce risk of falling. Assistance should be provided as needed for the woman when she ambulates to the bathroom.

Assess Woman's Discomfort—Use Comfort Measures. Many nursing actions can decrease the woman's discomfort. Positioning is important. The woman should assume the position that promotes relaxation and comfort. Lying on the side should be encouraged to decrease obstruction of gravid uterus on large blood vessels, facilitate renal blood flow, and promote more effective uterine contractions.

Back rubs enhance relaxation and stimulate circulation. Sacral support—applying firm, constant pressure with the palm of the hand on the lower curvature of the back—often decreases the discomfort. Effleurage, a rhythmic soft rubbing of the abdominal area in a circular fashion, may provide comfort. A cool cloth or facial sponge applied to the woman's forehead can decrease heat at that part of the body and decrease warmth and sweating. Attention focusing, as a form of distraction, is often useful. Dryness of the lips and mouth may be relieved by a lemon and glycerine sponge stick. When the membranes are ruptured, the bed linens should be changed frequently to decrease friction on the skin. If the woman lies on her back she should be observed for supine hypotension syndrome.

Administer Medication if Appropriate. As labor progresses, some women need medication so they can relax. Medication should not be given until the cervix is dilated to 4 cm or the labor is well established. It is important to chart the time and amount given. The woman's respirations and the fetal heart rate should be assessed before administration of medication and at frequent intervals afterwards to see if change occurs after giving the medication.

Assess Fetal Status. If electronic monitoring is not available for continuous monitoring of fetal heart rate (FHR), the FHR should be checked frequently. In particular, FHR should be checked immediately after rupture of membranes to assess for cord prolapse.

When a woman is on an electronic fetal monitor, the nurse should closely observe the FHR tracing. The nurse should report signs of fetal distress to the physician or midwife immediately. These signs are (a) loss of baseline variability, (b) variable or late decelerations that persist after maternal position change, or (c) persistent tachycardia (see Chapter 8). Also, meconium in amniotic fluid when the baby is in a vertex position should be reported (see Chapter 8).

Provision of Care During the Four Stages of Labor

FIRST STAGE (THREE PHASES)

Latent Phase

In the first phase of the first stage of labor, the woman is often excited that she is in labor (Table 12–2). For many women, a significant portion of the latent phase is spent at home. Her coping behaviors include smiling, laughing, talking, and crying. If she is unprepared and fearful about her labor experience, she may exhibit anxiety and concern. During this phase, the involuntary, intermittent contractions are usually mild. Because of this, cervical dilatation is slow (0 to 3 cm). The woman frequently has a desire to be independent, to participate, and to make decisions. Often she seeks information about her labor experience. Therefore, this period is an ideal time for instructing the woman about what is going to happen as labor progresses. The nurse can review the bodily sensations that will be felt and measures by which the woman can best help herself. If she can remain calm and use suggested breathing techniques, her labor will likely be shorter and present less discomfort (see Fig. 9–3).

Active Phase

During the active phase, the contractions become more frequent and intense. The woman usually experiences discomfort from the stretching and dilation of the cervix. Also, she may feel the pull of the supporting structures (ligaments) of the uterus. Her cervix dilates from 4 to 8 cm. Dependency is often manifested, and the woman desires constant companionship. She may begin to feel nauseated and physically uncomfortable. The woman's behavior frequently includes ill-defined doubts and fears. She may become quite restless. The significant other, if present, can be of assistance by rubbing her back, reminding her of breathing techniques, and encouraging her to rest between contractions. If the woman does not have a companion, the nurse should stay with her, if possible, and be her support person. Near the end of the active phase, it is important for the

nurse to talk slowly, clearly, and exactly to the woman and give her undivided attention.

Transition Phase

The transition phase is a difficult time for the woman. The contractions continue to become more frequent and intense. The woman feels discomfort from the stretching of the cervix (8 to 10 cm) to complete dilation. In addition, there is distention and stretching of the muscles of the pelvic floor and perineum. The woman should be instructed that labor's progress is not enhanced by increased intraabdominal pressure (bearing-down efforts) until cervical dilatation is complete. If bearing-down or "pushing" begins too soon, she needs to be told that the cervix can become edematous and impede labor. After complete cervical dilation, the fetal head (presenting part) descends, and the perineum begins to thin out and bulge. At this time, the woman may be asked to push to enhance the descent of the baby. When the baby's head can be seen, the term "crowning" is used. The baby's head is now near the outlet.

During the transition phase, the woman's behavior frequently changes. Her perceptual field is greatly narrowed and learning is difficult. She needs repetition on focusing and breathing techniques with each contraction, and she should be encouraged to rest between them. The woman's face often becomes flushed and beaded with perspiration. She may have a loss of inhibition and uncover herself. Frequently, she exhibits shaking and trembling of her lower extremities and states she cannot relax. The woman may show great fear and ask, "Am I going to be all right?" or state, "I can't go on."

Throughout the transition phase it is important for the nurse to keep the woman, and partner, informed about her progress and praise her for her efforts. The use of breathing techniques and comfort measures is very important during this phase. If medication is needed, it should be given a minimum of 1 hour before the anticipated birth of the baby. Because the woman desires a healthy baby, her discomfort tolerance may improve if informed why the drugs are withheld. During this phase some women demonstrate panic and uncontrollable behavior. They may be uncooperative and quite aggressive. It is important for the nurse

Text continued on page 214

STAGES OF LABOR	BEHAVIOR OF WOMAN	CHARACTERISTICS	INTERVENTION
First Stage *Main goals:* complete dilatation of cervix; descent of fetus			
Latent phase: 0–3 cm	Excited Sense of anticipation Sense of relief Happy Some apprehension	Uterine contractions mild (30–50 sec) May or may not follow regular pattern Abdominal discomfort Back ache Possible rupture of membranes "Show" (blood-tinged mucoid vaginal discharge)	Complete admission procedures Monitor maternal vital signs (BP, pulse, respiration, temperature) Monitor FHR Assess status of amniotic fluid (if membrane intact or ruptured) Observe voiding (time and amount) Assess coping ability (anxiety) Encourage walking (if membranes are intact) Encourage visiting, watching TV Encourage relaxation If lying down, change side positions every half hour Effleurage (if woman does not have significant other or wants caregiver to do it)
Active phase: 4–7 cm *Main goal:* descent of presenting part toward the cervical os (downward)	Apprehensive Ill-defined doubts and fears Desire for companionship Uncertain if she can cope with contractions	Uterine contractions stronger, longer, and more frequent (45–60 sec) Uterine contractions cause discomfort	Continue to monitor maternal vital signs and FHR every 15 min Assess status of amniotic fluid (if membrane intact or ruptured) Encourage voiding every hour Observe for full bladder Assess progress of labor (cervical dilatation) Provide comfort measures: Moisten lips or give ice chips Apply cool, damp cloth to woman's face Keep bed linens dry Effleurage Sacral support Oral hygiene Encourage significant other's support Inform woman (and significant other) about labor progress Administer medication, if ordered Explain electronic fetal monitor to woman Encourage woman to continue with focal point and breathing technique Protect woman from infection by frequent perineal care *Table continued on following page*

STAGES OF LABOR	BEHAVIOR OF WOMAN	CHARACTERISTICS	INTERVENTION
First Stage (Continued)			Protect woman from aspiration (if vomits)
			Protect woman from injury (if given medication)
Transition phase: 8–10 cm	Quite apprehensive	Uterine contractions stronger, lasting 60–90 sec, every 1–2 min apart	Continue nursing interventions from active phase
Main goal: Continued descent of fetus	Bewildered by intensity of contractions		Recognize this phase is difficult time for woman
	Irritable to touch	Amnesia between contractions	Caregiver or significant other needs to take charge: "Watch what I do"
	Frustrated and unable to cope with contractions if left alone	Cramps in legs	
		Generalized discomfort	Demonstrate breathing technique with each contraction
	Eager to have medication for pain	Hiccoughing and sometimes belching	DO NOT leave woman alone
	Unable to continue suggested breathing without being reminded	Marked restlessness and irritability	Accept behavior of throwing covers off, and so forth
		Nausea and/or vomiting	Encourage woman by telling her how well she is doing
	Unable to comprehend directions readily	Increased pain with contractions	Use touch relaxation
	Hot and cold flashes	Perspiration on upper lip and forehead (face)	Change Chux (pad) frequently
			Keep bed linen dry
		Increased dark, heavy vaginal show	Get blanket if woman feels cold
		Pulling or stretching sensation deep in pelvis	Use cold cloth to head when woman feels hot
		Rupture of membranes may occur (sometimes previously)	
		Severe, low back ache	
		Trembling of legs	
		Beginning of urge to push	
		Desire for medication; feels she "cannot go on"	
Second Stage	More involved with birth process	Full dilatation of cervix	Assess FHR after each contraction (if not on monitor)
Complete cervical dilatation (10 cm) to birth of baby	Relief baby is almost ready for birth	Contractions of 60–90 sec duration every 2–3 min, with urge to push	Assess contractions for frequency, duration and intensity
Main goals: descent of presenting part; fetal rotation; birth	Desire to push		Assess progress of labor
	Satisfaction with each push (when told baby is coming)	Increased vaginal show	When ready for delivery room, assist in transfer
	Complete exhaustion after expulsive contraction	Rectal and vaginal bulging with flattening of perineum	Set up for delivery (if not done); use sterile technique

STAGES OF LABOR	BEHAVIOR OF WOMAN	CHARACTERISTICS	INTERVENTION

Second Stage
(Continued)
	Unable to follow directions
	"Splitting" sensation due to extreme vaginal stretching as baby is born
	Desire to participate if prepared for childbirth
		Amnesia between contractions
		Gradual (or sudden) appearance of presenting part at vaginal opening
		Episiotomy may be done by physcian or nurse midwife
			Cleanse vulvar and perineal area using downward strokes (use hospital kit)
			Support woman (if no significant other present)
			Provide necessary materials and equipment (sterile gloves and so forth)
			Provide equipment for episiotomy repair
			Give immediate care to infant after birth
			   Dry infant
			   Assess infant; identify infant; place in warm incubator or on mother's abdomen
			   Apgar score by caregiver at 1 and 5 min
			Assess mother for hemorrhage (take BP, pulse, respirations)

Third Stage Placental stage *Main goals:* expulsion of placenta; prevention of hemorrhage	Exhausted but elated baby is born Eager to hear and see baby Sense of relief Hungry Thirsty	Contractions temporarily cease after birth Then 2–3 contractions to expel placenta Upward rise of uterus in abdomen Uterus assumes globular shape Visible lengthening of umbilical cord Trickle or gush of blood	Assess woman's vital signs (BP, pulse, respirations) Assess for excessive bleeding Provide materials for episiotomy repair After physician or nurse midwife is through, take woman's legs down from stirrups slowly and together (if legs were elevated to avoid muscle strain) Take mother to recovery room (if in traditional facilities Nursing assessment and intervention is directed toward prevention of hemorrhage

Fourth Stage
Immediate recovery period (1 hr)
Main goals: prevent hemorrhage; facilitate maternal-infant bonding (attachment)
	Exhausted but happy labor is over
	Eager to get acquainted with baby
	Hungry
	Thirsty
	Sleepy
		Rest	Assess:
			   Fundus location (height) and consistency (if not firm, massage and report)
			   Lochia amount, color, odor
			   Vital signs: BP, pulse, temperature
			   Perineum: episiotomy for edema, hematoma
			   State of hydration
			   Bladder: observe for distention
			   Fatigue and exhaustion (provide atmosphere for rest)
			If hospital policy allows, let mother get acquainted with baby; allow significant other to be with woman

to accept these maternal behaviors. On later communication with the woman, reference should not be made to negative behavior, but rather the nurse can state to the woman that she worked very hard during the end of her labor.

SECOND STAGE (BIRTH OF THE BABY)

Signs of Second Stage

The second stage of labor begins when the cervix is completely dilated (10 cm) and ends with the birth of the baby. As the head descends, the woman has the urge to push because of pressure of the fetal head on the sacral nerves and the rectum. The woman should be instructed to take one to three deep breaths, each followed by a cleansing breath to keep the oxygen and carbon dioxide in balance. Also, the woman may find it helpful to pull back on her knees while she exerts pressure. As she pushes, intraabdominal pressure is exerted by using her abdominal muscles. This additional pressure plus the labor contractions causes the baby's head to descend. Some women feel acute, increasingly severe pain with a splitting sensation. The perineum begins to bulge and flatten, and soon the baby's head appears. Some mothers will tell the nurse, "The baby is coming." When any of these signs appear, the nurse should realize that birth is about to occur. At this time, the woman will be in, or will soon be taken to, the delivery room.

Transfer to the Delivery Room

If possible, the delivery room is prepared ahead of time for the woman's arrival. The actual preparation of the delivery room will vary, but a few basic principles must be employed. Asepsis must be carried out to reduce the risk of maternal and infant infection. Whatever is to be introduced into the woman's birth canal should be kept as sterile as possible. In preparing the delivery room, the nurse should wear a cap to cover the hair and a mask to cover the mouth and nose. Using aseptic technique, the nurse assembles and arranges the sterile supplies in a convenient order (Fig. 12–3). During the delivery, the nurse should be knowledgeable in how to open sterile objects, forceps, and instruments and place them on a sterile table (Fig. 12–4). The nurse should know not to reach across a sterile table and that if a wet solution drops on a sterile table, that area is no longer sterile (Fig. 12–5). It is most important that the nurse correct any contamination. Most hospitals use a commercial delivery pack, which simplifies predelivery preparation.

Usually multiparas will be transferred to the delivery room when the cervix has dilated about

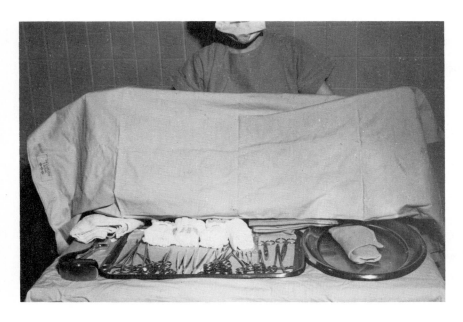

▲ **FIGURE 12–3**

Instruments arranged in a convenient order. At time of delivery, the nurse removes the sterile drape from the table. The nurse grasps the corners of the drape and brings the drape nearer to prevent leaning over sterile equipment.

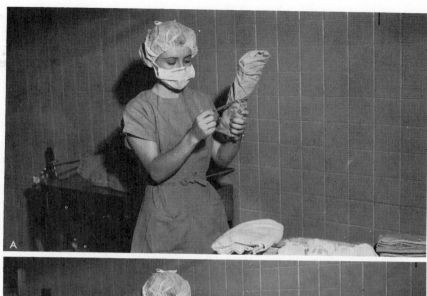

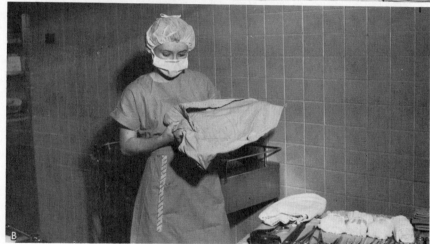

▲ FIGURE 12–4

A through **C**. Opening the outer
wrapper of delivery forceps.
*Illustration continued on
following page*

8 cm. Women having their first delivery may not
be transferred until the caput (back of the head)
is visible. Many hospitals now allow the significant
other in the delivery room, especially if that person
has attended childbirth classes. Partners should
be informed previously of the role that is expected
of them. They should be encouraged to coach the
woman throughout the birth experience.

Nursing Care in the Delivery Room

After the woman is taken to the delivery room,
the nurse assists her onto the delivery table (a
birthing chair is used in some hospitals). If she is
going to be placed in the lithotomy position, pads

or leggings are placed under her legs so her legs
do not come in contact with the cold metal stirrups. Both legs are lifted into the stirrups at the
same time to prevent strain on the pelvic ligaments
and muscles of the legs. By adjusting the delivery
table, the nurse brings the woman's buttocks near
the end of the table. The nurse cleanses the mother's abdomen, thighs, and vulva with a cleansing
solution (Fig. 12–6). Her abdomen and legs are
then covered with sterile drapes, and a drape is
placed under her buttocks.

Scrub suits, caps, masks, and shoe covers are
worn by all personnel in the delivery room. The
physician or nurse midwife conducting the delivery should have carried out appropriate hand
washing (surgical scrub) and put on a sterile gown

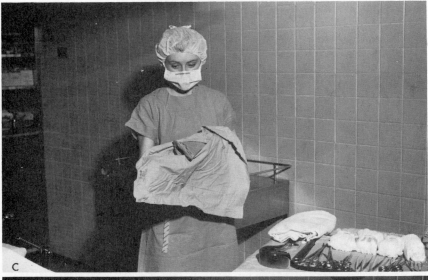

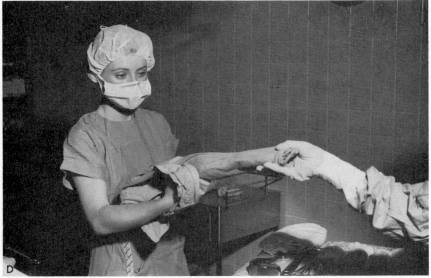

▲ **FIGURE 12–4** *Continued*

D. Holding onto the turned-back outer wrapper (so it does not touch sterile field), the nurse hands the physician the forceps, which are still in the sterile wrapper.

and gloves. Goggles are presently used in most hospitals to protect the health care provider from infection with AIDS and other STD infections.

Birth of the Baby

As the fetal head distends the perineum, the physician or nurse midwife applies gentle, steady, firm support on the head in the direction of the perineum in order to maintain flexion. Usually the

force of the next one or two contractions and maternal effort will deliver the head. After the head is delivered, the woman will be instructed to stop pushing. The physician or midwife will wipe the baby's face with gauze sponges and use a bulb syringe to suction first the mouth and then the nose (suctioning the nose first would cause the infant to gasp and aspirate amniotic fluid). The physician or midwife then checks the infant's neck for the umbilical cord. If the cord is present, it is usually long enough to be slipped over the

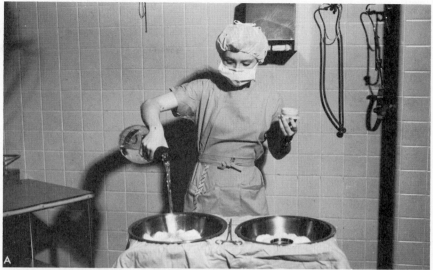

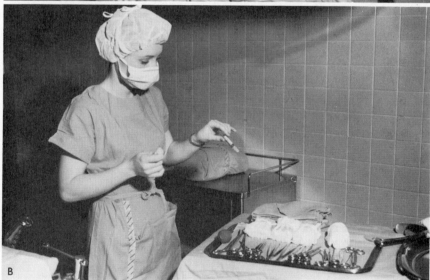

▲ FIGURE 12–5

Technique of adding sterile supplies without contaminating sterile setup. **A.** Adding sterile water to basins. **B.** Dropping sterile suture on table. Note that the nurse does not reach across the table.

Illustration continued on following page

head; however, it may be necessary to clamp and cut the cord first. Meanwhile, the head realigns itself with the shoulders (external rotation). The woman may be asked to bear down steadily with the next contraction to deliver the shoulders. Firm, steady pressure is applied to deliver the anterior shoulder, and the rest of the baby's body quickly follows. The baby is delivered, is dried with towels (to minimize the loss of heat), and often is placed on the mother's abdomen, after which the cord is clamped. If the husband/partner is present, it is ideal to allow him to participate in the experience of cutting the umbilical cord (Fig. 12–7).

Recording the Labor and Birth

An accurate record of the delivery is of medical and legal importance. Usually, hospitals have a prepared form that includes information such as the time of events and the premedication and anesthetics given. The events recorded are (a) time of birth, (b) position of the baby, (c) sex of the baby, (d) condition of the baby (Apgar scores at 1 and 5 minutes), (e) type of episiotomy, and (f) whether delivery was spontaneous or by forceps. In many hospitals, a copy of the record is kept with the infant's chart.

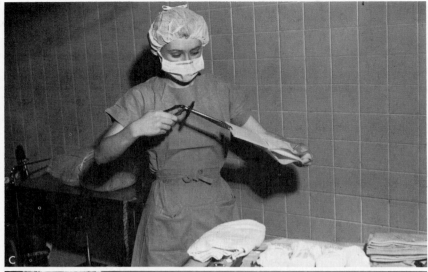

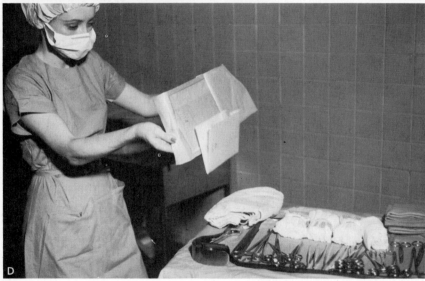

▲ **FIGURE 12–5** *Continued*

C and **D.** Two ways of adding gloves to table. **C.** Forceps is used, holding back the paper wrapper to prevent contamination. **D.** Method for dropping gloves directly from the outer wrapper.

POTENTIAL NURSING DIAGNOSES OF SECOND AND THIRD STAGES

- Altered comfort related to uterine contractions
- Altered comfort related to perineal trauma
- Impaired physical mobility
- Knowledge deficit related to effective pushing
- Ineffective neonatal airway clearance
- Ineffective thermoregulation related to infant's immature thermoregulatory system
- Knowledge deficit related to parent-infant interaction

THIRD STAGE

The third stage of labor begins after the birth of the newborn infant and ends with the expulsion of the placenta. After the delivery of the infant, the uterus rapidly shrinks. The placenta, however, does not decrease in size; thus, as the placental site becomes smaller, the placenta begins to buckle; it then separates, and as the uterus contracts it is expelled (see Chapter 10 for signs of separation). The third stage places the woman at risk for hemorrhage; therefore, assessment of the

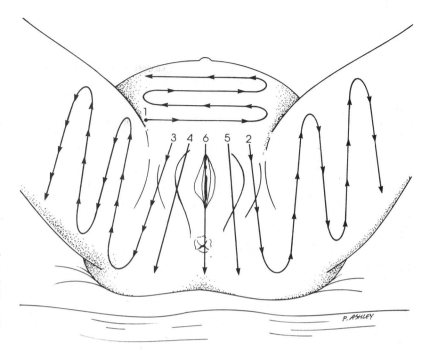

▲ FIGURE 12–6

Cleansing the perineum before delivery. The nurse follows the pattern of the numbered diagram, using prepared sponges or cotton balls for each area. Note the downward strokes, from the vagina toward the rectum.

amount of bleeding and the woman's blood pressure and pulse is important. The nurse records the time the placenta is expelled and whether it delivered spontaneously or was removed manually by the physician. An oxytocic drug (such as Pitocin) is given to the woman after the placenta is delivered. It causes the uterine muscles to contract and thereby reduces the amount of blood lost. Vital signs are taken, and frequently an ice bag is immediately applied to the perineum to reduce the amount of edema that occurs because of trauma and/or an episiotomy.

The woman shows relief, exhaustion, and an interest in the well-being of her baby. If the baby is normal, the woman usually relaxes and appears happy. She may show an emotional release by laughing or crying.

FOURTH STAGE (IMMEDIATE RECOVERY)

The fourth stage of labor is sometimes defined as the first hour after the expulsion of the placenta. It is the immediate recovery period. The woman is usually taken to the "recovery room," where she spends at least 1 hour before she is taken to the postpartum unit. The immediate postpartum period is a critical time for the woman's recovery. She is closely observed every 15 minutes during the first hour. The following assessments are made:

- Uterus: Assess the fundal height, location, and consistency. Massage the uterus and express clots. A soft and spongy uterus should be reported to the physician or midwife.
- Lochia: Vaginal discharge (rubra) saturating more than one pad in 15 minutes should be reported. Massage the uterus; attempt to expel clots.
- Bladder: Assess for distention every 30 minutes. If the bladder is full, the uterus will deviate to one side of the midline.
- Perineum: Assess the perineum for integrity. A hematoma will cause swelling or oozing from the episiotomy or laceration site and should be reported.
- Discomfort of perineum: Immediately apply ice to perineum to reduce edema owing to birth trauma or an episiotomy.
- State of hydration: Give oral fluids as tolerated. Provide nourishment if woman is hungry.
- Vital signs: Assess blood pressure, pulse,

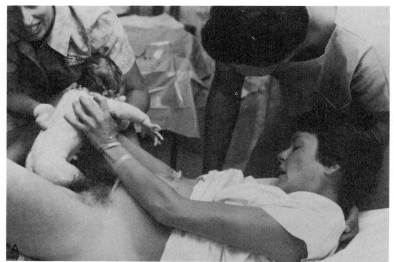

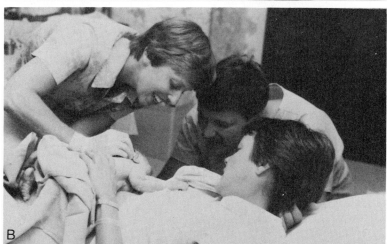

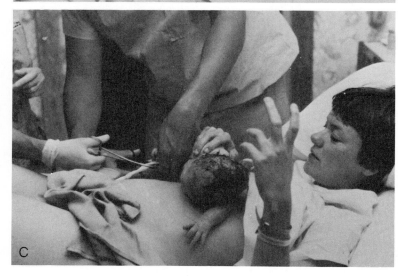

▲ FIGURE 12–7

A. Nurse midwife delivers infant. **B.** Baby is dried and placed on mother's abdomen. **C.** Father cuts cord. (Courtesy of Nancy Fleming, PhD, CNM.)

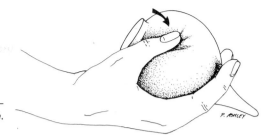

▲ **FIGURE 12–8**

Gentle suctioning of infant's mouth and nose using bulb syringe.
Note that the bulb syringe is compressed before insertion.

and respirations every 15 minutes for a minimum of 1 hour. Observe for potential signs of shock owing to excessive blood loss.

• Behavior: Assess for fatigue and provide atmosphere conducive to rest.

Provision of Initial Care to the Newborn by the Nurse

It is important that the nurse adhere to the CDC's universal precautions against STD transmission in the newborn. The immediate care of the newborn involves coming in contact with moist secretions and fluids, such as blood and amniotic fluid.

Shortly after birth, the newborn infant is placed in a radiant heated bed or incubator. The infant is wrapped in a warm blanket. If vital signs are normal, suction of the baby's mouth and nose is continued with a bulb syringe. The bulb syringe should be compressed each time before it is inserted in the mouth or nose (Fig. 12–8). When

suctioning, the nurse should take care not to traumatize the mucous membrane. Also, oversuctioning should be avoided because it deprives the infant of oxygen.

A cord clamp is placed about 1 to 1½ inches from the umbilicus, and the remainder of the cord is removed (cut). The cord is assessed for two arteries and one vein.

An Apgar score is obtained at 1 and 5 minutes to evaluate the infant's cardiorespiratory status (Table 12–3). The Apgar score consists of five observations: color, heart rate, respiratory effort, muscle tone, and reflex irritability. A value of 0 to 2 is given for each observation, and the values are then added, giving a total score. A baby in good condition would score 9 to 10. Most infants are not completely pink, because their hands and feet are usually blue. Therefore, a score of 9 is generally given. A score of 7 to 10 indicates a healthy baby who needs only brief oral and nasal suction to clear the airway. A score below 7 indicates that the infant requires immediate further attention by the physician (usually a pediatrician).

It is important to keep the infant dry in order to conserve body heat and prevent cold stress. In

TABLE 12–3. THE APGAR SCORING SYSTEM

	SCORE		
SIGN	0	1	2
Heart rate	Absent	Slow—below 100	Above 100
Respiratory effort	Absent	Slow—irregular	Good crying
Muscle tone	Flaccid	Some flexion of extremities	Active motion
Reflex irritability	None	Grimace	Vigorous cry
Color	Pale blue	Body pink, blue extremities	Completely pink

From Apgar, V. (1966). The newborn (Apgar) scoring system: Reflections and advice. *Pediatric Clinics of North America* 13:645.

some hospitals, a stockinette cap is placed on the infant's head to prevent heat loss. The infant is identified with bracelets that contain the mother's name, baby's date of birth, and sex of the baby. An identical bracelet will be put on the mother. Footprints from the baby and thumb- or index fingerprints from the mother are means of mother/infant identification (Fig. 12–9). The infant should not be removed from the delivery room until the identification is done. All states require that an antibacterial drug be used as prophylaxis against ophthalmia neonatorum. Formerly, silver nitrate 1% was used (and still may be used) to prevent a gonococcal infection of the eye, which can cause blindness. Presently, erythromycin ophthalmia ointment is used because it prevents not only a gonococcal eye infection but also chlamydial eye infection, which is a common problem today. A physical assessment is performed by the nurse or pediatrician to detect any abnormalities.

If the mother is going to breastfeed her baby, it is good to put the baby to breast right after delivery. This encourages mother–infant bonding.

Emergency Delivery by the Nurse (Without a Physician or Midwife)

Labor sometimes proceeds very rapidly; a physician or midwife may not be present, and the nurse may be the most qualified health professional present to deliver the baby. This type of delivery is most likely to occur in multiparous women, although it may also occur with oxytocin stimulation and with preterm infants.

The major concerns in an emergency delivery are to

- Remain calm and support the woman
- Provide cleanliness
- Control the birth of the baby

Calm. Reassuring the woman with a calm, confident approach will lessen her fear and anxiety. This approach will be helpful to a safe delivery.

Cleanliness. In a rapid delivery, events often happen so quickly that cleanliness is not the prior-

ity. However, efforts should be made to use clean linen and supplies. If the birth is in the hospital, the nurse working in the labor suite should be wearing sterile gloves before coming in contact with the fluids of the mother and baby to safeguard against transmission of infections. Often it is possible to quickly transfer the woman to the delivery room, where supplies and equipment are readily available.

Control of Birth. Controlling the rapid birth of the baby's head is the most important thing the nurse can do in the emergency delivery. This is important to prevent cerebral damage to the baby and lacerations to the mother. The mother should be encouraged to pant during the contraction to control her desire to push. Then, if possible, the nurse applies gentle pressure to the perineum and delivers the head between contractions. The rest of the baby's body usually follows with the next contraction. *The nurse should make no attempt to hold the baby's head back to prevent the birth.*

When the head appears, the nurse suctions the mucus from the baby's mouth and nose. Then she/he feels for the cord to make sure it is not around the baby's neck. If it is, the nurse attempts to slip it gently over the baby's head. If this cannot be done, the nurse should clamp the cord with two clamps and cut between them. Usually the head will rotate to the side (external rotation), and then the nurse can deliver the first shoulder by raising the infant's head gently; the other shoulder will deliver and the rest of the baby's body will slip out.

Immediately after birth, the baby should be dried off and wrapped in a dry, warm blanket. If the baby's color and respirations are good, he or she can be placed on the mother's abdomen. The sterile cord clamp can be put on the baby later and the cord cut with sterile scissors (using sterile technique to avoid infection).

The nurse then observes for signs of placental separation. When she is ready, the woman is asked to bear down with the next contraction to expel the placenta. After the placenta is expelled, the uterus is massaged to keep the uterus firmly contracted. The woman is observed for excessive bleeding. Her vital signs, quality of uterine firmness, and amount of vaginal bleeding are checked every 15 minutes for the first hour. If the birth of the baby takes place in the hospital and the wom-

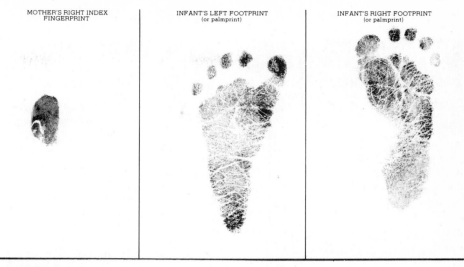

MOTHER'S RIGHT INDEX
FINGERPRINT

INFANT'S LEFT FOOTPRINT
(or palmprint)

INFANT'S RIGHT FOOTPRINT
(or palmprint)

▲ FIGURE 12–9

Index fingerprint of mother and footprints of baby are taken as a means of identification.

an's physician is absent, if possible some other physician should come to check the woman and infant and record that both are doing well. Also, as soon as the nurse has the opportunity, she/he should record the events as they took place, including the time of birth, sex of baby, and time of expulsion of placenta.

Alternative Birth Settings

Alternative birth settings include hospital birthing rooms, birthing centers, and home birth services (Fig. 12–10). They are designed, in principle, to emphasize the naturalness of childbirth.

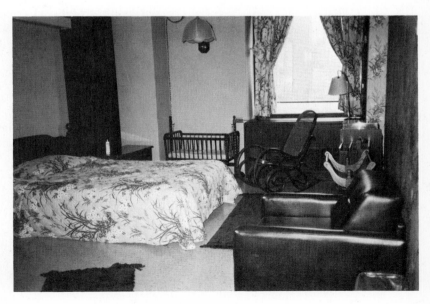

▲ FIGURE 12–10

Birthing room at the University of Illinois Hospital.

NURSING CARE PLAN 12–1

FIRST AND SECOND STAGES OF LABOR

Potential Problems and Nursing Diagnoses	Nursing Interventions
1. Anxiety related to whether true labor is occurring.	Explain to woman/couple that labor has started, cervix has begun to dilate.
2. Knowledge deficit related to early physical changes in process of labor.	Educate woman/couple about active labor process (uterine activity, possible rupture of membranes). Instruct woman to ambulate, if she feels comfortable and membranes are intact. Instruct to only have ice chips and no solid food during labor. Monitor intake and output.
3. Altered comfort related to increasing intensity of uterine contractions.	Observe woman's coping behavior. Coach woman to use pain relief measures (without medication if possible in beginning labor). Encourage use of relaxation techniques (music, low lighting) Provide sacral pressure during contractions. Encourage partner/significant other to coach patient on use of comfort measures.
4. Potential for injury and infection related to mother and infant.	Instruct woman to recognize need for protection from infection by frequently cleansing perineal region, frequently changing linen, and not letting persons with infection contact patient. Encourage side-lying position.
5. Knowledge deficit related to signs of second stage of labor.	Recognize sensations of second stage of labor as increased vaginal bleeding, feeling of pressure on rectum, and increased frequency and intensity of contractions.
6. Knowledge deficit related to potential birth of baby.	Communicate changes in status to patient. Explain pressure sensations; tell patient they are normal. Notify physician or midwife of changes. Allow woman to push, if cervix is completely dilated. Ensure patient, reinforce normalcy of changes in labor progress and that the birth of baby is imminent. Monitor fetal heart rate and relationship to maternal contractions.

Expected Outcomes

1. Woman verbalizes understanding of events of true labor such as opening of cervix (cervical dilatation).
2. Woman expresses understanding of changes that take place as labor proceeds. She recognizes why only fluids and no solid foods should be ingested during labor.
3. Woman participates in comfort measures to override the contractions.
4. Woman recognizes need to assume side-lying position during labor. She understands that nursing actions are to protect her from infection during labor.
5. Woman states confidence in her ability to go through the second stage of labor. She demonstrates the ability to take a cleansing breath before and after "pushing" with her contractions (after completely dilated).
6. Woman proceeds effectively as labor advances. She shows confidence in her abilities and constant support.

NURSING CARE PLAN 12–2

THIRD AND FOURTH STAGES OF LABOR

Potential Problems and Nursing Diagnoses	Nursing Interventions
1. Knowledge deficit related to third and fourth stages of labor.	Communicate changes in patient status. Explain need for episiotomy to reduce chance for laceration. Notify patient about medication injected to lessen pain to repair episiotomy. Encourage patient to push with contraction to expel placenta.
2. Knowledge deficit related to appearance of infant immediately after birth, and potential for hypothermia of infant.	Observe infant for color, cardiorespiratory function. Assess infant at 1 and 5 minutes for Apgar scoring. Dry infant and place infant in warm blanket in radiant heat bed. Show infant to mother, allow mother to hold infant. Describe infant with vernix caseosa, lanugo (fine hair), and slightly enlongated head.
3. Potential for infection related to contamination of sterile object on delivery table.	Notify physician and replace the unsterile with sterile field.
4. Alteration in parenting related to prolonged labor.	Provide skin-to-skin contact between mother and infant. Reinforce normalcy of infant. Encourage mother and father to touch and stroke baby.
5. Potential fluid volume deficit related to blood loss.	Monitor maternal vital signs every 15 minutes. Report excessive vaginal bleeding, boggy uterus, increased pulse rate, or decreased blood pressure.
6. Self-care deficit related to sleep and food intake.	Allow mother to rest. Provide oral fluids and solid food intake.

Expected Outcomes

1. Woman participates effectively in the third and fourth stages of labor.
2. Woman establishes eye contact while holding infant.
3. Patient recognizes need to keep drapes, instruments as sterile as possible to reduce risk of infection.
4. Woman touches and strokes the infant. She holds the infant close to chest and asks questions about the baby, to make sure it is normal.
5. Patient maintains normal pulse rate, blood pressure, status of uterus, and amount of bleeding.
6. Woman rests between nursing postdelivery assessments. She drinks fluids and eats solid food given to her. She shows appreciation for blanket for warmth. States she is feeling comfortable.

Frequently the nurse midwife, in collaboration with the physician, assumes the overall management of the birth as well as of the prenatal and postpartum care. However, some alternative birth settings are managed by the physician (without a nurse midwife). In these settings, the nurse assumes a variety of responsibilities, including childbirth education and assisting with the birth itself.

An important advantage of the alternative birth settings to the woman and family is that they have more control of the events surrounding the birth experience. The woman has an opportunity to decide on her activities during labor. She usually is allowed to vary her eating and drinking patterns and can select different positions for comfort during labor and birth. In addition, her companions are given the opportunity to participate more in the birth process. The woman and family, supported by the staff, treat the birth process as a normal physiological event. Some common obstetrical practices, such as artificial rupture of the membranes, intravenous administration of fluids, shaving of pubic hair, and administration of drugs, are discouraged in alternative birth settings. If complications occur, the woman is transferred to a hospital critical-care maternity unit.

IN-HOSPITAL BIRTHING ROOMS

An in-hospital birthing room is a hospital room or suite furnished to provide a home-like atmosphere conducive to the parents' participation in the birth. The woman stays in the same room for labor, birth, and recovery. In-hospital birthing rooms are used primarily for uncomplicated pregnancies. Some hospitals require that the couple have attended prenatal classes. Siblings can visit and get acquainted with the new infant shortly after birth. The hospital staff needs to believe in the philosophy that a home-like setting improves the birth experience and must be supportive to the family for the birthing room to be a success. If not, the birthing room will be used less frequently. A trend to have the mother in the same room for her labor, delivery, and recovery has increased the popularity of in-hospital birthing rooms.

OUT-OF-HOSPITAL BIRTHING CENTERS

Some families choose the out-of-hospital birthing center for maternity care. These centers combine a home environment with a short-stay, ambulatory, health facility with access to in-hospital obstetrical and newborn care. Their advantage over home birth is quick access to the hospital facility if needed. The programs usually provide comprehensive prenatal, birth, and postpartum care. The mother and infant stay in the facility for 4 to 12 hours after birth.

HOME BIRTH

The advantage of a home birth is that the woman is in familiar, comfortable surroundings during the labor and birth. If hospitalization is not required, some couples decide on home birth because it can be less expensive. However, the couple should know the risk factors in making the choice of a birth at home. Usually there is a lack of equipment to handle emergencies, and their home may be a distance from a hospital, if one is required.

The overall benefit and safety of home birth to the mother and baby must be considered in the couple's decision. It is important to have a backup system for home births, should an emergency occur that requires life-saving measures; for example, in an excessive hemorrhage.

References

American Academy of Pediatrics and American College of Obstetricians and Gynecologists (1988). *Guidelines for Perinatal Care*, 2nd ed. Washington, DC: Authors.

Apgar, V. (1966). The newborn (Apgar) scoring system: Reflections and advice. *Pediatric Clinics of North America*, 13:645.

Auvenshine, M. A., & Enriquez, M. G. (1990). *Comprehensive Maternity Nursing: Perinatal and Women's Health*, 2nd ed. Boston: Jones and Bartlett.

Carlson, J. H., Craft, C. A., McGuire, A. D., & Popkess-Vawter, S. (1991). *Nursing Diagnosis: A Case Study Approach*. Philadelphia: W. B. Saunders Company.

Dickason, E. J., Schult, M. O., & Silverman, B. L. (1990). *Maternal-Infant Nursing Care*. St. Louis: C. V. Mosby.

Doenges, M. E., Kenty, J. R., Moorhouse, M. F. (1988). *Maternal-Newborn Care Plans: Guidelines for Client Care*. Philadelphia: F. A. Davis.

Ladewig, P. W., London, M. L., & Olds, S. B. (1990). *Essentials of Maternal-Newborn Nursing,* 2nd ed. Redwood City, CA: Addison-Wesley Nursing.

Nichols, F. H., & Humenick, S. S. (1988). *Childbirth Education: Practice, Research, and Theory.* Philadelphia: W. B. Saunders Company.

Roberts, J. (1989). Managing fetal bradycardia during second stage of labor. *American Journal of Maternal-Child Nursing* 14:394–398.

Taubenheim, A. M., & Silbernagel, T. (1988). Meeting the needs of expectant fathers. *American Journal of Maternal-Child Nursing* 13:110–113.

Varney, H. (1987). *Nurse-Midwifery.* Boston: Blackwell Scientific Publications.

SUGGESTED ACTIVITIES

1. List the questions that are asked of the woman when she enters the labor suite.
2. Describe the admission care of a woman in labor.
3. Explain three nursing interventions for first, second, third, and fourth stages of labor.
4. List the five basic observations in the Apgar scoring system.
5. Discuss the care of the infant immediately after birth.
6. Describe alternative birth settings.

REVIEW QUESTIONS

A. Select the best answer to each multiple-choice question.

1. The longest stage of labor is the
   A. First
   B. Second
   C. Third
   D. Fourth

2. An assessment of uterine labor contractions includes all of the following EXCEPT
   A. Intensity
   B. Frequency
   C. Duration
   D. Dilatation

3. Normally the fetal heart rate ranges (in bpm) from
   A. 110-120
   B. 120-140
   C. 120-160
   D. 140-160

4. If the amniotic fluid is meconium stained, it is indicative of all EXCEPT
   A. Cephalic presentation with fetal distress
   B. Breech presentation with fetal distress
   C. Breech presentation
   D. Infection of fetus

5. During labor, the woman is NOT given solid food to prevent which of the following?
   A. Aspiration of food during vomiting
   B. Aspiration of particles if given an anesthetic
   C. Postbirth occurrence of pneumonia
   D. All of the above

6. To decrease a woman's discomfort during labor, a nurse may
   A. Provide sacral support
   B. Perform effleurage
   C. Apply cool cloth to face
   D. All of the above

7. To aid in the control of the advancing head and its delivery in a slow manner and to avoid laceration, the woman should be instructed to
   A. Give strong pushes with each contraction
   B. Push when the contraction begins
   C. Pant with contractions and voluntarily bear down between contractions
   D. None of the above

8. After the birth of the infant and after the cord is cut, the nurse notices a sudden gush of blood with a lengthening of the umbilical cord. This would indicate
   A. Laceration of the vagina
   B. Hemorrhage
   C. Separation of the placenta
   D. Uterine rupture

9. After the birth of the infant, the mother can be given Pitocin. This drug is classified as an
   A. Oxytocic
   B. Sedative
   C. Analgesic
   D. Amnesic

10. Alternative birth settings include
    A. In-hospital birthing rooms
    B. Home births
    C. Birth centers
    D. All of the above

Clinical Situation: Mary Martinez is admitted to the labor room in true labor. The history reveals that this is Mary's first baby and that she has had an uneventful pregnancy. She mentions that both she and her partner attended prenatal classes. Questions 11–15 refer to Mary.

11. The abdominal examination reveals the following information: Breech is felt in fundus, back on the left side of Mary's abdomen, directed anteriorly with the extremities of the fetus on the right side and the head firmly fixed in the pelvis. The presentation of the baby is
    A. ROA engaged
    B. LOA engaged
    C. LOA not engaged
    D. ROA not engaged

12. The abdominal examination reveals that the presenting part is
    A. Cephalic
    B. Breech
    C. Transverse
    D. Unknown

13. The vaginal examination reveals the presenting part to be −1 station. This means that the biparietal diameter of the head is
    A. At the level of the ischial spines
    B. Above the ischial spines
    C. Below the ischial spines
    D. None of the above

14. Mary's baby's fetal heart rate (FHR) is 130 beats per minute. This is
    A. Below normal limits
    B. Within normal limits
    C. Above normal limits
    D. None of the above

15. Mary's cervical dilatation is said to be 5 cm. This would place Mary in what phase of the first stage of labor?
    A. Latent phase
    B. Active phase
    C. Transitional phase

B. Choose from Column II the phrase that most accurately defines the term in Column I.

I

1. Latent phase _____
2. Active phase _____
3. Transition phase _____
4. Second stage _____
5. Third stage _____
6. Fourth stage _____
7. Pitocin _____
8. Hematoma _____

II

A. Hungry, thirsty, and sleepy
B. Sense of anticipation and happiness
C. Exhausted, but elated baby is born
D. Uterine contractions beginning to cause discomfort
E. Pant–blow breathing technique is used
F. Swelling or oozing from episiotomy site
G. Reduces blood loss
H. Trembling of legs and perspiration on face

UNIT V

THE POSTPARTUM PERIOD

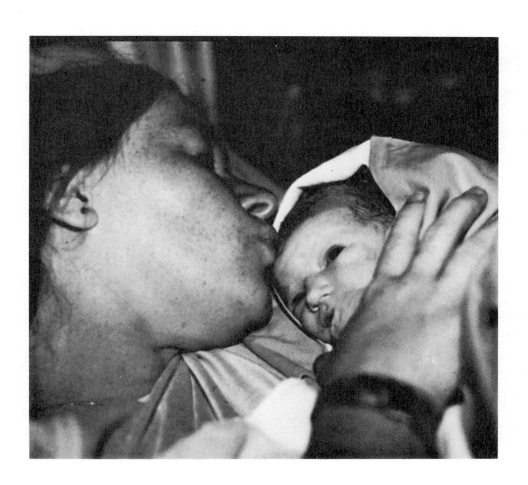

CHAPTER 13 _____

Chapter Outline

Physical Adjustments
    Involution of the uterus
    Changes in fundal position
    Uterine contractions: afterpains
    Lochia: vaginal discharge
    Vagina and perineum
    Vital signs
    Postpartum chill
    Postpartum diaphoresis
    Abdominal muscles
Adjustments of the Body Systems
    Circulatory system
    Urinary system
    Gastrointestinal system
    Endocrine system (including lactation)
Weight Loss
Postpartum Exercises
Psychological Adjustments
    Taking-in and taking-hold phases
    Attainment of the maternal role
    Postpartum blues

Learning Objectives

Upon completion of Chapter 13, the student should be able to
- Explain the involution of the uterus and describe changes in the fundal position.
- Explain the cause of afterpains.
- State the difference between a contracted and a relaxed uterus.
- Describe the color and appearance of lochia rubra, lochia serosa, and lochia alba.
- Describe the appearance of the vagina and perineum after delivery.
- Explain the importance of monitoring the vital signs during the first 24 hours.
- Name two nursing measures indicated when a woman has a postpartum chill.
- Recall postpartum diaphoresis and why it occurs.
- List the postpartum alterations in the circulatory system.
- List three factors that influence urinary retention after delivery.
- List three factors that contribute to postpartum constipation.
- List two significant events that occur as a result of changes in the endocrine system.
- Describe the major hormones involved in lactation.
- Sequence the lactation process.
- Identify the hormones responsible for milk production and milk ejection.
- List three factors that can inhibit the woman's milk supply.
- Describe the suppression of lactation.
- Explain the reasons for the woman's weight loss immediately after delivery.
- Explain ways to strengthen abdominal muscles.
- Identify Rubin's taking-in and taking-hold phases.
- List, in order, the stages of maternal role attainment.
- Explain the psychological alteration called "postpartum blues"

PHYSIOLOGICAL AND PSYCHOLOGICAL ADJUSTMENTS DURING THE POSTPARTUM PERIOD

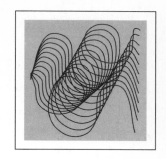

The postpartum period, or *puerperium,* is the interval from the birth of the infant until the woman's body returns to its nonpregnant state. Rapid physiological and psychological adjustments begin immediately after birth and continue for about 6 weeks.

The first 1 or 2 hours postpartum are sometimes called the *fourth stage* of labor. This time is very hazardous for the woman because of the dangers of *hemorrhage* and *hypovolemic shock.* For these reasons, the woman is observed closely in a recovery room, as discussed in Chapter 12, until she is free from the immediate danger and her condition is stabilized. After a minimum of 1 hour, if her condition is stable, she is moved to the postpartum unit.

After the initial dangers of hemorrhage and shock are past, the primary postpartum danger is *infection.* The nursing assessment, intervention, and evaluation during this period are geared toward prevention or reduction of hemorrhage and infection. In addition, care is given to promote the woman's natural physiological and psychological restorative processes. To accurately assess whether recovery is proceeding normally, the caregiver must know how, when, and why physiological and psychological adjustments occur.

Physical Adjustments

INVOLUTION OF THE UTERUS

Immediately after delivery, the placental site has a diameter of 8 to 9 cm, with open venous sinuses. Contractions of the uterine vessels act like living ligatures and compress the blood vessels, which control and reduce the amount of blood loss. A unique healing process called *exfoliation* enables the placental site to heal without scarring. In exfoliation, necrotic tissue is sloughed off, leaving a smooth surface of endometrial tissue. This sloughing off is an important part of the reparative process, because it ensures that future fertilized ova will implant in an unscarred uterus.

After birth, the uterus undergoes a rapid reduction in size and weight. The uterus weighs approximately 2.2 lb (1000 g) immediately after delivery. It decreases to 1.1 lb (500 g) during the 1st week and 12 oz (320 g) 2 weeks after delivery. The rate of decrease will vary with the size of the infant and the number of previous pregnancies. The decrease in the size of the uterus is known as *involution.* The primary cause of involution is the sudden withdrawal of estrogen and progesterone, which triggers the release of proteolytic enzymes into the endometrium. This release causes the protein material within the endometrial cells to be broken down into substances that can be secreted in the urine. The number of muscle cells does not change during involution, but rather the size of each cell is markedly reduced.

CHANGES IN FUNDAL POSITION

The *location* and *consistency* of the fundus (top of the uterus) are important nursing assessments. Immediately after delivery, the fundus of the uterus is approximately 2 cm (2 fingerbreadths) below the umbilicus. On external palpation, the uterus feels about the size of a large grapefruit and continues to decrease in size. It should be firm. Within about 12 hours after birth, the fundal height often rises to 1 cm (1 fingerbreadth) above

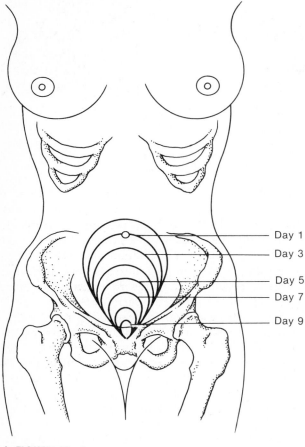

▲ **FIGURE 13–1**

Uterine involution showing changes in height of fundus. The height of the fundus decreases about 1 finger breadth (approximately 1 cm) each day. After 10 days, it recedes under the pubic bone and is no longer palpable.

the uterus. Each day postpartum, the uterus should be lower by 1 cm. At the end of the first week after delivery, the uterus is palpable at the pubic bone. Normally, after 10 days the uterus is no longer palpable (Fig. 13–1). When the uterus is higher than expected and is situated over to one side, distention of the bladder should be suspected (Table 13–1).

If the mother is breastfeeding, the release of oxytocin in response to suckling hastens the involution process. Also, some women receive an oxytocic drug, such as ergonovine (Ergotrate), to hasten involution (see Appendix B).

UTERINE CONTRACTIONS: AFTERPAINS

Uterine contractions are felt by the woman during the first few days post partum. In primiparas, the uterus generally remains in a state of tonic contraction (stays contracted), unless placental fragments remain in the uterus. In multiparas, the uterus has usually lost some of its muscle tone. Therefore, it relaxes and contracts rather than maintaining a sustained contraction. The contractions may be felt as marked cramping sensations, called *afterpains*. The release of oxytocin during breastfeeding stimulates the uterus to contract; therefore, the mother often notices afterpains when she nurses her infant.

LOCHIA: VAGINAL DISCHARGE

The vaginal discharge after delivery is called *lochia*. It contains blood from the placental site, particles of necrotic decidua, and mucus. Changes in color and amount of lochia occur as healing takes place at the site where the placenta was implanted. The quantity of lochia becomes moderate and then scant. The colors are indicated by the Latin words *rubra* for bright to dark red, *serosa* for pinkish to brownish, and *alba* for a creamy white color. Lochia rubra lasts for about 3 days, and lochia serosa continues for about 9 days. Lochia alba persists for about 2 additional weeks (Table 13–2).

The odor of lochia is characteristically "fleshy" or musty. An offensive, foul odor usually indicates infection. Continued lochia rubra or a recurrence of bright red vaginal discharge signifies possible retained placental fragments.

VAGINA AND PERINEUM

The vagina often appears edematous and bruised, and the opening in the vagina often gapes when intraabdominal pressure is increased, such as by coughing. By the third postpartum week the vagina reassumes the appearance of the nonpregnant state, with some relaxation of tissue, however. The pelvic floor muscles are overstretched and weak. The appearance of the perineum will vary greatly, depending on the type and extent of

TABLE 13–1. CHANGES IN UTERINE FUNDAL POSITION

TIME/DAYS	POSITION OF FUNDUS	LOCHIA
1–2 hr	Midway between umbilicus and symphysis pubis	Rubra
12 hr	At umbilicus or 1 cm above it	Rubra
3 days	3 cm below umbilicus (descent continues at 1 cm per day)	Serosa
10 days	Not palpable above symphysis	Alba

the episiotomy (cut in the perineum) or laceration. Usually, the soft tissues of the perineum are edematous and bruised.

VITAL SIGNS

Temperature. The woman's temperature during the first 24 hours after delivery may rise to 100.4° F (38° C) as a result of the exertion and dehydration of labor. After the first 24 hours, the woman should be afebrile, and any temperature above 100.4° F or higher suggests infection. Elevation over 100.4° F two times on any of the first 10 postpartum days (not including the first 24 hours) is referred to as *puerperal morbidity*. A short-term elevation on the second or third postpartum day can occur as a result of breast engorgement.

Pulse. The heart rate often decreases to a rate of 50 to 70 beats per minute (*bradycardia* or slow pulse) for the first 6 to 8 days postpartum. The drop in heart rate is attributed to a reduction in blood volume. An elevated heart rate may indicate undue blood loss, infection, pain, anxiety, or cardiac disease.

Blood Pressure. Blood pressure readings should remain stable after birth. Blood pressure decrease may be related to excessive blood loss. Blood pressure elevation, especially when accompanied by a headache, suggests pregnancy-induced hypertension and indicates the need for further evaluation (see Chapter 21).

POSTPARTUM CHILL

Commonly a woman experiences a shaking chill immediately after birth, thought to be related to a

TABLE 13–2. NORMAL AND ABNORMAL CHARACTERISTICS OF LOCHIA

LOCHIA/TYPE	TIME	NORMAL LOCHIA	ABNORMAL LOCHIA
Lochia rubra	Days 1–3	Bright red, bloody consistency; fleshy odor; temporary increase during breastfeeding and on rising	Numerous large clots; foul smell; saturation of perineal pad
Lochia serosa	Days 4–9	Pinkish brown; is of serosanguineous consistency	Foul smell; saturation of perineal pad
Lochia alba	Day 10 to approximately 3 wk	Creamy white; fleshy odor	Foul smell; persistent lochial discharge over 3 weeks; return to pink or red discharge

nervous response or to vasomotor changes rather than the coldness of the delivery/recovery room. If the chill is not followed by an elevated temperature, it is of no clinical concern. The woman should be covered by a warm blanket and reassured that the chill is a common experience after birth. After the first 24 hours, chill and fever indicate infection, and the woman should have further evaluation.

POSTPARTUM DIAPHORESIS

Diaphoresis (excessive perspiration) is common during both day and night. It is the woman's body's way of eliminating the excess fluid accumulated during pregnancy. This adjustment has implications for nursing care: Daily baths, frequent changes of clothing, and adequate fluid intake are necessary. It is suggested that clinical changes be discussed with the woman before they occur to decrease anxiety.

ABDOMINAL MUSCLES

The abdominal muscles are greatly stretched during pregnancy and lose much of their tone. Exercises, gradually but consistently performed, will help restore the muscle strength and tone. The striae (stretch marks) on the skin tend to become silvery and usually diminish but do not completely disappear.

Adjustments of the Body Systems

CIRCULATORY SYSTEM

Blood loss during delivery can cause an immediate decrease in blood volume post partum. In addition, extravascular fluid is mobilized and excreted. For the first 72 hours after delivery there is a greater decrease in plasma volume than in the cellular components of the blood, resulting in a slight increase in the hematocrit value. For the first 3 days post partum, there can be variation in the hematocrit value, hemoglobin level, and erythrocyte count. Because of these adjustments in the early postpartum period, the hemoglobin level and hematocrit value may be unreliable indicators of the red blood cell status or amount of blood lost during delivery. Laboratory blood values should be the same as prepregnancy values within 1 week post partum. As previously stated, there should be little or no change in blood pressure; however, a slow pulse is a common clinical postpartum finding (Table 13–3).

As discussed in Chapter 5, the increased hormone levels during pregnancy activate the blood coagulation factors. This effect persists during the postpartum period and, along with decreased activity, potential trauma, and sepsis, predisposes the woman to thromboembolitic disease (the occurrence of an embolus or thrombus). In order to decrease this risk, early and frequent ambulation is essential.

Varicose veins that have developed during the pregnancy usually diminish during the puerperium because the venous stasis that was caused by the gravid uterine compression (that is pressure of uterus on veins) decreases. In addition, there is a decrease in the progesterone level, which during pregnancy was largely responsible for a decrease in smooth muscle tone.

URINARY SYSTEM

Diuresis is noticeable during the first 24 hours post partum and may last as long as 5 days. By 5

HEMATOLOGICAL VALUES	NONPREGNANT	PREGNANT	SECOND DAY POST PARTUM
Hemoglobin	12–16 g/dl	11.5–12 g/dL	10.0–11.4 g/dL
Hematocrit	36–46%	35–42%	32–38%
White blood cells	5000–10,000/mm	5000–15,000/mm	14,000–16,000/mm

TABLE 13–3. LABORATORY BLOOD VALUES

days after birth the body's elimination of the 2 to 3 L of tissue fluid gained during pregnancy is complete. This process is also referred to as the reversal of the water retention during pregnancy. The urinary output in the early postpartum period can be great. It is not unusual for a mother who has just delivered to have an output of 1500 to 2500 ml within 6 hours. Tenderness (costovertebral-angle tenderness), fever, urinary retention, or dysuria with the urinary frequency signifies potential urinary infection. If the woman has any of these symptoms, further evaluation is necessary.

Urinary retention may occur after delivery because the bladder is often edematous and bruised. Other factors that contribute to urinary retention are a decreased sensitivity to fluid pressure with a full bladder, edema and bruising of the tissues around the urinary meatus, decreased sensation due to anesthesia, and an inability to void while in a recumbent position.

GASTROINTESTINAL SYSTEM

The woman is often hungry and thirsty after the birth of her infant. Frequently, she can have a light meal shortly after delivery, if nausea is not present. Postpartum constipation is common because of decreased gastrointestinal motility. Other factors that contribute to constipation are the effects of analgesia or anesthesia administered during labor, relaxed abdominal muscles, decreased solid food intake, cleansing via an enema during labor, dehydration, and perineal pain. Hemorrhoids (varicose veins of the rectum) frequently become more painful during the second stage of labor. Nursing assessment and intervention for constipation, perineal pain, and hemorrhoidal discomfort are discussed in Chapter 6. The appropriate nursing interventions should be implemented as soon as possible for patient comfort.

ENDOCRINE SYSTEM (INCLUDING LACTATION)

During pregnancy, the placenta produces several hormones. Prenatally, the woman has high levels of progesterone, estrogen, human chorionic gonadotropin, and human placental lactogen (hPL) (see Chapter 5). These hormones stimulate the development of the milk-producing component of the breasts. After delivery the levels of these hormones drop drastically. With this decrease, the *prolactin* level increases. The dramatic change in the endocrine system allows two significant events to occur: (a) lactation (milk secretion) begins as a result of suckling or manual stimulus, and (b) the menstrual cycle function returns.

Return to Menstruation

Most women who do not nurse their babies will menstruate 6 to 12 weeks after the infant's birth. Lactating mothers vary in the resumption of menses; some do not menstruate as long as they nurse their infants. Three to 6 months after delivery is the range for lactating mothers to begin menses. The frequency and duration of suckling stimulation, quantity of milk removed from the breasts, and amount of supplementary formula given the baby are all factors that affect when menstruation returns. In both nonlactating and lactating mothers, the first menstrual period flow is often greater than normal and frequently is anovulatory. However, the woman should be clearly reminded that it is possible to ovulate and to become pregnant before her first menstrual period after delivery.

Lactation Process

Lactation (the secretion of milk) is the end result of many interacting factors, including the development of the breast tissue (and duct system) primarily under the influence of hormones (estrogen, progesterone, and hPL). In addition, hPL stimulates the alveolar cells to begin lactogenesis (milk production), so that by the later part of pregnancy the breasts secrete *colostrum,* a yellow, premilk substance. After delivery, estrogen, progesterone, and hPL, prolactin-inhibiting agents, decrease rapidly, causing a brisk increase in prolactin secretion. Prolactin stimulates milk production, which is then enhanced by infant suckling.

Once lactation has been established, suckling is the most important stimulus for the maintenance of milk production. Infant suckling causes the pituitary gland to secrete prolactin and oxytocin.

By the third day after delivery, the prolactin effect on the breast tissue is evident, and the hormone is present in sufficient quantity to cause engorgement of the breasts, which is caused by a swelling of the blood vessels and lymphatics (note that engorgement is not an accumulation of milk). The breasts become distended, firm, tender, and warm. At this time, milk, which is thin and bluish, begins to replace the colostrum.

Colostrum. Early breastfeeding is beneficial to the infant. It allows the infant to receive colostrum (a creamy, yellow fluid) as well as stimulating the breasts to form milk. Colostrum provides the infant with passive immunity, having high levels of immunoglobulin (Ig) G and IgA. This type of antibody secretion appears to protect the infant against respiratory and gastrointestinal diseases. The immunity is significant, because the antibodies protect against *Escherichia coli,* to which the infants are regularly exposed and against which there is little or no natural immunity. It is important to note that IgA antibodies do not cross the placental barrier. Colostrum is also high in protein.

Milk Production and Ejection. Milk production and ejection are dependent on the infant's suckling stimulus or pumping of the breasts. Nerves

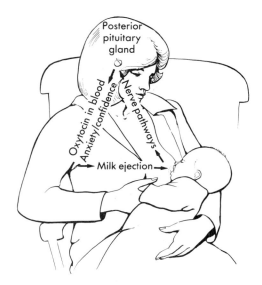

▲ FIGURE 13–3

Release and effect of oxytocin on lactation. (From Riordan, J. (1990). *A Practical Guide to Breastfeeding.* Boston: Jones and Barlett Publishing Co.)

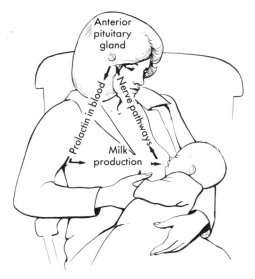

▲ FIGURE 13–2

Release and effect of prolactin on lactation. (From Riordan, J. (1990). *A Practical Guide to Breastfeeding.* Boston: Jones and Barlett Publishing Co.)

beneath the skin of the areola carry a message to the spinal cord, which transmits it to the hypothalamus. From the hypothalamus, a message is sent to the pituitary gland, stimulating the anterior and posterior areas of the gland to release prolactin and oxytocin, respectively (Figs. 13–2 and 13–3). Prolactin promotes milk production by stimulating the alveolar cells of the breasts. The infant's suckling on the mother's nipple releases oxytocin from the maternal posterior pituitary gland. This hormone increases the contractility of the myoepithelial cells; the contraction of the myoepithelial cells causes the flow of milk. The ejection of milk from the alveoli is caused by a neurohormonal mechanism (called the "let-down" reflex). From the alveoli, the milk travels to the lactiferous ducts and finally to the nipple.

Some mothers have described the let-down reflex as a tingling or prickling sensation during which they feel the milk "coming down." The let-down reflex can be stimulated by the mother's thinking about the infant and by the infant's suckling, presence, or crying. Other stimuli for the let-down reflex may be general, such as feeling the warm water during a shower. It is not unusual for the breasts to leak some milk before feeding time.

Positive emotions are important in successful breastfeeding. Negative emotions can inhibit the let-down reflex and thus the milk supply. The mother's lack of self-confidence, fear, embarrassment, or pain connected with breastfeeding may prevent the milk from being ejected into the duct system. Failure to empty the breasts frequently and completely also can decrease the milk production, because if milk accumulates and is not withdrawn, the buildup of pressure in the alveoli suppresses milk secretion.

Milk production is controlled by "supply and demand" after lactation is established. If milk production is diminished by stress or other negative emotions, breastfeeding every 2 to 3 hours may restore the milk supply. It is important that mothers understand that breast milk can look bluish and watery but still contain the important nutrients for the infant.

The Effect of Drugs on Breastfeeding. Drugs taken by the mother may be passed to the infant through the breast milk (see Appendix B). Certain drugs may inhibit lactation. Other drugs may affect the infant's physiological processes. The mother should be advised to tell the physician about all the drugs she is taking. Also, she should be given information about the potential effect of the medications on breast milk and possibly the nursing infant (Table 13–4).

Suppression of Lactation. If the woman does not wish to nurse her infant or if it is medically contraindicated, lactation can be suppressed by drugs (see Appendix B) or by discontinuing suckling and mechanical stimulus. The breasts will become distended, firm, and tender, but after 48 to 72 hours, lactation and discomfort will ease.

The administration of estrogens, androgens, or both is not recommended to suppress lactation. Studies have indicated that the use of estrogen or other hormones, such as lactation-suppressing drugs, can be linked to endometrial cancer. It is important for the caregiver to have the woman sign a consent form for these drugs, if they are given.

A recent drug, bromocriptine (Parlodel), has been made available as an alternative to estrogens and other hormones in the suppression of postpartum lactation. Bromocriptine acts to suppress lactation by preventing the secretion of prolactin. It is known to cause hypotension in some women.

Therefore, the woman's vital signs should be stabilized before the drug is administered. Bromocriptine may be given with meals to decrease the side effect of nausea.

Weight Loss

Immediately after delivery, the woman's weight decreases by about 10 to 12 lb (4.5 to 5.4 kg). This weight loss is accounted for by the removal of the infant, placenta, and amniotic fluid. An additional 5 lb (2.3 kg) is lost during the early postpartum period as a result of diuresis and diaphoresis.

During pregnancy, the woman's body stores 5 to 7 lb (2.3 to 3.2 kg) of fat for lactation needs. The mother who nurses her infant will gradually use this fat store over the first 6 months, and often she will return to her approximate prepregnancy weight. The woman who does not nurse her infant will tend to retain some of the excess weight gained during pregnancy. Therefore, women are encouraged to do postpartum exercises to lose the weight gained during pregnancy and increase the strength and tone of various muscles in their bodies.

Postpartum Exercises

In the postpartum period, fetal safety is no longer a concern. However, persistent maternal musculoskeletal and cardiovascular changes present potential problems. The hormonal effects on connective tissue will not be reversed until about 6 weeks post partum. Until that time, the risk of injury is still present. For the woman with an uneventful birth, deep breathing, Kegel exercises, and pelvic tilts can be started within the first or second postpartum day.

Whether exercise is permitted will depend on the woman's overall health, including lochia flow, fatigue, and discomfort. The fatigue level should be carefully monitored. Walking is an ideal exercise but in the beginning should be done in moderation. The woman's return to fitness activities such as jogging should be delayed for about 6 weeks, and the return should be gradual.

Table 13–4. DRUGS EXCRETED IN BREAST MILK THAT HAVE AN EFFECT ON THE INFANT

DRUG	EFFECT ON INFANT
Acetylsalicylic acid (aspirin)	Can interfere with blood clotting; infant must be observed for petechiae, bruises, and bleeding disorders
Alcohol	May cause drowsiness and depression and decrease mother's milk ejection reflex
Ampicillin	May cause diarrhea or increase susceptibility to thrush
Caffeine	May cause jitteriness, sleep disorders, and irritability
Chloramphenicol (Chloromycetin)	Infant does not excrete drug well, and it can accumulate
Cocaine	May cause cocaine intoxication
Coumarin	May cause bleeding disorders
Ergonovine maleate (Ergotrate)	May cause nausea and vomiting
Erythromycin	May cause infant under age of 1 mo to develop jaundice
Hydralazine hydrochloride (Apresoline)	May cause jaundice or electrolyte imbalance
Indomethacin (Indocin)	May cause convulsions
Marijuana	May impair RNA and DNA formation
Methadone	May cause depression or failure to thrive
Methyldopa (Aldomet)	May cause galactorrhea
Metronidazole (Flagyl)	May cause neurological disorders and blood dyscrasias
Narcotics	Can accumulate and cause addiction, depression, drowsiness, and poor feeding behavior
Nicotine (cigarette smoking)	May interfere with mother's milk production Infant can inhale smoke
Oral contraceptives	May decrease maternal milk
Streptomycin	May cause auditory and renal space disorders
Valium	May accumulate to high levels, increase neonatal jaundice, or cause drowsiness

The following are exercises for strengthening muscles and relaxation.

Abdominal Breathing. In a sitting or lying position (preferably with a pillow under her head), with arms near to or away from the body, the woman inhales deeply, using her abdominal muscles, then exhales slowly through pursed lips, tightening her abdominal muscles (Fig. 13–4A). This exercise strengthens the abdominal muscles.

Chin to Chest. While lying with a pillow under her head, the woman comfortably extends her legs, raises her head, and attempts to touch her chin to her chest; she then slowly lowers her head (Fig. 13–4B). This exercise strengthens abdominal muscles and releases tension.

Pelvic Tilt. The pelvic tilt is helpful for good postural alignment and to relieve strain on the lower back. It can be done in a sitting or standing position. With her arms stretched out, the woman tightens her abdominal and buttock muscles,

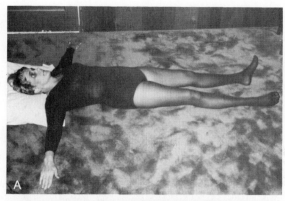

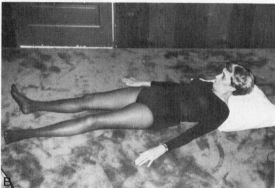

▲ **FIGURE 13–4**

A. Abdominal breathing. **B.** Chin to chest.

arches her back, and then flattens her back against the wall (if standing) or chair (if sitting). This exercise strengthens back muscles and lessens back discomfort (see Chapter 9).

Kegel Exercises. In performing Kegel exercises, the woman contracts the pelvic floor muscles. The woman pulls up her entire pelvic floor, as if trying to suck up water with her vagina. She then bears down, as if trying to push the imaginary water out. In doing this, she is using abdominal muscles also. The woman should feel a tightening of the muscles around the anal sphincter, vagina, and urethra. This is done to promote healing of perineal tissues, increase the strength of the muscles, and increase urinary control.

Arm Raising. While assuming a semirecumbent position, with arms extended away from body, the woman raises her arms in front of her until they are perpendicular to her chest, touches hands, then lowers arms slowly. The woman

should notice a tightening of the abdominal muscles.

Straight-Leg Lift. The woman assumes a semi-curled position (see Fig. 9–7) with one leg bent at the knee and the other extended with the foot flexed. She lifts the extended leg up as high as is comfortable (while inhaling), lowers the leg slowly to the floor (while exhaling), then repeats this with the other leg. This exercise promotes venous return and lessens tension.

Psychological Adjustments

Mood swings are common during the postpartum period. The rapid decline of hormones, such as progesterone and estrogen, contributes to emotional upsets. Other factors related to emotional reactions are conflict about the maternal role and personal insecurity. Women who have economic or family problems usually demonstrate more stress in response to motherhood. In addition, past fetal losses and pregnancy failures contribute to postpartum emotional problems. Physical discomforts such as a painful perineum, afterpains, breast engorgement, and fatigue all contribute to negative postpartum reactions.

TAKING-IN AND TAKING-HOLD PHASES

Maternal adaption has been described by Rubin as the taking-in phase and the taking-hold phase. The taking-in phase begins immediately after the birth and lasts for the first 2 days. During this time, the mother demonstrates dependent behavior. She needs nurturing and protecting. Her behavior can be characterized as passive and dependent. She accepts what is given, does what she is told, and awaits the caregiver's actions rather than initiating her own actions. She sleeps, eats heartily, and is concerned about the overall health of her infant. The mother often feels the need to review her labor and delivery several times to search for missing details. Working through these details ultimately prepares her for the next pregnancy. For the first few days the mother often is very talkative and sometimes exhibits euphoric speech. Her preoccupation with details about her

NURSING CARE PLAN 13–1

NURSING MANAGEMENT DURING POSTPARTUM ADJUSTMENT

Potential Problems and Nursing Diagnoses	Nursing Interventions
1. Pain related to uterine contractions (after-pains).	Explain to mother that contraction and relaxation of uterine muscles cause cramping sensations referred to as afterpains.
2. Knowledge deficit related to physical postpartum adjustments.	Educate mother that excessive sweating assists in the elimination of excess fluid accumulated during pregnancy.
	Educate mother about changes in the breast to prepare for lactation. Provide information of normal breast changes including engorgement, distention, firmness, and discomfort.
3. Knowledge deficit related to milk secretion and ejection.	Teach mother the importance of positive emotions and factors that inhibit milk production, if she plans to breastfeed her infant.
4. Alteration in tissue perfusion related to blood loss during birth.	Monitor mother's vital signs. Recognize that a slow pulse of 50 to 70 beats per minute is normal, due in part to the blood loss during birth.
	Assess and record skin color and blood pressure, at least once every 8 hours (after the initial 1-hour assessment).
5. Knowledge deficit related to restoration of muscle strength and tone.	Explain to mother that postpartum exercises strengthen and tone muscles. Also, postpartum exercises improve circulation and promote venous blood return. Explain to mother that improvement of local circulation promotes healing.
	Provide opportunity for mother to demonstrate abdominal breathing and pelvic tilt exercises.
6. Anxiety related to psychological adjustments.	Provide information about emotional changes that commonly occur during the postpartum period, such as feeling of dependence in caretaking activities and insecurity about attaining the mothering role.
	Instruct the mother that she may have mood swings and temporary feelings of depression, that she may exhibit crying behavior over minor matters, and that this behavior is normal.

NURSING CARE PLAN 13–1 *Continued*

NURSING MANAGEMENT DURING POSTPARTUM ADJUSTMENT

Expected Outcomes

1. Mother verbalizes understanding of the cause of uterine cramping or afterpains.
2. Mother expresses relief to know that excessive sweating is normal. She says she will ask for a gown or bed linen change when either is wet or damp.
3. Mother recognizes the value of positive emotions and verbalizes factors that inhibit adequate milk production.
4. Mother recognizes the need for frequent assessment of her pulse and blood pressure.
5. Mother verbalizes the importance of postpartum exercises and demonstrates her ability to do a pelvic tilt.
6. Mother shows relief that mood swings and crying behavior are accepted as normal.

birth experience may reduce her ability to concentrate on new information. The caregiver may need to repeat instructions during this period. Simply stated, the taking-in phase is the time when the new mother takes in care and support from others.

On the second or third postpartum day, the mother is ready to assert her independence and autonomy. This is the beginning of the taking-hold phase. She becomes the initiator and is ready to take charge of new responsibilities. She attempts to be a "good mother." There is a strong element of anxiety during this phase. She begins to perform some of the new tasks of mothering. Frequently she becomes exhausted in her new role, and her independent behavior dissolves into dependent behavior. At this time, her body is undergoing significant physical changes that contribute to her fatigue. Breast milk begins to appear, and if the mother is nursing, she may doubt her ability to successfully perform the task. She becomes concerned about her bowel and bladder functions and her body in general.

ATTAINMENT OF THE MATERNAL ROLE

More recently, studies have focused on the attainment of the maternal role. *Maternal role attainment* is the process by which the woman learns mothering behaviors and becomes comfortable with her identity as a mother. It is suggested that formation of maternal identity occurs with each newborn infant. As the bond between the infant

and mother forms, the mother and infant/child grow to know each other.

According to Mercer, maternal role attainment occurs in four stages. These four stages correspond to those identified by Rubin. In the *anticipatory stage,* which occurs during pregnancy, the woman looks to role models of how to be a mother. In the *formal stage,* which begins when the infant is born, the mother is still influenced by the guidance of others. The *informal stage* begins when the mother starts to make her own choices about mothering. She begins to find her own style of mothering. In the *personal stage,* the mother does what she is comfortable with in the role of mother. This stage occurs from 3 to 10 months after delivery. Social support, the mother's age, her personality traits, and her socioeconomic status all influence the mother's success in attaining the mothering role.

Some believe that today's new mothers tend to be less dependent and are better able to assume the self-care responsibilities because of factors such as the reduced amount of medications received during labor, early ambulation, rooming-in, and increased support from the father, significant other, or family.

The transition to motherhood is a complex behavioral process. Parents who are ill prepared for the changes in relationships, lifestyle, and roles associated with the integration of the new infant in the family will have more difficulty making the necessary transition. The level of the woman's maturity, minimal exposure of the mother to the baby in the case of small infants, lack of a support system, or ill health also can interfere with maternal role attainment.

POSTPARTUM BLUES

Because of hormonal changes, for some women the postpartum period is characterized by frequent instances of depression and crying over minor matters. The episodes are temporary and usually last for a short time. This type of depression is referred to as *postpartum blues* and continues until hormonal stability is reached. Mothers should be instructed that these feelings are experienced, to some degree, by most women and are not clinically significant. If a woman shows unusual or bizarre behavior, further evaluation should be done.

References

Ament, L. A. (1990). Maternal tasks of the puerperium reidentified. *Journal of Obstetric, Gynecologic, and Neonatal Nursing* 19:330–335.

Ladewig, P. W., London, M. L., & Olds, S. B. (1990). *Essentials of Maternal-Newborn Nursing*, 2nd ed. Redwood City, CA: Addison-Wesley Nursing.

May, K. A., & Mahlmeister, L. R. (1990). *Comprehensive Maternity Nursing: Nursing Process and the Childbearing Family*, 2nd ed. Philadelphia: J.B. Lippincott.

Mercer, R. T. (1985). The process of maternal role attainment over the first year. *Nursing Research* 34:198.

Rayburn, W. F., & Zuspan, F. P. (1982). *Drug Therapy in Obstetrics and Gynecology*. Norwalk, CT: Appleton-Century-Crofts.

Rubin, R. (1961). Puerperal change. *Nursing Outlook* 9:753–757.

Unterman, R., Posner, N., & Williams, K. (1990). Postpartum depressive disorders: Changing trends. *Birth* 17(3):131–137.

SUGGESTED ACTIVITIES

1. Recall the changes that occur in the uterus and appear in the uterine discharge during the first 7 days of the postpartum period.
2. Explain the expected range of the maternal pulse and temperature during the first 24 hours after birth.
3. Explain the process of lactation. Identify factors that influence the mother's success in breastfeeding.
4. Identify the common psychological alterations that occur during the postpartum period.

REVIEW QUESTIONS

A. Select the best answer to each multiple-choice question.

Clinical Situation: Nurse Joan Simpson is assigned to the postpartum unit. She recognizes the importance of knowing the normal postpartum changes that should occur and the deviations from the expected normal physical changes. An assessment of Ms. Johnson, 1st day postpartum, reveals the following: T = 100, P = 65, BP = 120/80; fundus is firm, 2+, and displaced to the right; lochia rubra is present; perineum is edematous; edges of episiotomy are well approximated. Questions 1 through 7 refer to Joan's postpartum assessment.

1. Joan's first action is to
   A. Call the physician about Ms. Johnson's increased temperature
   B. Apply ice pack to her perineum
   C. Assist her to void
   D. Record all findings of assessment but take no nursing action

2. Joan recognizes that Ms. Johnson's slow pulse rate of 50 to 60 bpm during the early puerperium
   A. Is indicative of shock
   B. Is a sign that infection is present
   C. Means that Ms. Johnson is dehydrated
   D. Is a transient phenomenon

3. Joan knows that the most common cause for Ms. Johnson's elevated temperature during the first 24 hours after delivery is
   A. Initiation of lactation
   B. Probable staphylococcus infection
   C. Mastitis
   D. Dehydration

4. Joan assesses Ms. Johnson's lochia. She knows that lochia proceeds as follows:
   A. Rubra, serosa, alba
   B. Serosa, rubra, alba
   C. Rubra, alba, serosa
   D. Serosa, alba, rubra

5. Joan checks Ms. Johnson's chart to see if she is Rh− or Rh+ to see if she should be receiving RhoGAM. Which statement regarding RhoGAM is false?

   A. It must be given intramuscularly within 72 hours after delivery to be effective

   B. It may be used prophylactically in Rh− women

   C. It should be given to an Rh− mother with an Rh− baby

   D. None of the above

6. Ms. Johnson is voiding large amounts of urine. This most likely is indicative of

   A. A postpartum cystitis

   B. Her body effort to return its water metabolism to normal

   C. An increased sensitivity of the bladder

   D. A nervous response

7. On the 2nd day postpartum Ms. Johnson tells Joan that each time she breastfeeds, she experiences some pain similar to the discomfort she had during labor. Joan explains that this pain is most likely indicative of

   A. Uterine atony

   B. Suppression of lochia

   C. Uterine involution

   D. Improper suckling by the baby

8. Thrombophlebitis is a complication in the postpartum period that usually can be reduced with

   A. Cesarean birth

   B. Early ambulation of postpartum women

   C. Aiding woman to prevent anemia

   D. Keeping blood loss to a minimum

9. Postpartum hemorrhage is bleeding in excess of

   A. 200 mL

   B. 300 mL

   C. 400 mL

   D. 500 mL

10. Immediately after a normal delivery, a nurse's assessment will reveal all of the following EXCEPT

    A. The uterus is below the umbilicus

    B. The uterus is firm

    C. The vaginal discharge is red in color

    D. The vaginal discharge is brown in color

11. Postpartum patients should be instructed that they will probably experience the following during the first 24 hours after delivery:

    A. Diaphoresis, hunger, thirst, and reduction in pulse rate

    B. Diaphoresis, hunger, and milk secretion

    C. Hunger, increased urine output, and increased pulse rate

    D. Increased pulse rate, increased temperature, and reduction in urinary output

12. A mother who plans to breastfeed her infant should be instructed in all of the following EXCEPT

    A. Not to take drugs unless they are approved by her physician

    B. To increase her fluid intake

    C. To increase her nonpregnant dietary requirement 500 calories

    D. To increase her nonpregnant dietary requirement 1000 calories

13. During the 1st and 2nd postpartum days, the common maternal psychological adaption is the

    A. Taking-in phase

    B. Taking-hold phase

    C. Letting-go phase

    D. Excitement phase

B. Choose from Column II the phrase that most accurately defines the term in Column I.

I

1. Lochia rubra _____
2. Lochia serosa _____
3. Lochia alba _____
4. Diaphoresis _____
5. Prolactin _____
6. Oxytocin _____
7. Lactation-suppressing drug _____
8. RhoGAM _____
9. Taking-hold phase _____
10. Taking-in phase _____

II

A. Obvious, excessive sweating
B. White vaginal discharge
C. Causes let-down reflex
D. Bright red vaginal bleeding
E. Enhances milk production
F. Decreases breast engorgement
G. Given to Rh− women
H. Maternal dependent behavior
I. Increases breast engorgement
J. Maternal independent behavior
K. Pinkish to brownish vaginal discharge

CHAPTER 14 _____

Chapter Outline

Arrangement for Postpartum Care
Physiological and Psychological Nursing Assessment
   and Intervention
      Vital signs
      Uterus
      Lochia
      Psychological assessment
Nursing Assessment of Comfort, Promotion of Health,
   and Self-Care Instruction
      Bath care
      Breast assessment: lactation and suppression of
        lactation
      Perineal care
      Elimination
      Lower extremities
      Ambulation
      Nutritional status
Postpartum Exercises
Resumption of Physical Activities
Resumption of Sexual Intercourse
Health Maintenance and Promotion of Health
      Danger signs to report
Promotion of Health for Future Pregnancies
      Rubella vaccine
      Rh_o (D) immune globulin (RhoGAM)
Family Planning
Sibling Adaptation
      Sibling visits
      Preparation for the additional family member
Discharge Examination, Commonly Given Instructions,
   and Medical/Nursing Follow-up Care

Learning Objectives

Upon completion of Chapter 14, the student should be
able to
- Identify two new tasks for new mothers that will affect
  the family unit.
- Describe different arrangements for postpartum
  care.
- Name four nursing diagnoses used in postpartum
  care.
- Explain bath care to the postpartum woman.
- Describe how to assess the postpartum woman's
  perineum.
- Explain instruction for self-care in applying an ice
  pack to the perineum and taking a sitz bath.
- Name three factors to include in education for self-
  care to improve elimination after delivery.
- Explain why assessment of the lower extremities is an
  important part of postpartum recovery care.
- List three reasons for early and frequent ambulation.
- Recall why the suppression of lactation in the non-
  nursing mother needs special attention.
- Explain the importance of the postpartum nutritional
  status in a nursing mother.
- Recall the importance of the perineal-tightening
  exercises.
- Outline the resumption of physical activities after
  childbirth.
- List two concerns women have about resumption of
  sexual intercourse.
- List four danger signs the woman should know to
  report to the physician, if they occur after she is
  discharged from the hospital.
- List two measures to promote the health of the fetus
  in future pregnancies and describe the teaching
  responsibilities of the nursing intervention.
- Describe sibling adaptation.
- Name three ways to prepare the older child for the
  new baby.
- Name five common postpartum instructions at discharge.

NURSING CARE DURING THE POSTPARTUM PERIOD

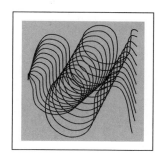

In the period after birth, called the *puerperium*, the mother is faced with many adjustments, physiological as well as psychological. Repair of injury to the birth canal, involution of the uterus, and return of the body's systems to the nonpregnant state are discussed in Chapter 13. The nursing assessments, interventions, and the woman's self-care are discussed in this chapter.

Clearly, the transition to parenthood is abrupt; the new responsibility for infant care comes suddenly. Parents often have limited preparation. In addition, because the woman usually has a short hospital stay, she is faced with an immediate need for instruction in both infant care and self-care.

The caregiver's main goals in postpartum care are to enhance the establishment of the family unit, assist and support the woman's return to the nonpregnant state, assess and identify deviations from the norm, educate the mother and family on care of the infant after discharge, and educate the mother on her own self-care. Special attention should be given to rest, nutrition, hydration, elimination, exercise, graduated activities, promotion of comfort, healing of tissues, and identification of early signs of complications.

The caregiver should understand the need for good medical aseptic technique during procedures, because the uterine cavity is easily accessible to microorganisms from the exterior. Also, the place where the placenta was attached is like an open wound and can be easily infected. Hence, the maternity unit is considered a "clean area" in contrast to other units of the hospital. In most institutions, the caregivers wear clean scrub dress attire in the maternity unit, and when they leave the unit they wear a laboratory coat or some type of a cover garment. This is in accordance with the hospital's infectious control committee's policy. In addition, health care providers should be free from infection. Caregivers who have an upper respiratory infection or a herpes lesion should not have direct contact with either the mother or the infant.

In order to reduce the potential risk of infection and maximize comfort, specific nursing actions are included in postpartum care. In addition, to make sure the mother's physiological and psychological restorative processes are within the normal range, assessments are conducted and recorded daily. This serial postpartum assessment allows the woman's body changes to be reviewed.

TASKS FOR NEW MOTHERS, FAMILIES, OR CAREGIVERS

- Form an attachment to the infant.
- Optimize the mother's physiological and psychological restorative processes.
- Instruct the mother about self-care.
- Develop infant caretaking skills.
- Develop a satisfactory relationship with the father that includes parenting.
- Develop a sense of a family unit when siblings are present.
- Alter the environment to meet infant and family needs.
- Make decisions regarding whether to have another pregnancy.
- Assess income and housing in relation to the additional family member.

Arrangement for Postpartum Care

If the mother gives birth in an alternative birthing unit, usually the mother and infant go home soon after birth (sometimes within hours). In the standard hospital setting, the mother plans to stay in the hospital for 1 to 2 days after delivery. The mother and newborn are cared for in either a traditional or a rooming-in arrangement. In the traditional arrangement, mothers and infants are kept in separate rooms, with the infants in nurseries except for feeding and viewing hours. In the rooming-in arrangement, present in many hospitals, the infant can room in with the mother most of the time. The physical and psychological assessment of the mother and the infant is essentially the same in either arrangement. However, the nursing interventions differ, particularly in the instruction of infant care. It is important that parent education become an integral part of nursing in both the traditional and rooming-in hospital settings (Fig. 14–1A).

First-time mothers should be encouraged to participate in rooming-in. The rooming-in plan provides learning opportunities for the mother because it permits closer and longer contact with the infant. Frequently, the father or significant other is permitted to visit the mother while she is with the infant. In addition, siblings sometimes are encouraged to visit their mother and get acquainted with the new infant. All visitors are instructed to wash their hands and, usually, to wear a gown before handling the infant.

In the rooming-in arrangement, the infant is kept at the mother's bedside or in an adjoining cubicle most of the day. If the mother desires to rest, her infant may be placed in the nursery for the night or for another specified period of time. While bathing the infant, the caregiver can answer the mother's questions about infant care. As the mother feels more confident, she is invited to participate in her infant's care. Rooming-in may not be desired by all parents. Some mothers, especially multiparas, welcome the rest period during which they will have limited direct responsibility for their infant's care. Others may feel too tired to have the infant at their bedside for extended periods of time. However, rooming-in,

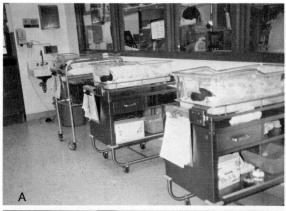
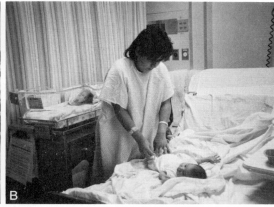
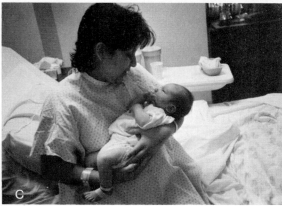

▲ FIGURE 14–1

A. Traditional nursery. **B.** Rooming-in at University of Illinois Hospital. **C.** Mother getting acquainted with her infant.

when available, offers a great learning experience (Fig. 14–1B and C).

Physiological and Psychological Nursing Assessment and Intervention

The caregiver should obtain as much information as possible on which to base nursing care for the woman during the postpartum period. The woman should be assessed immediately to establish a physical data base, including observation of the uterus, the lochia, the vital signs, the perineum, the breasts and nipples, hydration, the bladder, discomfort, the psychological status, and the general condition (Table 14–1).

Certain data should be obtained when the woman is transferred from the recovery room to the postpartum unit. This information includes the type of delivery, time of birth, analgesic or anesthetic received, amount of blood loss, interim from rupture of membranes to delivery, episiotomy incision or laceration, and any birth complications. In addition, the report should include the status of the infant with both the Apgar score and general appearance. As soon as possible, the wom-

an's record should be reviewed for pertinent data, including her prenatal course, laboratory findings, and any significant psychosocial information.

The data are used to plan for the woman's care. The caregiver can decide which nursing measures would be appropriate and which are to be given priority. The data can be used to formulate nursing diagnoses. Because many agencies use the NANDA (North American Nursing Diagnosis Association) list, physiological alterations form the basis of many postpartum diagnoses.

NURSING DIAGNOSES FOR POSTPARTUM CARE

- Altered pattern of urinary elimination
- Altered bowel elimination: constipation
- Altered tissue perfusion
- Anxiety
- Altered sexual patterns
- Impairment of skin integrity
- Self-deficit: bathing/hygiene
- Ineffective individual coping
- Knowledge deficit
- Pain
- Potential for infection
- Potential fluid volume deficit

TABLE 14–1. POSTPARTUM ASSESSMENT AND RECORDING

ASSESSMENT	RECORDING
Vital signs	Temperature, pulse rate, respirations, and blood pressure
Breasts and nipples	Signs of engorgement, tenderness, and lactation
Uterus	Fundal height, location, and consistency
Lochia	Amount, color, presence of clots, and odor
Perineum	Edema, hematoma, signs of episiotomy/laceration healing or signs of inflammation
Lower extremities	Edema, redness, tenderness, warmth, and positive Homan's sign
Voiding	Amount, frequency, and discomfort
Defecation	If or when patient had bowel movement
General condition	Color of skin and mucous membranes
Hydration	Amount of fluid intake
Ambulation	If patient was dizzy or faint when up and about; frequency of ambulation
Pain or discomfort	Location and degree of discomfort or pain
Psychological status	General attitude, sense of satisfaction, level of fatigue
Parenting	Mother's reaction to infant

It is important for the caregiver to establish a daily physical and psychological assessment of the woman. During this assessment, comfort measures, opportunity for rest, fluid and food intake, urinary output, condition of breasts, discomfort, vital signs, psychological status, and reaction to infant are evaluated.

For most women, the postpartal recovery is uneventful and is considered a healthy process. One must remember that every family has needs, although they may not be obvious when they are psychological or if there is a knowledge deficit.

VITAL SIGNS

The woman's vital signs are discussed in Chapter 13. After the first hourly assessment, it is important for the vital signs to be taken every 8 hours, more frequently if there is a deviation from the norm. An elevated temperature may occur during the first 24 hours because of dehydration, after which it should be about 98.6° F. As previously mentioned, a slow pulse rate is not of clinical significance and is related to a reduction in blood volume. The woman's blood pressure should remain stable after delivery. A change in the woman's vital signs should be reported to the midwife or physician.

UTERUS

The location, size, and consistency of the uterus are important nursing assessments. Before assessment of the uterus, the woman should void. This practice ensures that a full bladder is not causing the uterus to be pushed up or to one side (deviation from the midline). The caregiver should determine the relationship of the fundus to the umbilicus, as discussed in Chapter 13. Intervals for the assessment of the uterus immediately after birth (that is, the fourth stage of labor) are discussed in Chapter 13.

One hand is gently placed on the lower segment of the uterus to provide support, and the fingers of the other hand are placed on the top of the uterus (fundus) to determine the uterine location in fingerbreadths or centimeters (Fig. 14–2). The

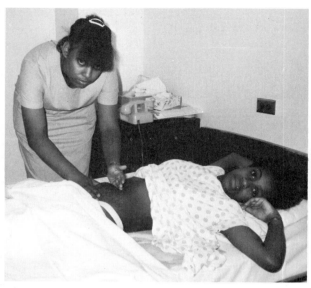

▲ FIGURE 14–2

Measurement of descent of fundus. Fundus is located at level of umbilicus.

position of the uterus is recorded either above or below the umbilicus. For example, the uterus is recorded as −2/u if it is located two fingerbreadths below the level of the umbilicus. If the fundus is located at the level of the umbilicus, it is recorded as 0.

The location of the uterus should be monitored at the beginning of every shift (every 8 hours). It should be monitored more frequently if problems of bogginess (sponginess owing to uterine relaxation) occur, the uterus changes position, lochia flow is heavy, or clots are present (see Chapter 13 for medication usage). Massage may stimulate the uterus to contract.

LOCHIA

Nursing assessment of lochia includes color, amount, consistency, and odor (see Chapter 13). The woman should be instructed that it is normal for some clots to be present because of blood pooling in the vagina. However, the passing of large clots is abnormal and should be reported immediately to the nurse for further evaluation.

The woman's pad-changing practice makes it difficult to determine the amount of flow. If the woman uses more than eight pads in 24 hours, she should be asked to leave a pad on for 20 minutes so the nurse can assess the amount of pad saturation.

PSYCHOLOGICAL ASSESSMENT

The woman's psychological behavior, including coping skills, should be assessed daily. Women exhibit dependent behaviors for the first 2 days. These behaviors become mixed with dependent and independent actions. By the third day, independent behaviors should be noticeable (Chapter 13). Depressive reactions, characterized by mood changes (postpartum blues), may be observed. The caregiver should assess, record, and report any abnormal findings. Also, the nurse should support the woman when she shares her emotional feelings.

The nurse should encourage the attachment process between the mother and infant (Chapter 16). The father also needs to interact with his infant. Fathers who attend expectant parent classes with their wives and participate in the birth of the infant usually begin the attachment process early.

Nursing Assessment of Comfort, Promotion of Health, and Self-Care Instruction

BATH CARE

The initial bath or shower may be taken after admission to the postpartum unit. Time spent helping with the bath or shower permits observation and patient instruction. Also, it provides comfort and protection against infection. The postpartum bath differs from routine baths given to hospitalized patients, because two areas of the woman's body are at greater risk for infections: the breasts and the perineum. If the woman had a cesarean birth, the abdominal incision would be an additional area susceptible to infection. The nurse should remain with the woman. If she feels dizzy, had a prolonged labor, had large blood loss, or exhibits unstable vital signs, additional caution is warranted.

Education for Self-Care. The postpartum woman should be instructed to begin her bath or shower by washing her breasts. Soap and water should be used sparingly. Some advise washing the breasts with clear water to decrease the drying of the skin and thereby reduce the risk of cracked nipples. The breasts should be washed in a circular manner from the nipple outward, after which they should be dried with a clean towel. If the mother is nursing, exposure of the breast to the air for approximately 15 minutes may be advocated.

The woman should be instructed not to rub her lower extremities vigorously because of the potential danger of emboli. She should be advised to have the call button readily available to her so she can get help quickly if she feels weak, faint, or dizzy.

BREAST ASSESSMENT: LACTATION AND SUPPRESSION OF LACTATION

The breasts should be assessed daily for tenderness, redness, warmth, firmness, and secretion whether or not the woman plans to breastfeed. The secretion changes from colostrum to milk. By the second or third day, the breasts become engorged, firm, and tender, and their venous pattern becomes prominent. By palpation, the breasts generally feel nodular (lumpy). As lactation is established, the nodules may be felt, and the milk-filled "sacs" will shift in position. If the woman is going to nurse, the nipples should be assessed for size and shape. The nipples should also be examined for erectility as opposed to inversions, cracks, and fissures. The breasts should then be palpated to determine if there is localized tenderness. The palpation technique used is the same as that used for self-examination of the breasts. The caregiver should assess the woman's knowledge of an adequate breast examination by observing the woman do it (see Chapter 25).

The woman who plans to nurse her infant should be taught ways to prevent her nipples from becoming sore or cracked. She should be instructed about changing the infant's position to

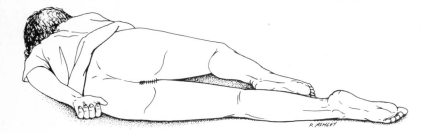

▲ FIGURE 14–3

Episiotomy is inspected with woman on her side and her upper leg forward.

change pressure points and breaking infant suction before removing the infant from the breast (see Chapter 19).

Breast care for the woman who is not nursing her infant includes assessment of engorgement and discomfort. The physician may prescribe a drug to suppress lactation (see Chapter 13 and Appendix B). Ice bags may be used to constrict the circulation, thus relieving the discomfort. A snug bra or binder may relieve some discomfort of breast engorgement. Pumping the breasts should *not* be done in a nonnursing mother because it stimulates the production of milk. Analgesic drugs may be required to reduce the woman's discomfort. A comparison of breastfeeding and bottle feeding is presented in Chapter 19.

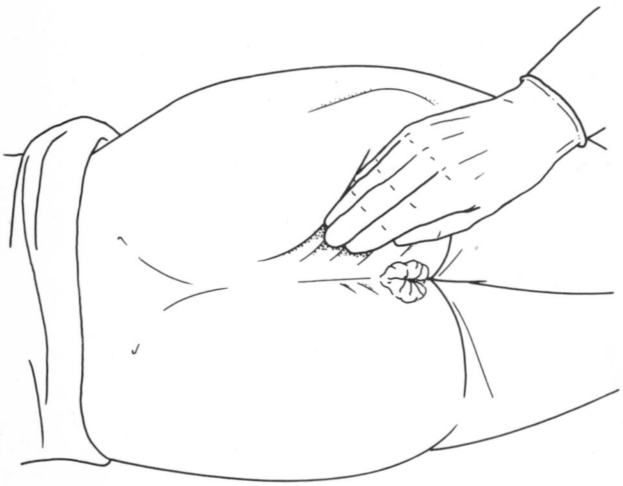

▲ FIGURE 14–4

Assessment of perineum with hemorrhoids. Nurse's gloved hand raises the upper buttocks to fully expose the anal area.

PERINEAL CARE

The aims of perineal care are to increase cleanliness and comfort, promote healing, and prevent infection. The importance of handwashing for both the caregiver and the woman cannot be overemphasized. The perineum should be assessed for unusual swelling, discoloration, and sharp pain, which would suggest that a *hematoma* is developing. A hematoma, collection of blood in the tissues, could be caused by the rupture of a blood vessel or a cut in a small vessel that is not sutured at the time of the episiotomy repair. The first clue of a hematoma is usually the woman's complaint of marked pain around her stitches. A developing hematoma needs to be reported to the physician because it requires surgical intervention.

Assessment of Intact Perineum or Status of Episiotomy

The perineum should be inspected daily as part of routine care. In addition to the type and amount of vaginal discharge, healing of the tissues should be assessed. If an episiotomy was performed, the woman should lie on her side with her upper leg forward so that the nurse can assess whether the stitches of the episiotomy are intact or separated and whether purulent drainage is present around the stitches (Fig. 14–3). It is important to identify infection early, should it occur. Hemorrhoids, if present, should be assessed for size, discomfort, and tenderness (Fig. 14–4). Measures to relieve hemorrhoidal discomfort include sitz bath, heat lamps, and medications. Hemorrhoidal discomfort decreases as edema is reduced and circulation is improved.

Education for Self-Care. The woman should be

instructed about the importance of good hygienic practice in perineal care. First, she should wash her hands before cleansing her perineum. Second, she should recognize the importance of stroking her perineum from front (symphysis pubis) to back (toward the anus) while washing. The bowel and fecal matter normally harbor many types of bacteria. If they remain in the bowel, the organisms are harmless, but if they are introduced into the vagina, urethra, or episiotomy area, a serious infection may result. Application of the peripad also should begin from front to back, with fingers touching only the edges and not the center of the pad. The same principle should be followed in applying ice packs and topical anesthetics to relieve perineal discomfort.

There are several methods of cleansing the perineum. Soap and water may be applied with a clean, disposable washcloth. The woman should be instructed to repeat perineal care after each bath, each voiding, and each bowel movement.

Application of Cold to the Perineum

An ice pack is frequently applied immediately after the episiotomy is repaired to reduce edema and numb the tissues, which promotes comfort. Inexpensive ice bags can be made by filling a disposable rubber glove with ice and then taping or securing the glove at the wrist area. An ice pack is most effective during the first 24 hours after delivery, when cold is most successful in preventing edema.

Education for Self-Care. The caregiver should instruct the woman about the purpose of the ice pack and how it can be prepared at home if swelling is present. She should be instructed to cover the ice pack with a Chux pad or washcloth to avoid an ice burn on her perineum.

Application of Heat to the Perineum

Heat is used to decrease the woman's discomfort. It increases circulation to the perineal area and thereby relaxes the tissues. Either moist or dry heat can be applied.

SITZ BATH

Sitz baths are commonly used to apply moist heat to the perineum. It provides comfort, promotes healing, and reduces the incidence of infection. Many hospitals supply a plastic, portable, sitz bath that fits inside the toilet. These baths are convenient for the woman to take as often as she wishes in the hospital and at home. If a sitz bathtub is used, it should be thoroughly cleansed between patients to prevent cross-contamination or transmission of infection.

Education for Self-care. The nurse should instruct the woman to cleanse the portable sitz bath or the tub before using it and have the temperature of the water at about 100° F. The water should not be above 105° F to prevent moist heat burn. She should be told to sit in the sitz bath for 15 to 20 minutes. Also, she should be instructed to use the call light if she begins to feel warm, dizzy, or faint. It is important that she use a clean towel to pat dry her perineum after the sitz bath and then use a clean perineal pad.

PERINEAL HEAT LAMP

Dry heat from a perineal lamp is helpful. It dries the perineal area and increases circulation to promote healing and comfort. The woman should be instructed first to cleanse the perineum to prevent drying of secretions in the area. She should be instructed that placement of the lamp is important. In the hospital or home, the lamp should be placed about 18 inches from the perineum and the lamp should contain a 60-watt (or lower) light bulb to avoid burns. A goose-neck lamp can be used in the home, if available. If a portable perineal heat lamp is used, the nurse should remember to never place it on the floor when not in use, because of contamination.

Application of Topical Anesthetics

Topical anesthetics are given to relieve perineal discomfort. Americaine and Dermoplast (benzocaine) sprays, Nupercaine ointment (dibucaine), or TUCKS are commonly used to relieve hemorrhoidal discomfort. Nurses should make sure to wash their hands after applying a topical medica-

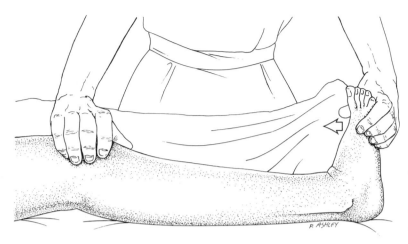

▲ FIGURE 14–5

Assessment of Homan's sign of the legs. While holding the woman's knee flat, the nurse dorsiflexes the woman's foot. Pain in the woman's leg is a positive Homan's sign.

tion on the patient, even though they used gloves as a universal precaution.

Education for Self-Care. The woman should be instructed to apply the topical medication after a sitz bath or after using the heat lamp. This is important because of the danger of tissue burn if the medication is used before the sitz bath. Also, the woman should wait 1 to 2 minutes to apply the vaginal pad, or much of the medication will be absorbed into the pad rather than staying on the perineal tissues.

ELIMINATION

After delivery, the caregiver should conscientiously monitor the woman's bladder status. A displaced uterus or a palpable bladder is a sign of urinary distention and requires nursing interventions. The caregiver should assess the frequency of urination, the amount of urine, or the inability to void. The woman must empty her bladder completely when she voids, or urinary stasis and infection can result.

The caregiver should obtain information about the woman's bowel elimination and elicit her concerns about it. Frequently, women fear that their first bowel movement will be painful and possibly damage the stitches of the episiotomy. Sometimes, a stool softener is given to lessen perineal discomfort during bowel elimination.

Education for Self-Care. The woman should be encouraged to have an adequate intake of fluids.

She should be encouraged to ambulate and use the bathroom, because this is more natural, more comfortable, and more conducive to normal functioning than using a bedpan. A proper diet, including an increase in fiber and fluid intake, along with exercise will assist the woman in regaining her regular bowel habit.

LOWER EXTREMITIES

The lower extremities (feet, legs, and thighs) should be assessed daily for warmth, tenderness, and a positive Homan's sign. For evaluation, the legs should be stretched out and relaxed. The foot is then grasped and sharply dorsiflexed (Fig. 14–5). No discomfort should be present. If pain is elicited, the woman has a positive Homan's sign, which should be reported to the nurse in charge or the physician. The pain is caused by inflammation of the vessels, which could be caused by thrombophlebitis. Skin temperature and edema of the legs, if present, should also be noted.

Education for Self-Care. The woman should be encouraged to ambulate frequently to promote good circulation. This reduces the risk of a thrombosis and infection during the postpartum period.

AMBULATION

Early and frequent ambulation is essential to reduce the risk of infection or thrombosis (clot formation). In addition, early ambulation lessens the chance that respiratory, circulatory, and urinary problems will develop. It also prevents or lessens constipation and promotes the rapid return of strength. Usually women ambulate soon after delivery, unless they have had spinal or general anesthetic.

When the woman gets out of bed for the first time, the caregiver should stay with her because she may become dizzy and faint. Women who have lost a large amount of blood are more apt to feel faint because of a decrease in blood volume.

Education for Self-Care. The woman should be instructed that if she becomes faint she should immediately call someone (using the call light), if possible. She should be instructed to ease into a chair and lower her head to her knees.

If the woman has been lying down for a period of time, there may be a sudden temporary gush of vaginal discharge (lochia) when she gets up. The color should be observed; if it is dark red, it most likely is normal. The woman should be instructed that this usually reflects her change in position. The vaginal discharge can pool in the recumbent position, then flow freely in the standing position. However, if the uterine flow continues, the woman should report it for further evaluation to rule out bleeding from other causes.

NUTRITIONAL STATUS

The caregiver's assessment of nutrition during mealtime provides an opportunity to observe the foods selected and avoided by the patient. Focusing on the foods eaten may help initiate a discussion of good nutrition. The woman should be encouraged to eat a well-balanced diet. If the woman is breastfeeding, she should increase her caloric intake 500 calories per day above the prepregnancy requirements. In addition, she should increase her fluid intake to 2000 to 3000 mL per day to increase her milk supply.

The hospital's dietitian should be informed of any cultural or religious beliefs that require specific foods. The woman should be encouraged to continue taking vitamins and her iron supplements. Laboratory values are often determined at the 6-

week postpartum examination to detect if anemia has persisted or developed.

Postpartum Exercises

Postpartum exercises are discussed in Chapter 13. However, one exercise, the Kegel exercise, is emphasized here because it is an important part of postpartum care.

The woman should be instructed to tighten her buttocks before sitting to lessen the discomfort and avoid direct trauma to the perineum. If the woman had a lateral episiotomy, lying on her side should be suggested for comfort. Often, it is more comfortable to lie on the same side as the episiotomy incision.

A perineal-tightening (Kegel) exercise should be encouraged to strengthen and tone the muscles of the pelvic floor. The woman should be instructed to contract the muscles as if stopping and starting the flow of urine during voiding. She should practice this exercise several times a day. The woman should be instructed that it is beneficial for her to continue perineal-tightening exercises throughout her life for the potential increase in sexual satisfaction and reduced risk of urinary incontinence.

Resumption of Physical Activities

Women frequently ask what they may and may not do once they are home. They should be advised to increase their activities gradually and avoid fatigue. The woman should be instructed to avoid heavy lifting, excessive stair climbing, and strenuous activity. She should be encouraged to take one to two naps daily, which may be most easily achieved if she rests when the baby sleeps. By the second week at home, light housekeeping may be carried out. Most women resume practically all activities by 4 to 5 weeks postpartum. However, it is customary to delay returning to work until after the 6-week postpartum examination. This allows potential problems to be identified before the woman goes back to work outside the home.

Resumption of Sexual Intercourse

Sexual intercourse can safely be resumed when lochia has ceased, the episiotomy incision has healed, and the woman feels ready. The time varies from 3 to 6 weeks. If the woman had an extensive episiotomy or a laceration, she may need to wait longer for the perineum to heal. The first postpartum intercourse will probably be somewhat uncomfortable. This is partly due to the dryness or diminished vaginal lubrication. Women should be instructed to use a water-soluble vaginal lubricant. Patience and gentleness by the partner are important factors for many women. A position that puts less strain on the woman's perineum is helpful (man on top, woman on top, or woman on her side). One of the positions may prove to be the most comfortable to her.

Health Maintenance and Promotion of Health

Health maintenance and promotion of health include postpartum activities previously discussed in this chapter, such as prevention of infection, promotion of comfort, and exercise. Most women experience an uneventful postpartum recovery. However, because some women will experience postpartum complications, all women should know signs to alert them to come back to the clinic or go to their physician for further evaluation. The following list of danger signs should be given to the woman at discharge.

DANGER SIGNS TO REPORT

The following danger signs should be reported to the physician, nurse, midwife, or clinic staff:

- Persistent, recurrent, or increased bright red vaginal bleeding with or without passage of blood clots
- Foul odor of the vaginal discharge
- Elevated temperature of 100.4° F (38° C) or higher on two consecutive readings at least 6 hours apart (puerperal morbidity)
- Localized pain, tenderness, or redness on the calves of legs
- Abdominal or pelvic pain or tenderness
- Painful, tender, or a localized reddened area of the breasts
- Cracked nipples with increased discomfort when nursing infant
- Unusual pain in the area of the episiotomy, with or without purulent drainage
- Painful urination

Promotion of Health for Future Pregnancies

RUBELLA VACCINE

Women who have a rubella titer of less than 1:10 may be given rubella vaccine during the postpartum period. This will protect their next fetus from fetal malformations. The caregiver should make sure that these women understand the purpose of the rubella vaccine and also that they must not get pregnant for the next 3 months. Counseling about the use of contraceptives is important to avoid pregnancy.

RH₀ (D) IMMUNE GLOBULIN (RhoGAM)

Women who are Rh− who meet specific criteria (Chapter 21) should receive RhoGAM within 72 hours for the health of the next child.

Family Planning

The woman or couple will need to discuss and make a decision about contraception before resuming sexual intercourse. The caregiver should provide information about family planning (Chapter

15) before the woman's discharge from the hospital. The woman or couple should be told about the clinics or groups that provide further information about contraception. Many public health departments have family planning clinics. In addition, some hospitals and private agencies conduct family planning services.

Sibling Adaptation

SIBLING VISITS

Recently, visits by siblings have been allowed in maternity units (Fig. 14–6). This policy contributes to family unity by promoting the acceptance of the new infant by the other children. For many years, state and local health department regulations prohibited children under 16 years from visiting patients in the hospital. These regulations were made to prevent the spread of infection. It is now known that the mothers and children benefit from seeing each other in the hospital setting. This arrangement can reduce the child's feelings of abandonment and reduce the anxiety,

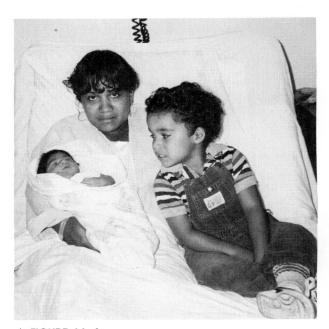

▲ FIGURE 14–6

Sibling visitation.

jealousy, and rivalry toward the new infant. It is possible that common negative reactions such as regression, attention seeking (acting out), and aggression toward the new infant are lessened by including the older child earlier in the acquaintance process, with less time separated from the mother.

PREPARATION FOR THE ADDITIONAL FAMILY MEMBER

There are many ways to prepare a child for an additional brother or sister, starting during the prenatal period:

- Encourage the child to feel the fetus move
- Give simple, concise explanations about the expected baby
- Take the child along on a prenatal visit to clinic or physician
- Make changes in sleeping arrangements before the birth of the baby
- Get a special new bed for the child
- Increase the involvement of the father with the child (seems to be directly related to better adjustment to separation from mother and baby)
- Give a gift to the child at the time of the baby's homecoming
- Involve the child in the baby's care whenever possible
- Praise the child for independent activities, such as getting dressed

Discharge Examination, Commonly Given Instructions, and Medical/Nursing Follow-Up Care

Before the woman is discharged, she often receives a physical examination by her physician or nurse midwife. In addition, she usually has an

NURSING CARE PLAN 14–1

NURSING CARE OF POSTPARTUM WOMAN AND FAMILY

Potential Problems and Nursing Diagnoses	Nursing Interventions
1. Self-care deficit related to hygiene and bathing.	Educate mother about the importance of bathing to provide comfort and protection against infection. Instruct mother about the importance of stroking from front to back, toward the rectum, to avoid contamination from the rectal area. Emphasize that this should be done during perineal care and placement of perineal pads.
2. Knowledge deficit related to application of heat to the perineum.	Explain how heat increases circulation to the perineal area and promotes comfort and healing. Instruct mother how to take a sitz bath under supervision and have her demonstrate the sitz bath technique.
3. Altered patterns of urinary elimination.	Monitor the intake and output. Report bladder distention. Palpate the uterus; if to the side of the midline, have mother empty her bladder. Assess the position of the uterus after voiding. Recognize that frequent small voidings are indicative of urinary stasis and infection can result.
4. Potential for infection.	Monitor the lower extremities for warmth and tenderness and potential infection of the vessels. Instruct mother to ambulate early and frequently to reduce the risk of a thrombosis. Ambulation increases the circulation in the lower extremities.
5. Anxiety related to increase in vaginal discharge.	Instruct mother that when she gets up after she has been lying down for a period of time, she may have a temporary increase in vaginal discharge. This usually reflects her change in position, which allows a free blood flow to occur.

NURSING CARE PLAN 14–1 *Continued*

NURSING CARE OF POSTPARTUM WOMAN AND FAMILY

6. Pain related to breast engorgement.	Monitor mother's breasts for engorgement and discomfort. Place ice packs and/or a supportive bra to relieve the discomfort. Instruct mother to not stimulate her breasts if she does not plan to breastfeed her infant.
7. Knowledge deficit related to resumption of physical activities.	Instruct mother that she can gradually increase physical activities but to avoid fatigue. Teach her to avoid heavy lifting and strenuous activity.
8. Knowledge deficit related to danger signs of hemorrhage or infection.	Educate mother about the danger signs to report, such as excessive bleeding or elevation of temperature after discharge.
9. Knowledge deficit related to preparation of family for new member.	Explain measures to reduce sibling jealousy and rivalry.

Expected Outcomes

1. Mother demonstrates correct procedure for self-care, including hygiene and bathing.
2. Mother communicates understanding of application of heat to the perineum and need for a sitz bath to promote healing and comfort.
3. Mother voices increased comfort after emptying her bladder. She also states she will report the number of times she voids in a 4-hour period.
4. Mother communicates understanding of early and frequent ambulation to increase circulation and reduce the risk of infection.
5. Mother acknowledges feelings related to increased vaginal discharge that occurs when she changes her position from lying down to standing. She appears relieved to have an explanation of the change in the amount of flow.
6. Mother expresses understanding of why breast engorgement occurs.
7. Mother expresses relief to know that on hospital discharge, she can gradually increase her physical activities, including some household chores that do not involve heavy lifting.
8. Mother communicates understanding of danger signs, such as excessive vaginal bleeding or a fever after hospital discharge.
9. Mother recognizes need to prepare siblings for the new baby to lessen jealousy.

KEY POINTS IN EDUCATION: POSTPARTUM INSTRUCTIONS

The following is a list of instructions commonly given to the postpartum woman when she is discharged from the hospital.

- HYGIENE: Tub baths, showers, and shampooing hair are permissible.
- ACTIVITY: Activity in moderation or not beyond the point of fatigue is recommended.
- SEXUAL INTERCOURSE: Sexual intercourse should be avoided until the episiotomy incision is healed. Gentleness and comfort are important.
- DOUCHING: No douching should be done for 6 weeks unless otherwise directed.
- VAGINAL PAD: A vaginal pad, not tampons, should be worn.
- BRASSIERE: A supportive brassiere should be worn by both nursing and nonnursing mothers for comfort.
- DIET: A well-balanced diet is encouraged. The nursing mother needs increased fluid intake and to drink 1 quart of milk a day.
- HEMORRHOIDS: Sitz baths should be taken and ointments applied as prescribed.
- EPISIOTOMY: Discomfort from the episiotomy incision can be relieved by sitz baths and prescribed medicated ointment.

- PRENATAL VITAMINS AND IRON: Vitamins and iron pills that were taken prenatally should be continued.
- POSTPARTUM EXERCISES: Postpartum exercises should gradually be increased, but not to the point of discomfort or fatigue.
- DANGER SIGNS: Any recurrence of bright red or excessive bleeding or a foul odor to vaginal discharge should be reported to the physician at once. An elevated temperature, prolonged abdominal or pelvic pain, pain in calf, or drainage of episiotomy should also be reported.
- 6-WEEK APPOINTMENT: A 6-week appointment is essential to detect an abnormal condition.
- FAMILY PLANNING: During the 6-week checkup, family planning, if desired, should be discussed.
- BREAST CARE: Nursing mothers should expose breasts to air and wash with water or very mild soap.
- POSTPARTUM UNIT PHONE NUMBER: The woman should be given the phone number of the postpartum unit and instructed to call if she has any questions, regardless of how simple.

exit interview with someone from the nursing team. The interview by the nurse gives the mother an opportunity to ask questions and discuss problems that she may have. Many maternity units and private physicians provide a printed advice list for their patients. The list addresses the common questions postpartum women have after they go home. It is important for the caregiver to discuss the list with the woman before she is discharged. The importance of the 6-week checkup by the physician or nurse midwife should be emphasized.

References

Brooten, D., Gennaro, S., Knapp, H., Brown, L., & York, R. (1989). Clinical specialist pre- and postdischarge teaching of parents of very low birth weight infants. *Journal of Obstetric, Gynecologic, and Neonatal Nursing* 18:316–322.

Fortier, J. C., Carson, V. B., Will, S., & Shubkagel, B. S. (1991). Adjustment to a newborn: Sibling preparation makes a difference. *Journal of Obstetric, Gynecologic, and Neonatal Nursing* 20:73–79.

Harrison, L. L. (1990). Patient education in early postpartum discharge programs. *American Journal of Maternal-Child Nursing* 15(1):39.

Hill, P. D. (1989). Effects of heat and cold on the perineum after episiotomy/laceration. *Journal of Obstetric, Gynecologic, and Neonatal Nursing* 18:124–129.

Kearney, M. H., Cronewett, L. R., & Reinhardt, R. (1990). Cesarean delivery and breastfeeding outcomes. *Birth* 17(2):97–103.

Ladewig, P. W., London, M. L., & Olds, S. B. (1990). *Essentials of Maternal-Newborn Nursing,* 2nd ed. Redwood City, CA: Addison-Wesley Nursing.

Martell, L. K. (1990). Postpartum depression as a family problem. *American Journal of Maternal-Child Nursing* 15(2):90–93.

May, K. A., & Mahlmeister, L. R. (1990). *Comprehensive Maternity Nursing: Nursing Process and the Childbearing Family,* 2nd ed. Philadelphia: J. B. Lippincott.

Moon, J. L., & Humenick, S. S. (1989). Breast engorgement: Contributing variables and variables amenable to nursing

intervention. *Journal of Obstetric, Gynecologic, and Neonatal Nursing* 18:309–325.

Spadt, S. K., Martin, K. R., & Thomas, A. M. (1990). Experiential classes for siblings-to-be. *American Journal of Maternal-Child Nursing* 15:184–186.

Stevens, K. A. (1988). Nursing diagnoses in wellness childbearing settings. *Journal of Obstetric, Gynecologic, and Neonatal Nursing* 17:329–335.

Walker, M., & Driscoll, J. W. (1989). Sore nipples: The new mother's nemesis. *American Journal of Maternal-Child Nursing* 14(4):260–265.

Unterman, R. R., Posner, N. A., & Williams, K. N. (1990). Postpartum depressive disorders: Changing trends. *Birth* 17(3):131–137.

SUGGESTED ACTIVITIES

1. Develop a teaching plan for mothers, including postpartum self-care and care of newborn infant.
2. Recall postpartum exercises that strengthen and improve muscle tone.
3. List ways to prepare siblings for the additional family member.

REVIEW QUESTIONS

A. Select the best answer to each multiple-choice question.

Clinical Situation: Mary Lawson, a 22-year-old gravida 1 para 1, gave birth to Walter, an 8½-lb, full-term infant. She is planning to breastfeed her baby. She had a 12-hour labor and an episiotomy with a 300-mL blood loss. As part of daily care, the nurse assesses the following to see if Mary is functioning normally on her second postpartum day.

1. Mary's fundus should be
   A. Firm and midway between the umbilicus and symphysis pubis
   B. Soft and at the level of the umbilicus
   C. Firm and at the level of the umbilicus
   D. Firm and two fingerbreadths below the umbilicus

2. Mary's lochia should have the following characteristic odor and color:
   A. Foul odor and dark brown
   B. Foul odor and reddish-brown
   C. Fleshy odor and pinkish-red
   D. Fleshy odor and bright red bleeding

3. Mary's perineum should be
   A. Edematous, painful to pressure, and displaying redness
   B. Edematous, painful to pressure, with episiotomy edges well proximated (close together)
   C. Displaying clear discharge
   D. Intensely painful in the episiotomy area, with clear drainage

4. Mary's breasts should be
   A. Soft and secreting milk
   B. Beginning to be somewhat firm and secreting colostrum
   C. Engorged and with no secretion of fluid
   D. Soft and with no secretion of fluid

5. Mary's urinary system demonstrates normal functioning by
   A. Voiding large amounts of urine but with no pain
   B. Voiding large amounts of urine but with pain
   C. Voiding small amounts of urine frequently
   D. Voiding small amounts of urine infrequently

6. When Mary picks up the baby to begin breastfeeding, she notices the spontaneous release of milk from her breasts. This response most likely is attributed to
   A. An overabundance of milk
   B. The let-down reflex
   C. Relaxation of the breast tissue
   D. Engorgement

Clinical Situation: Ms. Catalano, 25 years of age, married, gravida 1, had a baby girl weighing 8 lb. She had a 12-hour labor, spontaneous vaginal delivery, left mediolateral episiotomy, and a 350-mL blood loss. Ms. Catalano had her husband with her, as coach, during labor and birth. She plans to breastfeed her infant.

7. Ms. Catalano was asked to ambulate frequently after being moved to the postpartum ward for all the following reasons EXCEPT
   A. Promoting bowel function
   B. Promoting bladder function
   C. Promoting circulation
   D. Reducing diaphoresis

8. Ms. Catalano was instructed about breast care. She was told the most effective way to prevent sore nipples is
   A. To make sure the infant grasps most of the areola as well as the nipple while sucking
   B. At the end of nursing, to break the infant's suction by putting her finger in the corner of the baby's mouth
   C. To change the infant's position to alter pressure points on breast
   D. All of the above

9. The nurse's assessment for bladder care included all of the following EXCEPT
   A. Palpating uterus to see if it was displaced to one side
   B. Asking if she was voiding frequently and in small amounts
   C. Asking if she had burning on urination
   D. Asking if she had pain in her extremities

10. The nurse assessed Ms. Catalano's fundus daily to evaluate
    A. Rate of involution
    B. For infection
    C. Need for additional fluids
    D. None of the above

11. In regard to resumption of activities, Ms. Catalano was instructed to do all of the following EXCEPT
    A. Avoid heavy lifting
    B. Avoid excessive climbing of stairs
    C. Gradually increase activities but avoid fatigue
    D. Stay in bed most of the day

12. Ms. Catalano was instructed to report the following danger signs to her physician when she went home:
    A. Bright red bleeding, pain in calf, drainage from episiotomy incision
    B. Bright red bleeding, sweating, abdominal cramps
    C. Abdominal cramps, lack of appetite, tenderness in legs
    D. Temperature of 99° F, pinkish vaginal discharge, abdominal cramps

13. Sibling visitation is allowed in some maternity units. This policy assists children in all of the following EXCEPT
    A. Reducing their jealousy toward new infant
    B. Reducing anxiety about new family member coming home
    C. Reducing attention-seeking behavior
    D. Increasing negative reaction toward new infant

B. Choose from Column II the phrase that most accurately defines the term in Column I.

I

1. Engorgement _____
2. Involution _____
3. Postpartum blues _____
4. Perineal care _____
5. Postpartum exercises _____
6. Ambulation _____
7. Pinkish vaginal discharge _____
8. Massage of uterus _____
9. Cold application _____
10. Kegel exercise _____
11. Pelvic tilt _____
12. Sitz bath _____
13. Lactation _____
14. Rooming-in _____

II

A. Strengthens back and pelvic muscles
B. Psychological mood swing
C. Reduces risk of blood clot formation
D. Return of reproductive organs to nonpregnant state
E. Reduces edema and lessens discomfort
F. Perineal muscle-tightening exercise
G. Moist heat application to perineum
H. Snug bra relieves discomfort
I. Infant kept at mother's bedside
J. Third-day vaginal discharge
K. Stimulates contraction of uterine muscles
L. Lumps felt in milk-filled sacs of breasts
M. Wipe from front to back
N. Milk present in breasts

CHAPTER 15 _____

Chapter Outline

Contraception
    Oral contraceptives
    Intrauterine device
    Diaphragm
    Cervical cap
    Vaginal contraceptive sponge
    Spermicides
    Rhythm method
    Charting of cervical mucus changes (Billing's
      method)
    Condoms
    Coitus interruptus (penis withdrawal)
    Postcoital douche
    Lactation
Sterilization
    Male sterilization
    Female sterilization

Learning Objectives

Upon completion of Chapter 15, the student should be able to

- List the five types of contraception.
- Identify factors that influence the female's choice of contraceptive method.
- Describe the advantages and disadvantages of five types of contraception.
- Describe a method of contraception that reduces the risk of sexually transmitted diseases.
- Explain male sterilization.
- Explain female sterilization.

FAMILY PLANNING

Contraception

Contraception, control of a future pregnancy, has become a significant factor in health care. Although contraception has been practiced for a long time, recent developments have broadened the range of contraception methods available to couples. A woman or man has the right to be informed about the effectiveness, cost, conven-ience, shortcomings, and dangers of the various methods.

Some of the factors that influence the choice of contraception are personal acceptance of the method (for example, some women may feel un-comfortable having to touch the genitalia) and medical desirability (a medical problem such as hypertension can limit the use of a particular method). Other important factors are the conven-ience (for example, some select a method that will

---

KEY POINTS IN EDUCATION: USE OF CONTRACEPTIVES*

- Effectiveness does not protect the individual user.
- 3% failure rate for the pill will not protect the careless user, such as a 14-year-old girl, who is less likely to be compliant.
- 20% failure rate for a diaphragm need not discourage a careful, disciplined woman, in whom the failure rate would be less.
- Using two methods at once (for example, a diaphragm with a spermicidal barrier or a condom with spermicidal barrier) dramatically lowers the risk of accidental pregnancy provided they are used consistently.
- Failure rate of 12% for a condom is reduced to 2% with the use of a spermicidal barrier.

- Abstinence is the single most effective means of protecting against pregnancy.
- Using the IUD causes a 1.5- to 5-fold increase in the risk of pelvic inflammatory disease.
- Sterilization must be considered permanent.
- Benefits in addition to birth control:
  - Condoms protect against infections (for example, HIV).
  - Oral contraceptives ease menstrual discomforts.
- Having additional benefits from using the contraceptive often improves motivation to use method.
- Cost of contraceptive may impose financial problem (for example, monthly cost of oral contraceptives)

---

*Adapted from Hatcher, R. A., Stewart, F., Trussell, J., Kowal, D., Guest, F., Stewart, G. K., & Cates, W. (1990). *Contraceptive Technology 1990–1992*. New York: Irvington.

not interfere with sexual activity) and the religious, esthetic, and moral acceptability (the Roman Catholic Church, for example, approves of only abstinence or periodic abstinence, that is, the rhythm method or Billing's method). Affordability and effectiveness also influence the choice. The method chosen should be one with which the woman and man feel comfortable and will use in the correct manner. New products such as the vaginal sponge, the once-a-month pill, and under-the-skin implants are being developed and tested for effectiveness and side effects (Fig. 15–1).

ORAL CONTRACEPTIVES

Oral contraceptives (the pill) consist of two female sex hormones: estrogen and progesterone. By elevating the blood levels of these two hormones, the pill inhibits ovulation. The pill is the most effective of all birth control methods except permanent sterilization.

How the Pill Works

The pill prevents ovulation; therefore, it prevents pregnancy. There are three ways in which the pill prevents ovulation. First, estrogen levels are elevated, which prevents the ovum (egg) from developing to maturity. Second, greater progesterone levels cause the cervical mucus to thicken. This thickening prevents the sperm from entering the cervix. Third, the endometrium (lining of the uterus) changes, so a fertilized ovum would be less likely to implant there.

Types of Pills

The types of pills available differ in the amounts of estrogen and progesterone they contain. Both estrogen and progesterone have side effects, and in general, low doses of both in a pill will provide good effectiveness. Pills with this combination are usually prescribed.

There are two main types of pills available, the 21-day pill and the 28-day pill. The difference is in how they are taken. The 28-day pill is to help the woman establish a habit of taking a pill every day, so she will be less likely to forget to take it. If the woman uses the 28-day pill pack, no days are skipped between packages. If she uses the 21-

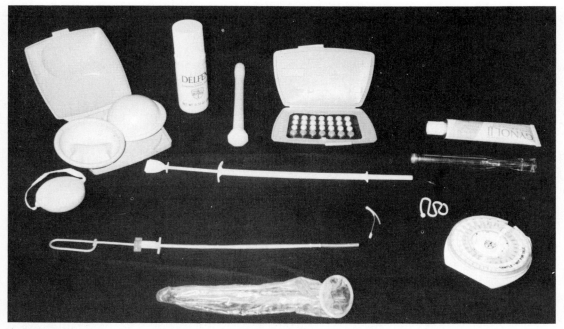

▲ FIGURE 15–1

Common methods of contraception.

day pack, she stops taking the pills for 1 week and then starts a new pack. Both the 21- and 28-day cycles allow breakthrough bleeding, which appears to the woman as a menstrual period.

The pill is very effective when it is taken as directed. The woman should take the pill at the same time each day. Sometimes, marking an X on the calendar each day when the pill is taken is a good memory device. If the woman forgets to take one pill, she should take it as soon as she remembers. If the woman forgets to take a pill on 2 consecutive days, she should take two pills each day for the next 2 days, then continue the regular schedule to catch up. If the woman forgets to take a pill 3 days in a row, she should wait 4 more days, making a full 7 days without the pill, then begin a new cycle of pills. Her elevated hormonal level of estrogen and progesterone will no longer be adequate. During this time, she should use an additional method of birth control, because she is no longer protected against pregnancy.

Side Effects

Certain minor but troublesome side effects are associated with taking the pill. These side effects include vaginal bleeding, nausea and vomiting, breast tenderness, weight loss or gain, migraine headache, cervicitis, thrombophlebitis, and mood swings. Frequently, these problems disappear after a woman has been taking the pill for 1 to 3 months. A change in dosage or a more appropriate balance in hormones is usually prescribed to relieve these side effects. Nausea and vomiting are related to the high estrogen content of the pill. A pill with a lower estrogen content may be prescribed. The cause of weight gain or weight loss has not been definitely established.

Contraindications for Taking Oral Contraceptives

There are several contraindications for taking oral contraceptives. These may become known by taking the woman's history. Oral contraceptives should not be prescribed if the following circumstances exist:

- History of heart disease

- History of thrombophlebitis or pulmonary embolus
- Impaired liver function
- Suspected cancer of breasts, uterus, or ovary or other possibly estrogen-dependent malignancies
- Hypertension
- Epilepsy
- History suggesting diabetes mellitus
- Age—over age 35 years, especially in a hypertensive or diabetic woman
- Excessive cigarette smoking, especially over 35 years of age (the pill is prescribed to healthy young women with no contraindications other than smoking one package of cigarettes per day; however, they should be informed about the increased risk of myocardial infarction, stroke, and thromboembolic injury)
- Pregnancy

The woman should be told to contact her physician or her clinic staff if she develops severe leg cramps, leg swelling, chest pain, coughing of blood, dyspnea (difficulty in breathing), severe headaches, dizziness, visual disturbances, or weakness or numbness of an arm or a leg.

Every woman should be examined by a physician, midwife, or clinic staff member after 3 months of taking the pill to help determine any possible complications. If she continues to take the pill, she should then be seen at 6-month intervals, at which times histories related to potential complications should be taken.

Other Considerations in Taking Oral Contraceptives

The woman who wants to become pregnant should discontinue taking oral contraceptives and use another method of birth control for a least 3 months before becoming pregnant. This step will decrease the risk of fetal abnormalities.

If a woman is nursing her baby, the hormones contained in the pill may decrease the milk production and also cross into the milk (see Appendix B). Therefore, birth control pills should not be taken during lactation unless the physician advises the woman to take them because a pregnancy, in her case, would be a greater risk.

The woman should be instructed to choose a backup method of birth control such as condoms or foam. The backup method should be handy in case the woman runs out of pills, forgets to take the pills, experiences danger signs and discontinues use of the pill, or wants protection from transmission of sexually transmitted diseases.

Morning-After Pill

The morning-after pill helps prevent pregnancy after unprotected sexual activity. To date, the risk of this method is high because of the very high level of estrogen that needs to be used. The action of the hormone is to keep the ovum from implanting. This method carries a high risk of teratogenic effects and malignant disease in a fetus conceived if the pill fails. Therefore it is not a routine method of family planning. This method has been used in cases of pregnancy resulting from rape.

INTRAUTERINE DEVICE

An intrauterine device (IUD) is a small, flexible object of various sizes and shapes. The IUD is made of plastic with a nylon thread at the end. The device is inserted into the uterine cavity by the physician or a specially trained nurse or nurse midwife during a pelvic examination (Fig. 15–2). IUDs come in two forms, medicated or nonmedi-

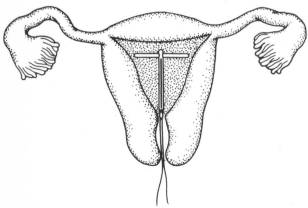

▲ FIGURE 15–2

Intrauterine device inside the uterine cavity.

cated. Currently, the Progestasert-T and the copper T are the only IUDs available in the United States. Although the Food and Drug Administration (FDA) continues to approve the sale and insertion of IUDs, some manufacturers of IUDs have voluntarily removed their products from the market because of liability issues.

The precise way in which the IUD prevents pregnancy is not fully understood. One possible mechanism is hinderance of implantation by making the uterus slightly irritable or by causing a slight inflammatory process at the implantation site. It is almost certain that the action occurs in the endometrial cavity.

The IUD is effective in about 97% of cases when it is retained for 6 months or longer. A woman is most likely to expel the IUD during the first 3 months after insertion. Therefore, many clinics suggest the use of an additional method of contraception during the first 3 months after IUD insertion. The woman should be taught how to feel for the string to determine that the IUD is still in place. The string should be checked before coitus or at least every week and during the menstrual period. To do this, the woman should first wash her hands, then insert her finger into the vagina until she touches the cervix. The cervix will feel similar to the tip of her nose. The string should be felt at the cervix. If the string seems longer or cannot be felt, she should see her physician or a member of her clinic staff to check the placement of the IUD or determine whether it has been expelled. Of course, if the IUD appears to be expelled, the woman should use an additional method of birth control.

Advantages

The IUD has fewer side effects than the pill. It is highly effective when it is inserted properly. Also, it can be easily removed if pregnancy is desired. The IUD is convenient because no precautions have to be taken before sexual activity (except checking for the string).

Disadvantages

The most common side effects of the IUD are uterine bleeding and painful cramps that lessen considerably after the first 3 months of IUD use. Also, there is a low risk of uterine perforation when the IUD is inserted. The menstrual period may last longer, and "spotting" or light bleeding between periods may be experienced for the first few months. The risk of a pelvic infection is about four times greater in women who use the IUD and does not decrease with continued use. The IUD tail is thought to be an excellent reservoir for infections that spread by traveling up the string to the ovaries and uterine tubes, causing pelvic inflammatory disease.

The most significant disadvantage is intolerance of the IUD; in some women it may act as a foreign body and be expelled spontaneously. Studies indicate that there is a 5% chance of pregnancy developing outside the uterus. The frequency of ectopic pregnancies (pregnancy in the tube) is increased with the use of the IUD.

Because the IUD must be inserted by trained personnel, the initial cost of inserting the IUD is high. Finally, this birth control method would not be appropriate for women who are not comfortable with touching the vagina.

Contraindications

The major contraindications to using the IUD include suspected pregnancy, history of pelvic infection, history of ectopic pregnancy, presence of uterine anomalies, postpartum endometritis during the preceding 4 weeks, and suspected uterine malignancy.

DIAPHRAGM

The diaphragm is a soft rubber or latex dome-shaped cup that is surrounded by a firm rim formed by a circular, rubber-covered spring. This device is made in various sizes and must be fitted by a physician or nurse with special training. The size must be changed if the woman's cervix changes.

The purpose of the diaphragm is to keep the sperm from entering the opening of the cervix. Diaphragm effectiveness is about 80% for the first year, and after 1 year the effectiveness increases

(to reach 88% to 98%) with proper use and with spermicidal jelly or cream.

Before the diaphragm is inserted, it should be filled with a spermicide (cream or jelly), which is placed in the shallow cup and completely covering the area around the rim. The device is squeezed together to allow its insertion into the vagina, where it then assumes its original shape. It covers the cervix, and part of it lies behind the pubic bone (Fig. 15–3).

The diaphragm may be inserted in the evening and left in during the night. However, if sexual intercourse is delayed more than 2 hours after insertion, the woman should place another application of contraceptive spermicide (cream or jelly) in the vagina without removing the diaphragm. The diaphragm should not be removed for 6 to 8 hours after sexual intercourse. Also, its position should be checked. The woman should be instructed not to douche for 6 to 8 hours after intercourse, because this action can dilute the spermicide and make birth control less effective.

After the fitting, the woman must have adequate opportunity to learn how to place and remove the diaphragm herself. The removal of the diaphragm is fairly simple. The woman can take it out by inserting her fingers into the vagina, holding the diaphragm under the rim or at the top of the rim, and removing it. The diaphragm should be cleaned immediately, with mild unscented soap and warm water; dried; and dusted with baby powder or cornstarch. It should be checked frequently for holes by holding it up to light or placing water in it.

Advantages

The woman needs to use the diaphragm only when she expects to have sexual intercourse. With proper care, the diaphragm can be used for about 1 year, which makes it an inexpensive method. Also, it does not interfere with sexual satisfaction.

Disadvantages

To be effective, the diaphragm must be used consistently and correctly. Even so, it is possible

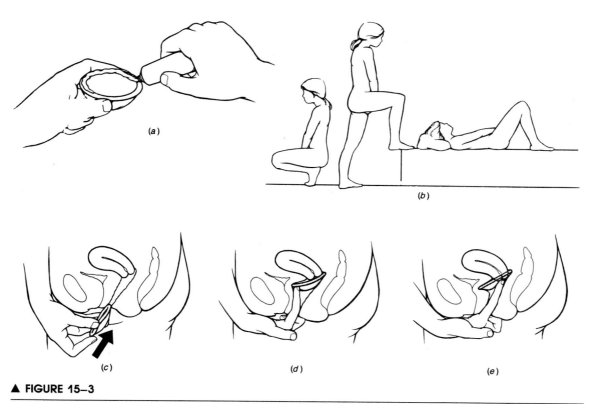

▲ **FIGURE 15–3**

Sequence of diaphragm insertion. *a.* Spermicidal cream is applied to rim and inner aspects of diaphragm. *b.* Three positions women may assume for the diaphragm insertion. *c.* Diaphragm is compressed and inserted the length of the vagina. *d.* With the posterior rim in the posterior fornix, the anterior rim is pressed upward behind the symphysis pubis with the index finger. *e.* Proper placement is determined by palpation of the cervix covered by the diaphragm. (From Butnarescu, G. F., & Tillotson, D. M. (1983). *Maternity Nursing.* New York: John Wiley & Sons. Copyright © 1983. John Wiley & Sons. Reprinted by permission of John Wiley & Sons, Inc.)

that a well-fitted and properly inserted diaphragm can become dislodged during intercourse.

The diaphragm must be inserted before intercourse, which may distract from the spontaneity of sexual foreplay. Also the size may need to be changed after the woman has had a baby, an abortion, or an excessive weight gain or loss (at least 10 lb). This method of contraception would not be right for women who do not like to put a device into their vagina. The woman should be informed of a low risk for toxic shock syndrome.

Contraindications

Although most women can use the diaphragm, if a woman has a severe prolapse of the uterus,

cystocele, or urethrocele she may not be able to be fitted properly. Also, she may find it more difficult to insert the device.

CERVICAL CAP

The cervical cap is like a large thimble made of rubber. It fits tightly over the cervix, where it is held in place by suction. The cervical cap is a barrier method of contraception similar to the diaphragm. A spermicide must be placed inside the dome of the cap, and it must not be removed for 6 to 8 hours after intercourse. Care for the cap is similar to that for the diaphragm. Although there has been limited experience with the cap, if used correctly, its effectiveness should be similar to that of the diaphragm.

Advantages

The advantages are similar to those of the diaphragm. Most users express satisfaction with its use. Its effectiveness depends on the woman's skill in inserting and removing the cap.

Disadvantages

The major drawbacks to use of the cap are possible effects of long-term exposure to secretions, spermicide, and bacteria that are trapped inside it. This problem increases the risk of toxic shock syndrome. The manufacturers specify times that a cap can and cannot be inserted and removed.

Contraindications

Contraindications in using the cervical cap include previous infections (history of toxic shock syndrome), cervicitis, or pelvic infections. Other contraindications include lack of medical personnel qualified to fit the cap or a woman's inability to learn the correct technique, an abnormal Pap smear, a cervical biopsy within the past 6 weeks, or full-term delivery within the past 6 weeks.

VAGINAL CONTRACEPTIVE SPONGE

The first vaginal contraceptive sponge was approved for use in the United States by the FDA in 1983. The sponge is a small, rounded one-size-fits-all polyurethane device that fits snugly over the cervix. The other side of the sponge has a loop used to remove the sponge from the vagina. Once in place, it provides protection for 24 hours. Sperm are destroyed by spermicide action.

Advantages

The sponge is convenient to use, and it may decrease the spread of sexually transmitted diseases (including gonorrhea and trichomoniasis) to the uterus. It is effective up to 24 hours without reapplication.

Disadvantages

Some women may have an allergic reaction or irritation from the spermicide or polyurethane material. Some have complained that the sponge absorbs too much of their vaginal secretions and thus creates dryness in the vagina. The risk of toxic shock syndrome is very low; nevertheless, patients using the sponge should be instructed about the danger signs of this syndrome.

SPERMICIDES

Spermicides are vaginal chemical contraceptives effective in two ways: the chemical property kills sperm, and the material containing the chemical acts as a mechanical barrier, blocking the entrance of the sperm into the cervix. Sperm thrive best at an alkaline pH of 8.5 to 9.0. Because the vagina loses its normal acidity during ovulation, chemical barriers are designed to keep the vagina slightly acid. In order for these effects to occur, the spermicide must be placed properly in the vagina. Spermicides come in several forms: foams, jellies, creams, and tablets or suppositories. Because spermicides do not require a prescription, they are readily available in drug stores and family planning clinics.

The effectiveness of spermicides depends on how well they are used and varies from 80% to 95%.

The foam, cream, or jelly preparation should be inserted while the woman is lying on her back. A full applicator of foam (jelly or cream) should be placed deep into the vagina. The woman should be instructed not to douche for 6 to 8 hours after intercourse, because douching will either remove the spermicide or dilute it so it is ineffective. Should the couple desire to repeat sexual intercourse 1 hour after the first application, another application of foam or jelly should be inserted into the vagina. Creams and jellies should be used only with another method of birth control such as a diaphragm or condom. Foam may be used alone as a contraceptive, but is better to use it in a combination with condoms.

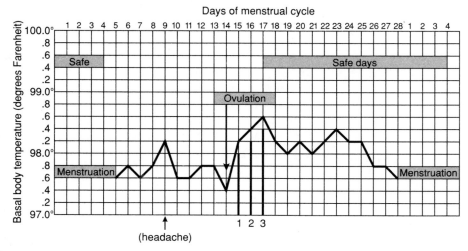

▲ FIGURE 15–4

Basal body temperature chart showing menstruation, ovulation, and nonfertile days.

Advantages

Creams, jellies, and foam add lubrication during sexual intercourse. Also, they give some protection against sexually transmitted diseases.

Spermicides can be purchased without a physician's prescription. Spermicides are a good backup for the woman who forgets her pill for more than 2 days.

Disadvantages

Some women are allergic to spermicidal foams, jellies, and creams. They can interfere with spontaneous sexual activity and may interfere with oral sex because of their unpleasant taste. They are often considered messy to use.

RHYTHM METHOD

The rhythm method is based on the concept that abstinence from intercourse during the fertile period of the woman's cycle (when ovulation occurs) will prevent pregnancy.

Ovulation can occur 12 to 16 days before the first day of the next menstrual period. The life span of the ovum is 24 hours, and the sperm can live as long as 72 hours. Intercourse must be avoided from 4 days before ovulation to 3 days after. A woman whose cycle occurs regularly at

28-day intervals would practice abstinence from day 10 through day 17 of her cycle.

The rhythm method's effectiveness can be increased by recording the woman's basal body temperature (BBT). This step requires that the woman record her temperature every day immediately on awakening and before any physical activity. Shortly after ovulation, the BBT rises 0.6° to 0.8° F. Temperature elevation for 3 days is fairly good evidence that ovulation has occurred and that the remainder of the cycle is a safe time for intercourse (Fig. 15–4). Some women notice a temperature drop about 12 to 24 hours before it begins to rise after ovulation, whereas others have no drop in temperature at all. A drop in BBT probably means ovulation will occur the next day. Another clue to ovulation is the changes in the vaginal secretions.

The one main advantage of the rhythm method over other methods of contraception is its acceptability to members of the Roman Catholic Church. However, the rhythm method is not very reliable. Stress, changes in environment, and minor illnesses can cause ovulation to occur earlier or later than anticipated. Also, infections, fatigue, and anxiety can cause the BBT to rise, unrelated to ovulation.

The safest way to use the rhythm method for birth control is to use a backup method for the first half of the cycle. One can usually assume that the fertile days are over on the evening of the third consecutive day that the BBT has risen and remained elevated.

CHARTING OF CERVICAL MUCUS CHANGES (BILLING'S METHOD)

Cervical mucus changes appear in recognizable patterns among most ovulating women. The observation of mucus changes is referred to as the Billing's method of birth control. Postovulation and near menstruation, the cervical mucus decreases and becomes scant, thick, cloudy, and white to yellowish. As ovulation approaches, the cervical mucus increases, becomes thinner, clear, and somewhat stretchy. At ovulation, the cervical mucus is abundant, clear, very thin, and very stretchy. A drop of this clear cervical mucus can be stretched between two slides (or fingers) into a thin strand that measures 6 cm or longer. This stretching is referred to as spinnbarkheit, and it enables the sperm to travel up through the cervix more easily (Fig. 15–5). Immediately before ovulation, during ovulation, and the 3 days after ovulation (the peak spinnbarkheit) are considered "fertile" times.

Cervical mucus also displays ferning during the fertile days. Ferning is well developed at ovulation, which occurs when the mucus is abundant, clear, elastic, and slippery. Ferning becomes minimal to absent postovulation to near menstruation.

In examining her cervical mucus, a woman must not confuse other substances in her vagina, such as semen, lubricants, spermicides, and suppositories, with midcycle secretions. The woman should not douche until the fertile period is over, to avoid washing out the mucus and concealing changes in discharge. The ferning or Billing's method is also accepted by the Catholic Church.

CONDOMS

Condoms are soft rubber shields that fit snugly over the erect penis. There should be a reservoir at the tip of the condom (either because it is made with one or because space is left when putting it on) in which the semen is collected. When a couple are using a condom, they must be extremely careful when removing the penis from the vagina, to prevent semen from spilling into the vagina or even onto the vaginal lips. The condom's effectiveness for the typical user is 88%. Its effective-

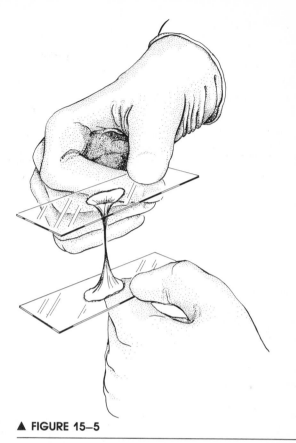

▲ **FIGURE 15–5**

Technique for determining the ability of cervical mucus to stretch. This stretching is referred to as *spinnbarkheit.*

ness depends on how it is used and whether it is used consistently.

Condoms do not require a prescription and are inexpensive. They are not reusable. Condoms come in many different styles: lubricated, colored, and ribbed to provide more stimulation for the female. Recently, condoms that are coated with spermicide as well as a lubricant were made available. If latex condoms cause genital irritation, condoms made from tissue from the lamb intestine can be used.

Advantages

The condom is an inexpensive and easily available method of birth control and can be obtained without medical prescription. The condom can be a reliable method of contraception if it is used properly and consistently. The effectiveness increases to 98% when condoms are used in combination with a vaginal spermicide. One aspect of safety of condoms is their contribution to the prevention of sexually transmitted diseases. However, the penis must be protected at all times during foreplay, which includes genital sex play. The use of the condom makes the male share responsibility for contraception.

Disadvantages

Sexual foreplay may be interrupted to apply the condom before vaginal penetration. In addition, a small number of men are allergic to rubber condoms, and the natural skin type does not provide protection against sexually transmitted disease. Condom breakage is a disadvantage. For men who have problems with erection, the condom is likely to be a poor contraceptive device.

Female Condoms

Extensive work is under way to produce an acceptable condom-like mechanical barrier for the woman to wear. Prophylactic, Inc., is testing a latex condom that may be worn as a G-string by a woman. A condom pouch is rolled up compactly, and when the penis first enters the vaginal vault, it pushes the condom pouch up into the vagina. The clinical trials are using latex twice as thick as the male condom and so far have indicated that sexual satisfaction is high.

COITUS INTERRUPTUS (PENIS WITHDRAWAL)

Coitus interruptus, withdrawal of the penis before ejaculation, is a very old and unreliable method of contraception. Preejaculatory secretions of the male frequently contain sperm (a small amount of the semen may be expelled before ejaculation), and precise male control is difficult to achieve.

POSTCOITAL DOUCHE

The postcoital douche is a very unreliable method of contraception. Because sperm are known to appear in the cervical mucus within a few minutes of an ejaculation, they can reach the site of the uterine tube within a short time. Once

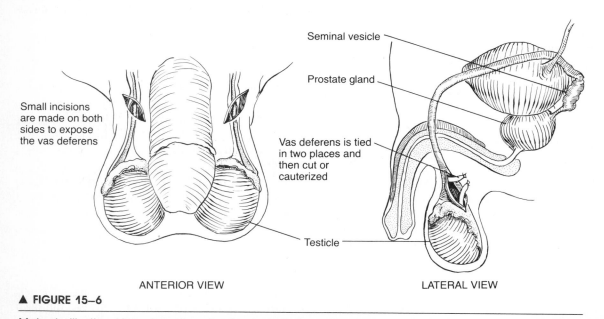

▲ FIGURE 15–6

Male sterilization. Vasectomy is a simple surgical procedure.

the sperm reaches the ovum, pregnancy is the potential result, and douching will not prevent it.

LACTATION

Lactation, nursing the baby, should not be recommended as a reliable form of contraception. However, studies have shown that whereas 50% of nonnursing mothers do not conceive for 4 months after the birth of a baby, 50% of nursing mothers do not conceive for 12 to 18 months after the birth of a baby. Therefore, nursing does have some influence on population control. If a woman nurses her baby approximately every 4 hours day and night, her protection from pregnancy is greater because her hormonal levels are kept more stable.

Sterilization

Sterilization (permanent contraception) may be selected by some couples for contraception, especially older parents, those who have medical problems, and those who are certain they do not want any more children. The men and women who desire surgical sterilization must be told that the operation is irreversible—an attempt to restore fertility has had some success in the male by microsurgery, but it is expensive. Because sterilization has legal implications, consent forms should be signed before the surgery is done.

MALE STERILIZATION

Vasectomy is the surgical cutting and tying of each vas deferens, the tubes that carry the sperm (Fig. 15–6). This blocks the passage of the sperm. The vasectomy is becoming more popular in the United States. It is often performed in the physician's office. Sperm can be present in the vas deferens for as long as 2 months after surgery. Therefore, an additional method of contraception should be used for that period of time. A vasectomy does not affect the male's pleasure in sexual intercourse.

FEMALE STERILIZATION

Female sterilization can be accomplished by several abdominal and vaginal procedures (Fig. 15–7). The fallopian tubes are plugged, ligated, or occluded by electrocautery. Clips or bands have the advantage of theoretically being removable if a return to tubal patency is desired. A postpartum laparoscopy may be done 1 to 2 days after delivery. Access to the uterus is gained through a small subumbilical incision in the abdomen. This can be performed later on an outpatient basis.

There are relatively few side effects to tubal sterilization other than mild postoperative pain. The woman should rest a few days and avoid heavy lifting for a week.

There is no change in hormones, because the ovaries are still intact. Some women show increased sexual interest because they no longer fear an unwanted pregnancy. However, some women who feel they were pushed into the sterilization by their husbands or for reasons of health or economics may have less interest in sex. They may mourn their loss of reproductive ability.

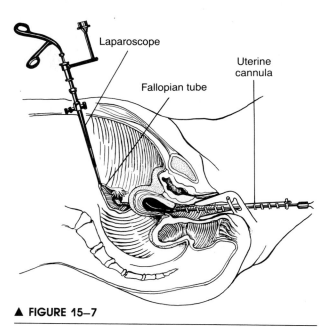

▲ **FIGURE 15–7**

Female sterilization. Laparoscopy is a common procedure.

NURSING CARE PLAN 15–1
FAMILY PLANNING

Potential Problems and Nursing Diagnoses	Nursing Interventions
1. Knowledge deficit related to contraceptive methods available.	Explain the contraceptive methods available and answer questions about each method. Specify each method's advantages and disadvantages.
2. Self-care deficit related to the selected method.	Provide instruction about the selected method in as much detail as required.
3. Anxiety related to use of a contraceptive method.	Provide a climate in which woman can openly discuss her concerns about using contraception and its effectiveness.
4. Noncompliance related to use of contraceptive method.	Instruct woman about the lack of effectiveness if method is not adhered to; for example, forgetting to take pills allows woman to become pregnant.

Expected Outcomes

1. Woman verbalizes an understanding of the contraceptive methods available.
2. Woman verbalizes the need to follow instructions in order to have protection from a pregnancy.
3. Woman states a relief to have concerns clarified. She feels more positive about using the method.
4. Woman states that noncompliance was the reason for the last pregnancy. Plans to mark calendar as a way to know that a pill was taken every day.

References

Auvenshine, M. A., & Enriquez, M. G. (1990). *Comprehensive Maternity Nursing: Perinatal and Women's Health*, 2nd ed. Boston: Jones and Bartlett.

Bobak, I. M., & Jensen, M. D. (1991). *Essentials of Maternity Nursing*, 3rd ed. St. Louis: Mosby Year Book.

Hatcher, R. A., Stewart, F., Trussell, J., Kowal, D., Guest, F., Stewart, G. K., & Cates, W. (1990). *Contraceptive Technology, 1990–1992*, 15th ed. New York: Irvington.

Ladewig, P. W., London, M. L., & Olds, S. B. (1990). *Essentials of Maternal-Newborn Nursing*, 2nd ed. Redwood City, CA: Addison-Wesley Nursing.

Loucks, A. (1989). A comparison of satisfactions with types of diaphragms among women in a college population. *Journal of Obstetric, Gynecologic, and Neonatal Nursing* 18(3):194–200.

May, K. A., & Mahlmeister, L. R. (1990). *Comprehensive Maternity Nursing: Nursing Process and the Childbearing Family*, 2nd ed. Philadelphia: J. B. Lippincott.

Monier, M., & Laird, M. (1989). Contraceptives: A look at the future. *American Journal of Nursing* 89:497–499.

SUGGESTED ACTIVITIES

1. Write a report on agencies in your local community that are concerned with family planning. Include in the report the medical services offered and the payment policies.
2. List the advantages and disadvantages of four different methods of contraception.

REVIEW QUESTIONS

A. Select the best answer to each multiple-choice question.

1. Oral contraceptives contain the following two hormones:
   A. Estrogen and progesterone
   B. Progesterone and prolactin
   C. Estrogen and follicle-stimulating hormone
   D. Estrogen and luteotropic hormone

2. Side effects of taking an oral contraceptive include
   A. Vaginal bleeding
   B. Nausea and vomiting
   C. Breast tenderness
   D. All of the above

3. Contraindications to taking oral contraceptives include
   A. Excessive cigarette smoking, hypertension, epilepsy
   B. Cigarette smoking, heartburn, nausea and vomiting
   C. Age 35 years or more, nausea and vomiting, and vaginal bleeding
   D. None of the above

4. Oral contraceptives are contraindicated in women with any of the following conditions EXCEPT
   A. Age over 35 years and cigarette smoker
   B. History of diabetes
   C. History of heart disease
   D. Vaginal bleeding during the cycle

5. A soft, dome-shaped contraceptive device that is inserted in the vagina is called a
   A. Condom
   B. Spermicide
   C. Diaphragm
   D. Rubber-covered ring

6. The sterilization procedure of the male is called
   A. Vasectomy
   B. Spermicide
   C. Tubal ligation
   D. None of the above

7. When instructing a woman about the use of a diaphragm, it is important to teach her that the diaphragm should be rechecked for correct size
   A. When weight gain or loss of 5 lb has occurred
   B. After each delivery
   C. Every 3 years routinely
   D. Every 5 years routinely

8. Ms. Wheeler is a 24-year-old gravida 1, para 1, with a history of severe migraine headaches and thrombophlebitis following the birth of her first baby. She wants a temporary method of birth control. Which method of contraception would you recommend?
   A. Birth control pills
   B. IUD
   C. Diaphragm with foam
   D. Foam alone

9. Contraceptive methods should be prescribed on the basis of
   A. Patient acceptance
   B. Availability
   C. Side effects
   D. All of the above

B. Choose from Column II the phrase that most accurately defines the term in Column I.

I	II
1. The pill _____	A. Soft, rubber shield
2. IUD _____	B. Withdrawal of penis
3. Spermicidal agent _____	C. Prevents ovulation
4. Diaphragm _____	D. Cauterization of tubes
5. Condom _____	E. Abstinence of coitus during fertile period
6. Rhythm method _____	F. Soft, rubber, dome-shaped cup
7. Coitus interruptus _____	G. Kills and mechanically blocks sperm
8. Tubal ligation _____	H. Prevents implantation

CHAPTER 16 _____

Chapter Outline

Early Contact
Sensual Responses
    Eye-to-eye contact
    Touch
    Voice
    Odor
    Entrainment
Factors That Influence Attachment
    Parental preconditions
    Prenatal assessment and intervention
    Hospital environment and practices
    Delivery assessment and intervention
    Postpartum assessment and intervention
    Parent–infant attachment in special circumstances

Learning Objectives

Upon completion of Chapter 16, the student should be able to

- List the factors that influence attachment.
- Outline factors that facilitate parent–infant attachment.
- Name factors that inhibit parent–infant attachment.
- List three parental preconditions that influence attachment.
- Explain two factors, present during pregnancy, that can inhibit attachment.
- Explain what a nurse can do immediately after birth to enhance parent–infant attachment.
- Identify three positive maternal–infant observations and three negative maternal–infant observations that can assist the nurse to develop an appropriate care plan.
- Identify two circumstances in which the risk of problems in attachment is high and in which the nurse can offer guidance and support.

PARENT–INFANT ATTACHMENT

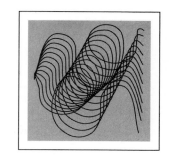

Attachment may be defined as the process that produces an affectional and emotional commitment between two individuals. This process begins during pregnancy, intensifies during birth and the early postdelivery period, and is consistent once established. *Bonding*, in the strict sense, relates to a tie from parent to infant and not the infant's attachment to the mother. In this text the term *attachment* will be used to refer to a two-way process between the parent and infant. A successful attachment process is important to lifelong mental and physical health. In the process, an exchange of feelings predicated by attractiveness and responsiveness occurs. Mutual satisfaction from the exchange leads to another exchange, and so on.

Early Contact

It has been shown that contact immediately after birth, including skin-to-skin contact between the infant and mother, has an important effect on the attachment process. Clearly, nurses need to encourage this contact. The study of bonding by Klaus and Kennell in 1982 has been instrumental in changing health care providers' attitudes and many hospitals' policies. Presently, mothers/parents are usually allowed to have contact with their infants right after birth. However, nurses need to reassure parents who desire but are unable to have early contact with their newborn that their emotional bond to their infant will not necessarily be weaker.

Sensual Responses

It is important for caregivers to recognize that the attachment process is strengthened through the use of sensual responses between the parent and child (Table 16–1).

EYE-TO-EYE CONTACT

During the first hour after birth from an unmedicated mother, a newborn infant is quite alert and is able to elicit a strong positive response from the mother by making eye contact with her. Some mothers make comments such as "When my baby looked at me, I fell in love with him" or "My baby just looked at me." Because of this parent–infant interaction, it is advisable for the nurse to withhold instillation of protective eye drops or ointment for a least 1 hour after birth. The dimming of lights may encourage infants to open their eyes, and parents should be encouraged to hold the newborn infant close enough to their face to stimulate eye-to-eye contact.

A mother should be instructed to hold the infant within 8 to 12 inches from her face and to continue to gaze at the infant (Fig. 16–1). This "en face" position encourages bonding or attachment. A shiny object may trigger the baby's interest. A 2-day-old baby can focus on and follow a moving object (see Fig. 18–18).

TOUCH

The first postbirth contacts between the mother and her infant usually appear in an orderly and

TABLE 16–1. MATERNAL–INFANT INTERACTIONS THAT OCCUR EARLY	
MOTHER TO INFANT	**INFANT TO MOTHER**
Touch	
Mother's touch progresses from fingertips to fingers to palms to encompass contact. Stroking and massaging may be observed.	Infant becomes quiet and relaxed with mother's touch and with the sensation of the heartbeat.
Eye-to-eye contact	
Mother looks, gazes, and takes in physical characteristics of infant she holds. She holds infant "en face" (a position in which the two can look into each other's eyes).	Infant can see mother's face and follow movement such as movement of finger (demonstrates knowing and caring to mother).
High-pitched voice	
Mother speaks to infant in a high-pitched voice. Often talks, coos, and sings to infant.	Infant responds to mother's high-pitched voice.
Hovers	
Mother hovers, maintains proximity, directs attention to, points to infant.	Infant responds to being held close and being cuddled.
Entrainment	
Infant's movement may reward mother to continue to speak to infant.	Infant becomes attentive to mother's voice and often moves in rhythm to her speech.
Assigns meaning to infant's actions	
Mother assigns meaning to infant's grasp reflex: "He or she is holding my finger."	As the mother shows positive responses to basic reflexes and behaviors, the infant reciprocates by becoming quiet and relaxed.
Claims infant as family member	
Mother claims infant by name and family characteristics.	As mother identifies infant as her own, love is felt and infant demonstrates positive behavior (sucks, smiles, and cuddles).

predictable pattern of touch. The mother usually begins with a fingertip exploration of the infant's head and extremities, within a short time uses her open palm to caress the baby's trunk, and then enfolds the infant in her arms. After the initial period of interaction, mothers begin to stroke, soothe, and quiet the infant by stroking the infant's back, picking up the infant, and holding the infant close (Fig. 16–2).

It is common for the infant to grasp the mother's finger (grasp reflex). Mothers feel this is a positive infant response and become encouraged to continue stroking the baby (this sets up a reciprocal positive reaction).

VOICE

The responses of the parent and infant to each other's voices are interesting. Many mothers are relieved to hear their baby's first cry. As the mother begins to comfort the infant, she usually uses a high-pitched voice, which causes the infant to become alert and turn toward the mother.

ODOR

Another behavior shared by parents and the infant is response to each other's odor. An infant

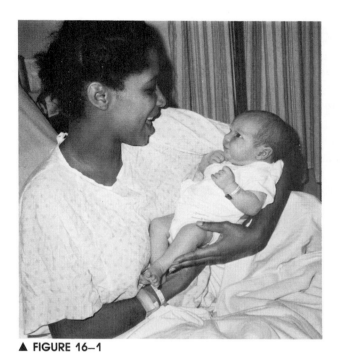

▲ FIGURE 16–1

Eye-to-eye (en face) contact between mother and infant facilitates attachment.

learns quickly to distinguish the odor of its own mother's breast milk. Mothers have been heard to comment about the smell of their babies when first born.

ENTRAINMENT

Klaus and Kennell found that in the first or second day after birth, newborns move in rhythm with the mother's speech. They called this characteristic *entrainment.* In their study, a baby moved in rhythm to the mother's voice as she slowly repeated ''pretty baby.'' On different occasions I have had my students repeat ''p-r-e-t-t-y b-a-b-y'' during the assessment of newborn infants. It has been interesting to see the positive interaction between the student and baby. It is believed that this shared rhythm elicits positive parent feedback that can begin to establish a healthy setting for effective communication.

The attachment process usually is progressive and changes over time. It is made easier with positive infant behaviors, some of which have been enumerated above. Others include sucking, smiling, clinging, and crying. In addition, an infant's response to stimuli, motor maturity, cuddlesomeness, consolability, defense movements, and self-quieting activities may encourage attachment.

Some negative behaviors can make the attachment process more difficult. Behaviors that elicit negative responses in some mothers include sleeping most of the time, hyperirritability or jerky movements when touched, exaggerated Moro's reflex, frequent crying with infrequent smiling, resisting holding and cuddling by crying and stiffening the body, and poor feeding. Even some caregivers label infants as unpleasant when they are irritable and resist being held (Table 16–2).

Every positive interaction between the mother and infant intensifies the attachment. The mother's claiming her infant as her own is enhanced through supportive caretaking. It is important for the caregiver to assess the mother's interest and ability in identifying and responding to the infant's visual, tactile, auditory, and verbal cues (Table 16–

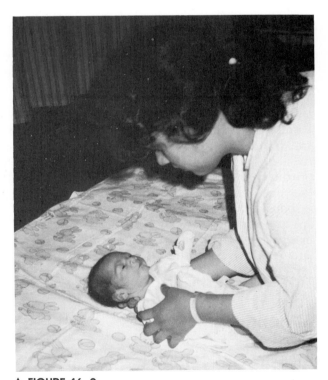

▲ FIGURE 16–2

Touch facilitates attachment.

TABLE 16–2. PARENT AND INFANT INHIBITING BEHAVIORS	
PARENT INHIBITING BEHAVIORS	**INFANT INHIBITING BEHAVIORS**
Visual Does not attempt to get infant's attention.	Has eyes closed or sleeps most of time.
Touch Provides little tactile stimulation for infant; moves away from infant.	Resists holding and cuddling by crying, stiffening body, or both.
Vocal Does not talk, vocalize, or sing to infant.	Cries frequently and for long periods of time.
Feeding Holds infant in an uncomfortable way during feeding. Does not burp infant.	Resists food offered. Does not suck effectively. Is fussy after adequate amount of feeding, providing no pleasurable reaction.
Clinging Does not show interest in grasp reflex or other clinging movements by infant.	Does not respond to parent's stimulation.
Consoling Finds it difficult to console or quiet infant in response to fussing or crying.	Is inconsolable or unresponsive to parenting (touch, voice, or being held).
Caring (genitalia) Shows distaste for cleaning infant's excretions.	Has frequent bowel movements.

3). Sensitivity to cues, or "reading the infant," is an important challenge for a parent. Parents who acquire this skill enjoy a feeling of competence and confidence in their own caretaking abilities. As a tie is formed between infant and parent, proximity is valued more highly. It can be said that one cannot love a "stranger"; therefore, the responses of the parent and infant to each other are important. They begin the acquaintance and inspire a commitment in the parents to care for and love their infant throughout their lifetime.

Factors That Influence Attachment

PARENTAL PRECONDITIONS

In addition to early contact between the parent and infant, other factors contribute to the process of attachment. A parent's emotional health and social support system, encompassing the mate, friends, and family, can be favorable preconditions for attachment. A parent who feels competent in caretaking skills is likely to feel secure and experience satisfaction in being with the infant. Conversely, a mother who is insecure, fatigued, and highly anxious with the infant may show maladaptive maternal behavior. The caregiver should be sensitive to parental behavior that can possibly cause a disturbance in the attachment process. Sometimes the grandparent may facilitate or hinder the attachment process. If the grandparent holds and cares for the infant more than the parent, the new parent may find it difficult to assume independence in caretaking.

Five preconditions have been said to influence attachment:

1. A parent's emotional health (including the ability to trust another person).

TABLE 16–3. ASSESSMENT TOOL FOR MATERNAL–INFANT INTERACTIONS

I. IDENTIFYING BEHAVIORS—The mother's observations and questions about her infant. Check if observed.
   A. Appearance and function
      1. Makes reference to size of the infant, e.g., "He is so little."   _____
      2. Inspects baby's body features, e.g., face, hair, fingers, feet, and genitals.   _____
      3. Verbally questions or makes comments on body functions, e.g., "Look, he is wet" or "Look at her yawn."   _____
      4. Asks questions pertaining to wholeness of baby, e.g., "Does she have all her fingers and toes?"   _____
   B. Appraisal of infant's condition
      5. Asks questions with specific reference to such things as skin, eyes, face, cord, and general color.   _____
      6. Asks questions about baby's condition, e.g., "Does he cry much?" and "How much weight has he gained?"   _____
      7. Makes statement that shows her awareness of change in the baby's condition, e.g., "Her color looks better today" or "Her skin does not look as dry today."   _____

II. TYPE OF INTERACTION—Method by which the mother begins to relate to her baby using visual, verbal, and tactile behaviors.
   A. Verbal contact
      1. Talks or sings to baby.   _____
      2. Speaks to infant's using his or her name (does not use "it" in reference to the baby).   _____
   B. Visual contact
      3. Has eye contact with baby's face.   _____
      4. Talks with baby when his eyes are open, e.g. "My baby is looking at me."   _____
      5. Tries to position baby to open her eyes.   _____
   C. Tactile contact
      6. Fingertip touch.   _____
      7. Palm of hand contact.   _____
      8. Touches extremities, feet, hands, or head.   _____
      9. Extends touch to trunk of baby's body.   _____
      10. Draws infant to her body.   _____
      11. Snuggles baby to body with cheek-to-cheek contact.   _____
      12. Increased contact with baby by kissing, cuddling, patting, and playing.   _____

III. CARETAKING BEHAVIORS—Mother's activities in baby care.
   A. Participation in baby's care
      1. Offers to feed baby.   _____
      2. Communicates baby's need and asks if she can do the task, e.g., "He is wet. Can I change him?"   _____
      3. Recognizes baby's needs, e.g. "Can I wipe the baby's face and nose?"   _____
   B. No participation in baby's care
      1. Does not feed baby or see if baby is wet.   _____
      2. Holds baby but performs no caretaking task.   _____
      3. Recognizes infant's needs but asks nurse to perform task, e.g., "My baby is wet."   _____

Table continued on following page

TABLE 16–3. ASSESSMENT TOOL FOR MATERNAL– INFANT INTERACTIONS Continued

IV. PLAN FOR HOME CARE—Mother's questions about baby's care after discharge.

1. Asks questions in preparation for home care, e.g., "What kind of soap should I use for her?" and "How often should I bathe him?"   _____

2. Makes reference to preparing for discharge, e.g., "I have all his clothes for him" and "I will have diaper service when the baby gets home."   _____

3. Makes reference to assistance in baby's care, e.g., "My mother is going to be with me to help me care for my baby."   _____

Note: This tool is designed to assist students to observe specific behaviors or interactions. Place an X next to the behaviors observed during mother–infant care.

2. A social support system encompassing mate, friends, and family.

3. A competent level of communication and caretaking skills.

4. Parental proximity to the infant.

5. Parent–infant fit (including infant state, temperament, and sex).

If one or more of these preconditions is not present or is less than desirable, skilled nursing intervention is necessary to prevent hindering the attachment process. Therefore, it is important that the caregiver obtain information through a history, interview, or observation to determine factors that can affect parental attachment (see Table 16–3). The nurse should be familiar with ways to encourage and strengthen attachment, such as early parent–infant contact and sensual responses.

PRENATAL ASSESSMENT AND INTERVENTION

The caregiver should be alert to the woman's attitude toward her pregnancy and the unborn infant. Sometimes the woman regrets being pregnant and feels very uncomfortable physically. She may state "I feel huge" and not think of the fetus as a human being. It is important to remember that women who initially regret their pregnancies can still establish a healthy relationship with their infant. However, the woman who has had difficulty incorporating the child as part of her psyche

during pregnancy may not be ready to adjust to the infant immediately after birth. The caregiver should be sensitive to those mothers who need more time to adjust to the birth of the infant.

HOSPITAL ENVIRONMENT AND PRACTICES

Caregivers should do their utmost to assist attachment among mother, father, and infant. Parents should be allowed to participate in decisions relating to prenatal care, labor, birth, and postpartum care. It is helpful if the hospital's facilities and practices are such that parents can choose the birth experience (for example, alternative birth settings) that satisfies their needs. After the birth, both mother and father should be encouraged to participate in the care of their infant, such as bathing, holding, and becoming acquainted with the infant's physical and self-quieting characteristics (Fig. 16–3).

DELIVERY ASSESSMENT AND INTERVENTION

Extended contact between parents and infant should be offered whenever possible. The parents' reactions to the infant and to each other should be observed. The mother should be observed for her interaction with her infant, such as what she says about the infant. Clues about negative mater-

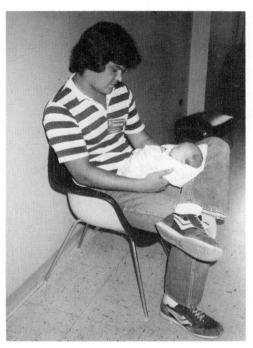

▲ FIGURE 16–3

The rewards of close early contact and continuing contact can be shared by both mother and father. Father and infant interact during father's hospital visit.

nal feelings should be observed and recorded by the caregiver.

POSTPARTUM ASSESSMENT AND INTERVENTION

Promoting the proximity (closeness) of mother and infant is perhaps one of the greatest and most exciting challenges for the caregiver. The caregiver is in a unique position to help the mother, evaluate her needs, and teach her about infant care and behavior.

The mother may be tired and concerned about her bodily needs, such as a painful episiotomy incision or uncomfortable-feeling breasts. The caregiver should provide appropriate comfort measures to the mother. Giving the mother pre-

scribed pain-relief medication may help her to rest and regain the physical energy lost during labor. If possible, the mother should be allowed to observe the caregiver perform a task before she attempts it herself. In addition, staying with the new mother until she feels comfortable undertaking the tasks alone is beneficial.

Coordination of resources in the community and hospital (i.e., social services) provides for better assessment and implementation of support when indicated. Mothers who consistently show limited or low-level attachment behaviors, such as holding the infant away from their body, not looking at the infant, lacking concern about feeding the infant, or lacking a desire to burp the infant, may require additional support and intervention provided by such services.

PARENT–INFANT ATTACHMENT IN SPECIAL CIRCUMSTANCES

Because of the uncertain outcome and the long-term separation, the birth of a preterm, sick, or malformed infant can affect the parent-to-infant attachment. Caregivers should be prepared to assist parents and work with them, so the parents can get acquainted with their infant and participate in infant care such as holding and feeding. The health care providers can offer support and guidance to meet the identified needs. Parents should be encouraged to call the staff and visit the infant frequently.

For many mothers who have had twins (or other form of multiple birth), attachment to more than one infant at one time is difficult. It is important to allow the parents to express their feelings regarding multiple births. Sometimes the attachment is enhanced by bringing both infants to the mother at the same time. This practice reinforces the reality of having twins. If one twin dies, the mother may find it difficult to become attached to the surviving infant while she is grieving. A caring attitude, showing patience and acceptance of parental behavior, is important in encouraging parent–infant attachment in such difficult situations.

NURSING CARE PLAN 16–1

PARENT–INFANT ATTACHMENT

Potential Problems and Nursing Diagnoses	Nursing Interventions
1. Altered parenting related to lack of knowledge.	Encourage participation in care, such as diaper changing, holding, and touching, whenever possible. Instruct parents how to bathe infant. Teach parents about infant's abilities and inabilities.
2. Altered parenting related to lack of self-confidence.	Encourage positive experience with infant, such as eye-to-eye contact and cuddling infant close to body.
3. Altered parenting related to infant's inhibiting behaviors.	Instruct parent that some infants are unresponsive to touch and being held.

Expected Outcomes

1. Parents verbalize knowledge about care-taking activities such as changing diaper and bathing infant.
2. Parents show increased signs of attachment by talking, smiling, touching, and cuddling baby.
3. Parents recognize that, at times, the infant is unresponsive to touch and not visually alert.

References

Auvenshine, M. A., & Enriquez, M. G. (1990). *Comprehensive Maternity Nursing: Perinatal and Women's Health,* 2nd ed. Boston: Jones and Bartlett.

Dickason, E. J., Schult, M. O., & Silverman, B. L. (1990). *Maternal-Infant Nursing Care.* St. Louis: C. V. Mosby.

Klaus, M. H., & Kennell, J. H. (1982). *Maternal-Infant Bonding.* 2nd Ed., St. Louis: C. V. Mosby.

Ladewig, P. W., London, M. L., & Olds, S. B. (1990). *Essentials of Maternal-Newborn Nursing,* 2nd ed. Redwood City, CA: Addison-Wesley Nursing.

May, K. A., & Mahlmeister, L. R. (1990). *Comprehensive Maternity Nursing: Nursing Process and the Childbearing Family,* 2nd ed. Philadelphia: J. B. Lippincott.

Mercer, R. T. (1985). The process of role attainment over the first year. *Nursing Research* 34:198.

SUGGESTED ACTIVITIES

1. Observe three mothers with their infants for 30 minutes each. Identify behaviors of both mother and infant that encourage the maternal–infant attachment process. List observed behaviors that are likely to produce negative maternal–infant responses.

REVIEW QUESTIONS

A. Select the best answer to each multiple-choice question.

1. Attachment involves
   A. Development of bonding between parents and infant
   B. Interaction between mother and infant
   C. Emotional and affectional commitment
   D. All of the above

2. Parental factors that contribute to the development of attachment include all of the following EXCEPT
   A. Social support system
   B. Emotional health
   C. Feeling of security
   D. Fatigue

3. The caregiver can promote the process of maternal attachment by all of the following EXCEPT
   A. Providing measures to decrease discomfort of episiotomy incisions
   B. Providing measures to decrease discomfort of breast engorgement
   C. Encouraging rest periods
   D. Suggesting that the mother hold her baby away from her body

4. Mothers should be instructed to hold their infants at what distance from their face for good eye-to-eye contact?
   A. 6 to 8 inches
   B. 8 to 12 inches
   C. 12 to 14 inches
   D. 14 to 16 inches

5. Mothers usually follow an orderly and a predictable pattern of touching their infants, which is as follows:
   A. First fingertip touch, followed by open palm touch, then enfolding infant in their arms.
   B. First open palm touch, followed by fingertip exploration, then pulling infant toward their body.
   C. First exploration of infant's body, followed by open palm touch, then touching of face and head.

6. A parental precondition that hinders attachment is
   A. Extended family support system
   B. Parental proximity to the infant
   C. Poor self-image
   D. Minimal to average financial assistance

B. Choose from Column II the pharase that most accurately defines the term in Column I.

I

1. Touch _____
2. Eye-to-eye _____
3. Proximity _____
4. Vocal _____
5. Clinging _____
6. Consolable _____

II

A. Infant response to high-pitched voice
B. Stimulation of infant's grasp reflex
C. Decrease in infant fussing and crying
D. Close infant–mother contact
E. Progression from fingertip to palmar touch
F. Hold infant in "en face" position

UNIT VI

THE NEWBORN INFANT

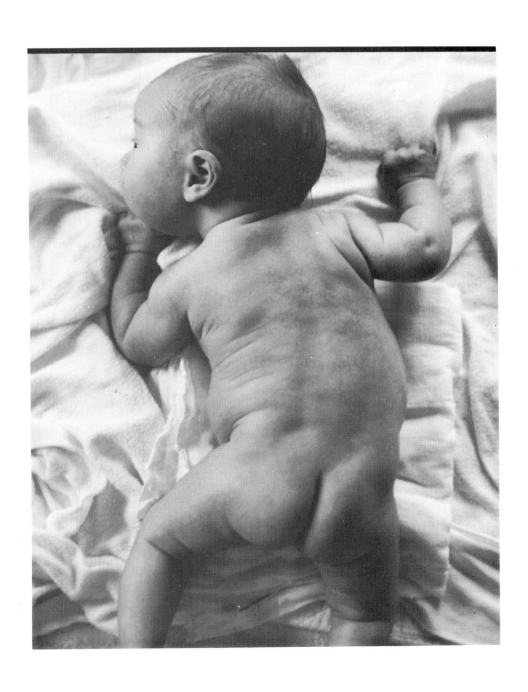

CHAPTER 17 _____

Chapter Outline

Respiratory and Circulatory Function
    Preparatory events to breathing
    Onset of breathing
    Changing from fluid-filled to air-filled lungs
    Opening up the pulmonary circulation
    Closing down the fetal structures
Gastrointestinal Function
Renal Function
Immunological Function
Hepatic Function
Neurological Function
Heat Production and Heat Loss
    Brown-fat metabolism
    General metabolism
    Cold stress
    Prevention of heat loss

Learning Objectives

Upon completion of Chapter 17, the student should be able to

- List four important infant adaptations to extrauterine life.
- Explain the importance of surfactant in the initial breathing of the newborn infant.
- Explain the process by which the fluid in the infant's lungs is replaced by air.
- Establish how the infant's pulmonary circulation opens up.
- Explain the closing down of three fetal circulatory shunts.
- Explain the initiation of gastrointestinal function.
- List two reasons for "air pocketing," the retaining of air in the upper stomach.
- Explain the significance of observing the infant's first stool.
- Explain the reason for the infant's deficiency of vitamin K.
- List two reasons for the infant's weight loss after birth.
- Explain why the newborn infant is susceptible to infections.
- Outline why the infant has the potential for an elevated bilirubin level.
- Explain why the newborn infant should be evaluated for oozing of blood from the cord and bleeding into the skin after birth.
- List a measure to prevent possible infant hemorrhage during the first few days of life.
- Identify the anatomical reason that basic reflexes are present after birth.
- Recall the location of brown fat and how it is used in infant heat production.
- List three reasons why the newborn infant should not be chilled or experience cold stress.
- Explain four ways to prevent heat loss in the newborn infant.

PHYSIOLOGICAL ADAPTATION OF THE NEWBORN TO BIRTH

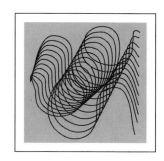

The newborn infant has to make important adaptations for the transition to extrauterine life. To live independently from the mother, the newborn infant must immediately establish pulmonary ventilation, that is, breathe on his or her own. This is accompanied by marked circulatory changes. These changes are smooth for most infants, but for others the process is problematic. The quality of the infant's life, not just survival, is at stake. The caregiver must understand the normal newborn adjustment in order to recognize the deviations from it (Table 17–1).

PHYSIOLOGICAL ADJUSTMENTS TO EXTRAUTERINE LIFE

- Quickly breathe and maintain respirations
- Replace fluid in the lungs with air
- Open up the pulmonary circulation and close the fetal shunts
- Allow pulmonary blood flow to increase and cardiac output (blood volume) to be redistributed
- Provide energy to maintain body temperature and support metabolic processes
- Dispose of waste products produced by food absorption and metabolic processes
- Detoxify substances entering from the environment

Respiratory and Circulatory Function

The respiratory and cardiovascular systems are required to quickly adapt to life outside the uterus.

When the cord is clamped, the placenta is cut off. The changes made by the lungs and heart are described below.

PREPARATORY EVENTS TO BREATHING

In utero, the infant's lungs are filled with fluid. This fluid is a combination of secretion of the alveolar cells of the lungs and some amniotic fluid. At birth, air must be substituted for the fluid.

Surfactant, a phospholipid, is produced by the lungs and prevents them from collapsing during exhalation after birth. In addition, surfactant reduces the surface tension of the lungs. This action is important because when the infant begins to breathe, less effort will be required to continue and maintain breathing. By 35 weeks' gestation, infants usually have sufficient surfactant to stabilize the alveoli of the lungs and reduce the possibility that atelectasis will occur. Many organs, like the lungs, are programmed for successful extrauterine life.

ONSET OF BREATHING

The first breath of the normal, full-term infant occurs within seconds after birth; by 30 seconds, the infant usually is breathing quite well. Many powerful stimuli send messages to the respiratory center of the infant's brain. The sensory stimuli that help respirations to begin are cold, touch, movement, light, and sound. Cooling and clamping of the umbilical cord are two powerful stimuli that influence the onset of respirations. Excessive

TABLE 17–1. IMPORTANT CHARACTERISTICS OF BODY SYSTEMS BEFORE AND AFTER BIRTH

BEFORE BIRTH	AFTER BIRTH
RESPIRATORY FUNCTION	
Lungs are filled with fluid.	Fluid is removed by chest squeeze during vaginal delivery and fluid absorption.
There is no air in lungs.	Air is pulled in with first breath to open lungs and establish functional residual capacity.
There is no movement of air in lungs.	Baby begins to breathe within 30 sec. Powerful stimuli (cold, touch, clamping of cord) help initiate breathing.
Respiratory rate is slower.	Respiratory rate increases 30–60 bpm because of greater need for oxygen.
Breathing pattern appears quite regular.	Baby has tendency for slight irregular respirations and slight apnea.
Temperature is warm and stable.	If the infant becomes chilled (cold stress), exchange and oxygen can be reduced.
Gas is exchanged through fetoplacental unit.	Infant must breathe on its own to get oxygen.
CIRCULATORY FUNCTION	
Pulmonary vessels are constricted.	Dilatation of vessels with increased blood flow to lungs. Increased oxygen to lungs.
Ductus arteriosus shunts blood to bypass lungs.	Ductus arteriosus begins to constrict and closes with increased blood flow to lungs and increased need for oxygen.
Ductus venosus shunts blood to bypass liver.	Ductus venosus constricts and becomes a ligament.
Foramen ovale allows flow from right atrium to left atrium.	Increased pressure in left atrium causes valve shunt to close.
GASTROINTESTINAL FUNCTION	
Fetus swallows amniotic fluid.	Baby voids. First stool is a sticky, dark-green meconium.
Abdomen remains unchanged.	Weak muscles make baby prone to abdominal distention.
No feeding is received.	Baby is prone to swallowing air during feeding and crying. Baby must be burped during and after each because of air pocketing.
No stooling occurs.	Active peristalsis in lower bowel causes baby to have frequent stools.
Stomach and bowel contents are sterile.	Stomach and bowel contents are sterile, but gastric contents become more acidic, which favors formation of vitamin K.
Basic taste sensations are present.	Baby has all basic taste sensations.
RENAL FUNCTION	
Fetus does excrete urine.	Baby voids to excrete waste products.
No weight loss due to urinary output occurs.	Baby has weight loss due to urine output and the passage of stools.
IMMUNOLOGICAL FUNCTION	
Before birth, fetus is in a sterile environment.	Baby comes in contact with many pathogenic organisms, thus is susceptible to infections.
	Baby has delicate skin and open sites vulnerable to infections, such as cord area.
	Handwashing and avoidance of cross-contamination are important in reducing infections.

TABLE 17–1. IMPORTANT CHARACTERISTICS OF BODY SYSTEMS BEFORE AND AFTER BIRTH *Continued*

BEFORE BIRTH	AFTER BIRTH
HEPATIC FUNCTION	
Liver is immature.	Liver function is hindered by deficiency in enzymes.
Production of vitamin K is limited.	Liver is often deficient in producing vitamin K, predisposing infant to hemorrhage during first few days of life. Vitamin K is administered to bring infant's clotting time within normal range.
NEUROLOGICAL FUNCTION	
Before birth, fetus has basic reflex.	Baby is born with basic reflexes (grasp, sucking, rooting, Moro, and tonic neck reflexes)
Neurological system is immature.	Neurological system continues to develop.

cooling, however, will interfere with breathing by increasing the need for oxygen and can produce acidosis. A lack of oxygen (hypoxia) at the tissue level will depress respirations rather than stimulate them. Because of this, it is very important to keep the infant warm.

CHANGING FROM FLUID-FILLED TO AIR-FILLED LUNGS

During vaginal birth, the infant's head is delivered first, then the thoracic cage. The chest area, made up of cartilage and bones, is compressed, promoting drainage of fluid from the lungs. Before the chest is delivered, almost half of the fluid is forced out. As the chest returns to its natural position, the infant pulls or sucks in air (20 to 40 mL) without having to make any effort of its own. The lung expansion creates the negative intrapleural pressure, which is maintained throughout life. The fact that the lung is already distended with fluid greatly reduces the pressure necessary to open the airways.

The infant who is delivered by cesarean birth does not experience chest compression followed by chest recoil and thus is at greater risk for respiratory distress. However, there are other mechanisms by which the lung is cleared after the vaginal squeeze. Some of the fluid is absorbed by the lymphatic vessels, and the rest of the fluid is removed by the pulmonary capillaries. If the fluid

is not removed, the infant will experience labored breathing, respiratory distress, or both.

With the first breath, *functional residual capacity* (FRC) is established. This means there is air left in the lungs after expiration. With the establishment of FRC, the second, third, and subsequent breaths do not require as much pressure; with each breath respiration becomes easier.

OPENING UP THE PULMONARY CIRCULATION

As the lungs take over the job of providing oxygen and clearing waste products (carbon dioxide), the amount of blood sent to the lungs, or *pulmonary circulation,* increases. In utero, only about 10% of the blood goes to the lungs, because of the fetal structure (shunts) and a high resistance to blood flow that is the result of vasoconstriction and thick pulmonary arterioles. In addition, the lungs before birth are only partially expanded and rather noncompressible because of fluid. At birth, with the onset of breathing, expansion of lungs, and clearing of fluid, the pulmonary circulation quickly changes to a low-resistance, high-flow, systemic resistance system.

The newborn infant's respiratory rate is 30 to 60 breaths per minute, compared with the adult rate of 14 to 16 breaths per minute. The reason for the higher respiratory rate is the infant's greater need for oxygen. Clinically, the infant is observed to have shallow, sometimes irregular respirations, with a tendency for apnea or transitory cessation in breathing.

If they do not receive enough oxygen, newborn infants are able to use glycogen (the form in which glucose is stored in the body) for metabolism. This permits the infant to tolerate longer periods of anoxia (less oxygen in the tissues) than an adult can tolerate. However, unchecked anoxia will lead to respiratory distress.

If the flow of blood to the lungs does not rapidly increase, clinical problems usually occur, and resuscitation is often required. Because of this, emergency equipment should be available. Adequate ventilation and oxygenation are two of the most important aspects of infant resuscitation.

EMERGENCY EQUIPMENT NEEDED IN CASE PULMONARY CIRCULATION DOES NOT ADAPT

- Overhead radiant warmer
- Heated, humidified oxygen
- Suction and suction catheters (size 8 French for preterm infants and 10 French for term infants)
- Wall suction set for 40 to 80 mm Hg
- Ventilation bag and manometer
- Intubation equipment, including laryngoscope (size 0 for preterm infant and 1 for term infant)
- Endotracheal tubes
- Oxygen mask with neck piece
- Gloves, tape, replacement bulb for laryngoscope
- Drugs, intravenous fluids, or blood volume expanders

Chilling of the infant, called *cold stress,* should be avoided, because it can restrict both the systemic circulation (blood going throughout the body and back to the heart) and pulmonary circulation (blood going from the right side of the heart, to the lungs, and back to the left side of the heart). In other words, cold stress can decrease the delivery of oxygen to the tissues and cause carbon dioxide retention, reducing gas exchange. In addition, if pulmonary circulation adjustments are not made quickly at birth, fetal-type circulation will persist, and blood will continue to be shunted around the lungs, which can be fatal.

Normal arterial blood gas values are shown in Table 17–2.

CLOSING DOWN THE FETAL STRUCTURES

Foramen Ovale

The *foramen ovale* is an opening between the right and left atria of the heart. It functions like a one-way valve for blood flow. After clamping of the umbilical cord, a large stream of blood from the placenta is cut off. As a result, the pressure of the left side of the infant's heart becomes greater than that of the right side, and the foramen ovale closes. This change, in effect, is a reversal of the previous pressure gradient. The foramen ovale functionally closes about 1 minute after birth. The anatomical closure takes place in about 2 weeks. However, it may take much longer for the septa to fuse together (see Chapter 4).

Ductus Arteriosus

The *ductus arteriosus* shunts blood from the pulmonary artery to the aorta, bypassing the lungs. As the pulmonary arterioles dilate in response to the increased oxygen needs of the lungs, the ductus arteriosus constricts and completely closes. The functional closure of the ductus arteriosus occurs about 15 hours after birth. The anatomical closure occurs at about 3 weeks.

It is important to note that the ductus arteriosus can dilate (reopen) during the first several weeks

TABLE 17–2. NORMAL ARTERIAL BLOOD GAS VALUES

VALUE	RANGE
pH	7.35–7.45
Arterial oxygen pressure (PaO_2)	54–95 mm Hg
Carbon dioxide pressure ($PaCO_2$)	35–45 mm Hg
Bicarbonate (HCO_3)	22–26 mEq/L
Oxygen saturation (O_2)	95–100%

after birth. If the infant experiences a decrease in (blood flow) pressure or oxygen, there may be a return to fetal-type circulation, with a reopening of the ductus arteriosus. This is referred to as patent ductus arteriosus and can lead to right side heart failure and pulmonary congestion. If the ductus arteriosus does dilate, unoxygenated blood will go through the pulmonary artery into the aorta and general circulation.

Ductus Venosus

The *ductus venosus* is a structure (shunt) that allows most oxygenated blood to bypass the liver and enter the inferior vena cava in utero. The clamping of the cord at birth cuts off the umbilical venous blood flow, which greatly reduces the flow of blood through the ductus venosus. It then constricts, closes anatomically in about 2 weeks, and becomes a ligament. The mechanics for the closure are unknown.

Summary

It is important that the caregiver understand the basic mechanisms behind the closure of the fetal structures or shunts. Understanding the pressure changes within the heart and changes in the blood flow pattern will help the caregiver recognize a temporary problem, congenital heart defect, or lack of closure of one of the circulatory fetal structures, and determine appropriate management.

Gastrointestinal Function

In utero, the fetus's gastrointestinal (GI) tract is relatively inactive. Amniotic fluid is swallowed, which provides a source of water that can be reabsorbed for body use. If an infant has an upper GI tract obstruction, water absorption is hindered and excessive amniotic fluid often develops.

The infant's first stool, *meconium,* is a combina-tion of intestinal gland secretions, bile, unconjugated bilirubin, and debris swallowed from amniotic fluid. Meconium is sticky but becomes even more tenacious if pancreatic secretions are lacking, such as occurs in cystic fibrosis. If the fetus becomes distressed or hypoxic before birth, the anal sphincter often relaxes, and meconium is passed. This will stain the amniotic fluid green. If meconium is aspirated into the fetal lungs, it can pose a threat to the infant's airway and cause pneumonia or respiratory distress syndrome.

At birth, the stomach has poor musculature, making the infant prone to abdominal distention. The infant has weak cardiac and pyloric sphincters and experiences bouts of reversed peristalsis. Because of these factors, the infant has a tendency for mild regurgitation or slight vomiting and "air pocketing," the retaining of air in the upper part of the stomach. Air can enter the stomach quite easily when the infant is crying or feeding. Air pocketing is avoided by burping the infant frequently during and at the end of feedings. At birth, the stomach is able to hold approximately 20 ml or less of fluid. Overfeeding will also cause the infant to regurgitate or "spill over" the amount given. Peristalsis is increased in the infant's lower bowel, which causes frequent stools. The newborn infant averages five to six stools daily. Absence of a stool within 48 hours after birth is indicative of an intestinal obstruction; therefore, the occurrence of the first stool is significant. Explanations to the mother about why vomiting occurs, why the baby needs to be burped, and why the baby has frequent stools will reduce the mother's anxiety in caring for her infant.

At birth, the infant has most of the enzymes needed to digest proteins and simple sugars; however, digestion of fat is more difficult. In general, breast milk is easier for the infant to digest than formula, although the sugar and protein content of formula is made as similar as possible to that of human breast milk.

At birth, the stomach and bowel contents are sterile and neutral in pH. This initial pH prevents the growth of the normal bacterial flora of the stomach and intestines. Because vitamin K is dependent on the bacterial flora for its formation, infants often have a deficiency of this vitamin. Therefore, vitamin K is usually given shortly after birth. The gastric contents become more acidic after birth.

Newborn infants have all four taste sensations (acid, sweet, salt, and sour) at birth. They often react strongly to odors. They are able to suck, swallow, and breathe simultaneously during feeding. The tongue has an up-and-down movement (retrusion reflex) at birth, and at about 3 months of age lateral movement is possible. Newborn infants suck on everything placed in their mouths.

Renal Function

At birth, the infant's kidneys are functionally mature enough to excrete waste products, which involves filtering of substances from the blood through the glomeruli. Because the infant has a lower than normal clearance of sodium chloride and urea, pink spots (uric acid crystals) in the urine may be observed on the diaper after voiding.

Newborn infants can lose as much as 10% of their body weight during the first few days of life. One reason for this is that 80% of infants' distribution of body water is extracellular (compared with 55% in adults), which makes them prone to dehydration. In addition, the infant loses weight in the passage of stools, which figured into the birth weight.

Immunological Function

Whereas the fetus lives in a sterile intrauterine environment, the newborn infant is in contact with hordes of pathogenic organisms. Thus, the newborn infant is very susceptible to infections. The amount of passive immunity derived from the placental transfer of maternal antibodies is a crucial determinant for the infant's ability to have an active response against organisms such as bacteria, viruses, and molds.

The newborn infant derives some passive immunity from the mother in the form of immunoglobulin (Ig) antibodies. This immunity gives protection against diphtheria, tetanus, and polio for 3 to 5 months. Because IgM antibodies do not cross the placenta, the infant does not have protection against infectious diseases, such as toxoplasmosis, rubella, cytomegalovirus, herpes simplex, and against other diseases such as syphilis. This group of infections is often called "torch infections."

The infant's susceptibility to infections is the result of delicate skin and fewer opsonins (substances in the blood that coat foreign particles so they can be recognized and destroyed). Handwashing and avoidance of cross-contamination are important while caring for the infant.

Hepatic Function

During the first week of life, the liver is hindered in its functions primarily because of a deficiency in enzymes. Because of a deficiency in the enzyme glucuronyl transferase, the liver has an inadequate ability to convert bilirubin from an indirect fat-soluble compound to a direct, water-soluble compound that can be excreted. Therefore, visible jaundice (called physiological jaundice) is seen in many infants by the second or third day. Bilirubin is toxic, especially to the infant's central nervous system. Therefore, assessment of the bilirubin level is important in infant care.

The liver also is not fully capable of regulating blood sugar. Consequently, hypoglycemia is common. Glycogen stored in the liver is often low in infants who have had a stressful birth, who have had asphyxiation at birth, who have experienced cold stress, who are premature, or who have diabetic mothers.

The liver often is deficient in the production of prothrombin, which is dependent on the production of vitamin K. As previously mentioned, the formation of vitamin K depends on the bacterial flora of the GI tract, and these flora are absent at birth. As they become established, gastric acidity increases. Vitamin K deficiency predisposes the newborn to hemorrhage during the first few days of life. Oozing from the umbilicus, bleeding into the skin (ecchymosis), and bloody stools should be reported to the physician for further evaluation. A preventive measure against bleeding is the intramuscular administration of 1 mg of vitamin Kl.

In clinical studies, administration of vitamin K to the mother before the baby is born is proving to be beneficial because the vitamin K metabolites received by the baby from the mother are absorbed more easily than vitamin K given directly to the baby after birth.

Neurological Function

At birth, all of the neurons of the cerebral cortex are present. As the infant grows they increase in size and complexity. All of the infant's sensory processes are myelinated (that is, nerves are insulated for conduction of nerve impulses), but the motor processes are not. The newborn infant has several basic reflexes, such as the grasp, Moro, and tonic neck reflexes (see Chapter 18). As myelination continues and the cerebral cortex takes over voluntary control, the basic reflexes will disappear. If they are absent at birth or are prolonged in their appearance, the infant may have a neurological problem.

Heat Production and Heat Loss

The fetus is kept in a stable, ideal temperature within the uterus. In contrast, after birth, the infant's environment can vary tremendously. When exposed to a cool environment, the newborn infant requires additional heat. The physiological mechanisms that increase heat production are referred to as *thermogenesis*. These include increased basal metabolic rate (BMR), muscular activity, and chemical thermogenesis called nonshivering thermogenesis.

BROWN-FAT METABOLISM

Nonshivering thermogenesis is an important mechanism of heat production unique to the newborn. It uses the infant's storage of brown adipose tissue (also called brown fat). Brown adipose tissue is the primary source of heat used in the cold-stressed infant. It is found between the scapulas, in the axillas, around the neck and thorax, behind the sternum, and around the kidneys and adrenal glands (Fig. 17–1). Brown fat constitutes 3% to 6% of the newborn's total weight. Brown fat receives its name from its dark color, which comes from its rich supply of blood and nerves. The nerve supply initiates metabolic activity. Brown-fat deposits are used within the first 3 months after birth.

Hypoxia (lack of oxygen) and certain drugs may prevent the infant's metabolism of brown fat.

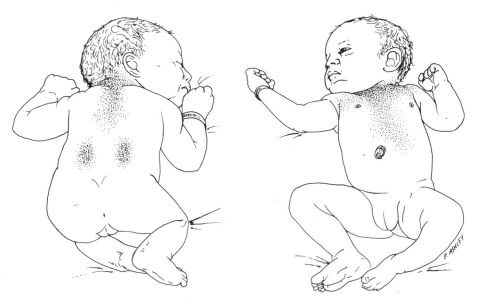

▲ **FIGURE 17–1**

Distribution of brown adipose tissue in the newborn infant.

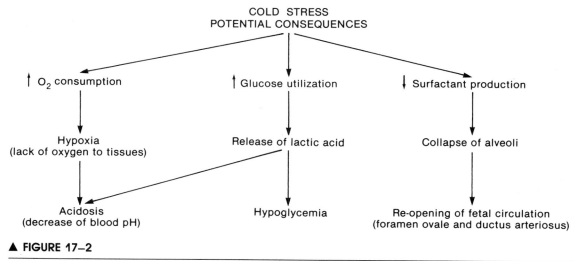

COLD STRESS
POTENTIAL CONSEQUENCES

↑ O₂ consumption   ↑ Glucose utilization   ↓ Surfactant production

Hypoxia   Release of lactic acid   Collapse of alveoli
(lack of oxygen to tissues)

Acidosis   Hypoglycemia   Re-opening of fetal circulation
(decrease of blood pH)   (foramen ovale and ductus arteriosus)

▲ FIGURE 17–2

Cold stress and potential consequences.

GENERAL METABOLISM

Changes in the infant's BMR in response to warming or cooling of the infant's body usually take 12 to 14 hours. Thus, the general metabolism is not effective if the infant is cooled immediately after delivery. In the older infant or child, the increase in the BMR will increase the level of the thyroid hormone, which will cause vasoconstriction. This action will cause a "goose-pimple" effect *not* seen in newborn infants.

The normal infant is able to respond to a slight decrease in temperature with an increase in BMR. However, an environmental drop of 2° is sufficient to cause double oxygen consumption by the term infant. The preterm infant may be unable to stabilize its temperature without a great increase in oxygen consumption and use of brown fat. As mentioned in Chapter 12, immediately after birth, infants are dried and kept warm by use of a radiant heater or an incubator to reduce heat loss.

COLD STRESS

When the infant is chilled or experiences cold stress, a chain of events takes place that can be harmful or even prove fatal (Fig. 17–2). Cooling the infant has an adverse effect on oxygen consumption, use of glucose, blood pH, surfactant production, fetal circulation, and bilirubin level.

Oxygen Consumption

In an attempt to maintain a normal temperature during cold stress, the infant's body initiates brown-fat and general metabolism. These changes increase oxygen consumption. The infant whose body temperature is 95°F (35°C) will require almost twice as much oxygen as will the infant whose temperature is 98.6°F. To maintain a "neutral thermal environment," in which the infant's oxygen consumption and metabolic rate are minimal, it is necessary to keep the infant's temperature between 97.7°F and 98.6°F (36.5°C and 37°C).

Calories—Use of Glucose

Cold stress also affects the rate at which the infant uses calories. More important, the rate at which glucose (stored as glycogen in the liver) is metabolized is also increased. During cold stress, the infant may deplete glycogen stores and be-

Some drugs given to the mother during labor may cause a prolonged metabolic effect, resulting in infant hypothermia (lower temperature).

come hypoglycemic. Hypoglycemia is defined as a blood glucose level of 35 mg/dL or less for the term infant and 25 mg/dL or less for the preterm infant during the first 72 hours after birth. Hypoglycemia requires the administration of glucose. Oral dextrose in water may be given with a follow-up blood glucose (Dextrostix) test. Untreated hypoglycemia may result in brain damage.

Blood pH

During cold stress, the infant metabolizes both brown fat and glucose. When fat is burned, fatty acids are released into the bloodstream. In addition, without sufficient oxygen, glucose releases lactic acid in the blood. The accumulation of lactic acid and fatty acids makes the blood more acidic and decreases the pH. A low pH means the infant is acidotic, and acidosis can result in death. The acid–base homeostasis refers to the maintenance of pH in the normal range. The normal pH is between 7.35 and 7.45; a pH of less than 7.35 can be very detrimental to the infant if uncorrected.

Surfactant Production

Surfactant, as previously stated, is necessary for the expansion of the lungs and maintenance of breathing after birth. Surfactant is made continuously and is secreted onto the surfaces of the air sacs (alveoli) of the lungs. Production is greatly inhibited by cold stress. If cold stress is allowed to continue over a period of time, the alveoli will collapse, and respiratory distress will result.

Reopening of Fetal Circulation

When pulmonary constriction and hypoxia (diminished amount of oxygen in tissues) are allowed to continue, fetal structures such as the ductus arteriosus and foramen ovale may reopen. This condition causes the infant to become cyanotic (blue) and require additional oxygen (ventilation).

Bilirubin

During cold stress, the fatty acids that are released by the brown fat often combine with albumin. With fewer albumin sites available to bind with bilirubin, the infant becomes more prone to develop hyperbilirubinemia. Hyperbilirubinemia, referred to as *kernicterus,* can damage the central nervous system.

PREVENTION OF HEAT LOSS

The major reason for heat loss immediately after birth is the evaporation of water (amniotic fluid) on the skin of the infant. Therefore, it is essential that the infant be dried as soon as possible. To prevent heat loss to cold air or cold surfaces, the infant should be placed in a dry, warm blanket. As soon as the blanket becomes wet, it should be replaced with another dry, warm one. The infant can be placed in a warm incubator or next to the mother's skin. If the infant is placed in an incubator, the incubator should be away from an outside wall.

Nonvital procedures, such as bathing and physical examinations, should be done after the body temperature and respirations are stabilized. Newborn infants' temperature may be as low as 96.8°F (36°C) at birth. Adjusting to extrauterine existence may take 6 to 12 hours, after which the temperature should stabilize at approximately 98.2°F (37.4°C).

Evaporation

Evaporation is the cooling effect derived from the loss of moisture from the skin (Fig. 17–3). The temperature of an infant wet from amniotic fluid will drop quickly after birth. Over a 10-minute period, it is possible for the infant's temperature to drop 2° to 3°F. For this reason, it is extremely important to immediately dry the infant. This step includes drying the head, which is a large surface area of the body. A stockinette cap is placed on the baby's head in many hospitals to reduce heat loss.

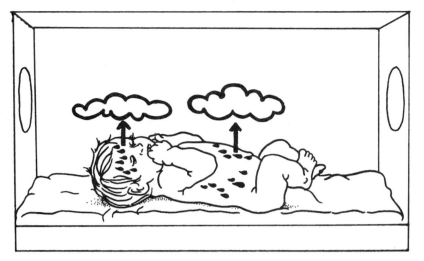

▲ **FIGURE 17–3**

Evaporative heat loss depicted in the conversion of skin water to vapor. Heat consumed in this process is lost from the infant's body surface. (From Korones, S. B. (1986). *High-Risk Newborn Infants*, 4th ed. St. Louis: C. V. Mosby.)

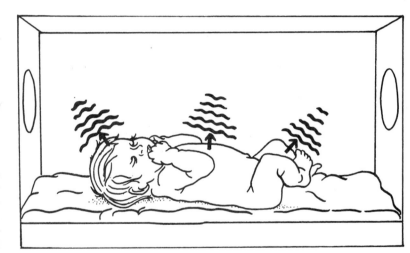

▲ **FIGURE 17–4**

Convective heat loss is indicated as the transfer of heat from body surface to cooler ambient air in the incubator. (From Korones, S. B. (1986). *High-Risk Newborn Infants*, 4th ed. St. Louis: C. V. Mosby.)

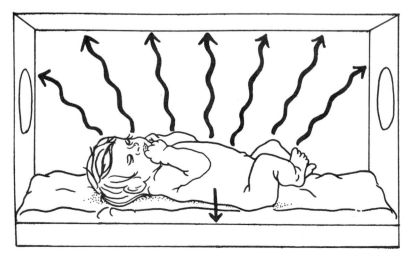

▲ **FIGURE 17–5**

Radiant heat loss is shown as the transfer of heat from body surface directly to cooler incubator wall, regardless of the temperature within the incubator. (From Korones, S. B. (1986). *High-Risk Newborn Infants*, 4th ed. St. Louis: C. V. Mosby.)

Conduction

Heat loss through conduction occurs when the infant has direct contact with cold objects. Therefore, it is important to place the infant, wrapped in a prewarmed blanket, in a heated crib. The caregiver should remember that heat can easily be lost by weighing the infant on a cold scale.

Convection

Heat loss through convection occurs through the flow of air (Fig. 17–4). Infants are likely to lose heat if they are born in a room where the lower temperature of the air carries heat away from their bodies. This may take place in an air-conditioned room.

Radiation

Radiant heat (radiation) occurs when an infant is placed near a cold surface, such as an outside window or a cold wall (Fig. 17–5). The caregiver should remember that the infant will lose heat to the cooler surface. This is why, as mentioned earlier, the incubator should not be placed near the outside wall.

Summary

Temperature regulation of the newborn is maintained by balancing the amount of heat produced with the amount of heat lost. If the amount of heat loss exceeds the amount of heat produced, the body temperature will fall. It is difficult for the newborn infant to maintain a stable body temperature. Frequently at birth, the infant's temperature will fall 2° to 3° below the in utero temperature. This can be very upsetting to the infant's condition and can cause physiological problems that will require additional days of hospitalization.

References

Auvenshine, M. A., & Enriquez, M. G. (1990). *Comprehensive Maternity Nursing: Perinatal and Women's Health,* 2nd ed. Boston: Jones and Bartlett.

Bobak, I. M., & Jensen, M. D. (1991). *Essentials of Maternity Nursing,* 3rd ed. St. Louis: Mosby Year Book.

Dickason, E. J., Schult, M. O., & Silverman, B. L. (1990). *Maternal-Infant Nursing Care.* St. Louis: C.V. Mosby.

Ladewig, P. W., London, M. L., & Olds, S. B. (1990). *Essentials of Maternal-Newborn Nursing,* 2nd ed. Redwood City, CA: Addison-Wesley Nursing.

May, K. A., & Mahlmeister, L. R. (1990). *Comprehensive Maternity Nursing: Nursing Process and the Childbearing Family,* 2nd ed. Philadelphia: J.B. Lippincott.

Wilkerson, N. N. (1988). A comprehensive look at hyperbilirubinemia. *American Journal of Maternal-Child Nursing* 13:360–364.

SUGGESTED ACTIVITIES

1. List the physical factors that are involved in the initiation of infant breathing.
2. Identify three changes that occur after birth in the infant's body systems.
3. Explain ways in which the infant loses heat from the body after birth. Suggest nursing interventions to prevent the infant's heat loss.

REVIEW QUESTIONS

A. Select the best answer to each multiple-choice question.

1. A transition to extrauterine life requires the newborn to
   A. Replace the fluid in the lungs with air
   B. Open up the pulmonary circulation and close down fetal shunts
   C. Quickly breathe and maintain respirations
   D. All of the above

2. The following fetal structures close after birth:
   A. Foramen ovale
   B. Ductus arteriosus
   C. Ductus venosus
   D. All of the above

3. After birth, the infant's liver has a decreased ability to do all of the following EXCEPT
   A. Conjugate bilirubin so it can be excreted
   B. Regulate sugar; therefore, hypoglycemia is common
   C. Produce prothrombin; therefore, less vitamin K is produced
   D. Prevent erythema toxicum

4. After birth, one of the first nursing measures regarding infant care is to dry the infant in order to
   A. Stimulate circulation
   B. Prevent heat loss
   C. Make the infant more pleasant for the mother to hold
   D. Stimulate the infant's reflexes

5. During the birth process, which one of the following is VERY significant to the infant's adaptation to extrauterine life:
   A. Squeeze of thorax, chest recoil, and establishment of functional residual capacity (FRC)
   B. Tactile stimulation, decrease in blood volume, and opening up of air sacs
   C. Mottled skin appearance, cyanosis of feet, and cyanosis of hands
   D. Tactile stimulation, cyanosis of hands, and chest recoil

6. Baby Jones has a heart rate of 140. She is crying and her muscles are well flexed. She had a vigorous cry when her footprints were taken. Her hands exhibit acrocyanosis. The Apgar score is
   A. R
   B. 8
   C. 9
   D. 10

7. Factors that initiate the transition of fetal circulation to adult (mature) circulation include all of the following EXCEPT
   A. Change in peripheral vascular resistance
   B. Lung expansion with fall in pulmonary vascular resistance
   C. Change in right and left atria pressure relationship
   D. Lack of increase in oxygen exchange in lungs

8. When the infant is experiencing cold stress the following may occur:
   A. Increased oxygen consumption, hypoglycemia, and milia of skin
   B. Hypoglycemia, hypoxia, and intracardiac shunting
   C. Increased oxygen consumption and decreased glucose consumption
   D. Aggravation of respiratory distress and vomiting

B. Choose from Column II the phrase that most accurately defines the term in Column I.

I

1. Brown fat _____
2. Nonshivering thermogenesis _____
3. Regurgitation _____
4. IgM antibodies _____
5. Glucuronyl transferase _____
6. Bilirubin _____
7. Vitamin K deficiency _____
8. Evaporation _____
9. Conduction _____
10. Convection _____
11. Radiation _____

II

A. Substance toxic to brain cells
B. Compensatory heat production mechanism
C. Do not cross placenta for infant protection
D. Special adipose tissue able to produce heat
E. Necessary for transfer of bilirubin to water-soluble form that can be excreted
F. Increased by reverse peristalsis
G. Predisposes infant to hemorrhage
H. Heat loss through cool flow of air
I. Heat loss directed toward cold surface
J. Heat loss due to moisture on skin
K. Heat loss due to direct contact with cold object

CHAPTER 18 _____

Chapter Outline

General Appearance
Vital Signs
    Heart rate
    Respirations
    Temperature
    Blood pressure
Physical Characteristics
    Skin
    Head
    Neck and chest
    Abdomen
    Bladder
    Genitals
    Anus
    Spine
    Extremities
Neurological Assessment
Activity and Awareness

Learning Objectives

Upon completion of Chapter 18, the student should be able to
- Describe the assessment of the infant's resting posture.
- State the normal range of the infant's heart rate, respirations, and temperature. Explain reasons for variations in each.
- Explain the appearance and location of milia, mottling, vernix caseosa, and lanugo.
- Describe two factors that cause jaundice in the newborn.
- Explain how to measure the infant's head, chest, and abdomen.
- Define molding, caput succedaneum, and cephalohematoma.
- Describe the assessment of the anterior and posterior fontanelle.
- Recount the assessment of the infant's face and eyes.
- Explain the cause of chemical conjunctivitis and subconjunctival hemorrhage.
- Identify areas of the mouth that should be assessed and what the findings might be.
- Describe how to assess the infant's neck and chest.
- Explain what is included in the assessment of the abdomen.
- Describe phimosis and the procedure that is done to correct it.
- Outline the assessment of the extremities. Describe a simian crease.
- Explain the significance of gluteal creases that are not symmetrical.
- Identify infant movements that may indicate seizure activity.
- Recall four different infant awake and sleep states.
- Describe the quiet-alert state. Explain why this state is the best time to test the infant's responses.

NURSING ASSESSMENT OF THE NEWBORN

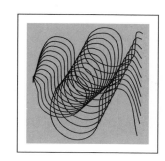

Nursing assessment of the newborn includes observation, inspection, auscultation, palpation, and percussion. The assessment is not done in a single examination, but in a series of examinations. A complete assessment of the newborn includes detailed evaluation of all body systems. Observation of such things as skin color, type of respirations, temperature, activity, and feeding problems alerts the examiner to the health status of the newborn.

The first assessment takes place immediately after birth, usually in the delivery room, and is aimed at identifying life-threatening conditions that demand prompt attention. A more complete examination is performed after the infant has had an opportunity to adapt to extrauterine life. A head-to-toe examination is done, including measurements of head and chest to provide baseline data that will be used for comparison with future assessments. The caregiver should remember to wear gloves in the assessment of the infant. Also, because the infant loses heat quickly, it should be exposed only as necessary, unless a radiant heat bed is being used. It is best to perform the examination about 1 hour after feeding to minimize interference with gastrointestinal functioning. Excessive handling soon after feeding could cause the infant to regurgitate or vomit.

General Appearance

The resting posture and spontaneous movements can best be evaluated before the infant is disturbed. Flexion and symmetry can be observed while the infant is resting. Spontaneous movements may provide subtle clues to potential central nervous system problems. Noticeable jerky or jit-

tery movements many indicate excessive electrical discharge from the neurons or a metabolic disorder, such as hypoglycemia, hypocalcemia, or hypoxia; neurological damage; or drug addiction. Repetitive blinking or pedaling movements of the lower limbs may represent seizure activity caused by injury at birth. Prolonged or excessive tremors may indicate hyperactivity and should be reported to the physician for further evaluation. Frequently a heel stick is done to determine the blood glucose level using a Dextrostix (Fig. 18–1). It is important to stick the lateral aspect of the heel to avoid the medial plantar artery crossing the heel. Hypoglycemia is present if the blood glucose level is 35 to 40 mg/100 mL or less.

The infant's cry should be loud and lusty. If the infant is observed to have a high-pitched cry, central nervous system damage or drug addiction may be present.

Vital Signs

Vital signs should be taken when the infant is quiet or resting. The heart rate and respiratory rate will be much faster if the infant is fussing or crying than when in the quiet state.

HEART RATE

The infant's heart rate varies with activity. When the infant is in deep sleep, the rate can be as low as 100 beats per minute (bpm). When the infant is crying, the heart rate can go up to 180 bpm (range, 120 to 160). The heart rate is determined using a stethoscope and listening to the apical beat

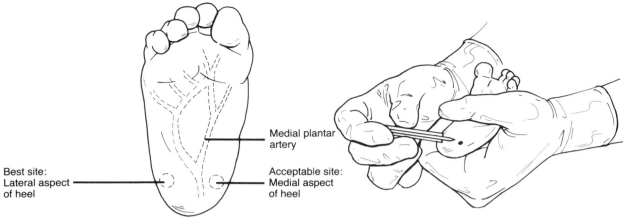

▲ **FIGURE 18-1**

Best locations for heel stick to obtain a sample for blood glucose levels. The lateral aspect of the heel should be used, thus avoiding the medial plantar artery. Before performing the stick, warm the infant's heel for 3 to 5 minutes, then cleanse the selected site with alcohol and blot dry with sterile gauze.

at the precordial region, which is two finger-breadths below the left nipple (at the fourth inter-costal space and to the left of the midclavicular line). The two femoral pulses (in the groin region) should be evaluated (Fig. 18–2). The absence of a femoral pulse suggests a coarctation stricture of the aorta. A weak or slow pulse may indicate decreased cardiac output and should be reported to the charge nurse or physician.

RESPIRATIONS

A newborn's respirations are irregular and ab-dominal or diaphragmatic in character. Typically, the range is from 35 to 60 breaths per minute, with an average of 40. The respirations, like the pulse rate, vary with activity. A persistent rate of 45 or more breaths per minute is often considered abnormal. Movements of the chest and abdomen

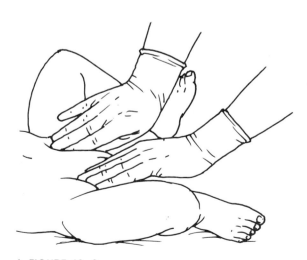

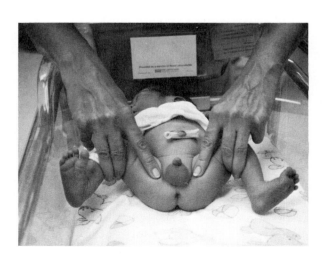

▲ **FIGURE 18-2**

Palpating a femoral pulse. The pulse is palpated simultaneously on both sides with tips of fingers.

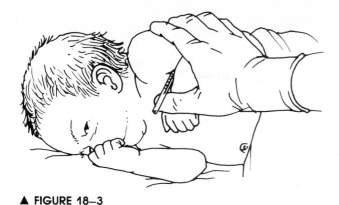

▲ FIGURE 18–3

Taking axillary temperature.

should be synchronized. A lag in inspiration, represented by a "seesaw" movement of chest and abdomen, is a sign of respiratory distress. Other signs of respiratory distress are pulling of the chest wall in the rib or sternal area on inspiration; use of intercostal muscles, giving rise to sternal retractions; marked flaring of the nostrils; or grunting noises during respirations.

TEMPERATURE

The infant's temperature drops immediately after birth. The internal organs are poorly insulated, and the skin is relatively thin. In addition, the infant's heat-regulating center has not yet matured. The infant's body rapidly reflects the temperature of the environment.

The newborn is unable to maintain or raise body temperature by shivering; instead, efforts to increase body temperature are aided by a special tissue called brown fat (Chapter 17). Immediately after birth, a thermal sensor is usually applied to the skin to monitor the temperature until it is stabilized (4 to 6 hours).

The newborn's temperature is most frequently measured in the axilla (Fig. 18–3). The normal range of the axillary temperature is 97.7°F to 98.6°F (36.5°C to 37°C). If a rectal temperature is taken, the caregiver should support the infant's legs during the entire procedure to prevent injury due to sudden or unpredictable movements (Fig. 18–4).

An elevated temperature can occur from dehydration, too much clothing, and infection. Sub-

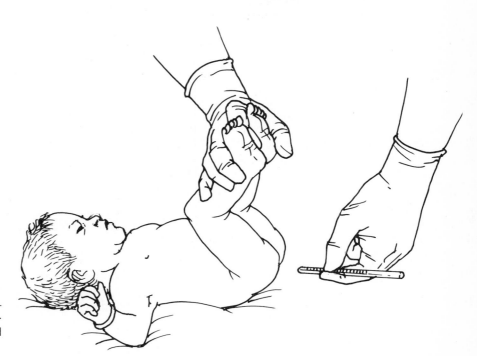

▲ FIGURE 18–4

Support of legs for rectal temperature. Support is continued during entire procedure.

TABLE 18–1. NURSING ALERT: VITAL SIGNS

AREA ASSESSED	NORMAL FINDINGS	VARIATIONS—POSSIBLE PROBLEMS
Heart rate	Apical pulse is 120 to 160 bpm	100 (sleeping) to 180 (crying); may be irregular for brief period, especially after fussing or crying Persistent fast pulse—170 means respiratory distress syndrome (RDS)
Femoral pulse	Femoral pulses are equal and strong	Weak or absent femoral pulse indicates coarctation of aorta
Respirations	40/min; tend to be shallow, irregular when fussing or crying	Persistently over 45 means RDS; apnea or pause in respirations for 15 seconds may occur
Blood pressure	75/42–80/46 mm Hg	Varies with activity level; may provide clue for hypotension or congenital heart problem
Temperature	Axillary is method of choice Rectal to check for patent anus Thermal sensor for continuous temperature	Below normal may reflect heat loss, infection, or dehydration

normal temperatures in infants can be the result of metabolic disturbances and infections. An environmental temperature that is too high can increase the infant's temperature; one that is too low can decrease the temperature. Because the infant is not able to perspire effectively (the sweat glands do not fully function), overheating can cause the infant to break out in a pinpoint, reddish rash that is often referred to as *prickly heat* or *miliaria*.

BLOOD PRESSURE

Blood pressure, if not taken routinely, is taken at least in infants in distress, in infants whose circulatory adequacy is questionable, and in preterm (premature) infants. It should be measured with a 1-inch cuff. The average blood pressure at birth is 75/42 to 80/46 mm Hg. A Doppler blood pressure device greatly improves the accuracy of the reading. A systolic reading may be obtained by noting the pressure when palpating the return of the brachial pulse, if other methods are not available (Table 18–1).

Physical Characteristics

SKIN

The skin provides a visible record of the newborn's health status. The skin is inspected for characteristics related to the full-term, preterm, or postterm infant. Some of the clinical findings are common and not significant; however, they are of concern to parents (Table 18–2). Other findings are important and should be reported to the physician.

Texture. In a well-hydrated newborn infant, the skin is often dry because it has to become accustomed to the dry air rather than the wet, amniotic fluid that surrounded it in utero. By the second or third day the skin often becomes flaky, and cracks are noticeable, particularly around the ankles. The epidermis is thin and delicate and thus can be easily irritated.

Turgor. The well-hydrated infant has good skin turgor or elasticity. When the skin is pinched, it quickly returns to its previous position. If the infant is dehydrated, the skin returns slowly to the original position.

Milia. Milia are small, raised, white spots representing distended sebaceous glands. They appear on the chin, nose, and forehead and disappear spontaneously within a few weeks. The mother should be instructed not to prick these pimple-like spots (Fig. 18–5).

Mottling. Mottling is a lacy pattern of dilated blood vessels under the skin. It may last for a few days to several weeks and represents general circulatory instability. It may be related to temporary fluctuation in skin temperature (seen when the infant is exposed to cold air) or, if persistent, may be associated with a serious cardiac illness.

TABLE 18–2. NURSING ALERT: ASSESSMENT OF SKIN		
CLINICAL FINDING	**NORMAL ASSESSMENT**	**VARIATIONS—POSSIBLE PROBLEMS**
Texture	Smooth, dry; may have cracks in hands and feet	Generalized cracks; very dry skin indicates dehydration
Turgor (elasticity)	When skin is pinched it quickly returns to original position	When skin in pinched, it slowly returns to original position. Associated with dehydration
Milia (distended sebaceous glands)	Small raised white spots on chin, nose, and forehead	Will disappear spontaneously
Vernix caseosa	Yellowish white, greasy substance Deposits thickest in creases	Absent in postmaturity Excessive in prematurity
Erythema toxicum	Red rash, often blotchy; peak is 24–48 hr	Skin delicate and sensitive Specific cause unknown
Petechiae	Bluish red spots caused by minute capillary breakage during birth	Fresh or numerous petechiae suggest hemophilia or infection
Jaundice	Yellow color due to bilirubin Normally occurs second or third day, then level decreases Press skin or sternum or assess color of gums or sclera of eyes	Increased bilirubin level can damage central nervous system
Lanugo	Fine hair on shoulders, upper back, and forehead	Varies in amount; absent in postmaturity; excessive in prematurity
Mongolian spots	Bluish purple spots frequently on back, shoulders, and buttocks Common in darker skinned people	Varies in amount Will fade in 1–2 years
Acrocyanosis	Bluish discoloration of hands and feet Lips, gums, and tongue should be pink	Represents sluggishness in peripheral circulation Differentiate from generalized cyanosis
Birthmarks	Stork bites are red and flat and found on upper eyelids, back of neck, and midforehead Port-wine stain indicates hemangioma	Will disappear with blanching Will not disappear

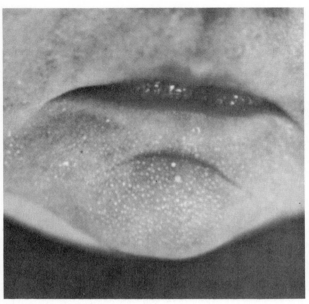

▲ FIGURE 18–5

Milia are tiny sebaceous cysts commonly found on the chin or across the bridge of the nose. They disappear within a few weeks after birth. (Courtesy of Mead Johnson Laboratories, Evansville, Indiana.)

Pallor. A pale skin is significant and should be reported to the physician. It may represent anemia, shock, asphyxia, or edema.

Vernix Caseosa. Vernix caseosa is a thick, yellowish-white sebaceous deposit that covers the body of the fetus and protects the skin from the watery environment in utero. At birth, some infants are covered thickly, whereas others may have deposits only in their body creases. Some of the vernix is removed during the initial bath; however, if the skin is rubbed to remove the vernix, irritation may result.

Erythema Toxicum. Erythema toxicum is a normal finding and is harmless but may be of concern to the mother. It has a red, rash-like, often blotchy appearance. It may appear suddenly, usually over the trunk and diaper area but possibly widespread. The peak incidence is in the first 24 to 48 hours of life. The cause is unknown, and no treatment is necessary. Sensitivity to the environment is suspected. The caregiver should explain to the parents that the infant's skin is delicate and may be sensitive even to soft clothing.

Petechiae. Petechiae are pinpoint, bluish-red spots. Often they are caused by the breakage of minute capillaries during birth. Frequently they are seen over the trunk and face of the infant. They are increased when the umbilical cord has been around the neck. Usually, petechiae fade within 24 to 48 hours. Fresh or numerous petechiae may suggest a blood disease (hemophilia) or an infection. Also, they may be associated with drugs such as aspirin taken by the mother. Fresh petechiae appearing after birth should be reported immediately to the physician.

Jaundice. About the second or third day (28 to 36 hours) after birth, the skin of some infants appears yellow, or jaundiced. Jaundice is a result of the breakdown of an excessive number of red blood cells that are not needed after birth. This type of jaundice is often referred to as "physiological jaundice," and it quickly disappears. Another reason for jaundice is a deficiency in the enzyme *glucuronyl transferase,* which is necessary to convert the insoluble, indirect bilirubin into a direct, water-soluble bilirubin that can be excreted. In addition, it is due to an immature liver's inability to excrete bilirubin. A laboratory test to determine the level of bilirubin is usually performed, because it is possible for brain damage to occur when hyperbilirubinemia occurs. Laboratory reports that support the diagnosis of hyperbilirubinemia include:

- An increase in serum bilirubin level of more than 5 mg/dL in 24 hours.
- In full-term newborns, a serum bilirubin level greater than 12 mg/dL, which represents the upper limit of peak concentration of physiological jaundice.
- In low-birth-weight newborns, a serum bilirubin level of 15 mg/dL.

Pathological hyperbilirubinemia is discussed in Chapter 24. Jaundice that occurs early, during the first 24 hours, is likely to be pathological. A technique to assess jaundice is to blanch or press the infant's skin over the sternum or observe the mucous membranes of the gums or the sclera of the eyes for a yellow tint.

Lanugo. Lanugo is a soft growth of fine hair that is often observed on the shoulders, back, and forehead of the newborn. It is more prevalent in premature infants. Lanugo disappears in a few weeks after birth.

Mongolian Spots. Mongolian spots are bluish-purple spots over parts of the infant's body. They vary in size and shape and frequently are seen over the back, shoulders, and buttocks. They are caused by the presence of large, branching chromatophore cells lying beneath the epidermis. They are common in Asian and black infants and newborns of other dark-skinned races. They are harmless and gradually fade during the first or second year of life, although they have been known to last up to 6 years of age. Explaining this to parents will help alleviate their concerns.

Acrocyanosis. Acrocyanosis represents a sluggishness in the infant's peripheral circulation. It is a bluish discoloration of the hands and feet and may be present in the first 2 to 6 hours after birth. If the central nervous system is adequate, the blood supply should return quickly when the skin is blanched with a finger.

The nurse should assess the mucous membranes of the lips, gums, and tongue, which should be pink. It is important for the caregiver to differentiate poor circulation in the palms and soles caused by acrocyanosis from generalized cyanosis, which indicates a pathological condition. Generalized cyanosis may be caused by respiratory distress, anoxia, anemia, pneumonia, or some congenital heart defects.

Birthmarks. Telangiectatic nevi ("stork bites") are hemangiomas that appear as flat red areas commonly on the upper eyelids, back of the neck, and midforehead. Apparently the result of skin capillary dilatation and abnormal thinness of the skin, they are more common in light-complexioned infants. They disappear with blanching, because the blood is drained from the engorged capillaries. These marks have no clinical significance and fade by the first or second year of life. An explanation about their disappearance is important to the mother.

A "strawberry" mark is usually single and may be slightly raised (like a slice of strawberry). Sometimes this type of birthmark will enlarge and then regress. In most cases, it will disappear by 7 years of age.

The birthmark that is of concern is the *port-wine stain* or *nevus*. Nevi vary in shape and location. These birthmarks do not disappear. If the area of discoloration is large and noticeable, as on the face, it may cause cosmetic difficulties. Cosmetic surgery may be done at an older age to remove the nevus (Table 18–2).

Harlequin Color Change. When the harlequin color change is present, the examiner will notice a color difference running the length of the body (from the forehead). One half of the body is paler than the other half. This discrepancy is not clinically significant.

HEAD

The newborn's head is large compared with its body and represents about one-fourth of the total body length. The average head circumference is 13.2 to 14.8 inches (33 to 37 cm). The infant's head circumference either equals or exceeds by 1 inch the circumference of the chest. If the head circumference is more than 4 cm greater than that of the chest, a serial assessment for increased intracranial pressure or possible hydrocephalus is indicated.

The shape of the infant's head varies depending on the type and length of labor. The heads of breech-born newborns and those born by elective cesarean are characteristically round because pressure was not exerted on them during birth. However, infants born head first, vaginally, often have an elongated head.

Skull

Molding and Caput Succedaneum. Molding and caput succedaneum are normal findings at birth. Molding, overlapping of the bones of the head, occurs as a result of head compression during the birth process. It disappears within about 2 to 3 days. Caput succedaneum is a diffuse, edematous swelling of the soft tissues of the scalp (Fig. 18–6). It can be palpated as a soft, fluctuant mass that may cross over the suture lines. Caput succedaneum is absorbed and requires no treatment.

Cephalohematoma. Cephalohematoma is caused by a collection of blood under the cranial bone. It is confined to a particular bone, usually the parietal (Fig. 18–7). It may be unilateral or bilateral and does not cross the suture line. This swelling occurs on the second or third day. Its disappearance may take as long as 6 weeks. It

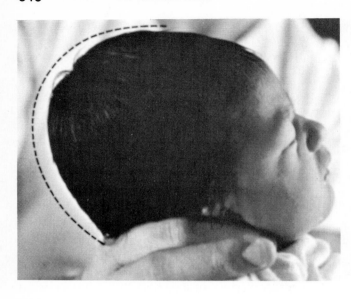

▲ FIGURE 18—6

Caput succedaneum. (Courtesy of Mead Johnson Laboratories, Evansville, Indiana.)

usually results when trauma occurs to small blood vessels of the periosteum. This finding is more common when the mother has had a prolonged or difficult labor. With excessive bleeding, the infant may experience anemia. In addition, as the blood is absorbed, the infant's bilirubin may rise to a dangerous level; therefore, this problem requires medical management.

Fontanelles and Sutures. The infant has an

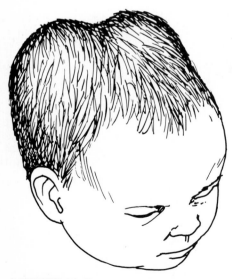

▲ FIGURE 18—7

Bilateral cephalohematoma.

anterior and a posterior fontanelle, which are known as "soft spots." The *anterior fontanelle* is the largest and is called the *bregma*. It is diamond shaped and formed by the juncture of the cranial bones. The anterior fontanelle should be palpated to determine if it is bulging or depressed (sunken). When the infant cries, coughs, or vomits, the anterior fontanelle may bulge. When the infant is quiet, it should not be elevated but should be level with the sutures. A bulging anterior fontanelle while the infant is quiet is indicative of increased intracranial pressure. A depressed fontanelle is indicative of dehydration. A large fontanelle may be present in an infant who has retarded bone growth. The anterior fontanelle closes at about 18 months of age.

The *posterior fontanelle* is triangle shaped. It is located between the occipital and parietal bones. It closes when the infant is about 2 months old. Late closure of the fontanelle may indicate hydrocephaly. Because parents are often concerned about touching the infant's soft spots, they should be informed that the fontanelles are covered with layers of protective tissue so that they can be touched and washed.

Face

The infant's chin usually is somewhat recessed, and the nose is often flattened from in utero

TABLE 18–3. NURSING ALERT: ASSESSMENT OF THE HEAD		
AREA ASSESSED	**NORMAL FINDINGS**	**VARIATIONS—POSSIBLE PROBLEMS**
Shape and size	Elongated in vaginal head-first birth	Shape depends on type and length of labor
	Breech birth—head is round Cesarean—head is round	No pressure on head in breech birth
Molding	Molding (overlapping of bones) is common	Severe molding is present in difficult birth; assess for neurological damage
Caput succedaneum	Caused by edema of soft tissues	Usually disappears within a few days
Cephalohematoma	Caused by collection of blood under cranial bone; usually is confined to parietal bone (does not cross suture lines)	Absorption of blood can increase bilirubin
Anterior fontanelle	Diamond-shaped; should not be bulging when infant is quiet	Bulging when quiet indicates increased intracranial pressure
		Sunken or depressed anterior fontanelle suggests dehydration
		Large fontanelle suggests growth retardation
Posterior fontanelle	Triangular	Reassure parents that "soft spots" on both fontanelles can be touched and washed and will close
Circumference	Head circumference (12.5–14.5 inches) is 1 inch greater than chest circumference	If head circumference is greater than 1 inch of chest circumference, hydrocephaly is indicated
Portion of body	Head is ¼ of body size	Small head is indicative of microcephaly

pressure. The cheeks show a fullness due to an accumulation of fat, which makes up the "sucking pads." These pads allow the infant to have a strong sucking reflex. The face is sensitive to touch. The infant's facial movements should be symmetrical (the same on both sides). Occasionally, a facial nerve is damaged owing to a prolonged labor or a forceps delivery. A facial paralysis, if present, may be temporary; sometimes nerve damage is permanent. The parent should be informed about the possible outcome (Table 18–3).

Eyes

The eyes of the white infant are slate-blue or gray. Scleral color tends to be bluish because of its relative thinness. Dark-skinned infants tend to have darker eyes at birth. The newborn infant's eye color is not established until about 3 months of age, and it may change during the first year of life.

The infant's eyes should be checked for equality, pupil size, reaction of pupils to light, blink reflex to light, and inflammation of the eyelids. In addition, the nurse should assess whether the red reflex is present in the retina, because an absence may indicate congenital cataracts.

Angle of Slant. The angle of slant from the inner to outer canthus (a mongolian slant) should be assessed. A slant up or down from the inner to the outer canthus is associated with trisomy 21 (Down's syndrome).

Setting-Sun Sign. The setting-sun sign is caused by retraction of the upper lid and is seen in infants with hydrocephalus.

Strabismus and Nystagmus. When the infant is alert, the eye movements should be smooth and in unison. In *strabismus*, there seems to be a crossing of the eyes. *Nystagmus* is a twitch rather than smooth movements. It is a common uncoordinated eye movement. As the muscles develop, nystagmus will usually disappear.

Short Palpebral Fissure. Short palpebral fissure (lower eyelid) is associated with fetal alcohol syndrome. Infants with this syndrome also have a depressed, broadened nasal bridge, thin upper lip (fishmouth appearance), and short nose.

Optical Blink. The normal infant is sensitive to bright lights and loud noises. When a bright light is placed toward the infant, a protective blink occurs.

Pupil Reaction. The pupils' reaction to light is part of the physical examination. Using a penlight or ophthalmoscope, the caregiver should note how pupil size reacts to light (constriction or dilation of 1 to 2 mm). The pupils should react equally to the light. No reaction of the pupils indicates increased intracranial pressure or hemorrhage.

Chemical Conjunctivitis. Chemical conjunctivitis may appear a few hours after placing silver nitrate drops in the eye to prevent *ophthalmia neonatorum*. A purulent drainage may appear in some infants' eyes as chemical conjunctivitis. This drainage is the same as would appear in an infec-tion. The use of erythromycin ointment instead of 1% silver nitrate has lessened the incidence of chemical conjunctivitis.

Subconjunctival Hemorrhage. Subconjunctival hemorrhage appears in about 10% of newborns as a result of changes in pressure during passage through the birth canal. The hemorrhagic areas are usually small; if they seem to be enlarging, further assessment should be done.

Cataract. Congenital malformations of the eyes include cataracts and glaucoma. Cataracts vary from a pinpoint size to the total involvement of the lens.

Vision. Vision is more advanced in the newborn than was previously thought. Infants are myopic and see best at a length of about 8 to 12 inches. The ability of infants to follow objects is called *visual tracking*. Infants can focus on an object for about 10 seconds. They can discriminate between simple and complex patterns and prefer simple ones. Newborns also prefer highly contrasting colors, such as black and white, and colors of medium intensity, such as medium pinks, yellows, and greens. They sometimes focus on a

TABLE 18–4. NURSING ALERT: ASSESSMENT OF EYES

AREA ASSESSED	NORMAL FINDINGS	VARIATIONS—POSSIBLE PROBLEMS
Placement	Eyes on parallel plane	Slant, except in Orientals, is associated with Down's syndrome (trisomy 21)
Color	Blue or slate-blue gray	Lack of pigmentation (albinism)
	Color not established until 3 mos of age	
Movement	Strabismus appears as crossing of the eyes	As mucles develop, strabismus should disappear
	Nystagmus is twitching rather than smooth movements	Nystagmus lessens as infant's focus improves
Optical blink	Blink with bright light	Absence of blink associated with central nervous system (CNS) damage
Pupil reaction	Pupils react to bright light	Unequal or lack of pupil change suspicious of CNS damage
	Eyes should constrict or dilate	
Chemical conjunctivitis	Due to silver nitrate	Irritation of conjunctiva (temporary)
		Purulent drainage should be cultured
Subconjunctival hemorrhage	Small hemorrhages due to pressure during birth	Large areas of bleeding should be evaluated
Vision	Myopia (sees best 8–12 inches)	If infant does not focus or follow object, assess for vision damage
	Infant can follow object (visual tracking)	

bright, shiny object. Infants prefer a formed image to an unformed one; thus, one of the strongest stimuli for the newborn is the human face. The mother should be instructed to make eye-to-eye contact with the infant as a means of establishing maternal to infant bonding or attachment (Table 18–4).

Nose

The infant's nose is relatively flat. Because the infant breathes through the nose and not through the mouth, obstructions of mucus or an atresia cause varying degrees of difficult breathing. It is important that the infant has patent (open) nares. Sneezing is common in infants to clear their nasal passages. The newborn infant can identify odors such as the odor of breast milk.

Mouth

The infant's mouth should be assessed for palate closure, presence of teeth, and infection. A *cleft palate* (lack of closure of the palate) can be assessed by placing a gloved finger in the infant's mouth. At the same time, the strength of the sucking reflex can be assessed. *Epstein's pearls*, which are small white nodules resulting from an accumulation of epithelial cells, are commonly found on both sides of the hard palate. They disappear a few weeks after birth. The presence of teeth is rare; if they are found, they often have to be removed because the roots are poorly formed, and the teeth tend to become loose and can be aspirated.

If the tongue appears large and protruding, the infant should be further evaluated, because this is one characteristic of Down's syndrome. *Thrush*, a fungal infection caused by *Candida albicans*, is sometimes picked up in the mother's vaginal secretions during birth. It appears as gray-white patches on the tongue and mucous membranes. The patches can be distinguished from curdled milk if they cannot quickly be removed. It is important for caregivers to wash their hands after handling an infant with thrush so as not to spread the infection to other infants.

The *sucking reflex* is stimulated when the infant's mouth is touched. Sucking movements occur when an object, such as the nipple, is placed in the infant's mouth. A poor sucking reflex may result from respiratory depression, central nervous system damage, drug addiction of the mother, or prematurity. The *rooting reflex* is well developed and can be elicited by stroking the corner of the infant's mouth. If the normal infant should turn the head toward the stimulated side, this is noted as a positive rooting reflex.

Ears

In observing the infant's ears, the nurse should evaluate their formation, their position, and the amount of cartilage present. In addition, the infant's ability to hear should be assessed. The infant should respond to the ringing of a bell or a human voice by grimacing and moving the body. Risk factors associated with poor hearing include maternal rubella infections during pregnancy and congenital defects of the ear.

The relationship of the position of the ear to the outer canthus of the eye is another important assessment. Low-set ears can be indicative of a chromosomal abnormality (Fig. 18–8). In a full-term infant, the cartilage is well developed (Table 18–5).

NECK AND CHEST

Neck

The newborn has a short neck, creased with skin folds. Because the muscle tone is not well developed, the infant's neck cannot support the full weight of the head. Therefore, the head lags when the infant is pulled from supine to sitting position. The mother should be instructed to support the infant's head by placing her hand behind the neck, so the head will drop back only slightly.

The neck should be palpated for masses or injury to large muscles. The clavicles are assessed for evidence of fractures, which may occur with a difficult delivery of the shoulders. Adequacy of range of motion and neck muscle function is determined by placing the head in various directions.

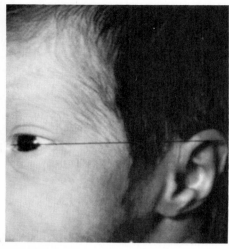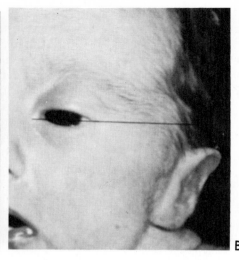

A   B

▲ FIGURE 18–8

A. Normal position of the newborn's ears. B. Low-set ears. (Courtesy of Mead Johnson Laboratories, Evansville, Indiana.)

TABLE 18–5. NURSING ALERT: ASSESSMENT OF NOSE, MOUTH, AND EARS

AREA ASSESSED	NORMAL FINDINGS	VARIATIONS—POSSIBLE PROBLEMS
Nose	Nose is quite flat	
	Nares are patent (open)	Obstructions such as mucus or atresia cause varying degrees of difficult breathing
	Newborn infant is a "nose breather"	
	Sneezing is way to clear nasal passage	
Mouth	Mouth should be assessed for palate closure	Lack of closure is called a cleft palate
	Teeth, if present, should be removed due to poor root formation	Newborn infant's teeth can come loose and be aspirated
	Epstein's pearls are small white nodules that will disappear	None
	Tongue is free moving	Large and protruding tongue is characteristic of Down's syndrome
	Thrush, a fungal infection	If white patches cannot be removed it is probably thrush
		Caregiver should frequently wash hands and be careful not to spread infection to another infant
	Sucking reflex is strong	If weak, assess for prematurity or central nervous system damage
	Rooting reflex is well developed	If absent, assess other reflexes for normality
Ears	Correct placement is line drawn from outer canthus of eye to top of ear	Low-set ears can be indicative of chromosomal abnormality
	Cartilage well formed in full-term infant	Poorly formed cartilage is found in preterm infant
	Hearing is present	Infant should respond to noise; loss of hearing may be due to maternal infection (rubella)

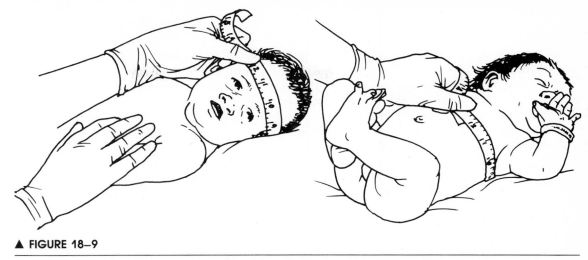

▲ **FIGURE 18–9**

A. Measuring head circumference of the infant. **B.** Measuring chest circumference of the infant.

Chest

The chest is somewhat barrel shaped. Protrusion of the lower part of the sternum, called the *xiphoid cartilage,* is common. The chest's circumference is taken as a baseline measurement for respiratory expansion. It also provides an indicator of what the head circumference should be. The chest is measured at the nipple line and averages about 1 inch less than the head (Fig. 18–9).

The position and distance between the nipples and the size of breast tissue are important measurements. At term, the infant has a breast tissue mass of 5 cm or more. The distance between the nipples is about 8 cm. A wide distance between the nipples may be indicative of a congenital defect. Breast engorgement is common in both the male and female infants because of hormones received from the mother before birth.

Breath sounds are listened to by the nurse and the physician. They should be clear and demonstrate the moving of dry air in and out. The presence of noise (rales or crackles) is an indication of fluid in the chest. Heart rates can be as rapid as 180 bpm and fluctuate a great deal with changes in the level of activity from quiet to crying. The normal range of heart rate is 120 to 160 bpm. The apical heart rate should be taken with a stethoscope for a full minute. The heart sounds are heard best toward the lateral half of the left side of the chest. A detection of the louder sound in another position on the chest can indicate a murmur or an abnormality. The nursing assessment of the chest should include observation for breathing difficulties, grunting, apnea episodes, retractions, and cyanosis.

ABDOMEN

The newborn infant's abdomen is cylindrical, with slight rounding. The abdomen moves with

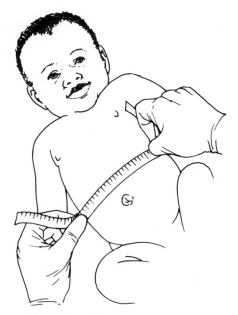

▲ **FIGURE 18–10**

Measuring the abdominal circumference above the umbilicus.

the chest during respiration. If the abdomen looks distended, a measurement of the abdominal circumference may be taken (Fig. 18–10). A shiny and stretched abdomen is abnormal. It can be indicative of infection, tracheoesophageal fistula, or a congenital obstruction. No masses should be palpable.

The umbilical cord should contain two arteries and one vein, which should be assessed immediately after birth. A single artery is associated with congenital anomalies. The cord begins to dry within 2 hours after birth and is shriveled and darkened by the second or third day and sloughs off by 7 to 9 days. It is important for the caregiver to observe the cord for any signs of bleeding or infection. Frequently the umbilical cord projects beyond the skin and appears as if it were an umbilical hernia. It is important to instruct the mother that the protrusion is skin and it will slowly disappear or invaginate (Table 18–6).

BLADDER

The infant's first voiding should be noted and charted to make sure that the urinary system is functioning properly. The urine should be nonoffensive, with only a mild color. A foul odor indicates infection.

TABLE 18–6. NURSING ALERT: ASSESSMENT OF NECK, CHEST, AND ABDOMEN

AREA ASSESSED	NORMAL FINDINGS	VARIATIONS—POSSIBLE PROBLEMS
Neck		
Shape	Neck is short with creases	Abnormal appearance may reflect abnormality
Muscle tone	Muscle tone not well developed	Excessive lack of muscle tone in prematurity
	Head lag when newborn is pulled to sitting position (support head)	More pronounced in preterm infant
Clavicles (assess for fracture)	Straight and intact	Potential fracture in difficult delivery
Chest		
Shape	Chest almost circular or barrel shaped	Funnel shape may be due to respiratory distress or malformation
Circumference	Circumference averages 1 inch less than head; circumference is measured at nipple line	
Breast tissue	At term, breast tissue is easily felt, 5 cm or more	Breast tissue is limited in preterm infants
Nipple placement	Nipples are prominent and symmetrically placed	Wide distance between nipples is indicative of congenital defect
Breast engorgement	Breast engorgement is common in both sexes	
Breath sounds	Breath sounds should be clear; demonstrates dry air moving in lungs	Presence of noise (rales) indicates fluid in chest, possible respiratory distress syndrome
Abdomen		
Contour	Rounded, no distention	Abdominal distention is indicative of infection or obstruction
Umbilical cord	Umbilical cord should contain 2 arteries and 1 vein	Single artery is associated with congenital anomalies
	Cord dries, darkens, and sloughs off by 7–10 days	Purulent drainage from cord indicates infection

GENITALS

Female Infants

The sex of the infant should be clearly differentiated. The labia majora usually cover the labia minora in full-term female infants. Sometimes the labia minora are more prominent than the labia majora, such as in premature infants. A hymenal tag that protrudes from the vagina is common. It will disappear in a few weeks. There may be a milky white, mucoid, vaginal discharge caused by maternal hormones. Sometimes the discharge is slightly pink in color. Some refer to this vaginal discharge as *pseudomenstruation.* Smegma, a white cheeselike substance, is often seen under the labia minora.

Male Infants

The male penis is inspected for the position of the urinary opening, which should be at the tip of the penis. An opening of the urinary meatus in the undersurface is referred to as *hypospadias,* and an opening of the urinary meatus on the upper surface is called *epispadias.* These conditions may interfere with the urinary stream. In most male infants, the foreskin adheres to the glans penis; this is called *phimosis.* If the foreskin cannot be retracted beyond the urethral opening, a circumcision may be done. The circumcision is also done for other reasons, such as reducing the risk of infection and religious belief. The value of routine circumcision is debated among pediatricians at present.

The male testes are usually descended by birth in full-term infants. If the testes are undescended (cryptorchism), further assessment should be done to see if there is an inguinal hernia. In the preterm infant, undescended testicles are expected.

ANUS

The anus is assessed to see if it is open, has good muscle tone, and includes an anal sphincter. An open anus will allow the passage of meconium stool; therefore, charting and reporting the first infant stool is important. Obstruction must be considered if the infant has not had a stool in the first 24 hours of life (Table 18–7).

TABLE 18–7. NURSING ALERT: GENITALS AND ANUS

AREA ASSESSED	NORMAL FINDINGS	VARIATIONS—POSSIBLE PROBLEMS
GENITALS		
Female		
General appearance	Labia majora covers labia minora in full-term infant	Labia minora prominent in prematurity
Discharge	Vaginal blood-tinged discharge caused by maternal hormones (pseudomenstruation)	Will disappear in 1–2 days after birth
Male		
General appearance	Urinary meatus at tip of penis	Undersurface of penis (hypospadias) Upper surface of penis (epispadias) Both associated with other anomalies
Tight foreskin	When foreskin adheres to glans penis, it cannot be retracted	Circumcision (surgical removal of portion of foreskin)
Testes	Testes are usually descended in full-term infant	Testes are undescended in premature infant
ANUS		
Patency	Anus should be open and allow passage of stool	Lack of passage of stool in 24 hr indicates potential obstruction
Stools	Assess for change in stool pattern from meconium to milk stool	Stools that are hard and dry indicate dehydration

SPINE

The infant's spine should be assessed for dimples, masses, hair tufts (a few hairs), and spinal curvatures. A healthy spinal response is an incurving of the spine directed toward the stroked or stimulated side. This response indicates neural intactness. The gluteal and popliteal folds (creases) of the hips should be symmetrical on both sides. If the skin folds appear different and there is limited abduction (movement away from the midline), further evaluation should be done to rule out the possibility of a congenital dysplasia of hip (Fig. 18–11).

EXTREMITIES

The extremities should be assessed for extra or missing digits, deformities, palmar creases, and absence of femoral pulses. The presence of extra digits, called *polydactyly*, on the hands and feet may occur as a hereditary trait. Polydactyly is more common in the black population. Usually, the extra digit only needs to be ligated or tied off, and it will slough off. Each infant has its own individual pattern of palmar creases. However, a *simian crease*, a single line, is associated with Down's syndrome. The examiner should note if the feet are in a normal position or if there is any deformity, such as club foot. Some orthopedic deformities are much easier to correct if they are found early.

When examining the extremities, the caregiver should assess the presence of strong femoral pulses, both of which can be felt at the same time. Absence of a femoral pulse is indicative of a heart defect, specifically coarctation of the heart (Table 18–8).

Neurological Assessment

The neurological assessment is conducted to determine the intactness of the infant's nervous system. It is most effective when performed 24 or more hours after birth. At this time the effects of the birth process and maternal medications will have decreased. It is important to get baseline information on general behaviors including resting posture, cry, quality of muscle tone, muscle activity, and state of alertness.

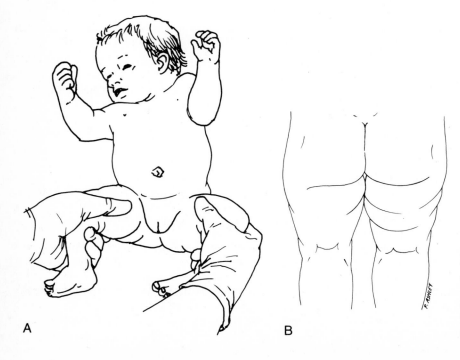

A   B

▲ **FIGURE 18–11**

Assessment of the gluteal and popliteal folds of hips. The folds should be symmetrical. **A.** Limitation of abduction. **B.** Asymmetry of skin folds.

TABLE 18–8. NURSING ALERT: ASSESSMENT OF EXTREMITIES

AREA ASSESSED	NORMAL FINDINGS	VARIATIONS—POSSIBLE PROBLEMS
Number of digits (intactness)	All fingers and toes should be present	Absence of fingers or toes indicates potential chromosomal defect Webbing of digits is abnormal
Femur	Assess for hip dysplasia	Click heard; femoral head is overriding acetabulum
Femoral pulses	Femoral pulses should be felt at same time	Absence of femoral pulses is indicative of congenital heart problem
Bone structure	Assess for normal bone structure	Bone deformity such as club foot
Creases	More than one palm crease	Simian crease (single crease) is associated with Down's syndrome
	Gluteal creases should be equal	Unequal gluteal creases indicate hip dysplasia
Joints	Joints should move freely	Spasticity may be due to cerebral palsy

Infant tremors are common; however, they must be assessed to make sure they are in the normal range of severity and are not convulsions. Infant seizures may consist of excessive blinking, chewing, or swallowing movements. Whether the infant's spontaneous movements are smooth or jerky and whether both sides move equally well are significant evaluations. Lack of good muscle tone may be due to central nervous system immaturity, seen in preterm infants.

Some basic reflexes demonstrate neurological function and an intact central nervous system (Table 18–9) and (Fig. 18–12).

Activity and Awareness

The nurse observes the newborn infant for variations in alertness and activity during the first 24 hours of life. From birth to the first 30 to 60 minutes, the infant is alert, has its eyes open, and responds to stimuli. Heart rate and respirations are somewhat higher during this period. The first hour after birth is ideal to begin the parent–infant bonding process, because the mother and infant can have eye-to-eye contact (Fig. 18–13). For this reason, silver nitrate eyedrops that cause irritation should be withheld until the infant is taken to the "transition" nursery.

After the 30 to 60 minutes, the infant frequently goes into a deep sleep and sometimes shows irregular breathing (Fig. 18–14). During this time the heart rate decreases to 120 to 140 bpm, and the breathing rate decreases to 50 to 60 respirations. During the next 2 to 4 hours, the newborn is often awake and alert, has sucking movements, and may secrete mucus from the mouth. The infant's body temperature should begin to stabilize at about 98° F. Respirations and heart rate may fluctuate. After 4 to 6 hours, the infant's vital signs should stabilize.

Six states of consciousness or awareness have been identified in the newborn infant; reactions vary markedly as the infant passes from one state to another.

The sleep states vary from *regular (deep)* sleep to *irregular (light)* sleep. When infants are in regular sleep, they have almost no body movements except "startle." Breathing is regular, and there are no eye movements. When infants are in irregular sleep, they have rapid eye movements (REM sleep). Eye movements can be seen through the eyelids. This is the best time to test the infant's hearing (Fig. 18–15).

The awake states include *drowsy (semidozing)*, *quiet-alert, active-alert,* and *fussing* to *crying.* In the drowsy state of awareness, the infant is sensitive

Text continued on page 325

TABLE 18–9. NURSING ALERT: ASSESSING REFLEXES AND SPECIAL SENSES OF THE NEWBORN INFANT

REFLEX OR SPECIAL SENSE	NORMAL FINDINGS	PRESENCE, DURATION, AND POTENTIAL PROBLEMS
Reflex		
Moro's (startle)	Elicited by sudden jarring, sudden movement, or a loud noise. Infant's response is extension and abduction of extremities, with a fanning of the fingers forming a C followed by flexion of arms in an embracing motion.	Persistence of Moro's reflex past 6 mos may indicate brain damage. Strongest in first 2 mos. Asymmetric (unequal) Moro's reflex can be due to an injury to clavicle or to the brachial plexus (the response of one side will differ from the other).
Grasp	Infant will grasp any object that touches its palm. Infant can hold on momentarily.	Fades at about 2 mos. It is replaced by a voluntary movement by 8 mos.
Plantar reflex	When the sole of the infant's foot is stimulated the toes will curl downward.	
Babinski's	Can be elicited by stroking one side of the sole upward or across the ball of the foot. The infant's response is hyperextension or fanning of the toes.	Absence in full-term infant is indicative of a spinal cord defect. Disappears after 1 yr.
Tonic neck	Can be elicited (when infant is on its back). When the infant's head is turned quickly to one side, the extremities on that side extend, and those on the opposite side flex. This is sometimes called the "fencing position."	Disappears by 4 mos. Absence in full-term infant indicates neurological problem.
Stepping	When the infant is held upright and one foot touches a flat surface, the infant will step out with opposite foot.	Disappears after 4 wks. Absence in full-term infant may indicate neurological problem.
Trunk incurvation	When the infant is in a prone position, stroking the spine causes the infant's trunk to turn to the stimulated side.	Absence of this reflex may indicate central nervous system (CNS) damage. Disappears at about 4 wks.
Crawling	When the infant is placed in the prone position, he/she will push up and attempt to crawl.	Disappears at about 6 wks.

TABLE 18–9. NURSING ALERT: ASSESSING REFLEXES AND SPECIAL SENSES OF THE NEWBORN INFANT *Continued*

REFLEX OR SPECIAL SENSE	NORMAL FINDINGS	PRESENCE, DURATION, AND POTENTIAL PROBLEMS
Reflex *Continued*		
Pupillary	Elicited by shining bright light. Infant response is constriction of pupil.	Continues throughout life. Unequal constriction or fixed, dilated pupil requires further assessment. It is indicative of CNS damage.
Sucking	Can be elicited by placing nipple or gloved finger in infant's mouth. Sucking is also stimulated by touching the lips.	Continues through 6 to 8 mos.
Rooting	Touching the cheeks or lips causes the infant to turn the head toward the stimulus.	Lasts until 6 mos.
Gag	On stimulation of the uvula, as during suctioning and sometimes during feeding, reverse peristalsis occurs.	Gag reflex continues throughout life.
Special Sense		
Sight	At birth, the infant can focus on an object 8 to 12 inches from the face and 4 to 6 inches above or to the side. Infants have preferences for human faces, moving objects, and bright, shiny colors.	Newborn's visual alertness enhances eye-to-eye contact and maternal to infant attachment. Provides means for parent–infant interaction.
Hearing	Responds to a variety of sounds, especially the range of the human voice. Can locate the general direction of a sound.	The human voice provides a means to console the upset infant (response demonstrates the value of this stimulus to the infant).
Touch	Infant responds to touch used as a consoling means. An infant's lips are very sensitive to touch.	An infant can be soothed by touch, progressing from a crying to an active-alert or sleep state.
Smell	Infants can smell sweet and sour odors. An infant can distinguish the mother's breast odor from other odors.	

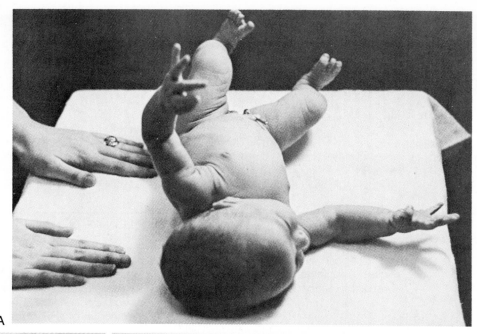

A

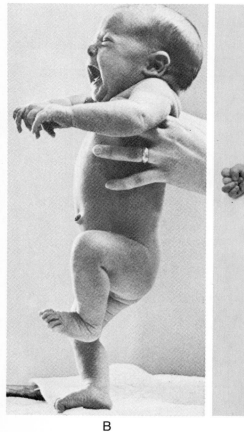

B

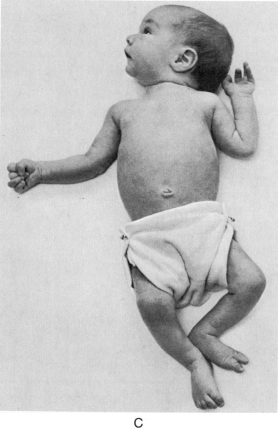

C

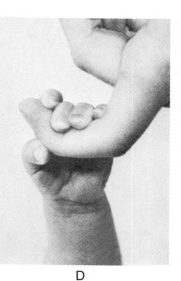

D

▲ FIGURE 18–12

A. Moro reflex. **B.** Stepping reflex. **C.** Tonic neck reflex. **D.** Grasp reflex. (Courtesy of Mead Johnson Laboratories, Evansville, Indiana.)

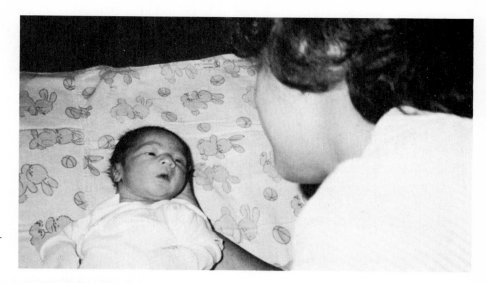

▲ **FIGURE 18–13**

Infant gazes intently at mother.

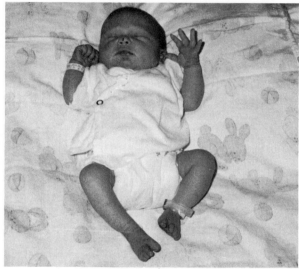

▲ **FIGURE 18–14**

The sleep state.

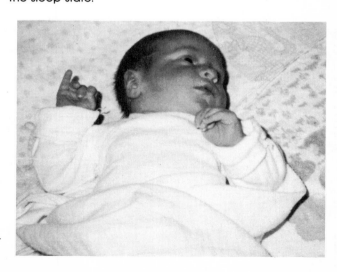

▲ **FIGURE 18–15**

The quiet-alert state.

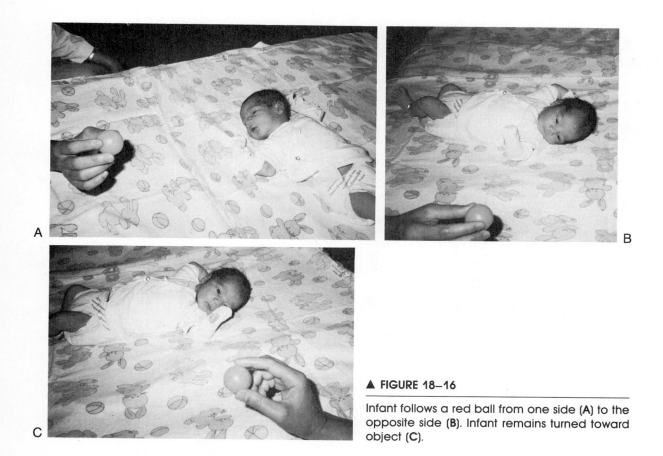

▲ FIGURE 18–16

Infant follows a red ball from one side (**A**) to the opposite side (**B**). Infant remains turned toward object (**C**).

to stimuli, sucks, smiles, and makes smooth movements. In the quiet-alert state, the infant has a bright look and can focus attention on sources of stimulation (visual and auditory) with a minimum of motor activity (Fig. 18–16). This is the best time to test the infant's responses. During the active-alert state, the infant has considerable body movements, and the heart rate increases. When the infant is in the fussing or crying state, reactions to stimuli are often violent, and the infant can become very fatigued. For this reason, mothers are encouraged to pick up their infants when they cry.

References

Auvenshine, M. A., & Enriquez, M. G. (1990). *Comprehensive Maternity Nursing: Perinatal and Women's Health*, 2nd ed. Boston: Jones and Bartlett.

Bobak, I. M., & Jensen, M. D. (1991). *Essentials of Maternity Care*, 3rd ed. St. Louis: Mosby Year Book.

Ladewig, P. W., London, M. L., & Olds, S. B. (1990). *Essentials of Maternal-Newborn Nursing*, 2nd ed. Redwood City, CA: Addison-Wesley Nursing.

May, K. A., & Mahlmeister, L. R. (1990). *Comprehensive Maternity Nursing: Nursing Process and the Childbearing Family*, 2nd ed. Philadelphia: J.B. Lippincott.

Sherwen, L. M., Scoloveno, M. A., & Weingarten, C. T. (1991). *Nursing Care of the Childbearing Family*. Norwalk, CT: Appleton & Lange.

SUGGESTED ACTIVITIES

1. Briefly describe the newborn infant's general appearance.
2. Discuss the normal range of the newborn's vital signs, including heart rate, respiratory rate, and temperature.
3. List four physical clinical findings commonly observed on the newborn infant's skin.
4. List four reflexes present in the newborn infant.
5. Discuss the newborn infant's activity state during the first 24 hours of life.

REVIEW QUESTIONS

A. Select the best answer for each multiple-choice question based on the situation given.

Clinical Situation: Baby Susan (female, weight 7 lb 3 oz, Apgar score of 8 at 1 minute and 9 at 5 minutes) was born by a normal, spontaneous, vaginal delivery. She cried immediately after birth. Her muscle tone was good, respirations were 30/minute, and heart rate was 140 bpm. Her head was slightly elongated owing to the birth process. She had noticeable vernix caseosa and lanugo on her skin. In addition, acrocyanosis was observed on her hands and feet. Her eyes were open and focused on caregivers. Baby Susan was dried, wrapped in a warm blanket, and placed in a heated crib. The nurse secured identification bands around her wrist and ankle; administered vitamin K, 1 mg, intramuscularly, in her left thigh; and placed two drops of silver nitrate in each eye. Baby Susan was taken to the transitional nursery for a 2-hour observation period to closely assess her cardiorespiratory adjustment. The pediatrician gave baby Susan a complete physical examination, which confirmed that she was normal. After the examination, baby Susan was taken to the regular nursery. Questions 1 through 13 refer to baby Susan.

1. A white, cheesy material, noticeable on baby Susan, protected her skin before birth while she was surrounded with fluid. It is called
   A. Caput succedaneum
   B. Lanugo
   C. Vernix caseosa
   D. Mongolian spots

2. The infant's respirations vary with activity. The normal range (in respirations per minute) of baby Susan is
   A. 20–30
   B. 20–40
   C. 30–40
   D. 30–60

3. Baby Susan's head is elongated owing to pressure during the birth process. Elongation is referred to as
   A. Molding
   B. Milia
   C. Cephalohematoma
   D. Bulging fontanelles

4. It is important to palpate baby Susan's anterior and posterior fontanelles because the assessment may indicate
   A. Bulging fontanelles due to increased intracranial pressure
   B. Sunken fontanelles due to dehydration
   C. Large fontanelles due to retarded bone growth
   D. All of the above

5. The nurse knows the following about baby Susan's vision:
   A. She can see best at a length of 8 to 12 inches
   B. She can follow objects, which is known as visual tracking
   C. She prefers high-contrast colors, such as black and white
   D. All of the above

6. Baby Susan's breathing is normal. She
   A. Breathes through nose, irregularly and quietly
   B. Breathes through mouth, regularly and quietly
   C. Breathes through mouth, irregularly and quietly
   D. Breathes through nose, with seesaw respirations and noise

7. When the corner of baby Susan's mouth is touched, she turns her head toward the stimulated side. This reflex is called
   A. Sucking
   B. Rooting
   C. Babinski's
   D. Tonic neck

8. Baby Susan's ears are assessed for
   A. Formation, position, ability to hear
   B. Formation, position, ear wax
   C. Position, rooting reflex, ear wax
   D. Ability to hear, rooting reflex, Moro's reflex

9. Baby Susan's anus is examined for
   A. Muscle tone
   B. Reflex response
   C. Patency
   D. None of the above

10. Baby Susan's hands are examined for
    A. Extra digits
    B. Missing digits
    C. Simian crease
    D. All of the above

11. Baby Susan's resting posture is observed. Normal posture or movements include
    A. Jittery movements
    B. Flexion of all four extremities
    C. Repetitive blinking
    D. None of the above

12. When baby Susan's mother places her hand in Susan's palm, the baby takes hold of it momentarily. This is called the
    A. Rooting reflex
    B. Sucking reflex
    C. Moro's reflex
    D. Grasp reflex

13. The reflex that causes baby Susan to respond to a sudden movement of the crib by drawing up her legs and bringing her arms forward and upward is called
    A. Babinski's
    B. Moro's
    C. Rooting
    D. Tonic neck

The nurse's assessment of the newborn infant is very informative about the infant's condition. The nurse should know when the infant is having difficulty making the adjustments to extrauterine life. Questions 14 through 18 relate to normal infant adjustments and problems for further evaluation.

14. If a nurse sees 8-hour-old baby Martinez gagging and turning cyanotic, she should
    A. Give oxygen to the infant
    B. Alert the physician
    C. Lower the infant's head
    D. Aspirate the oral and nasal pharynx

15. At 14 hours of age, baby Martinez is assessed by the nurse for the characteristics of his head and skin. Which observation should be reported to the physician?
    A. Molding and edema of the head
    B. Lanugo on shoulders and upper back
    C. Pallor when quiet or sleeping
    D. Cracking of the skin, particularly noticeable on the hands and feet

16. At 18 hours of age, the following vital signs are noted while baby Martinez is sleeping. Axillary temperature is 97.8°F, respiratory rate is 60, pulse is 180, color is pale. What is your assessment?
    A. Normal but only for a quiet, sleeping infant
    B. Normal but only for the 1st day of life
    C. Not normal but probably caused by the low temperature
    D. Not normal and shows warning signs for an impending illness

17. The nurse assessess the breathing pattern of baby Martinez. She is aware that the normal breathing pattern for a full-term infant is predominantly
    A. Shallow and irregular respirations
    B. Diaphragmatic with chest lag
    C. Chest breathing with nasal flaring
    D. Abdominal with synchronous chest movements

18. The average apical pulse range of a full-term quiet, awake newborn is
    A. 80–110 bpm
    B. 100–120 bpm
    C. 120–140 bpm
    D. 150–180 bpm

19. When taking the newborn infant's apical pulse rate immediately after the baby has been crying, it is important that the nurse be aware that the healthy newborn's heart rate can go as high as
    A. 150 bpm
    B. 160 bpm
    C. 180 bpm
    D. 200 bpm

20. Shortly after birth, the nurse should prevent the infant from developing hypothermia due to evaporation by
    A. Warming the crib and blanket
    B. Turning on the overhead radiant heat lamp
    C. Wiping amniotic fluid off the baby with a warm blanket
    D. Preventing drafts on the baby

B. Choose from Column II the phrase that most accurately defines the term in Column I.

I

1. Caput succedaneum _____
2. Erythema toxicum _____
3. Cephalohematoma _____
4. Acrocyanosis _____
5. Milia _____
6. Lanugo _____
7. Mongolian spots _____
8. Strabismus _____
9. Epstein's pearls _____
10. Femoral pulse _____
11. Female mucoid discharge _____

II

A. Sluggish peripheral circulation
B. Fine hair noticeable on shoulders and back
C. Small, white, distended sebaceous glands
D. Cross-eyed appearance due to poor muscle control
E. White nodules occurring from accumulation of epithelial cells
F. Absence suggests coarctation of heart
G. Collection of blood under cranial bone
H. Pink rash with hive-like elevations
I. Diffuse edema over scalp's soft tissues
J. Purple spots commonly found over infant's buttocks and sacrum
K. Result of maternal hormones

CHAPTER 19

Chapter Outline

Immediate Care
    Clearing the airway
    Clamping the cord
    Evaluating cardiorespiratory function
    Regulating the environment
    Identifying the infant
    Protecting the infant from eye infection
    Recording information about the birth and baby
Transitional or Observational Nursery
Regular Nursery or Rooming-In
Prevention of Infection
Promotion of Safety
Parent Instruction
    Daily care of the infant
    Bath instruction
    Positioning and holding the infant
    Nasal and oral suctioning
    Nail care
    Circumcision
    Temperature assessment
    Stools and voiding
    Infant activity
    Infant feeding
Birth Registration
Discharge and Follow-Up Care
Summary

Learning Objectives

Upon completion of Chapter 19, the student should be able to

- Explain the immediate care of the newborn infant.
- Describe the differences in care between the regular nursery and rooming-in.
- Name five nursing measures that protect the infant from infection.
- List three nursing measures that promote safety.
- Describe infant bath instruction to parents.
- Demonstrate three ways to hold the infant.
- Demonstrate the proper way to suction the infant with a bulb syringe.
- Describe parent instruction of infant nail care.
- Describe the care of an infant after circumcision.
- Explain how to take an infant's temperature.
- Recall parent instruction about infant stools and voiding.
- Explain normal infant activity.
- List four things a mother can do to encourage the infant to breastfeed.
- Identify four basic breastfeeding skills that the mother should know if she plans to nurse her infant.
- Describe how to teach the mother to burp her infant.
- Compare the content of human milk with cow's milk.
- Explain the discharge plan of care. List five aspects of infant care that the mother should understand before discharge.

NURSING CARE OF THE NEWBORN INFANT

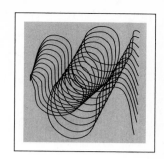

The nursing care of the newborn is directed toward promoting the physical well-being of the infant and supporting the family unit. Immediate care of the infant takes place in the birth room and transition nursery. Because numerous physiological adaptations begin right after birth (see Chapter 17), immediate care is a very important part of infant care. The first goal is to help the newborn make the transition to extrauterine life. Close observation is required to determine if this transition is going smoothly. The second goal is to promote the health status of the newborn. The third goal is to teach the parents and/or family members how to care for the new infant.

Knowledge of the infant's adjustments in the transition to extrauterine life and an accurate physical assessment of the newborn are essential for the nurse to plan the newborn's individualized care. The physiological adjustments of the newborn are discussed in Chapter 17, and the complete assessment of the newborn is discussed in Chapter 18. The nurse often is the key person to assess the parents' need for information, support, and instruction about the newborn's care. This chapter focuses on the promotion of the newborn infant's health and the provision of instructions to the parents regarding the care of their new baby.

Immediate Care

Immediately after birth, the newborn infant is faced with risks such as heat loss and aspiration of fluid and the challenge of functioning in a new environment. Nursing care is directed toward the infant's well-being. Some of the newborn's needs must be met in the birth room. Before anything else is done, the infant is immediately dried and placed in a preheated radiant heat bed (Fig. 19–1).

Universal precautions should be followed in performing the immediate care of the infant. These are listed in Table 19–1.

CLEARING THE AIRWAY

The infant's face should be wiped after the delivery of the head to prevent aspiration of fluid. The physician or midwife gently suctions the infant's mouth with a soft bulb syringe (Fig. 19–2), then suctions the nose. The order is important because by stimulating the nasal mucosa, it is possible to cause a reflexive inhalation of pharyngeal material, thus causing aspiration of meconium fluid. As the infant is born, his or her body is held slightly downward to assist the drainage of secretions. After the cord is cut, the infant is placed on the mother's abdomen or in a radiant heat bed. If the infant's airway needs further attention, a pediatrician (or other appropriate personnel) may insert a tube into the larynx to provide an open airway; this procedure is called *intubation*. Secretions, if present, are removed by suctioning the trachea. If the contents are greenish, positive meconium aspiration is indicated, and the infant is observed carefully for respiratory distress.

CLAMPING THE CORD

The cord is clamped tightly to prevent blood loss. There are several types of cord-clamping devices. If the infant's mother is Rh−, the cord may be left longer for future medical interventions.

TABLE 19–1. NURSING ALERT: CENTERS FOR DISEASE CONTROL UNIVERSAL PRECAUTIONS FOR NEONATAL NURSES

1. Health care workers should use appropriate barrier precautions to prevent exposing their skin and mucous membranes to blood and body fluids.
   A. Gloves and protective skin coverings (gowns, plastic aprons) should be worn when handling newborn infants before and during first bath.
   B. Gloves should be worn during venipuncture, heel stick, and intravenous needle insertions.
   C. Gloves should be worn when applying pressure to stop bleeding after venipuncture, heel stick, and intravenous needle insertions.
   D. Gloves should be worn when changing diapers and when collecting (and testing) urine and stool samples.
   E. Gloves should be worn when suctioning infants.
   F. All nurses should carry a clean pair of gloves in their pocket to quickly put on hands in emergency situations.
   G. Eye goggles or face masks should be worn during procedures that are likely to cause splashing, such as infant's first bath, and during circumcision.
2. Hands, skin surfaces, eyes, and mucous membranes should be washed immediately if contaminated with body fluids.
3. Precautions should be taken to prevent injuries caused by needles or other sharp instruments.
   A. Needles should not be recapped, bent, or broken after use. They should be placed directly into a puncture-resistant container.
   B. Heel-stick lancets should be disposed of immediately into a puncture-resistant container.
   C. Reusable, sharp instruments such as circumcision instruments should be placed in puncture-resistant containers for transport to reprocessing unit/department.
4. Resuscitation bags and infant masks should be available for infant care to minimize need for mouth-to-mouth resuscitation.
5. If aspiration is necessary, adaptors should be used to connect mucus-trap catheters to wall suction. Manual suction devices such as the DeLee Mucus Trap should no longer be used to aspirate mucus.
6. Health care workers who have exudative lesions or dermatological areas not intact should refrain from all direct contact with patient and patient equipment until condition resolves.
7. Because the patient's history and laboratory test cannot reliably identify individuals with hepatitis, human immunodeficiency virus infections, and other blood-borne infections, the U.S. Department of Health and Human Services recommends the above universal body substance precautions.

Adapted from Centers for Disease Control (1990). *HIV/AIDS Surveillance Report, November.* Atlanta, GA: Centers for Disease Control.

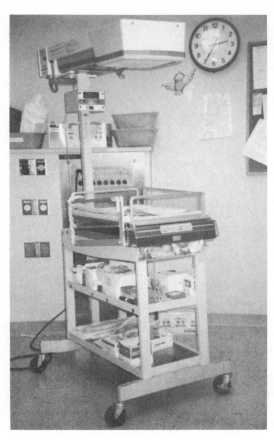

▲ FIGURE 19–1

Radiant heat bed to help stabilize the infant's temperature.

Cord blood is routinely sent to the laboratory to identify the immediate blood status of the infant. After the cord is clamped, it is cut; the infant may be placed either on the mother's abdomen or in the radiant heat bed.

EVALUATING CARDIORESPIRATORY FUNCTION

The cardiorespiratory function is evaluated immediately after birth. The Apgar score is determined at 1 and 5 minutes as a method of evaluating the infant's physical condition (see Chapter 12).

REGULATING THE ENVIRONMENT

One of the most important functions of the nurse in taking care of the infant is to prevent cold stress (see Chapter 17). When excess heat loss occurs, the infant may develop problems such as hypoglycemia, acidosis, and respiratory distress. A *neutral thermal environment* should be provided in order for the infant's oxygen consumption and metabolic rate to be minimal. If the infant's temperature stays between 97.7° F and 98.6° F, heat loss from the skin will be minimized.

Immediately after birth the greatest heat loss is from the infant's being wet with amniotic fluid. Therefore, the first important nursing measures are to dry the infant, including the head, and place it in a prewarmed, dry blanket, covering the head of the infant with a stocking cap (Chapter 12).

IDENTIFYING THE INFANT

Adequate identification of the newborn infant is required by hospital policy. The American Acad-

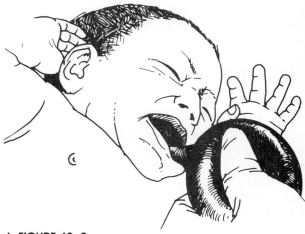

▲ FIGURE 19–2

A bulb syringe should be readily available to suction mucus from the infant's mouth and nose during the first 24 hours after birth. The bulb is compressed before insertion, then released to create sufficient suction to remove mucus.

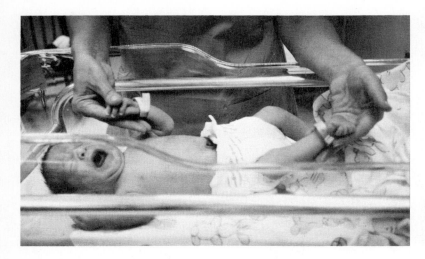

▲ **FIGURE 19–3**

Identification bands on the infant's wrist and ankle.

emy of Pediatrics recommends that the infant be identified while still in the delivery room. Usually, duplicate identification bands are placed on the infant's wrist and ankle (Fig. 19–3). The information on them includes the mother's full name, hospital admission number, sex of the infant, and date and time of birth. In addition, many hospitals take the infant's foot- or palm prints along with the mother's fingerprint. Throughout the hospital stay, it is essential to verify the identity of the newborn, by comparing the numbers and names on the identification bracelets of the mother and infant, before giving the baby to the mother.

PROTECTING THE INFANT FROM EYE INFECTION

The infant can acquire a serious eye infection called *ophthalmia neonatorum* when passing through an infected birth canal. The infection is due to either gonorrhea or chlamydia. Because the gonorrhea infection can cause blindness, most states require that a medication, such as one drop of 1% silver nitrate, be placed in each eye (Fig. 19–4) or that erythromycin ointment be used. Erythromycin ophthalmic ointment is commonly used today because it produces less eye irritation and also destroys the chlamydia organism. It is recommended that the eye prophylaxis be delayed 1 hour after birth to allow the infant unimpaired eye contact with the parents.

RECORDING INFORMATION ABOUT THE BIRTH AND BABY

The initial recording on the newborn infant's chart begins in the birth room. The record should include the Apgar score, time of birth, sex, description of cry, color, obvious abnormalities, and resuscitation measures. The dose of medication the mother received and the time it was received should also be noted. The interval between the

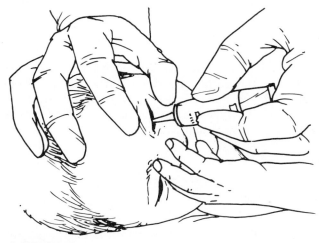

▲ **FIGURE 19–4**

The nurse administers either erythromycin ophthalmic ointment or silver nitrate solution in each eye to prevent eye infection.

rupture of membranes and the type of delivery is also significant information to be recorded. The admitting nurse in the transitional nursery should review the recorded information for potential problems.

Transitional or Observational Nursery

In many hospitals, the newborn infant is transferred from the delivery room to a transitional nursery for close observation during the critical period of physical adjustment to extrauterine life (Fig. 19–5). The infant frequently is kept in this nursery for 2 to 4 hours or until the heart rate and respirations have stabilized. Then the infant is admitted to a regular nursery or to the mother's room for rooming-in.

The newborn infant is weighed when he or she enters the immediate-care nursery (Fig. 19–6). The infant also receives an initial bath and cord care; the head and chest circumferences are measured;

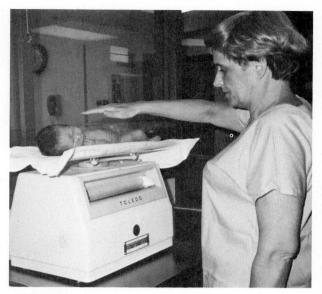

▲ **FIGURE 19–6**

When weighing the infant, the nurse keeps one hand ready to take hold if the infant becomes active.

and vitamin K is administered to prevent intracranial bleeding and to improve the clotting time of the newborn's blood. Vitamin K is given intramuscularly in the midanterior thigh, where the muscle development is adequate. The newborn is placed in a warm crib or radiant heat bed. A physician or nurse further assesses the infant for gestational age (see Chapter 20) and any deviations from normal. Often the temperature is monitored continuously for the first 2 to 4 hours or until stable with a thermal sensor placed on the infant's abdominal skin.

The initial bath includes washing the hair, which is often matted with dried blood accumulated by passing through the birth canal, and removing the heavy deposits of vernix caseosa. A complete water bath often is not given because it would increase heat loss. During all baths—first partial, first complete, and all later baths—caregivers should wear gowns and rubber gloves for protection against infection (see Table 19–1).

The infant's temperature may be taken once, rectally, to see that the anus is patent (open). The infant's pulse and type of respirations are important; they should be monitored and recorded. This is the most likely time for the infant to show problems in breathing or respiratory distress.

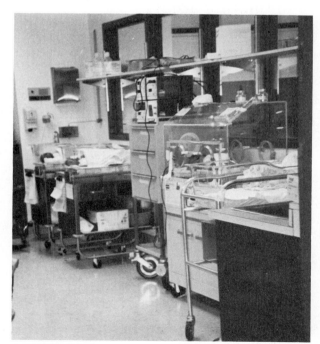

▲ **FIGURE 19–5**

Transitional nursery.

Regular Nursery or Rooming-In

After the infant's physical condition has stabilized, the infant is moved to a regular nursery or a rooming-in facility next to the mother. During the rest of the hospital stay, caregivers do what they can to prevent the infant from infection, provide comfort, meet the infant's physical needs, and promote parent–infant attachment (see Chapter 16).

Prevention of Infection

The newborn infant is susceptible to infection and must be protected from it. During the first days of life, extra care must be taken to reduce the newborn's risk of infection. Cracks in the skin, particularly on the hands and feet, and the umbilical cord area are areas especially subject to infection.

MEASURES TO PROTECT THE INFANT
FROM INFECTION

- Persons who have direct contact with the infant (caregiver and others) should be required to do a 3-minute scrub (up to the elbows) at the beginning of each shift.
- Caregivers should wear a clean scrub gown each day before entering the nursery or caring for the infant.
- Caregivers should wash their hands again before touching the common nursery equipment or touching another infant (to avoid cross-contamination of objects).
- Caregivers should wash their hands after touching a soiled surface, such as the floor or one's hair or face.
- Outside visitors to the maternal–newborn unit should wash their hands and put on gowns before coming in contact with either the infant or equipment. This includes fathers, other nurses, laboratory technicians, physicians, and housekeepers.
- Any person who has an infection should not be admitted to the maternal–infant area.
- Every infant should have his or her own

individual unit, including equipment and clothing.
- The umbilical cord area and broken skin should be assessed daily for redness, warmth, or purulent discharge.
- An infant suspected of infection should be semiisolated or removed from the nursery (depending on the type of infection).

In addition to the preceding measures to guard against infection, the number of infants placed in one nursery should be limited—ideally to six—to reduce exposure of many infants to one other. In some traditional nurseries the infant is wrapped with an outside cover (over the blanket) when taken to the mother. This technique may limit contamination, but may also limit the mother's acquaintance with her infant; mothers should be encouraged to explore their infants. Most maternal–infant units stress the importance of a complete change of the mother's bed linens each day as a protection for the infant. In addition, teaching the mother to wash her hands before touching the infant is an essential part of parent instruction.

Promotion of Safety

Protection of the newborn infant includes regulation of the room temperature as well as observation of the infant for normal versus abnormal behavior. To ensure infant safety, most hospitals will not allow the mother to carry her infant from her room to the nursery. Also, parents should be instructed, before discharge, to obtain an infant car seat for vehicle transportation. In several states parents are required by law to use an infant car seat. Parents should be instructed in ways to protect their infant from injury.

PRECAUTIONS TO PROMOTE INFANT
SAFETY

- Infants in the nursery should never be left unattended.
- Infants should never be left unattended on the table or on a weighing scale (see Fig. 19–6).
- Infants should be held for bottle feedings. Bottles should never be propped because of

the potential for spitting up, aspirating, and choking. Propped bottles may also lead to otitis media (ear infection).

- Infants should not be allowed to lose body heat. The environmental humidity and heat should be carefully controlled. Ideal humidity and temperature are 50% and 75° F, respectively.
- Infants should be placed on their side after feeding to prevent aspiration of regurgitations.

Parent Instruction

Parent instruction is an important part of newborn care. The nurse may demonstrate holding, suctioning, and bathing of the infant and then observe the mother perform each procedure. In-dividual instruction is beneficial; it may be followed up with group classes and discharge planning to verify the mother's knowledge when she leaves the hospital. Follow-up calls after discharge lend additional support by providing another opportunity for parents to have their questions answered.

DAILY CARE OF THE INFANT

It is important to keep a record of baseline data to provide information about the infant's progress. The daily record includes assessments of feedings, output (stool and urine), vital signs, general appearance (color, skin condition), and infant behavior (crying, contentment, and irritability).

Each day the newborn is assessed and weighed, and its temperature is taken. The infant is cleansed as needed and kept in dry clothes. In some nurs-

KEY POINTS IN EDUCATION: BATHING THE NEWBORN

- Assemble all the articles needed for the bath before beginning, to avoid chilling the infant.
- Sponge baths are given until the cord is off and well healed to avoid infection (usually about 7 to 10 days). After the cord is off the infant can be given tub baths.
- Test the water with your elbow. It should be warm but not hot (98° to 90°F).
- Cleanse the eyelids with moistened cotton balls, wiping from the inner canthus outward. A separate cotton ball (or corner of a clean washcloth) should be used on each eye.
- Assess the infant's nostrils. If there is milk curd or mucus in them, remove it with a small, moist piece of cotton or swab.
- Wipe the infant's face with a moist washcloth or cotton ball.
- Mild soap can be used for the rest of the bath; however, some physicians recommend clear water to avoid drying the infant's skin further.
- Wash the infant's hair with mild,

unscented soap and rinse with warm water. The "soft spots" can be washed, because they are well protected. The hair can be combed at the end of the bath.
- Remove the shirt and inspect and wash the hands, arms, and axillae. The axillae might have vernix caseosa that can be wiped off.
- At this time, the creases in the neck can be assessed for secretions; this is done by gently tilting the infant's head back. It is important to keep the creases clean to avoid skin irritation.
- Inspect the cord for redness and drainage. Cleanse it with a cotton swab soaked in 70% alcohol.
- Turn the infant on the abdomen and inspect and wash the infant's back.
- Remove the diaper. Cleanse the feet, legs, groin, genitalia, and buttocks. The female genitalia should be wiped from front to back to avoid contamination. (The genital/anal area should be bathed last).
- Dress the infant quickly to avoid chilling the infant.

eries, the infant's cord is wiped with an alcohol swab each day to hasten drying of the cord (triple dye, an antibacterial solution, is applied to the cord in the transition nursery). Most nurseries use disposable diapers; with these it is important to keep the diaper lower than the cord so that air can get to the cord to dry it. Also, this will keep the plastic material of the diaper from covering the cord, creating a potential source of irritation.

BATH INSTRUCTION

Sponge baths are given until the cord is off and well healed. Then the infant may have a tub bath. Preferably, baths should be given before feedings. The bath provides an excellent opportunity for infant assessment. Ideally, in the rooming-in unit, the bath should be given first with the mother as an observer and then with her as a participant. In some hospitals the bath is given at night, when there is less activity of visitors and hospital procedures. The caregiver should wash her/his hands before beginning care, after changing a diaper with an infant's stool, and before caring for another infant to avoid cross-contamination, thus reducing the risk of infection. Each infant should have an

individual unit with a thermometer, linens, and such objects as a comb and bulb syringe for suctioning. Maternity units vary in their bathing techniques, but the principles remain the same.

POSITIONING AND HOLDING THE INFANT

Confidence in performing infant care can be encouraged in parents by giving them an opportunity to hold their infants and allowing them to ask questions about different methods of positioning and holding the infant. It is important to teach the parent that the newborn infant has limited control of the head, although when prone the infant may raise the head slightly and briefly. Because of this, parents should be instructed that the infant must be placed on a firm crib mattress.

Whenever the infant is lifted up and held, the head must be supported, because the head is larger than the rest of the body and the neck muscle strength is not well developed. There are three basic ways to hold the infant (Fig. 19–7). The *cradle hold* is frequently used during feeding. The infant's head is cradled in the bend of the holder's elbow. This hold permits eye-to-eye contact, provides a sense of closeness and warmth,

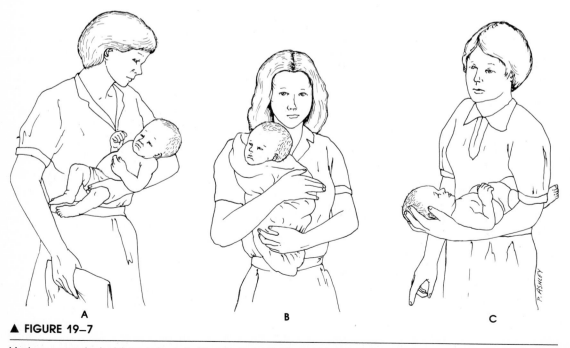

▲ **FIGURE 19–7**

Various ways to hold an infant: **A.** Cradle hold. **B.** Upright hold. **C.** Football hold.

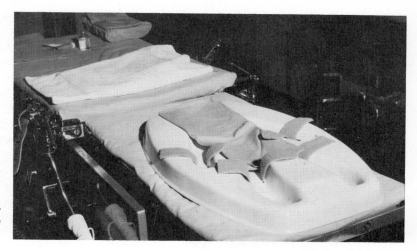

▲ **FIGURE 19–8**

Circumcision board prepared to receive infant.

and frees one of the holder's hands to reach for objects needed, such as the formula bottle. The *upright position* is a way to hold the baby and feel secure in supporting the head, upper back, and buttocks. It is an ideal position for burping the infant. In the *football hold,* about half of the infant's body is supported by the holder's forearm, and the head and neck rest in the palm. This hold is ideal for shampooing and breastfeeding. However, it leaves the infant's head somewhat unprotected.

A combination of basic infant holds is often used to provide warmth and closeness, allow eye-to-eye contact, and feed the infant.

NASAL AND ORAL SUCTIONING

During the first few days of life, the newborn has increased mucus, and gentle suctioning with a bulb syringe may be indicated. The nurse can demonstrate the use of the bulb syringe in removing mucus from the mouth and nose (a procedure described previously). Parents should repeat the demonstration before discharge. They should be instructed to thoroughly wash the syringe after each use.

NAIL CARE

The nails of the newborn infant are rarely cut in the hospital. However, the mother should be instructed how to cut the nails at home. Within a week the nails separate from the skin and often

break off. If the nails are long, and the baby scratches himself or herself, the nails should be trimmed. The nails should be cut straight across and with a blunt-ended scissors. It is advisable that the nails be cut while the baby is quiet or asleep.

CIRCUMCISION

Circumcision is the surgical removal of the foreskin of the penis (Fig. 19–8). Currently, pediatricians are questioning performing this practice on a routine basis. There is general agreement that it should be performed in cases of *phimosis,* in which the foreskin cannot be retracted. It is usually done on the basis of religious, cultural, social, and family traditions.

Written consent from the mother is necessary

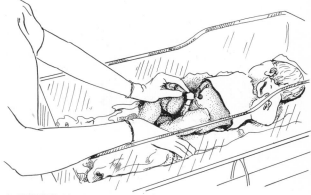

▲ **FIGURE 19–9**

Nursery nurse inspects petroleum jelly (Vaseline) dressing for evidence of bleeding.

before the procedure is done. The infant who is circumcised must be watched closely for a few days for bleeding and for infection (Fig. 19–9). Immediately after the circumcision, a sterile gauze with petroleum jelly (Vaseline) is wrapped around the penis to form a pressure bandage. If bleeding occurs, it should be reported to the physician. This bandage is removed in a few hours. Each time the diaper is changed, petroleum jelly on a sterile gauze should be reapplied to the penis. This procedure prevents the diaper from sticking to the penis. The circumcision wound usually heals in 3 to 5 days.

TEMPERATURE ASSESSMENT

The caregiver should demonstrate to the parents how to take rectal and axillary temperatures (see Chapter 18). A return demonstration by the parents is a good way to assess their understanding. Parents should be shown how to shake down the thermometer and how to read the degree of temperature. If the temperature is taken rectally, the rectal thermometer should first be well lubricated with petroleum jelly. The infant should be supine and the legs should be held with one hand, with the rectum exposed. The baby should not be left alone.

The axillary temperature is taken by placing the thermometer under one of the infant's arms, making sure that the thermometer is within the armpit for 3 minutes. The parents should be instructed that they need to take the temperature only if the infant shows signs of illness.

STOOLS AND VOIDING

Babies may void six to eight times a day. Voiding less than five times a day may indicate that the baby needs more water or fluids. The parents should be familiar with the frequency, color, and consistency of stools. The first stools are dark green which might alarm the parents. On about the third or fourth day, the baby's stools may become slightly liquid and yellowish-green; these are referred to as the transitional (from meconium to milk) stools. Formula-fed babies may have constipated stools that are quite firm and well formed, whereas breastfed babies have softer stools and void more frequently, usually with each feeding.

INFANT ACTIVITY

The newborn infant demonstrates different sleep–wake patterns at different times (see Chapter 18). The parents need to be instructed what is normal. If the newborn cries continually, the cause should be identified. The newborn may be comforted by holding, rocking, and cuddling. If the newborn is quiet all the time, without crying or fussing, assessment for lethargy needs to be done. Parents need to be instructed about the importance of parent–infant attachment. They need to be familiar with behaviors that enhance and those that inhibit positive infant behavior (see Chapter 16).

INFANT FEEDING

The newborn infant is normally fed glucose in water within 4 hours after birth. This feeding is

KEY POINTS IN EDUCATION: INSTRUCTION ABOUT INFANT STOOLS

- Breastfed babies void more frequently; their stools are yellow and less well formed than the stools of formula-fed babies.
- Formula-fed babies may have three to four stools a day, which are yellow to yellow-brown and more formed than those of breastfed babies.
- Less than two stools a day may indicate constipation, and water intake should be increased. Offer water between feedings two to three times a day.
- Liquid stools indicate the possibility of diarrhea. If liquid stools continue, the baby should be taken to a clinic or seen by a private physician. Any stool that is green and leaves a water ring on the diaper is significant and should be reported to the physician or clinic.

done to maintain adequate glucose levels and to prevent dehydration. Most infants lose 3% to 10% of their birth weight during the first few days of life. Within about 3 days after birth, the infant will begin to gain weight; the birth weight is usually regained by 10 days.

Because it is very common for the infant to vomit or spit up after the first feeding, the infant should be observed during the first feeding to decrease the risk of aspiration. Often, infants are taken to their mothers for feeding as soon as they are admitted to the regular nursery. If the mother is in a rooming-in facility, feeding, particularly breastfeeding, occurs as soon as the infant has stabilized.

Breastfeeding

The mother who wishes to breastfeed her infant should be encouraged and assisted by the caregiver. The mother should be instructed to wash her hands and have clean nipples for the infant. She should be shown various positions in which she can nurse her infant (Figs. 19–10 and 19–11). Using different positions can provide comfort for the mother, and also the pressure points of the infant's suckling will differ, which will lessen the chance of sore nipples. In addition, she should be taught how to break the infant's suction (Fig. 19–12).

The mother should be taught the basic breast-feeding skills: (a) stimulating the rooting reflex, (b) judging the amount of areola the infant needs to have in the mouth, (c) breaking the suction before taking the infant from the breast, (d) burping the infant, and (e) keeping the breast tissue away from the infant's nose during sucking. The current thinking is not to limit the nursing time. It is important to start with the alternate breast at each feeding. This practice will minimize the trauma to the nipples and stimulate milk secretion. Mothers can remind themselves which breast to begin with by placing a safety pin in the clothes on that side. Lactation and the let-down reflex are discussed in Chapter 14.

As more information about human breast milk has become available, the number of women interested in breastfeeding has increased. Some hospitals have a nurse lactation specialist available for the mothers. In addition, many hospitals have classes for breastfeeding mothers. The La Leche League, an organization that promotes breastfeeding, is active in most communities. Members of the organization will assist mothers with concerns or problems about breastfeeding. The advantages and disadvantages of breastfeeding are as follows:

ADVANTAGES OF BREASTFEEDING

- Breast milk is safe and always fresh.
- Breast milk is readily available.
- Breast milk contains a variety of antiinfection factors and immune cells.

KEY POINTS IN EDUCATION: BREASTFEEDING TECHNIQUES

- Before putting the infant to breast, the mother should manually express a few drops of colostrum. This will make the nipple stand out, so the infant can hold the nipple back in its mouth.
- The mother should stroke the infant's cheek with the nipple. The infant will turn toward the nipple and usually open the mouth. If the infant missed the nipple, the process is begun again.
- Nursing begins with the opposite breast from the last nursing period. Breasts are alternated during feeding. After the third day, it is important to have the infant empty the first breast completely before changing to the other breast.
- Before taking the infant off the breast, the mother should break the suction by putting a finger in the corner of the infant's mouth or by pushing downward on the infant's chin.
- While the infant is suckling, it is necessary to keep the breast away from the infant's nose. Because infants are nose breathers, they will let go of the nipple if they cannot breathe.

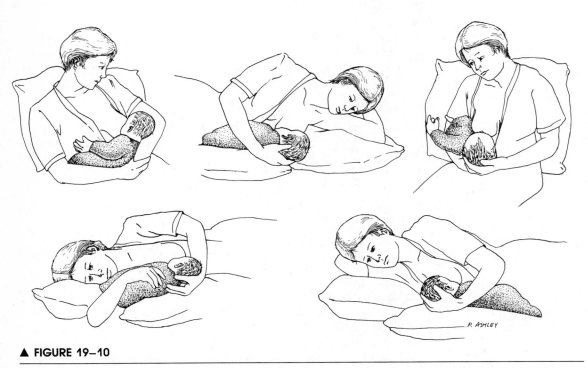

▲ **FIGURE 19–10**

Changes in breastfeeding position to facilitate breast emptying and prevent sore nipples.

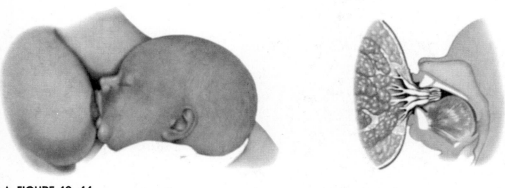

▲ **FIGURE 19–11**

The infant's mouth should cover the majority of the areola to compress the ducts and lessen tension on nipples. (From Ross Laboratories Clinical Education Aid No. 10. Courtesy of Ross Laboratories, Columbus, Ohio.)

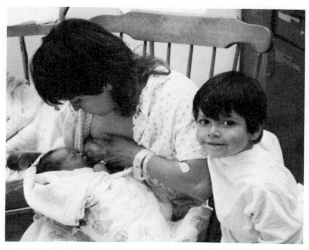

▲ FIGURE 19–12

Pressing a finger against the corner of the baby's mouth to release suction.

- Breast milk is the least allergenic food for the infant.
- Breastfeeding promotes good jaw and tooth development.
- Breastfed infants are less likely to be overfed; therefore, they are less likely to be obese.
- Breastfeeding usually costs less than feeding with the commercial infant formulas (even with the mother's increased nutritional needs).

DISADVANTAGES OF BREASTFEEDING

- Adolescent mothers and working mothers may not return to school or jobs.
- Mothers who must pump their breasts may find it undesirable or inconvenient.
- Some mothers are embarrassed by breastfeeding or breast exposure.

OTHER CONSIDERATIONS

- Unlike commercially prepared formulas with iron added to the formula, breast milk is low in iron. Therefore some physicians order iron supplementation at the first well-baby visit. However, the need for iron supplementation is still controversial because the iron in breast milk is well absorbed and the infant's iron stores appear sufficient for 6 months, as shown by hemoglobin values.
- An oral supplement of 0.25 mg of fluoride daily is recommended for the breastfed infant because the fluoride content of human milk is low. Fluoride provides protection against tooth decay.

Bottle Feeding

Many infants are given commercially prepared formulas, which are made as similar as possible to breast milk. Because this form of packaging is expensive, another type can be recommended for home use. An infant formula may be made by using evaporated milk, water, and a sweetener (Karo syrup). The mother should be given a detailed booklet on the preparation of formula. The booklet is free on request from the formula companies Ross Laboratories (Columbus, OH) and Mead Johnson Company (Evansville, IN). Two methods of preparing formula are the aseptic method and the terminal method. In the aseptic method, all the supplies (bottles, nipples, and so forth) are washed and *sterilized* (boiled for 5 minutes) at the same time. An automatic dishwasher may be used if available. The bottles, caps, and nipples are removed with tongs from the kettle or sterilizer. A sterilized measuring pitcher is used to determine the appropriate amount of water and formula to go into each bottle. Bottles are refrigerated until needed.

In the terminal method, after the equipment is washed, the formula is prepared according to the directions. Bottles are filled with the formula, and the nipples are inverted into the bottles with the caps loosely applied. The bottles are placed in 2 or 3 inches of water in a large kettle or bottle sterilizer. The kettle is covered, and the bottles are boiled for 25 minutes. The bottles are removed when cool, the lids are tightened, and the bottles are stored in the refrigerator. The formula should be stored at a temperature of less than 50° F (10° C).

TYPES OF FORMULAS

- Concentrated—Requires dilution with water
- Ready-to-use that requires measuring into bottles

KEY POINTS IN EDUCATION: BOTTLE FEEDING TECHNIQUES

- The bottle's nipple should be placed on the top of the infant's tongue.
- The entire nipple should be full of milk at all times to keep the infant from swallowing air.
- The size of the nipple hole should be just big enough that the milk flows in drops when the bottle is inverted. When the nipple hole is too large, the infant can eat too fast and regurgitate or overeat.
- The infant should be held close to the mother's body and be cuddled to facilitate bonding. Stroking and talking during feeding promote pleasure and relaxation for infant and mother.

- The infant should be burped at the middle and end of the feeding.
- Bottles should *never be propped*. The infant can aspirate the formula. In addition, the infant lying in a horizontal position can develop otitis media (ear infection).
- Milk should not be saved for the next feeding if the infant does not empty the bottle. Organisms will grow, and the infant can develop diarrhea (infection). The leftover formula can be used for cooking.

- Ready-to-use that is sold in disposable bottles (most expensive type)
- Powder form—Requires mixing with water according to label instructions
- Evaporated milk formula—Least expensive; because of possible bacterial contamination and improper measurement, special instructions are given for parents who choose this method.

Mothers may have many questions about bottle feeding their infants. They may wonder if the infant is feeding too slowly or too fast. They also may question how much to feed the infant. It is easier for the formula-fed infant to be overfed and become obese, which is not desirable for the infant's health. When teaching a mother how to bottle-feed her infant, the caregiver should emphasize the following points.

After feeding, the infant's diaper should be changed, if necessary, and the infant should be placed on its right side or abdomen to sleep. While the infant is in the hospital, the amount of formula taken is recorded. The infant may take only 1 oz the first day, and 2 or 3 oz the second and third days of life.

Comparison of the components of cow's milk with those of human milk gives a clue to formula preparation. Cow's milk has more protein; therefore, it has to be diluted. In the process of the dilution, more carbohydrates (sugar) are added to

formula. Although commercial infant formulas provide satisfactory alternatives to breast milk, cow's milk does differ in the following ways.

COW'S MILK VERSUS HUMAN MILK: COMPARISON OF CONTENTS

- Protein—The protein content of human milk is lower. Human milk contains more lactalbumin (cow's milk contains more casein), which reduces the curd formation in the infant's gut.
- Fat—The fat in human milk is easier to digest and absorb than the fat in cow's milk.
- Lactose—The lactose (sugar) content of human milk is significantly higher than that of cow's milk.
- Iron—Iron content is low in human milk. It often is added to cow's milk formula.
- Immune cells—The immune cells are a unique component of human milk. They include antibodies to intestinal microorganisms that may protect the infant from gastrointestinal infections.

As previously stated, feeding the infant should be an enjoyable and a pleasurable task for both the infant and the parent (Fig. 19–13). It is a time when the parent and infant can get to know each

The checklist should include knowing how to prevent infection, promote safety, bathe the infant, hold the infant, suction the infant if necessary, perform circumcision care if appropriate, take the infant's temperature, check for normal stools and voiding, check for normal infant activity and crying and sleep pattern, and feed the infant.

The parents should be aware that hospital nursing staff are available by telephone 24 hours a day for additional support during the first few days at home with their newborn. Routine well-baby visits should be encouraged. If appropriate, the first clinic appointment should be scheduled at the time of discharge.

Summary

Throughout this chapter, emphasis has been placed on continuous observation and assessment of the newborn and the planning of care that centers around the infant's needs. In addition, parent instruction and discharge planning should be an integral part of the plan. Developing a written plan that incorporates nursing diagnoses and expected goals is important to assess the adequacy of the infant's care as well as to assess the family's ability to perform the care after the infant is discharged. The following list of nursing diagnoses applies to the newborn and family.

NURSING DIAGNOSES

- Ineffective airway clearance related to mucus obstruction
- Hypothermia related to body heat loss
- Potential for infection related to newborn's susceptibility to pathogens
- Knowledge deficit related to safety
- Knowledge deficit related to lack of experience in infant care
- Altered urinary elimination related to circumcision
- Knowledge deficit related to taking infant's temperature and reading the thermometer
- Constipation related to decrease in number and consistency of infant stools
- Altered nutrition: less than body requirements related to limited nutrient/fluid intake
- Altered parenting related to the need to integrate the new infant into the family unit

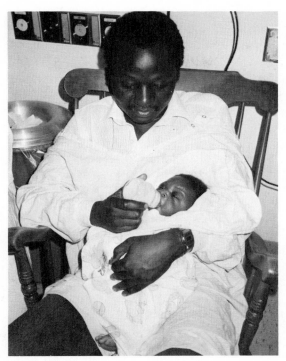

▲ **FIGURE 19–13**

Father bottle-feeding his infant. Note the nipple is filled with milk to keep the infant from swallowing air.

other. The caregiver plays an important role in assisting the mother in either breastfeeding or bottle feeding her infant. Instruction, including discussion of common concerns, will help the parents to smoothly assume one of their new tasks of parenting.

Birth Registration

Each state has a department of vital statistics in which all births are registered. A clerk from the medical records department of the hospital usually comes to the maternity unit to obtain information for the birth certificate. It is then sent to the department of vital statistics.

Discharge and Follow-Up Care

The discharge plan of care should include assessing the parents' knowledge of infant care. A checklist is useful to see if parents understand the necessary caregiving methods before discharge.

NURSING CARE PLAN 19–1

THE NORMAL NEWBORN

Assessment	Potential Problems and Nursing Diagnoses	Nursing Interventions
1. Assess breathing.	Ineffective airway clearance related to mucus obstruction.	Suction mouth and nose with bulb syringe to remove mucus and prevent aspiration. Instruct mother how to use bulb syringe for oral and nasal suctioning. Instruct parents to position infant with head to side after feeding to prevent spitting up of milk from obstructed breathing.
2. Assess temperature.	Hypothermia related to body heat loss.	Keep infant dry and warm and avoid chilling effect and lowering temperature. Postpone infant's bath after birth until its temperature is stabilized. Measure axillary temperature every 3 to 4 hours when infant has a temperature lower than 97.7° F. Prevent exposure to drafts and maintain warm environment.
3. Inspect cord.	Potential for infection.	Keep the cord clean and fold plastic portion of diaper below cord. Allow air to reach cord. Wash hands before touching cord area. Use medication (triple dye) to prevent infection.
4. Inspect skin.	Potential for infection related to status of skin.	Recognize that infant is susceptible to infection through cracks in skin. Enforce practice of caregiver and parents washing their hands before touching infant.
5. Observe infant safety.	Knowledge deficit related to safety.	Provide instruction to parents to never leave infant unattended. Instruct parents to place infant on firm mattress in crib.
6. Observe infant care.	Knowledge deficit related to care requirements of infant.	Instruct parents how to bathe, diaper, and hold infant. Teach comfort measures (burp, rock). Instruct parents about normal and abnormal stools. Explain that common skin lesions will disappear without special treatment.

NURSING CARE PLAN 19–1 *Continued*

THE NORMAL NEWBORN

Assessment	Potential Problems and Nursing Diagnoses	Nursing Interventions
6. Observe infant care. *Continued*		Discuss environmental needs of infant (clothing, room temperature, visitors). Explain the importance of reciprocal interaction in the attachment process. Teach parents to observe for signs of illness (fever, poor feeding, weight loss, vomiting, diarrhea, excessive crying).
7. Observe voiding.	Altered urinary elimination related to circumcision.	Instruct parents about the potential problem of infant voiding due to pressure of bandage over urinary meatus.
8. Observe stools.	Constipation related to decreased number of stools.	Teach parents normal infant stool pattern. Less than two stools a day indicates potential constipation and need for increased fluid intake.
9. Note eating pattern.	Nutrition: less than body requirements.	Teach parents how to successfully breastfeed or bottle-feed infant. Explain the importance of fluid and nutrient intake. Explain the importance of infant's comfort while feeding (position, burping to get rid of air).
10. Observe parent–infant interaction.	Altered parenting related to inexperience and inadequacy.	Provide opportunity for parents to get acquainted with infant by holding, cuddling, and touching infant. Discuss normal infant behavior with parents, including reflexes. Discuss ways to promote positive parent–infant reciprocal reactions (eye-to-eye contact, talking to infant). Answer parents' questions about infant's response to verbal, auditory, and tactile cues. Discuss sleep and awake states with parents, including the amount of sleep infants require. Assist parents as necessary to feel comfortable with infant.

Nursing Care Plan continued on following page

NURSING CARE PLAN 19–1 *Continued*
THE NORMAL NEWBORN

Expected Outcomes

1. Infant will maintain an open, clear airway and breathe without difficulty. Parents demonstrate proper use of the bulb syringe and verbalize the importance of the infant's having an open airway.
2. Infant is warm, and temperature is stable.
3. Cord is clean, dry, and healing.
4. Infant skin is intact except for superficial cracks in hands and feet.
5. Parents verbalize importance of never leaving infant unattended and having a firm crib mattress.
6. Parents demonstrate bathing, diapering, and holding infant.
7. Infant voids after circumcision.
8. Parents demonstrate knowledge that lack of fluid intake can cause infant constipation.
9. Parents verbalize how to properly feed infant, including position and burping.
10. Parents discuss ways to promote positive parent–infant interactions.

References

Auvenshine, M. A., & Enriquez, M. G. (1990). *Comprehensive Maternity Nursing: Perinatal and Women's Health,* 2nd ed. Boston: Jones and Bartlett.

Bobak, I. M., & Jensen, M. D. (1991). *Essentials of Maternity Nursing,* 3rd ed. St. Louis: Mosby Year Book.

Bryant, B. G. (1984). Unit dose of erythromycin ophthalmic ointment for neonatal ocular prophylaxis. *Journal of Obstetric, Gynecologic, and Neonatal Nursing* 13:83–87.

Care of the infant born exposed to human immunodeficiency virus. (1990). *Obstetrics and Gynecology Clinics of North America* 17:637–649.

Johnstone, H. A., & Marcinak, J. F. (1990). Candidiasis in the breastfeeding mother and infant. *Journal of Obstetric, Gynecologic, and Neonatal Nursing* 19:171–173.

Jones, M. B. (1990). A physiologic approach to identifying neonates at risk for kernicterus. *Journal of Obstetric, Gynecologic, and Neonatal Nursing* 19:313–318.

Ladewig, P. W., London, M. L., & Olds, S. B. (1990). *Essentials of Maternal-Newborn Nursing,* 2nd ed. Redwood City, CA: Addison-Wesley Nursing.

Meier, P., & Wilks, S. (1987). The bacteria in expressed mothers' milk. *American Journal of Maternal-Child Nursing* 12:420–423.

Minchin, M. K. (1989). Positioning for breastfeeding. *Birth* 16(2):67–73.

Sherwen, L. N., Scoloveno, M. A., & Weingarten, C. T. (1991). *Nursing Care of the Childbearing Family.* Norwalk, CT: Appleton & Lange.

Shirago, L., & Bocar, D. (1990). The infant's contribution to breastfeeding. *Journal of Obstetric, Gynecologic, and Neonatal Nursing* 19:209–215.

Tolentino, M. B. (1990). The use of Orem's self-care model in the neonatal intensive-care unit. *Journal of Obstetric, Gynecologic, and Neonatal Nursing* 19:496–500.

Walker, M. (1989). Functional assessment of infant breastfeeding patterns. *Birth* 16(3):140–147.

SUGGESTED ACTIVITIES

1. List three nursing activities included in the immediate care of the newborn infant.
2. Explain four ways to protect the newborn infant from infection.
3. Demonstrate, using a doll, how to give a newborn infant an inspection sponge bath.
4. Demonstrate, using a doll, three ways to hold an infant.
5. Name four things a mother should be taught if she plans to breastfeed her infant.
6. List five things a mother should be taught if she plans to bottle feed her infant.

REVIEW QUESTIONS

A. **Select the best answer to each multiple-choice question.**

1. Ms. Castillio asks if her baby can see. Select the most appropriate answer the nurse could give her.
   A. A baby's eye muscles are weak, so the baby cannot look at an object for more than 2 or 3 minutes at a time
   B. At first the baby possibly sees white and black objects
   C. A baby can follow a light just like an adult can
   D. A baby can focus on an object about 8 to 12 inches away, such as the mother's face

2. The mother should be instructed to gently handle the baby after feeding. Because the cardiac sphincter of the esophagus has decreased tone during the newborn period, the infant is more likely to have one of the following
   A. Projectile vomiting
   B. Regurgitation of feeding
   C. Cyanosis with each feeding
   D. Heart beat irregularities

3. Ms. Castillio states she is afraid to wash her baby's hair because she might injure the "soft spot." The nurse should instruct the mother that
   A. There is an old wives' tale about this but it is incorrect
   B. The soft spot will be filled in in a few weeks
   C. There is no problem because a tough membrane covers the area
   D. If afraid, do not wash the baby's head

4. Ms. Castillio has chosen to breastfeed her baby. The nurse observes the first feeding to assess
   A. Maternal self-confidence with the technique
   B. Infant's ability to coordinate sucking, swallowing, and breathing
   C. Infant's interest in sucking
   D. Adequate amount of intake

5. Ms. Castillio should be instructed that the most important action to protect her baby from infection at home is
   A. Limit visitors until her baby is 3 months old
   B. Wear a face mask when she feels tired and may be getting a cold
   C. Maintain good personal hygiene and handwashing
   D. Offer her baby water two times a day

6. Baby J, 2 days old, is circumcised. Which of the following should be part of his postcircumcision care?
   A. Apply petroleum jelly, which acts as a lubricant to help prevent irritation from the diaper
   B. Keep the wound clean to prevent contamination of the incision
   C. Observe for bleeding from the surgical site for the first 12 to 24 hours
   D. All of the above

7. The nurse should be familiar with what is considered normal in the newborn. Which of the following observations would *not* require prompt notification of the physician?
   A. Failure to have a meconium stool during the first 24 hours of life
   B. Failure to void during the first 24 hours of life
   C. A pink or rust-colored stain on the diaper after voiding
   D. All of the above

8. The nurse administers vitamin K during the period immediately after birth because of all the following EXCEPT
   A. A newborn's liver is immature
   B. A newborn lacks intestinal bacteria with which to synthesize vitamin K
   C. A newborn is susceptible to intracranial hemorrhage
   D. A newborn has an increased clotting time

9. Intramuscular injections are always given to a newborn infant in the midanterior thigh because
   A. Circulation is more effective at this site
   B. Muscle development is more adequate at this site
   C. It is easier to give an injection to the infant at this place
   D. Other sites do not absorb medication well

10. If a newborn infant shows generalized cyanosis, which one of the following needs to be considered?
    A. Glucose levels
    B. Environmental temperature
    C. Cardiac function
    D. Gestation age

11. Baby Brown's mother is concerned about his weight loss during the first 2 days of life. The nurse instructs the mother that
    A. Weight loss reflects a fluid imbalance
    B. Weight loss can range from 5% to 10% in healthy infants
    C. Weight loss of 15% is acceptable
    D. All of the above

12. Baby Brown's mother asks the nurse about the bluish color of the palms of his hands and the soles of his feet. The nurse explains that this is a common and temporary condition called
    A. Acrocyanosis
    B. Erythema neonatorum
    C. Lanugo
    D. Vernix caseosa

13. Bluish hands and feet in the first 12 hours of life indicate
    A. Lack of adjustment to environmental temperature
    B. Delayed vasodilation in the extremities
    C. Hyperglycemia
    D. Low hemoglobin levels

14. Erythromycin ointment is placed in baby Brown's eyes. The nurse explains to his mother that the purpose of the medication is to
    A. Destroy infectious staphylococcus
    B. Destroy infectious streptococcus
    C. Destroy gonococcal and chlamydia organisms potentially acquired from the birth canal
    D. Remove the exudate from the eyes

15. All of the following measures are taken to protect the newborn infant from infection EXCEPT
    A. Handwashing before giving care to infants
    B. Not caring for infants if the caregiver has an infection
    C. Limiting the time the infant is taken out of the nursery to be with the mother
    D. Providing each infant with its own individual unit, including equipment and clothing

16. Protection of the infant includes all of the following EXCEPT
    A. Attending infant while it is on a table or scale
    B. Placing infant on side or abdomen, in crib, after feeding
    C. Avoiding extremes in room temperature in the nursery
    D. Allowing the infant to feed in bed with a bottle of formula secured by a rolled diaper

17. Special instructions the nurse can give the mother concerning the infant's sponge bath include all of the following EXCEPT
    A. Wiping the eyes from inner canthus outward
    B. Clearing the infant's nostrils with a moist, twisted piece of cotton
    C. Washing the infant's anal-genital area before rest of body
    D. Avoiding chilling the infant during the bath

18. A breastfeeding mother should be instructed in all of the following EXCEPT
    A. Placing the infant in different positions while nursing in order to change suction pressure points
    B. Breaking the suction before taking the infant off the breast
    C. Allowing the infant to suck on only one breast during each feeding
    D. Keeping the breast tissue away from the infant's nose

19. Advantages of breastfeeding over formula feeding include all of the following EXCEPT
    A. Breast milk contains immune cells
    B. Breastfeeding promotes jaw development
    C. Breastfeeding is more likely to make the infant obese
    D. Breastfed infants are less likely to be overfed

20. Teaching a mother how to bottle-feed her infant includes all of the following EXCEPT
    A. The nipple should be filled with milk to avoid swallowing air
    B. If nipple holes are too large, the infant can eat too fast and regurgitate the formula
    C. While giving the formula, the infant should be held close and cuddled
    D. Formula left in the bottle can be saved for the next feeding

21. Whereas commercial formulas provide satisfactory alternatives to breastfeeding, cow's milk differs from human milk in all of the following ways EXCEPT
    A. Protein content in human milk is lower
    B. Fat in human milk is easier to digest
    C. Iron in human milk is low but is often added in formulas
    D. Sugar content in human milk is lower than in cow's milk

22. If the infant is formula fed, which would be the most effective way to meet the infant's psychological needs?
    A. Give the formula after a bath
    B. Hold the infant while feeding
    C. Diaper infant before and after feeding
    D. Burp infant frequently during the feeding

B. Choose from Column II the phrase that most accurately defines the term in Column I.

I

1. Cradle hold _____
2. Circumcision _____
3. Neutral thermal environment _____
4. Daily newborn record _____
5. Eye cleansing _____
6. Female hygiene _____
7. Aseptic method of formula preparation _____

II

A. Wipe from inner canthus outward
B. Infant's head is placed in bend of elbow
C. Recording of feeding, voiding, stools, and general appearance
D. Surgical removal of foreskin of penis
E. Wipe from front to back
F. All equipment is sterilized at same time
G. Way to minimize heat loss

PROBLEMS

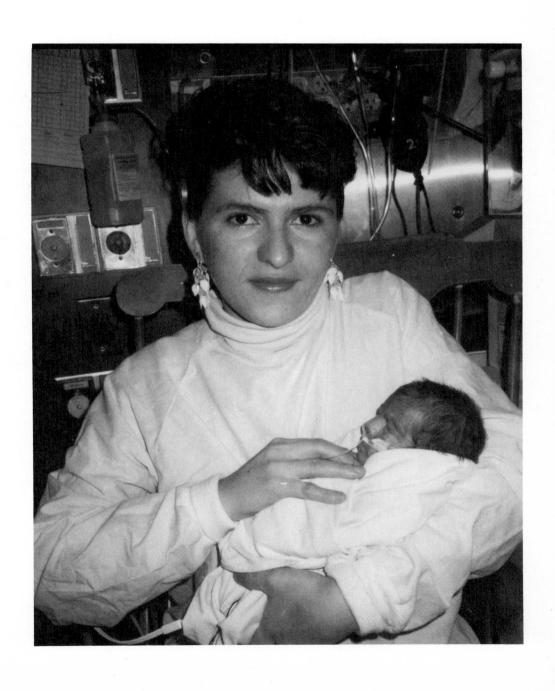

CHAPTER 20 _____

Chapter Outline

Determination of Gestational Age
    Small-for-gestational-age infant
    Large-for-gestational-age infant
    Postterm infant
    Preterm (premature) infant
        Body systems
        Care of the preterm infant

Learning Objectives

Upon completion of Chapter 20, the student should be able to

- Describe the determination of gestational age.
- Recall the causes of intrauterine growth retardation.
- Describe the postterm infant.
- Describe the preterm infant's immaturity.
- Describe the care of the preterm infant.
- Outline the needs of parents who have preterm infants.

THE NEWBORN INFANT AT RISK

Previously, infants were classified at birth as premature or term on the basis of weight alone. Infants who weighed less than 2500 g (5.5 lb) were considered premature. This classification is unsatisfactory because it does not indicate maturity. We now know that many infants are born at term but are low in birth weight. Prematurity (preterm delivery), birth weight, and body system maturity are not all related. The clinical problems may be quite different in an infant who is born at term weighing 4.5 lb from those of an infant whose gestational age (in utero) is 36 weeks and who weighs the same. Because of this possibility, a more precise system of terminology has evolved. The newer classification of infants at birth, based on gestational ages and birth weights, is as follows:

- *Preterm* or *premature*—An infant born before the end of 37 weeks' gestation, regardless of weight
- *Term* or *full-term*—An infant born between 38 and 42 weeks' gestation, regardless of weight
- *Low birth weight*—Any infant at birth who weighs less than 2500 g or 5.5 lb
- *Small for gestational age* (SGA)—Any newborn infant whose weight is below the 10th percentile, (according to intrauterine growth curve), regardless of gestation
- *Appropriate for gestational age* (AGA)—Any newborn infant whose intrauterine growth has been normal (according to intrauterine growth curve) for that length of gestation
- *Large for gestational age* (LGA)—Any infant born whose weight is above the 90th percentile (according to intrauterine growth curve) regardless of gestation

- *Intrauterine growth retardation*—Fetal growth retardation for any reason
- *Postterm*—An infant born after 42 weeks' gestation, regardless of weight

Determination of Gestational Age

The ability to assess gestational age of the infant after birth has opened a new avenue of anticipating and preventing many illnesses of newborns. Thus, the two parameters, birth weight and gestational age, have helped in better infant care (Fig. 20–1). It must be noted, however, that the clinical findings are interpreted as plus or minus 2 weeks compared with the expected date of confinement as based on an "accurate" menstrual history.

There are several scoring systems available to help one arrive at the baby's gestational age (Table 20–1). Although the scoring systems are not identical, they all use growth and maturity criteria as indicated by physical and neuromuscular signs. The examiner assigns a score for each characteristic, such as genital development (Figs. 20–2 and 20–3). It is important to note that infants can vary in size and weight, yet be the same gestational age (Fig. 20–4).

SMALL-FOR-GESTATIONAL-AGE INFANT

An SGA infant is a newborn who is at or below the 10th percentile (according to intrauterine growth curves) on the newborn classification chart. An SGA infant may be preterm, term, or postterm. Other terms used to designate the

Text continued on page 360

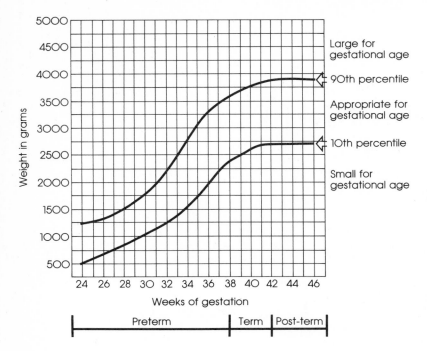

Weight in grams

5000
4500
4000
3500
3000
2500
2000
1500
1000
500

24 26 28 30 32 34 36 38 40 42 44 46

Weeks of gestation

Preterm | Term | Post-term

Large for gestational age

90th percentile

Appropriate for gestational age

10th percentile

Small for gestational age

▲ FIGURE 20–1

Classification of newborn infants by birth weight and by gestational age. The weights and gestational ages are plotted on the graph. The infant, at birth, is then classified as large for gestational age, appropriate for gestational age, or small for gestational age. (Redrawn from Battaglia, F. C., & Lubchenco, L. O. (1967). A practical classification of newborn infants by weight and gestational age. *Journal of Pediatrics* 71:161.)

TABLE 20–1. PHYSICAL FINDINGS AND SCORING SYSTEM THAT CORRELATE WITH BALLARD'S SCORING SYSTEM*

Posture

With the infant supine and quiet, score as follows:

Arms and legs extended	0
Slight or moderate flexion of hips and knees	1
Moderate to strong flexion of hips and knees	2
Legs flexed and abducted, arms slightly flexed	3
Full flexion of arms and legs	4

Square Window

Flex hand at the wrist. Exert sufficient pressure to get as much flexion as possible. The angle between the hypothenar eminence and the anterior aspect of the forearm is measured and scored as illustrated. Do not rotate the wrist.

Arm Recoil

With infant supine, fully flex the forearm for 5 seconds. Then fully extend arm by pulling on hands and releasing. Score as follows:

Remains extended or random movements	0
Incomplete or partial flexion	2
Brisk return to full flexion	4

Popliteal Angle

With infant supine and pelvis flat on examining surface, flex leg and fully flex thigh with one hand. With the other hand, extend the leg and score the angle attained as illustrated.

Scarf Sign

With infant supine, draw infant's hand across the neck and as far as possible across the opposite shoulder. Assistance to the elbow is permissible by lifting it across the body. Score the location of the elbow as follows:

Elbow reaches opposite anterior axillary line	0
Elbow between opposite anterior axillary line and midline of thorax	1
Elbow at midline of thorax	3
Elbow does not reach midline of thorax	4

Heel to Ear

With infant supine, hold infant's foot with one hand and move it as near to the head as possible without forcing it. Keep pelvis flat on examining surface.

*See Figure 20–2. Adapted from Klaus, M. H., & Fanaroff, A. A. (1973). *Care of the High-Risk Neonate*. Philadelphia: W. B. Saunders Company.

Neuromuscular Maturity

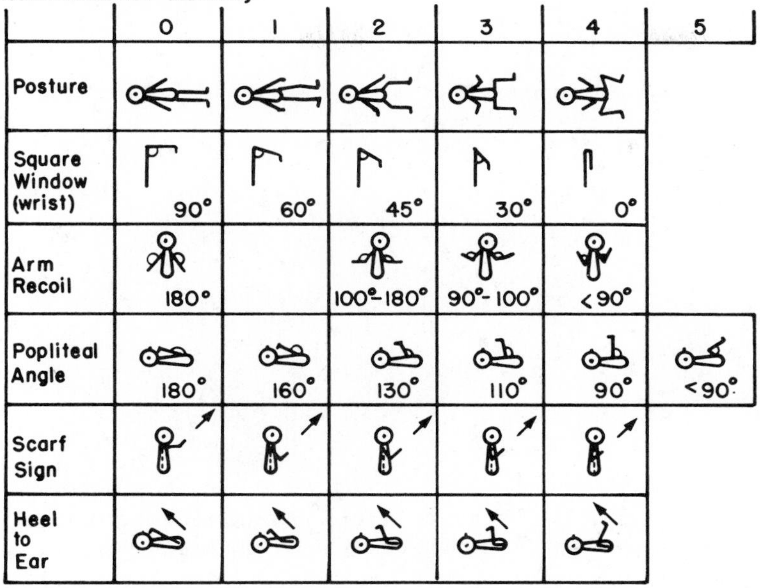

	0	1	2	3	4	5
Posture						
Square Window (wrist)	90°	60°	45°	30°	0°	
Arm Recoil	180°		100°–180°	90°–100°	<90°	
Popliteal Angle	180°	160°	130°	110°	90°	<90°
Scarf Sign						
Heel to Ear						

PHYSICAL MATURITY

Skin	gelatinous red, transparent	smooth pink, visible veins	superficial peeling &/or rash few veins	cracking pale area rare veins	parchment deep cracking no vessels	leathery cracked wrinkled
Lanugo	none	abundant	thinning	bald areas	mostly bald	
Plantar Creases	no crease	faint red marks	anterior transverse crease only	creases ant. 2/3	creases cover entire sole	
Breast	barely percept.	flat areola no bud	stippled areola 1–2 mm bud	raised areola 3–4 mm bud	full areola 5–10 mm bud	
Ear	pinna flat, stays folded	sl. curved pinna; soft with slow recoil	well-curv. pinna; soft but ready recoil	formed & firm with instant recoil	thick cartilage ear stiff	
Genitals ♂	scrotum empty no rugae		testes descending, few rugae	testes down good rugae	testes pendulous deep rugae	
Genitals ♀	prominent clitoris & labia minora		majora & minora equally prominent	majora large minora small	clitoris & minora completely covered	

MATURITY RATING

Score	Wks
5	26
10	28
15	30
20	32
25	34
30	36
35	38
40	40
45	42
50	44

▲ FIGURE 20–2

Ballard's assessment of gestational age. (Modified with thanks to Dr. J. Ballard. From Klaus, M. H., & Fanaroff, A. A. (1986). *Care of the High-Risk Neonate,* 3rd ed. Philadelphia, W. B. Saunders Company.)

Premature Infant

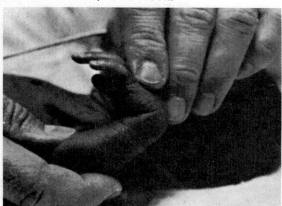

Full-term Infant

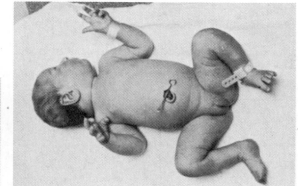

RESTING POSTURE The premature infant is characterized by little, if any, flexion in the upper extremities and only partial flexion of the lower extremities. The term infant exhibits flexion in all four extremities.

Premature Infant, 28-32 Weeks

Full-term Infant

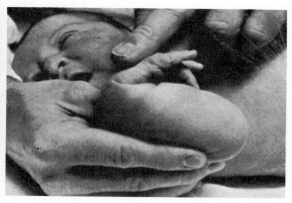

WRIST FLEXION Flex the wrist, applying enough pressure to get the hand as close to the forearm as possible. Measure the angle between the hypothenar eminence and the ventral aspect of the forearm. (Care must be taken not to rotate the infant's wrist.) The premature infant at 28 to 32 weeks' gestation will exhibit a 90° angle. With the full-term infant it is possible to flex the hand onto the arm.

▲ **FIGURE 20–3**

Examples of tests to determine gestational age. Photographs show tests described in Figure 20–2. (From Sullivan, R., Foster, J., & Schreiner, R. L. (1979). Determining a newborn's gestational age. *American Journal of Maternal—Child Nursing.* 4(1):33–45. Use of photograph courtesy of Dr. Richard Schreiner.)

Flex extremities and hold

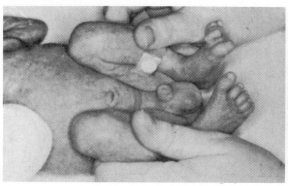

Response in Premature Infant

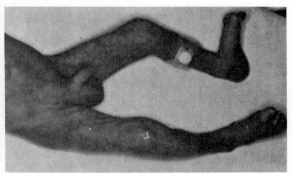

Extend

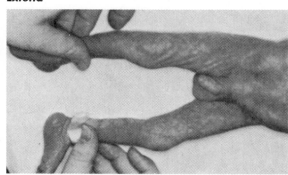

Response in Full-term Infant

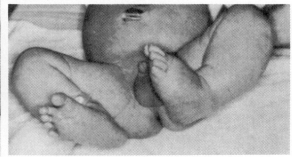

RECOIL OF EXTREMITIES Place the infant supine. To test recoil of the legs, (1) flex the legs and knees fully and hold for 5 seconds, (2) extend by pulling on the feet, (3) release. To test the arms, flex forearms and follow same procedure. In the premature infant, response is minimal or absent; in the full-term infant, extremities return briskly to full flexion.

Premature Infant

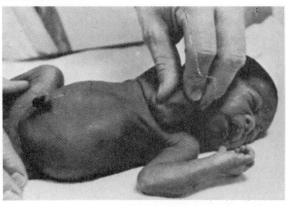

Full-term Infant

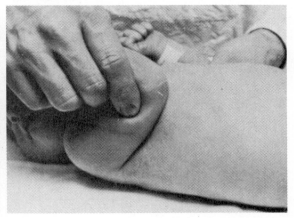

SCARF SIGN Hold the baby supine, take the hand, and try to place it around the neck and above the opposite shoulder as far posteriorly as possible. Assist this maneuver by lifting the elbow across the body. See how far across the chest the elbow will go. In the premature infant, the elbow will reach near or across the midline. In the full-term infant, the elbow will not reach the midline.

▲ **FIGURE 20–3** Continued

Illustration continued on following page

Premature Infant

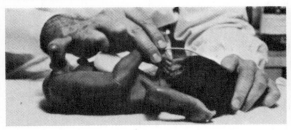

Full-term Infant

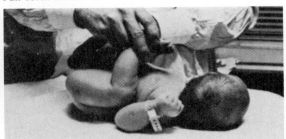

HEEL TO EAR With the baby supine and hips positioned flat on the bed, draw the foot as near to the ear as it will go without forcing it. Observe the distance between the foot and head as well as the degree of extension at the knee. In the premature infant, very little resistance will be met. In the full-term infant, there will be marked resistance; it will be impossible to draw the foot to the ear.

Premature Infant

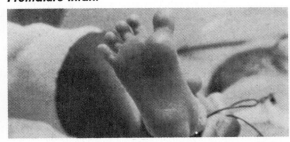

Full-term Infant

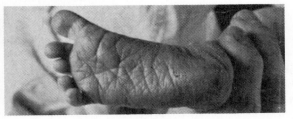

SOLE CREASES The sole of the premature infant has very few or no creases. With increasing gestational age, the number and depth of sole creases multiply, so that the full-term baby has creases involving the heel. (Wrinkles that occur after 24 hours of age can sometimes be confused with true creases.)

Premature Infant

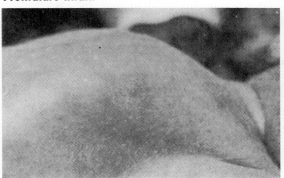

Full-term Infant

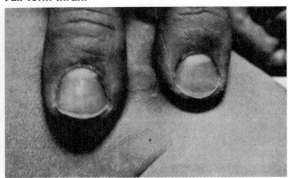

NIPPLES AND BREAST In infants younger than 34 weeks' gestation, the areola and nipple are barely visible. After 34 weeks the areola becomes raised. Also, the infant of less than 36 weeks' gestation has no breast tissue. Breast tissue arises with increasing gestational age due to maternal hormonal stimulation. Thus, an infant of 39 to 40 weeks will have 5 to 6 mm of breast tissue, and this amount will increase with age.

▲ **FIGURE 20–3** *Continued*

Premature Infant, 34-36 weeks

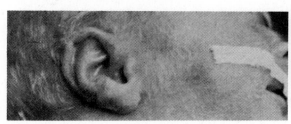

Full-term Infant

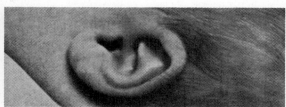

EARS At less than 34 weeks' gestation, infants have very flat, relatively shapeless ears. Shape develops over time so that an infant between 34 and 36 weeks has a slight incurving of the superior part of the ear, the term infant has incurving of two-thirds of the pinna, and an infant older than 39 weeks has incurving that continues to the lobe. If the extremely premature infant's ear is folded over, it will stay folded. Cartilage begins to appear at approximately 32 weeks so that the ear returns slowly to its original position. In an infant of more than 40 weeks' gestation, there is enough ear cartilage that the ear stands erect away from the head and returns quickly when folded. (When folding the ear over in this portion of the examination be certain that the surrounding area is wiped clean, or the ear may adhere to the vernix.)

Full-term Male

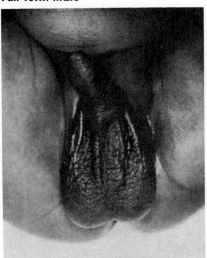

Premature Male

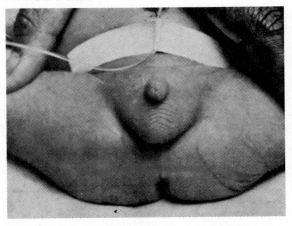

MALE GENITALIA In the premature male the testes are very high in the inguinal canal and there are very few rugae on the scrotum. The full-term infant's testes are lower in the scrotum, and many rugae have developed.

▲ **FIGURE 20–3** Continued

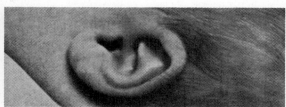

Illustration continued on following page

Premature Female

Full-term Female

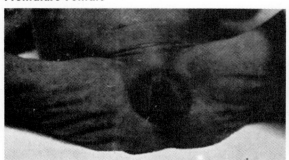

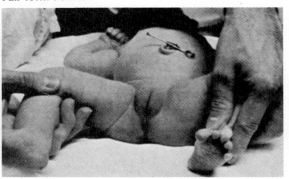

FEMALE GENITALIA When the premature female is positioned on her back with hips abducted, the clitoris is very prominent and the labia majora are very small and widely separated. The labia minora and the clitoris are covered by the labia majora in the full-term infant.

▲ **FIGURE 20–3** *Continued*

growth-retarded newborn include *intrauterine growth retardation* (IUGR) and *small for date* (SFD). In this discussion, SGA and IUGR are used interchangeably.

The incidence of SGA infants is 3% to 7% of all pregnancies. The mortality of SGA infants is about eight times higher than that of normal infants.

A number of factors can cause the infant to undergo IUGR. Some infants are incompletely developed owing to some insult to the embryo early in development. These infants are sometimes called *hypoplastic* SGA infants. They are not equipped with all of the cells for normal growth potential. Some organs, even the brain, can be affected by an early insult to the embryo or fetus. Identified causes for IUGR include genetic defects, maternal rubella, maternal drug ingestion, and maternal chronic malnutrition.

The infant with IUGR may have all the cells and normal growth potential, but development may have been restricted owing to some unfavorable condition. Maternal diseases that cause an inade-

▲ **FIGURE 20–4**

Three infants, same gestational age, weigh 600, 1400, and 2750 g, respectively, from left to right. (Reproduced by permission from Korones, S. B. (1986). *High-Risk Newborn Infants*, 4th ed. St. Louis, C. V. Mosby.)

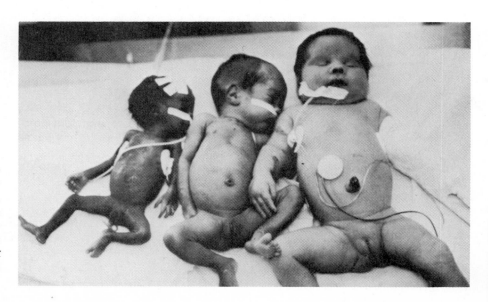

quate blood supply can cause poor fetal nutrition. Conditions in the woman that result in an impaired vascular blood supply are likely to result in an infant who is SGA. Pregnancy-induced hypertension, chronic hypertension, diabetes with vascular involvement, cigarette smoking (causing vasoconstriction), and maternal drug use (such as cocaine use) can have an adverse effect on the nourishment of the infant. They can decrease growth potential, and the infant will be SGA.

Twins (multiple births) are usually small. If the twins share the same placenta, one twin at birth is often much smaller and anemic.

Table 20–2 lists the problems (and their causes) for which SGA infants are at risk.

Physical Appearance

On first inspection, many of the SGA infants show physical characteristics that suggest impaired intrauterine growth. The head might seem large, but its circumference is normal or near normal. It is the chest and abdominal circumfer-

TABLE 20–2. PROBLEMS AND RISK FACTORS IN SMALL-FOR-GESTATIONAL-AGE INFANTS	
PROBLEM	**RISK FACTOR**
Asphyxia	Chronic hypoxia in utero
Meconium aspiration	In utero hypoxia leading to relaxation of anal sphincter and passage of meconium
Hypoglycemia	Poor liver glycogen stores
Hypothermia	Diminished subcutaneous fat and large body surface
Intraventricular hemorrhage	Fragile vessels
Polycythemia	Physiological response to in utero chronic hypoxia stress
Hypocalcemia	Calcium depletion secondary to birth asphyxia
Maternal factors that cause low birth weight or hypoxic stress	Vascular complications due to pregnancy-induced hypertension, advanced diabetes, smoking, poor nutrition, use of drugs

ences that are reduced owing to decreased subcutaneous fat. The adipose tissue and muscle mass over the cheeks, buttocks, and thighs are diminished. Because the body length is usually normal, the infants appear thin and long. They often have "worried faces" because the faces are thin; they look like little old people. The skull's sutures are frequently wide apart as a result of impaired bone growth; thus, the infant's fontanelles are often large and somewhat sunken.

Behavior

Most SGA infants are more active than expected for their size. This observation is especially true if one contrasts them with preterm infants. The cry of an SGA infant is vigorous and may be impressive in relation to size. The SGA infant has a strong sucking response, in contrast with weak sucking response in the preterm infant. The SGA infant will often eat well and gain weight more quickly than the premature infant. The overall impression of vigor and well-being may be misleading. The infant's wide-eyed, alert facial expression may be due to chronic hypoxia (lack of oxygen). The SGA infant is also prone to hypoglycemia because the glycogen stores are frequently inadequate or depleted. The SGA infant is also more apt to have asphyxia due to meconium aspiration. Because of such potential complications, the caregiver needs to closely observe the SGA infant.

LARGE-FOR-GESTATIONAL-AGE INFANT

The infant who weighs 4000 g or more at birth is referred to as LGA. The diabetic woman who does not have advanced vascular changes is likely to have a large infant. The large infant often poses a mechanical problem during delivery and, after a prolonged labor, is delivered by cesarean birth. LGA infants are often sluggish, hypotonic, and hypoactive at birth. If the infants have diabetic mothers, they are prone to hypoglycemia; therefore, they need blood glucose level assessments (Nursing Care Plan 20–1).

Table 20–3 lists the problems (and their causes) for which LGA infants are at risk.

TABLE 20–3. PROBLEMS AND RISK FACTORS IN LARGE-FOR-GESTATIONAL-AGE INFANTS

PROBLEM	RISK FACTOR
Asphyxia	Chronic hypoxia in utero
Meconium aspiration	Acute or chronic hypoxia in utero
Polycythemia	Physiological response to in utero chronic hypoxic stress
Birth injuries	Cephalopelvic disproportion
Increased incidence of cesarean birth	Large size

POSTTERM INFANT

The postterm infant (postmature) is born after 42 weeks' gestation. Many are large, but they can be small by virtue of a progressive decrease in placental function. In other words, the placenta does not function as well after 40 weeks' gestation, or placental insufficiency develops. Because of the progressive degeneration of the placenta, the fetus does not receive adequate oxygen and nutrients. The fetus may use up some of the subcutaneous fat and when born will look thin, with loose skin. Often, the skin is cracked and dry, with a parchment-like texture. This infant is at risk for hypoxia, meconium aspiration, and asphyxia. Caregivers should closely observe all postterm infants, regardless of size.

Table 20–4 presents the problems (and their causes) for which postterm infants are at risk.

PRETERM (PREMATURE) INFANT

The most common factor associated with neonatal death is prematurity. The preterm infant is one who is born before the end of 37 weeks' gestation. An infant may be born much earlier than 37 weeks' gestation and still live, but it may be very poorly developed to survive outside the uterus. The preterm infant's skin is often wrinkled, delicate, and thin. Usually, the skin is covered with lanugo. The preterm infant is thin, has a little subcutaneous fat, and has prominent fon-

tanelles and suture lines of the skull. The cry is weak, matching the frail appearance.

Body Systems

The preterm infant has several physical problems that need to be taken into consideration during care. In fact, because these infants require a great deal of special attention, they are often transferred to a regional hospital that has a high-risk intensive-care unit for preterm infants. If it is not possible to transfer the mother before delivery, a transport team of physicians and nurses may be available to bring the infant to the regional center. Before and during the transfer, the infant is given resuscitation as needed, is given oxygen, is kept warm, and is protected from infection.

Respiratory System. The preterm infant's respiratory system is functionally and structurally immature. Because of incomplete development of air sacs and surfactant deficiency, the preterm infant often develops respiratory distress (see Chapter 24). In addition, the preterm infant is subject to apnea (periods of nonbreathing).

Temperature Regulation. The preterm infant's heat loss is greater than that of a full-term infant, and the ability to produce heat is limited. The infant has a lack of subcutaneous fat (brown fat) and has feeble muscular activity. The surface area is relatively large in proportion to body weight.

TABLE 20–4. PROBLEMS AND RISK FACTORS IN POSTTERM INFANTS

PROBLEM	RISK FACTOR
Asphyxia	Chronic hypoxia in utero
Meconium aspiration	In utero hypoxia leading to relaxation of anal sphincter and passage of meconium
Hypoglycemia	Resulting from depleted glycogen stores
Polycythemia	Increased red cell production in response to hypoxia
Birth trauma	Large size (diameters)
Congenital anomalies	Cause unknown
Seizure activity	Hypoxic insult

Cardiovascular System. The preterm infant has a tendency toward persistent fetal circulation. Because of a problem in lung expansion and an inability to establish alveolar stability, as a result of surfactant deficiency, the infant may have a delayed closure of the ductus arteriosus or a re-opening of the fetal circulation. High oxygen tension in the blood is essential to the opening up of the pulmonary system and a closing down of the ductus arteriosus (see Chapter 4). In addition, the preterm infant may have problems in the closing of the foramen ovale. All of this creates lung hypoperfusion for the preterm infant. Hypoperfusion results in less gas exchange and waste-product removal. For this reason, blood gas determinations are done frequently.

Digestive System. The preterm infant has a weak sucking reflex, delayed stomach emptying, and reduced intestinal motility. Therefore, abdominal distension, rigidity, and failure to absorb food can occur. Preterm infants are prone to hypoxia, and, because less blood is shunted to vital organs, they can be damaged. The intestinal cells damaged by hypoxia stop secreting mucus and can be invaded by bacteria, which can be fatal. As a result of ischemia of the bowel, the infant becomes predisposed to necrotizing enterocolitis.

Liver and Metabolic Function. Because preterm infants have reduced glycogen, fat, vitamin, and mineral (especially calcium) stores at birth, they are faced with problems of hypoglycemia and hypocalcemia. Some of the clinical signs are twitching, convulsions, and a high-pitched cry.

Poor clearance of bilirubin and decreased feeding reduce the removal of bilirubin in the intestines. In addition, the preterm infant is more subjected to cold stress, which releases free fatty acids. The excess fatty acids compete for albumin binding sites, which displaces bilirubin (see Chapter 17). More simply stated, the preterm infant is at a higher risk for hyperbilirubinemia.

Renal System. The preterm infant has problems with water retention, edema, and poor drug clearance. There is also a reduced ability to concentrate urine or conserve water; therefore, preterm infants are more likely to become dehydrated.

Immune System. The preterm infant did not stay in utero long enough to receive passive immunity from the mother. These infants are very susceptible to infections. Sepsis or infection accounts for a high percentage of death in premature babies. Protection from infection is essential.

Care of the Preterm Infant

Prevention of Infection. Caregivers must be aware of the preterm infant's high susceptibility to infection and must do everything possible to protect against it. It is important to practice strict asepsis in all procedures. Nurses who have an infection or who recently cared for a patient with an infection should not care for the preterm infant. Meticulous hand washing, sterilization of supplies and equipment, and maintenance of individual technique (hand washing after handling each infant and before proceeding to next infant) should be practiced. In addition, any preterm infant who is potentially infectious should be immediately isolated from the other infants.

Respiratory Support. The preterm infant frequently needs oxygen, because the atmospheric content (concentration of 21%) is insufficient. Preterm infants who have difficulty in breathing may be placed on mechanical machines to assist them. The ideal arterial oxygen tension or pressure (Pa_{O_2}) is 60 to 80 mm Hg. If the infant has much less arterial oxygen tension, cell death can occur.

Prolonged periods of hyperoxygenation (PO_2 levels above 90 to 100 mm Hg) can be dangerous to the infant and produce oxygen toxicity. Oxygen toxicity can cause vasoconstriction in the vessels of the retina, resulting in a condition called *retrolental fibroplasia* that can lead to blindness.

A relatively new noninvasive monitoring system, called *transcutaneous oxygen tension monitoring* ($TcPO_2$), has been helpful in closely observing the infant's oxygen needs. Arterial blood gas samples are still required, but not as often. If the infant remains on supplemental oxygen over 60 mm Hg for a period of time, a thickening of the alveolar sacs can develop, with the occurrence of atelectasis. Therefore, the amount of oxygen is reduced and the infant is weaned from supplemental oxygen as soon as weaning is tolerated by the infant.

Preterm infants frequently have periods of apnea (nonbreathing) of 15 seconds or more. They are usually placed on an apnea monitor and are

NURSING CARE PLAN 20–1

SMALL-FOR-GESTATIONAL-AGE NEWBORN INFANT

Potential Problems and Nursing Diagnoses	Nursing Interventions
1. Impaired gas exchange related to meconium aspiration.	Suction as needed. Give oxygen before suction. Auscultate breath sounds. Perform chest physiotherapy as ordered.
2. Potential for injury related to hypoglycemia.	Observe, record, and report signs of hypoglycemia: jitteriness, seizure activity, lethargy, apnea, and cyanosis.
3. Ineffective thermoregulation related to decreased subcutaneous fat.	Monitor temperature with skin probe or axillary temperature every 1 to 2 hr. Minimize heat loss by warming and humidifying oxygen; keeping skin dry; adjusting incubator or radiant heat bed to maintain skin temperature; avoiding cold surfaces. Monitor signs for cold stress, such as decreased temperature, pallor, and lethargy.
4. Altered nutrition: less than body requirements.	Promote growth by caloric intake of 120 to 150 calories/kg/day. Supplement gavage or nipple feedings with intravenous therapy (per order) until oral intake is sufficient for growth. Monitor daily weight.
5. Impaired tissue integrity.	Monitor broken skin sites for adequate healing. Observe broken skin sites for potential infection.
6. Potentially altered parenting related to prolonged hospitalization.	Include parents in the infant's care. Encourage parents to visit or call frequently. Provide opportunities for parents to ask questions about the infant's progress and care.

Expected Outcomes

1. Infant's respirations are between 35 and 50 per minute, with no cyanosis, sternal retractions, or nasal flaring.
2. Infant's Dextrostix value is 50 mm/dL. Infant does not show jitteriness, seizure activity, or lethargy.
3. Infant's temperature remains stabilized between 97° F and 98° F.
4. Infant is able to begin to take oral feedings.
5. Assessment shows the infant's skin to be intact.
6. Parents come to visit the infant, and the mother gives the infant an oral feeding.

carefully observed. Stimulation usually restarts their breathing.

Maintenance of Body Temperature. The maintenance of a constant neutral thermal environment, discussed in Chapter 17, is essential to the preterm infant's survival. Full-term infants can modify their body temperatures by increasing muscular activity and by adopting a more flexed position. The flexed position minimizes the surface area from which heat is lost and allows the blood to go to the major organs. Preterm infants have little to no muscular activity. In addition, they remain in the extended position because of their lack of muscle tone; thus, their heat losses are greater.

The preterm infant is usually placed in a radiantly heated bed or incubator. Also, a skin thermistor probe is used to monitor the infant's temperature.

Nutritional Needs. The premature baby has an increased need for calories for energy and growth. The last 3 months in utero are the most effective time for the storage of glycogen and fat. Therefore, an infant born several weeks before term has a limited amount of subcutaneous fat (brown fat) and glycogen. In order to assist the infant in gaining weight, the nutritional needs are calculated every 12 to 24 hours on the basis of clinical information. If the mother wants to breastfeed her infant, she usually is encouraged to express her milk manually and provide a supply to the nursery. When the infant is able to breastfeed (very small infants can do so), the mother should be urged to come to the nursery when possible to nurse her infant.

Preterm infants who are unable to bottle-feed or breastfeed may be fed by a nasogastric or nasojejunal tube until their reflex is strong enough to suck on a nipple. Feedings can be given by continuous, interrupted, or bolus infusion. It is very important that preterm infants be fed with great care. They are given small amounts slowly, with frequent rest and burping. Overfeeding can be dangerous to these infants, because it may cause regurgitation and aspiration. It is important to remember that the gag reflex is weak, and these infants may aspirate fluid (milk) into their lungs. Nonnutritive suckling opportunities assist preterm infants in taking early oral feedings.

The caregiver should keep an accurate record of the exact amount of formula taken at each feeding as well as the infant's response to the feeding. This information is used in evaluating the infant's progress.

Needs of Parents of Preterm Infant

The reaction of parents to a preterm birth has been described as an acute emotional crisis. They must progress through some psychological tasks. First, they often experience anticipatory grief and begin to prepare for the death of the infant. Second, they must face the realization that they have a preterm infant and accept that they had no control over the failure to deliver a full-term infant. Usually, the next task is to resume the process of relating to the infant or begin to establish the attachment process. After the initial attachment, they are faced with the problem of learning about the special care needs of preterm infants and how they differ from the needs of full-term infants. Perhaps the two components of the mother-to-infant interaction that are affected most by having the preterm infant in the high-risk nursery (separated from the parents) are the sensory or touch component and the care-taking component. The caregiver can do much to help the parents overcome these problems. Parents should be encouraged to come to the nursery as soon as it is possible to learn about their infant. The parents should be given assistance in touching the infant and doing whatever they can in caring for the infant. If possible, when the infant is discharged, the public health nurse or the nurse from the Visiting Nurses' Association can help the parents with the infant's care. Parents are usually reassured to know that this help is available. In addition, the parents can always call their physician or clinic staff if necessary.

References

Beckholt, A. P. (1990). Breast milk for infants who cannot breastfeed. *Journal of Obstetric, Gynecologic, and Neonatal Nursing* 19(3):216–220.

Brooten, D., Brown, L. P., Munro, B. H., York, R., Cohen, S. M., Roncoli, M., & Hollingsworth, J. (1988). Early discharge and specialist transitional care. *Image: Journal of Nursing Scholarship* 20(2):64–68.

Dickason, E. J., Schult, M. O., & Silverman, B. L. (1990). *Maternal-Infant Nursing Care.* St. Louis: C.V. Mosby.

Gennaro, S., Brooten, D., & Bakewell-Sachs, S. (1991). Post-discharge services for low-birth-weight infants. *Journal of Obstetric, Gynecologic, and Neonatal Nursing* 20(1):29–35.

Kling, P. (1989). Nursing interventions to decrease the risk of periventricular-intraventricular hemorrhage. *Journal of Obstetric, Gynecologic, and Neonatal Nursing* 18(6):457–464.

Ladewig, P. W., London, M. L., & Olds, S. B. (1990). *Essentials of Maternal-Newborn Nursing,* 2nd ed. Redwood City, CA: Addison-Wesley Nursing.

May, L. A., & Mahlmeister, L. R. (1990). *Comprehensive Maternity Nursing: Nursing Process and the Childbearing Family,* 2nd ed. Philadelphia: J.B. Lippincott.

McCormick, A. (1984). Special considerations in the nursing care of the very low birth weight infant. *Journal of Obstetric, Gynecologic, and Neonatal Nursing* 13(6):357–363.

Merenstein, G. B., & Gardner, S. L. (1989). *Handbook of Neonatal Intensive Care,* 2nd ed. St. Louis: C.V. Mosby.

Miller, E. P., & Armstrong, C. L. (1990). Surfactant replacement therapy. *Journal of Obstetric, Gynecologic, and Neonatal Nursing* 19:14–16.

Null, S. (1989). Nursing care to ease parents' grief. *American Journal of Maternal-Child Nursing* 14(2):84–89.

Sherwen, L. N., Scoloveno, M. A., & Neingarten, C. T. (1991). *Nursing Care of the Childbearing Family.* Norwalk, CT: Appleton & Lange.

Sullivan, R., Foster, J., & Schreiner, R. (1979). Determining a newborn's gestational age. *American Journal of Maternal Child Nursing* 4(1):38–45.

Weibley, T. T. (1989). Inside the incubator. *American Journal of Maternal-Child Nursing* 14(2):96–100.

SUGGESTED ACTIVITIES

1. List five infant physical characteristics that are used to determine gestational age.
2. Identify four physical problems that commonly occur in preterm infants.
3. Explain common emotional reactions when parents have a preterm infant.

REVIEW QUESTIONS

A. Select the best answer to each multiple-choice question.

Clinical Situation: Baby Michael is born at 34 weeks' gestation, weighs 2 lb 10 oz, and is 36 cm long. At 1 minute, his color is blue, heart rate is 110 bpm, and respirations are slow and irregular. He shows some flexion of his extremities and cries on stimulation. He is immediately dried, aspirated with suction, and placed in a heated bed. At 5 minutes, his color improves, and his respirations increase. The pediatrician, who was present at the birth, decides that baby Michael should be taken to the intensive care, high-risk nursery so he can be monitored closely for any untoward problems. Baby Michael's mother is informed that she can go to the nursery to see him when she is able. She is also told that she would be able to touch or hold her baby after his physical condition stabilizes.

1. At 1 minute after birth, the pediatrician gives baby Michael an Apgar score of
   A. 5
   B. 7
   C. 9
   D. 10

2. Baby Michael is
   A. Preterm
   B. Term
   C. Postterm
   D. None of the above

3. Baby Michael's physical characteristics are in accordance with his gestational age (refer to text). They are
   A. Wrinkled, thin skin
   B. Lanugo on back and shoulders
   C. Limited subcutaneous fat
   D. All of the above

4. Baby Michael is more likely to have all of the following EXCEPT
   A. Tendency toward persistent fetal circulation
   B. Inadequate voiding
   C. Limited ability to produce body heat
   D. Development of respiratory distress

5. Baby Michael's parents' reactions are likely to include all of the following EXCEPT
   A. Anticipatory grief
   B. Acceptance in having a preterm infant
   C. Concern about learning special care needs for their infant
   D. Concern about baby Michael's future handicaps

6. During gestation, the lungs of the fetus reach the point of maturity at which the fetus can be born with minimal respiratory difficulty. A preterm infant is likely to have respiratory distress syndrome if it is born before
   A. 28 weeks' gestation
   B. 32 weeks' gestation
   C. 35 weeks' gestation
   D. All of the above

7. The most common factor associated with neonatal death is
   A. Birth injury
   B. Prematurity
   C. Congenital malformations
   D. Metabolic diseases

8. Full-term newborns, even those with low birth weight, should have
   A. Labia majora that are in contact with one another
   B. At least one testis in the scrotum
   C. Finger nails that extend to or beyond the fingertips
   D. All of the above

9. The small-for-gestational-age infant is at risk for
   A. Asphyxia due to chronic hypoxia
   B. Hypothermia due to diminished subcutaneous fat
   C. Hypocalcemia due to calcium depletion secondary to birth asphyxia
   D. All of the above

10. The postterm infant is at risk for
    A. Birth trauma if large in size
    B. Hypoglycemia resulting from depleted glycogen stores
    C. Seizure activity related to hypoxia in utero
    D. All of the above

B. Choose from Column II the phrase that most accurately defines the term in Column I.

I

1. Square window _____
2. Arm recoil _____
3. Scarf sign _____
4. Heel to ear _____
5. Posture _____
6. Ear _____
7. Plantar creases _____
8. Genitals _____
9. Skin _____
10. Lanugo _____

II

A. Movement of foot toward ear
B. Extension and release of arm
C. Movement of hand toward opposite shoulder
D. Flexion of hand at wrist on forearm
E. Fine hair commonly observed on shoulders and back
F. Extent of coverage of sole creases
G. Degree of flexion or extension of extremities
H. Cartilage formation and recoil response
I. Prominence of clitoris and labia minora
J. Degree of visible vessels and observed transparency

CHAPTER 21 _____

Chapter Outline

Pregnancy-Induced Hypertension
    Risk factors
    Major symptoms
    Physiological changes
    Assessment and intervention
Hyperemesis Gravidarum
    Assessment and intervention
Diabetes Mellitus
    The diabetic woman during pregnancy
    The effect of diabetes on pregnancy
    The effect of pregnancy on diabetes
    Assessment and intervention
Heart Disease in Pregnancy
    Assessment and intervention
Rh Incompatibility
    Assessment and intervention
ABO Incompatibility
Bleeding Disorders
    Abortion
    Ectopic (extrauterine) pregnancy
    Hydatidiform mole (gestational trophoblastic disease)
    Placenta previa
    Abruptio placentae
    Disseminated intravascular coagulation
Infections During Pregnancy
    Rubella
    Toxoplasmosis
    Tuberculosis
    Urinary tract infections

Learning Objectives

Upon completion of Chapter 21, the student should be able to
- List five causes of high-risk pregnancies and name the three leading causes of maternal mortality.
- Determine the difference between preeclampsia and eclampsia.
- Name four factors that increase the risk for pregnancy-induced hypertension.
- Identify three signs that a pregnant hypertensive woman should report immediately to her physician.
- Name one drug commonly given to women with preeclampsia. Name the antidote for toxicity from it.
- Explain hyperemesis gravidarum in pregnancy.
- List causes of bleeding early and late in pregnancy.
- Name three causes of spontaneous abortion.
- Describe ectopic pregnancy.
- Describe placenta previa and name the characteristic symptom. Name two complications.
- List two types of abruptio placentae.
- List five nursing measures in the care of a woman who is hemorrhaging.
- Explain the cause of coagulation defects in pregnancy.
- List three ways diabetes mellitus affects pregnancy, and explain the importance of rigid control.
- List four aspects of self-care for the diabetic woman.
- Discuss heart disease in pregnancy.
- Explain the process of isoimmunization, including Rh factor and ABO incompatibility.
- Describe rubella and its consequences in pregnancy.
- Name the changes that occur in pregnancy that predispose the woman to urinary tract infections.
- List three self-care measures for a pregnant woman with urinary tract infection.

Health Problems That Complicate Pregnancy

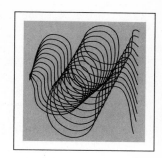

Health problems during pregnancy may pose a threat to the woman and her infant. Several factors can be detected at the beginning of pregnancy. Pregnancies characterized by such problems are termed *high-risk pregnancies*. Most of the causes of high-risk pregnancies are listed in Table 21–1. For women whose pregnancies are at risk, prenatal care provides necessary health teaching for promotion of health and prevention of illness. Prompt identification, assessment, and management of the problems are essential to effect the successful outcome of the pregnancy and the well-being of the infant.

The focus of this chapter is on preexisting medical disorders and problems unique to pregnancy. The three complications that are the leading cause of maternal death are hypertension, hemorrhage, and infection. Hypertension, hemorrhage, and nonpuerperal infections are discussed in this chapter, and puerperal infection is discussed in Chapter 23.

Pregnancy-Induced Hypertension

Pregnancy-induced hypertension (PIH) is the most common hypertensive disorder in pregnancy. Preeclampsia and eclampsia are types of PIH. A progressive disorder found only in pregnancy, *preeclampsia* is characterized by (a) hypertension with (b) proteinuria and/or (c) generalized edema after 20 weeks' gestation. *Eclampsia* means "convulsion." If a woman has a convulsion, her condition is then defined as eclampsia, which is the most severe form of PIH. Most of PIH (preeclampsia or eclampsia) is seen in the last 10 to 12 weeks of pregnancy. PIH usually ends after the birth of the infant; however, it may be seen 24 to 48 hours after the delivery. If hypertension is found before 20 weeks' gestation, it is most likely due to a preexisting elevated blood pressure or chronic hypertension.

RISK FACTORS

The exact cause of PIH is unknown. The incidence of PIH is about 6% of all pregnancies. There are several risk factors that are associated with an increase in PIH:

- Adolescence
- Age over 35 years
- Lower socioeconomic class
- Poor nutrition
- First pregnancy
- Family history of hypertension
- Chronic hypertension
- Diabetes mellitus
- Multiple pregnancy
- Hydatidiform mole
- Hydramnios (excessive amniotic fluid)
- Rh incompatibility (with profound fetal edema)

MAJOR SYMPTOMS

During an uneventful pregnancy, the blood pressure remains normal, and there is no protein in the urine. Most pregnant women have edema of the lower extremities (dependent edema) owing to pressure of the gravid uterus on the inferior vena cava and the relaxation of the smooth muscle

TABLE 21–1. CAUSES OF HIGH-RISK PREGNANCIES

General
- Maternal age of 15 years or younger or 35 years or older
- Either nulliparous or para 5 or more
- Nonwhite
- Unmarried
- Low socioeconomic group, limited education
- Start of prenatal care after 27 weeks of pregnancy, or fewer than 5 prenatal visits made before birth

Obstetrical
- Infertility
- Previous abortion
- Premature or low-birth-weight infant
- Previous excessive size infant
- Postterm, beyond 42 weeks
- Previous cesarean section
- Incompetent cervix
- Uterine anomaly
- Contracted pelvis
- Abnormal presentation
- Rh −, sensitized
- Polyhydramnios
- Preeclampsia
- Multiple pregnancy

Medical
- Anemia
- Sickle cell anemia
- Hypertension
- Diabetes
- Thyroid disease
- Venereal disease
- Cervical neoplasia
- Urinary tract infection
- Psychiatric or neurological problem, or both
- Other medical conditions

Other
- Nutritional deficits
- Smoking
- Drug abuse or alcohol abuse

in the blood vessels. Edema of the face and hands, however, is a warning sign, because it characterizes the generalized edema of PIH. This sign is often noticed first by a weight gain of more than 2 lb per week. Protein in the urine demonstrates reduced kidney function, which is of concern.

Hypertensive disorders of pregnancy vary in severity. The clinical findings will also vary, which makes the caregiver's assessment very important in the management of the condition. Because the woman may feel well, she often does not understand the need for close monitoring of her condition to assess her health status. Some women with PIH or preeclampsia are comparatively symptom free and may have little or no noticeable peripheral

edema after bed rest. Therefore, a blood pressure 30 mm Hg above normal and a diastolic pressure 15 mm Hg above normal is a diagnostic sign. Clearly, a woman whose blood pressure rises from a baseline of 108/72 to 138/87 during pregnancy should be carefully and frequently observed. A screening test called the "roll-over test" has some predictive value in determining patients who are likely to develop PIH during pregnancy (Table 21–2). The identification of patients who will subsequently develop preeclampsia makes this test worthwhile even though false-positive tests occur.

The baseline blood pressure often is not known because many women, especially those seen in prenatal clinics, seek care later in pregnancy. It is for this reason that the arbitrary blood pressure level of 140/90 is significant. It is very important to remember that a mild form of PIH may rapidly progress to a severe form, and possibly to eclampsia (convulsions). In severe cases of preeclampsia, generalized edema is apparent, and there may be pitting edema over the lower extremities, abdominal wall, face, hands, and sacral area. The condition is characterized by a sudden weight gain of 2 lb (0.9 kg) or more per week and daily 24-hour urinary protein level of 300 mg or more. The woman may also experience frontal headache, blurred vision, nausea, vomiting, hyperactive reflexes, oliguria (diminished secretion of urine), an elevated hematocrit level (due to hemoconcentration and hypovolemia), and epigastric pain.

PHYSIOLOGICAL CHANGES

The primary physiological disorder in PIH is peripheral arteriolar vasoconstriction and vaso-

TABLE 21–2. THE ROLL-OVER TEST

Procedure:
1. Measure blood pressure with patient in the lateral recumbent position until stable.
2. Roll patient to supine position.
3. Measure blood pressure immediately.
4. Repeat blood pressure in 5 min while supine.

Positive test: An increase of 20 mm Hg or more in the diastolic blood pressure at the 5-min reading

Negative test: An increase of less than 20 mm Hg in diastolic blood pressure at the 5-min reading

spasm, leading to alterations in many maternal organ functions. Vasospasm in the arterioles leads to an increase in blood pressure level and, ultimately, a decrease in blood flow to the uterus and placenta. A clinically significant alteration also occurs in the kidneys. Renal vascular changes cause a lowering of the renal blood flow, a lowering of the renal glomerular filtration rate, and consequently proteinuria. Changes in the central nervous system may include cerebral edema, which causes headaches and visual disturbances. As the condition progresses in severity, hyperactivity of the deep tendon reflexes develops. Hepatic alterations include enlargement of the liver and tension on the liver capsule. These alterations cause epigastric pain, which may precede eclampsia.

Severe preeclampsia and eclampsia have been associated with serious complications, such as cerebrovascular accidents (stroke), acute renal failure, abruptio placentae, disseminated intravascular coagulation, and fetal and maternal death. The HELP (hemolysis, elevated liver enzymes, and low platelet count) syndrome is found in about 10% of severe preeclampsia cases. In women who exhibit the HELP syndrome, the onset of eclampsia may be abrupt.

ASSESSMENT AND INTERVENTION

One goal of prenatal care is to detect the signs of PIH early, before the condition progresses. For this reason, recording the woman's weight, taking her blood pressure, and performing urinalysis (for protein) are of utmost importance during each prenatal visit. In addition, asking the woman questions about subjective signs, such as swelling of face or fingers, frontal headache, or epigastric pain, is significant. Examples of nursing diagnoses that should be considered in the care of the woman with PIH are listed in Nursing Care Plan 21–1.

NURSING DIAGNOSES

- Fluid volume excess related to water retention and impaired sodium excretion
- Altered tissue perfusion related to vasoconstriction of glomeruli, resulting in decreased kidney function

- Potential for injury related to vasoconstriction and vasospasm of cerebral blood vessels, resulting in oxygen depletion, possible convulsions, and possible placental separation
- Knowledge deficit related to PIH, its treatment, and implications for the woman and her infant
- Ineffective individual coping related to reduction in physical activities
- Anxiety related to unknown outcome of pregnancy and baby
- Altered family processes related to the need for additional rest, sleep, and reduction in activities
- Ineffective denial with inability to accept illness
- Noncompliance because elevated blood pressure, pulse, and protein in urine do not seem significant to woman
- Anxiety related to close monitoring of PIH and hospitalization

Education for Self-Care

The management of PIH depends on the severity of the symptoms, the philosophy of the physician, and the understanding and *compliance* of the patient. Careful teaching and guidance regarding the condition are very important to the woman, her infant, and her family.

In early PIH, if the woman is well informed and conscientious in carrying out the medical and nursing instructions (that is, reports headaches, visual disturbances, epigastric pain, or development of significant edema), management may be done on an outpatient basis. However, many physicians prefer to hospitalize patients until symptoms are controlled. Management is directed toward reducing edema and hypertension and restoring normal kidney function. The nurse should help the woman and the family to understand the importance of controlling mild PIH.

Sufficient bed rest, while lying on the left side, is an important part of the management because it increases both the renal and placental blood flow, which in turn decreases edema and blood pressure. A high-protein diet is helpful, and sodium should not be restricted (however, an excessive intake of foods with high amounts of sodium,

NURSING CARE PLAN 21–1

MANAGEMENT OF THE WOMAN WITH PREGNANCY-INDUCED HYPERTENSION

Potential Problems and Nursing Diagnoses	Nursing Interventions
1. Fluid volume excess related to water retention, impaired sodium retention.	Monitor sudden weight gain, edema, elevated blood pressure, and protein in urine. Assess reflexes for hyperactivity.
2. Potential for injury related to potential seizure activity.	Monitor neurological changes such as headache and/or blurred vision. Assess for epigastric discomfort.
3. Altered tissue perfusion related to arteriolar spasms with decreased oxygen to fetus.	Monitor fetal heart rate by electronic fetal monitoring. Recognize possible poor perfusion of placental/fetal unit. Report late decelerations in fetal heart rate.
4. Knowledge deficit related to PIH and potential injury to self and fetus.	Discuss implications of PIH for mother and fetus. Explain importance of treatment measures.
5. Ineffective coping related to reduction in physical activity.	Acknowledge woman's feelings about bed rest and reduced activity.
6. Anxiety related to the unknown outcome of pregnancy.	Explain that usually symptoms improve with treatment. Explain the necessity for close monitoring to reduce risk of complications.

Expected Outcomes

1. Edema decreases in woman's hands and face; elevation in blood pressure decreases.
2. Frontal headache disappears, and no other neurological signs are present.
3. Fetal heart rate pattern returns to normal.
4. Woman verbalizes understanding of the implications of illness for herself and her infant.
5. Woman communicates feelings about bed rest and recognizes the need for it.
6. Woman expresses confidence in caregiver's ability to care for her.

KEY POINTS IN EDUCATION: MANAGING MILD PREGNANCY-INDUCED HYPERTENSION

The woman should be instructed that to modify mild PIH, she must

- Recognize that bed rest is essential
- Rest on the left side
- Eat a high-protein diet
- Reduce anxiety
- Take medication if prescribed by the physician

- Keep prenatal visits (usually 2 times a week)
- Report to the clinic or physician immediately if any of following symptoms appear: headache, epigastric pain, visual disturbances, or edema of the face or hands

TABLE 21–3. NURSING CARE RELATED TO MILD TO MODERATE PREGNANCY-INDUCED HYPERTENSION (PIH)

NURSING INTERVENTIONS	RATIONALES
Bed rest—woman is to stay in bed except when specifically permitted to get up.	Bed rest promotes increased diuresis; decreases blood pressure and edema.
Daily weighings—done at the same time each day, preferably in early morning with empty bladder.	Weight change indicates increase or decrease in fluid retention.
Blood pressure read every 2–4 hr.	Blood pressure increase is indicative of greater severity of disease.
Listen to fetal heart rate frequently or monitor FHR continuously with fetal electronic monitor.	Assess for fetal well-being or fetal compromise.
Check urine for protein every 4 hr.	Assess for decreased kidney function.
Assess 24-hr fluid intake and hourly urinary output.	Assess for adequate kidney function.
Inspect and palpate woman's face, extremities, and sacrum for edema (and extremities when in bed).	Assess for fluid retention.
Test for deep tendon reflexes (knee jerk) for hyperactivity.	Assess for muscle and nerve irritability.
Inquire about presence of headache, visual disturbance, and epigastric pain.	Check for signs that are indicative of increasing disease severity.
Assess for signs of labor.	Assess for signs of labor progression, such as frequency of contractions.
Assess anxieties and concerns.	Anxiety can increase the blood pressure.
Attempt to reduce sensory stimulation.	Reduce neuromuscular irritability.
Check high-protein dietary intake.	Provide appropriate nutrients.
Assess need for sedation.	Sedation is given to provide rest and thereby reduce blood pressure.
Check for completeness of emergency tray or equipment in woman's room and for antihypertensive drugs.	Have all necessary equipment readily available for emergency.

such as pickles, olives, and potato chips, should be discouraged). Sometimes, a sedative is ordered to make resting easier for the woman.

Attention should be given to the woman's emotional and physical support while at home. Bed rest may be difficult for a mother to get if she has small children. The fact that the woman usually feels well makes education especially important in getting her to take the precautions that will help her avoid hospitalization.

Hospital Care

When a woman with PIH is hospitalized, the ideal regimen is rest in a quiet room. The goals for care are to maintain the functioning of the woman's body systems and to keep her as quiet and nonstimulated as possible. This plan reduces the neuromuscular irritability and the potential for convulsions. For some women, the presence of a supportive person is helpful. Efforts should be made to reduce her anxiety. Anxiety can further increase her blood pressure level. Often, women are prescribed complete bed rest, with medications administered to prevent seizures. If medications are administered, the side rails are raised to prevent the patient from falling out of bed. The need for nursing assessment is continuous. Nursing care is shown in Table 21–3.

Medications for Pregnancy-Induced Hypertension

Medications used in the treatment of progressing severity of PIH include sedatives, antihyper-

TABLE 21–4. NURSING ALERT: ADMINISTRATION OF MAGNESIUM SULFATE (MgSO$_4$)

Use
To prevent convulsions.

Action
Blocks neuromuscular transmission.
Decreases neuromuscular irritability.
Causes slight peripheral vasodilation, reduces edema in brain, and may increase perfusion.

Contraindications
Drug is excreted through kidneys—not given if woman has kidney impairment.
Drug toxicity.

Maternal side effects
Most side effects are related to magnesium toxicity: sweating, warmth, flushing, nausea, slurred speech, confusion, and kidney and circulatory collapse.

Administration
Intramuscular (IM) or intravenous (IV).
IV by infusion pump is preferred to control dosage. Loading dose is 3–4 g of MgSO$_4$ in 5% dextrose and water over a 20-min period. Maintenance dose is 1–2 g/hr
For IM, use z tract because MgSO$_4$ is very irritating to tissues

Nursing considerations
Assess vital signs every 15 min.
Assess urine output every hour.
Check reflex response every hour.
Monitor fetal heart rate (FHR) continuously.

Withhold drug due to toxicity if:
Reflexes are dull or absent.
Respiratory rate is under 12/min.
Urinary output is less than 30 mL/hr.

Effects on fetus/newborn
Drug readily crosses placenta.
Decrease in FHR variability.
Tachycardia.
Low Apgar scores.
Newborn hypotonia.
Respiratory depression.

NOTE. Calcium gluconate is an antagonist (antidote) to MgSO$_4$. One to 3 g of calcium gluconate should be readily available when administering MgSO$_4$.

tensives, and anticonvulsants. Magnesium sulfate (MgSO$_4$) is the drug of choice to modify hypertensive symptoms. This drug depresses the conduction of nerve impulses and decreases the hyperreflexia commonly seen in preeclampsia. MgSO$_4$ also has some vasodilating effects, which tend to lower the blood pressure and increase the blood flow to the kidneys and uterus. In addition, because MgSO$_4$ has a depressing effect on the central nervous system, it serves as an anticonvulsant. MgSO$_4$ can be given intramuscularly or through an intravenous infusion pump. It is very irritating to the tissues; therefore, if given intramuscularly, the z-tract technique should be used. MgSO$_4$ can build up to a toxic level in patients, characterized by loss of deep tendon reflexes (knee jerk), depression of respirations, and lowered pulse rate. It should be withheld or discontinued if the reflexes are poor or absent, respirations are less than 12 per minute, heart rate is markedly decreased, or the urine output is less than 30 mL/hour. Calcium gluconate, an antidote to MgSO$_4$, should be readily available to counteract depressant effects if necessary (Table 21–4). A woman who is receiving MgSO$_4$ should never be left alone.

Emergency Care

Emergency equipment and drugs should be kept in the patient's room. These include a plastic airway; a padded tongue blade; oxygen and suction equipment; ophthalmoscope; and medications such as MgSO$_4$, calcium gluconate, and cardiac stimulants.

Fortunately, convulsions occur in only 5% of PIH patients. However, every nurse should know that a rise in blood pressure level, severe headache, abdominal pain, apprehension, twitching, and hyperirritability of the muscles often precede a convulsion. As soon as a convulsion manifests itself, a plastic airway or, if hospital policy allows, a padded tongue blade or a rolled washcloth should be placed in the woman's open mouth between her teeth to prevent her from biting her tongue and to help to maintain an open airway. If possible, the patient's entire body and head should be turned to the side to prevent aspiration of mucus and vomitus into her lungs. During the periods of rigidity and muscle contraction, the woman's body should be restrained only enough to keep her from hurting herself or from rolling out of bed. If possible, the sides of the bed should be padded with pillows. Labor may progress rapidly at this time, and infants have been born suddenly during a convulsive episode. Whenever the woman shows signs of a possible convulsion, the physician should be notified immediately, an assessment of the woman and the fetal heart rate should be done, and specific orders should be carried out.

When the convulsions are controlled, labor may be induced or a cesarean birth performed, if the woman does not go into labor spontaneously. In any case, termination of the pregnancy is the only cure for PIH or preeclampsia and eclampsia. Nursing care at this time includes continuous monitoring of the woman and fetus. All stimuli, such as noise and bright lights, should be reduced to lessen electrical charges to neurons of the nervous system. Frequent monitoring of vital signs is important. It is important to remember that the woman can have a convulsion after birth and 1 to 2 days postpartum (rarely after 48 hours). Therefore, continual assessment is necessary until her condition has stabilized.

Hyperemesis Gravidarum

As discussed in Chapter 6, many pregnant women experience nausea with or without vomiting in early pregnancy. This symptom is more apparent when the woman rises in the morning, probably because of the effect of increased hormone levels on an empty stomach. Because the occurrence is more common in the morning, it is referred to as "morning sickness." It usually disappears about the twelfth week, as the woman's body becomes accustomed to the tremendous hormonal changes within it.

When vomiting persists, however, causing serious dehydration, starvation, and excessive weight loss, the condition is called *hyperemesis gravidum* (excessive vomiting of pregnancy). No single cause has been identified, but there is evidence that the physiological alterations of pregnancy contribute to it, especially the higher hormonal levels and the metabolic disturbances during pregnancy. In addition, psychological factors can be involved.

ASSESSMENT AND INTERVENTION

When dehydration occurs, the woman is usually hospitalized. Intravenous administration of fluids is started immediately. These fluids contain glucose, electrolytes, and vitamins. Correcting fluid and electrolyte imbalances is important in the treatment. All oral intake of food and fluids is stopped until the woman can retain fluid in small amounts. Sedation may be given; however, drugs are kept at a minimum because of potential damage to the fetus. Necessary treatment is carried out to prevent irreversible damage to the woman's vital organs. Heartburn and reflux esophagitis should be treated symptomatically. Usually there is rapid improvement, and the pregnancy is carried to term. However, in rare cases, pregnancy has to be terminated.

Caregivers play an important role in the management of patients with hyperemesis gravidarum, because visitors are sometimes restricted until the woman's condition improves. The nurse who is caring for a woman with hyperemesis gravidarum should maintain a cheerful, optimistic attitude and exhibit patience and understanding. Discussion of food should be avoided until the woman can tolerate eating. The nursing assessment should include listening to the woman's conversation for clues to what triggers her nausea or vomiting. Usually after 48 hours' hospitalization, the woman's condition has improved, and she is able to tolerate small amounts of dry food. Later, she is given a low-fat diet.

Diabetes Mellitus

Diabetes mellitus is an endocrine disorder of carbohydrate metabolism that results from inadequate production and use of insulin. Specifically, it is due to a faulty functioning of the islets of Langerhans, ductless glands within the pancreas. This results in a deficient production of insulin. Usually, insulin is released into the bloodstream in just the right amount and at just the right time to allow the glucose in the blood to be used by the body. During pregnancy, physiological changes affect the glucose–insulin relationship. Therefore, a pregnant woman who is a diabetic is considered at high risk.

Diabetes or impaired glucose tolerance that first appears during pregnancy is called *gestational diabetes*. If the woman has gestational diabetes, the routine urinalysis will show an excess of glucose; this condition is called *glycosuria*. Diet usually controls gestational diabetes, and insulin injections may not be needed. The symptoms of diabetes may disappear a few weeks after the birth of the infant. However, as many as 35% to 50% of patients with gestational diabetes will show further deterioration of carbohydrate metabolism in the next 15 years of life.

There are characteristic signs and symptoms of diabetes mellitus. When these symptoms appear, further evaluation should be done to diagnose or rule out diabetes from the differential diagnosis.

SIGNS AND SYMPTOMS OF DIABETES

- Hyperglycemia (excess glucose in the blood)
- Glycosuria (excess glucose in the urine)
- Polyuria (frequent urination)
- Polydipsia (excessive thirst)
- Polyphagia (excessive hunger)
- Weight loss

Polyuria is the result of water's not being reabsorbed by the renal tubules owing to the osmotic activity of glucose. Frequent urination predisposes the woman to polydipsia by tissue hydration. Polyphagia is caused by tissue loss. Breakdown of tissue occurs because of the cells' inability to use blood glucose. Weight loss is the result of the body's using fat and muscle tissue for energy.

THE DIABETIC WOMAN DURING PREGNANCY

Pregnancy is associated with many physiological alterations that affect the maternal–fetal glucose–insulin relationships. The changes and effects are as follows:

- Decrease in maternal glucose and amino acids.
  The fetus draws on maternal glucose and amino acids for energy and protein synthesis.

- Increase in insulin secretion.
  Placental hormones antagonize insulin; thus, more insulin has to be secreted to meet the nonpregnant level.

- Increase in maternal ketones.
  Acetone in maternal blood and urine caused by woman's incomplete oxidation of fat (upset in acid–base balance).

THE EFFECT OF DIABETES ON PREGNANCY

A pregnant woman who is a diabetic has a higher incidence of complications. Maternal complications may arise from metabolic, vascular, and infectious problems. The most widely used risk assessment for complications was developed by Dr. Priscilla White (Table 21–5).

Fetal complications include premature birth, congenital anomalies, metabolic alterations, stillbirths, large-for-gestational-age infants, and respiratory distress. Polyhydramnios (excessive amount of amniotic fluid) is also associated with diabetes. Both maternal and fetal complications can be minimized with careful medical, nursing, and dietary management.

Insulin levels can be unchanged or lower in early pregnancy but higher in the second half of pregnancy or late pregnancy. In addition, insulin levels can increase more rapidly after eating in a pregnant woman than in a nonpregnant woman.

Despite the potential hyperinsulin state in the second half of pregnancy, glucose tolerance is impaired and the woman has a tendency toward hypoglycemia (decreased blood glucose level). Some factors that influence the maternal insulin instability are increased insulin levels, increased placental and fetal use of glucose, decreased hepatic production of glucose, and decreased renal reabsorption of glucose. As pregnancy continues, the fasting level of blood glucose declines. The glucose tolerance test (GTT) standards are adjusted to correct for these physiological responses.

During pregnancy, the effects of insulin-antagonistic hormones (progesterone, estrogen, and human placental lactogen) are increased. The effects are more pronounced in the second half of pregnancy, because the concentration of the hormones is greater.

THE EFFECT OF PREGNANCY ON DIABETES

The fetus and placenta constantly use nutrients, such as glucose and amino acids, from the mother. The secretory mechanisms of the fetal pancreas are immature and do not play a role until the third trimester. With prolonged maternal hyperglycemia, fetal hyperinsulinemia owing to hyperplasia of the fetal islets of Langerhans can occur. The high fetal blood glucose levels that occur in response to high maternal blood glucose concentrations can result in macrosomia (large infant). In addition, the infants often have delayed lung maturity because of the insulin-antagonist effect of hormones on the maturing lung. This effect explains why respiratory distress is a common complication in infants born of diabetic mothers.

Diabetes results in a wide range of effects that differ in severity. In pregnancy, conditions vary from gestational diabetes to severe diabetes. As already mentioned, gestational diabetes results in abnormal GTT and usually is managed by diet alone. As one would expect, the perinatal complications are increased according to the severity and duration of maternal diabetes. Instruction should include the importance of monitoring exercise; exercise such as walking after a meal can decrease the rise in blood sugar after that meal.

ASSESSMENT AND INTERVENTION

Obtaining an adequate history is very important in identifying potentially and overtly diabetic pregnant women. When screening for the possibility

TABLE 21–5. WHITE'S CLASSIFICATION OF DIABETES IN PREGNANCY

CLASS	CHARACTERISTICS	INSULIN DEPENDENT
A	Abnormal glucose tolerance with normal fasting blood glucose levels. Glucose tolerance returns to normal after termination of pregnancy.	No
B	Onset of diabetes mellitus prior to pregnancy and after 20 years of age. Disease has been present for less than 10 years.	Yes
C	Onset of diabetes mellitus occurred between ages 10 and 19 and has a duration of 10–19 years	Yes
D	Onset of diabetes mellitus occurred before 10 years of age and has been present for more than 20 years. Peripheral vascular disease, retinal changes, and hypertension are present.	Yes
E	All of the characteristics of Class D, plus calcification of pelvic vessels.	Yes
F	All of the characteristics of Class E, plus neuropathy	Yes

From White, P. (1974). Diabetes mellitus in pregnancy. *Clinics in Perinatology* 1:331.

of diabetes, the nurse should ask questions concerning family history of diabetes, unexplained stillbirths, neonatal deaths, and congenital abnormalities. Women who are obese, who have had infants weighing more than 9 lb, or who have had hydramnios (excessive amniotic fluid) are also at a greater risk for diabetes.

The caregiver should explain the extreme importance of good observation and prenatal care. In addition, the caregiver should instruct the woman about the importance of dietary management.

Diabetic management during pregnancy is extremely important. Strict control of blood glucose levels requires the woman to keep a record of her urine or blood glucose, undergo periodic sampling and testing of blood, maintain a proper diet, and self-administer insulin. To achieve strict control, the diabetic woman should receive instruction from the dietitian along with the nurse and physician. Frequently, women with diabetes are hospitalized two to three times during their pregnancy for adequate assessments of their condition. The nurse can assist the woman to prepare for this type of care.

The woman taking an oral hypoglycemic agent (oral insulin) should be instructed to DISCONTINUE ORAL HYPOGLYCEMICS when she plans to become pregnant or immediately after she becomes pregnant. Oral hypoglycemic drugs are contraindicated during pregnancy because they can cross the placenta and stimulate the fetal pancreas to produce increased amounts of insulin, resulting in hyperinsulinemia. Women who need insulin must receive it by injection. A mixture of intermediate-acting (NPH) and short-acting (regular) insulin is used to adjust to the woman's individual needs. These needs will vary during her pregnancy.

A rigid control of serum glucose levels (normal range = 80 to 120 mg/dL) and the avoidance of ketoacidosis (elevation of acetone bodies) are the goals of medical and nursing care throughout pregnancy. The change in blood glucose levels and the necessary insulin dosage are best assessed by determination of blood glucose values by venipuncture. Capillary glucose values obtained by "finger stick" or Dextrostix can be done at home or in the hospital. Home monitoring can be effectively performed by the woman with equipment such as the "One-Touch" machine to check blood glucose levels. Urinary glucose values are less reliable because the renal threshold for glucose is decreased during pregnancy.

Insulin requirements may either decrease or remain the same during the first half of pregnancy; however, they usually increase during the second half of pregnancy when the insulin-antagonistic effect of hormones becomes apparent. The nurse should assess caloric intake, nausea and vomiting, and the woman's activity and exercise levels when changing the insulin dosage.

NURSING DIAGNOSES

- Knowledge deficit related to metabolic disorder, self-testing, and meaning of results
- Nutrition: Less than body requirements related to potential for imbalance of nutrients necessary for insulin intake
- Potential for injury to fetus and woman related to hyperglycemia or hypoglycemia
- Potential for infection related to alterations in the urinary tract during pregnancy
- Potential for injury to fetus related to uteroplacental functioning
- Altered family processes related to woman's need to be hospitalized during pregnancy
- Noncompliance related to need for close monitoring and additional prenatal visits

Medical and Nursing Management During Labor and Birth

Control of the blood glucose level during labor and delivery is achieved by intravenous infusion of dextrose with intermittent or continuous insulin therapy or administration of regular insulin. Frequently, diabetic women are hospitalized 1 week before delivery for evaluation of their condition. The method of delivery depends on the maturity and size of the fetus and the control of the woman's diabetes. Sometimes, a cesarean section is necessary because of the possible mechanical difficulty of delivering a large infant. During labor and delivery, insulin requirements are frequently evaluated.

Medical and Nursing Management During the Postpartum Period

After the delivery of the baby and placenta, insulin requirements drop dramatically for 24 to 72 hours. These values then rise to slightly less than the prepregnancy values. The decline in insulin requirement immediately post partum is due to the dramatic decline in the level of pregnancy hormones. Insulin needs will return to the prepregnancy level within 6 weeks after the birth of the infant.

Breastfeeding usually decreases insulin requirements, despite the increase in caloric intake. However, for both breastfeeding and nonbreastfeeding mothers, regular insulin dosage needs to be adjusted every 6 hours. This need will continue during the immediate postpartum period. Insulin

KEY POINTS IN EDUCATION: SELF-CARE IN DIABETES

- Symptoms of hypoglycemia and ketoacidosis: The pregnant diabetic woman must be able to recognize symptoms that indicate a change in glucose levels. She should be instructed to check her capillary blood glucose level to see if it is above or below normal. In addition, she should always carry a snack as a fast source of glucose. She should be advised to drink milk when possible to avoid a rebound of hyperglycemia.
- Travel: If insulin is required, the woman should keep it refrigerated, if possible while she is traveling. A bracelet should be worn that identifies the woman as being diabetic.
- Cesarean birth: The woman should be instructed that the possibility of a cesarean birth is increased.
- Hospitalization: The woman should be instructed that she may be hospitalized two to three times during her pregnancy to evaluate glucose levels and adjust her insulin level.
- Fetal monitoring: The woman should be instructed that fetal status will be assessed periodically during pregnancy.
- Smoking: The woman who smokes should be instructed about the harmful effects of smoking on both the maternal vascular system and the development of the fetus.
- Strict adherence to diet: The woman should understand that during pregnancy, for the well-being of the fetus, she must adhere to her diet.
- Careful monitoring of glucose levels at home: The woman should be instructed that reliability in her daily record of glucose levels is important in her care.
- Careful monitoring of exercise.

preparation, including different types, is discussed in Appendix B.

Heart Disease in Pregnancy

Physiological changes that occur in pregnancy make the diagnosis of certain forms of cardiovascular disease difficult. Pregnant women frequently complain of dyspnea, dizzy spells, and even faintness. Edema in the lower extremities and visible neck veins are commonly found in pregnant women. Certain findings, however, may indicate heart disease in pregnancy. These symptoms include severe dyspnea, faintness on exertion, and chest pain on exertion. Signs of heart disease are cyanosis, clubbing, diastolic murmurs, cardiac arrhythmias, and loud systolic murmurs.

ASSESSMENT AND INTERVENTION

Because pregnancy increases the heart's work load, physical exertion frequently is restricted in women with heart disease. Women who have some forms of heart disease, such as mitral stenosis, tolerate pregnancy poorly, especially with more than minimum physical exertion or activity. Additional rest is needed during pregnancy, and some women may require bed rest for the last part of the pregnancy. All women who have heart problems should get at least 9 to 10 hours of sleep and take rest periods during the day. This means that they should get someone to assist them with their housework and take care of the children at home.

It is important to counsel the pregnant woman with heart disease to avoid infection. She should avoid exposure to persons who have upper respiratory infections (colds and sore throats). Excessive weight gain also places additional strain on the woman's heart, so it is important for her to follow a carefully planned nutritional program, which may include limiting excess sodium in her diet. She should consult the dietitian in every clinic visit. The dietitian as well as a cardiologist should be part of the health care team. Women with heart disease should especially be encouraged to discontinue smoking during pregnancy, if this is a habit.

During labor, cardiac activity is increased; therefore, oxygen should be readily available. To minimize the exertion of the second stage of labor, the obstetrician may perform a low forceps delivery. All precautions should be taken to reduce the chance of infection during the labor and birth process. After delivery, the woman should be closely monitored for signs of cardiac distress. Frequently she is kept in the hospital for a few extra days to make sure she is able to make the necessary postpartum physiological adjustments.

MANAGEMENT OF CARDIAC DISEASE DURING PREGNANCY

- Activity restriction
- Close observation during pregnancy, labor, birth, and the postpartum period
- Additional sleep and rest
- Infection control
- Diet modification
- Team approach

Rh Incompatibility

At the beginning of prenatal care, the woman should be tested to determine whether she is Rh+ or Rh−. If she is Rh−, the father of the baby should have an Rh determination done as well. If the father is Rh−, all of their children will be Rh−, and there will not be a problem of incompatibility. However, if he is Rh+, there is a good possibility that the children will be Rh+, because the Rh+ gene is dominant and the Rh− gene is recessive. It is true that not all Rh+ men are homozygous for the Rh factor. In other words, a man may carry an Rh+ (dominant) gene and an Rh− (recessive) gene and be heterozygous. Thus, the offspring will have a chance of being Rh+ or a chance of being Rh−.

The problem of Rh incompatibility arises when an Rh− woman becomes pregnant by an Rh+ man and then carries an Rh+ fetus. When some of the Rh+ red blood cells from the fetus cross the placental barrier and enter the woman's bloodstream, the Rh+ red blood cells become antigens and stimulate the formation of antibodies against the Rh+ cells (Fig. 21–1).

Once the woman produces antibodies in her blood, she will always have them. In subsequent pregnancies with Rh+ fetuses, some of these antibodies will enter the circulation of the fetus. These antibodies will attack and destroy the fetus's red blood cells. The destruction of red cells produces anemia in the fetus, and in severe cases, referred to as *erythroblastosis fetalis,* fetal death can occur.

Maternal Rh sensitization (isoimmunization) can occur in other ways. The woman can become sensitized during a blood transfusion (with Rh+ blood), during an abortion of an Rh+ fetus, through amniocentesis, during ectopic pregnancy, from bleeding complications during the last trimester of pregnancy with an Rh+ infant, and during the time of placental separation immediately after birth of an Rh+ infant. The Rh− woman can be sensitized during pregnancy and/ or pregnancy complications only when she is carrying an Rh+ infant.

When a woman has a history that might lead to possible development of antibodies, she is carefully monitored during her pregnancy. Because transplacental hemorrhage is possible during pregnancy, Rh_o (D) immune globulin (RhoGAM) is often administered prophylactically at 28 weeks' gestation to prevent sensitization, if the woman has *not* been previously sensitized.

Postpartal management includes giving the Rh− mother who has no antibody titer (negative indirect Coombs test indicates nonsensitization) and who has delivered an Rh+ baby (negative direct Coombs test) an intramuscular injection of RhoGAM. She must receive RhoGAM within 72 hours after delivery of the baby so that she does not have time to produce antibodies to fetal cells that entered her bloodstream when the placenta separated. The administration of RhoGAM gives temporary passive immunity to the mother, which prevents the development of permanent active immunity (antibody formation) that would result in isoimmunization.

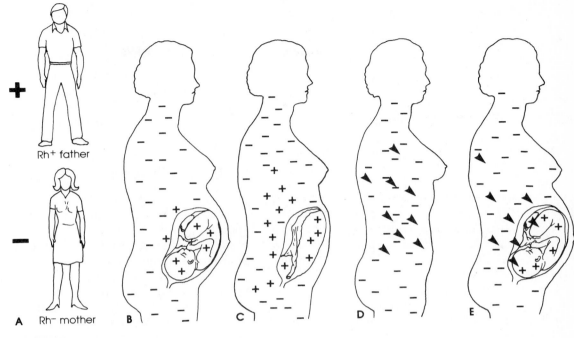

▲ **FIGURE 21–1**

Rh isoimmunization. **A.** Rh− mother and Rh+ father. **B.** Pregnant with Rh+ fetus. Some Rh+ fetal blood enters the mother's blood. **C.** During separation of placenta, further inoculation of mother by Rh+ red blood cells occurs. **D.** Mother becomes sensitized to Rh+ blood and develops Rh+ antibodies. Mother now has titer or positive Coombs test. **E.** During subsequent pregnancy with Rh+ fetus, maternal anti-Rh+ antibodies enter fetal circulation and cause hemolysis of fetal red blood cells.

NURSING ALERT: FACTS ABOUT Rh SENSITIZATION

- The potential for sensitization occurs when an Rh− woman and an Rh+ man conceive a fetus that is Rh+.
- If the woman becomes sensitized, her body will produce antibodies to her fetus's Rh+ blood.
- Tests used to detect antibody formation or sensitization:
  a. An indirect Coombs test is done on the mother's blood to measure the amount of Rh+ antibodies.
  b. A direct Coombs test is done on the baby's blood to detect antibody-coated Rh+ red blood cells.
- Depending on the results of laboratory test, the following interventions are considered:
  a. When the mother's indirect Coombs test is negative, she is given RhoGAM within 72 hours after birth of baby.
  b. When the mother's indirect Coombs test is positive and the Rh+ baby has a positive direct Coombs test, RhoGAM is not given; however, the baby is carefully monitored for potential hemolytic disease.
  c. It is currently recommended that RhoGAM be given at 28 weeks' gestation (prenatally) to reduce the potential fetal Rh+ cell reaction in the Rh− mother's bloodstream.
  d. RhoGAM should be administered after each amniocentesis, abortion, or ectopic pregnancy, and within 72 hours or less after birth of an Rh+ infant.
  e. Rh− mothers should be instructed about the process of Rh sensitization and the

importance of prophylactic injection of RhoGam.

f. Previous history of an Rh− mother's offspring outcome is important to the caregiver.

ASSESSMENT AND INTERVENTION

During the prenatal care, the nurse should explain what Rh− and Rh+ means. Also, the nurse should teach the woman how Rh sensitization takes place and the importance of receiving RhoGAM after each abortion, after an ectopic pregnancy, and if an amniocentesis is done. The nurse should also discuss the purpose of RhoGAM given at week 28 of pregnancy, if she is not already sensitized.

The caregiver should provide emotional support to the mother who is sensitized to the Rh factor. The mother should be told that there are ways to treat the infant, should the infant require special care (see Chapter 24).

ABO Incompatibility

Maternal–fetal blood incompatibility may also occur when the mother has type O blood and the infant is type A or B. This condition is referred to as *ABO incompatibility*. It usually is a less serious complication than Rh incompatibility.

In blood types, there are two kinds of antigens, A and B. In type O blood neither antigen is present. Therefore, when the fetus inherits A or B blood from the father and the mother has type O blood, fetal blood may cross through the placenta and cause the mother to be sensitized to antigens foreign to her blood type. The most common ABO incompatibility occurs when the mother is type O and the infant is type A or B. ABO incompatibility can affect the first-born infant, usually with jaundice, within the first 24 hours. After birth, antibodies may be detected by the Coombs test. To date, there is no immunoglobulin such as RhoGAM to counter the antibody formation in the sensitized mother.

Bleeding Disorders

Bleeding during pregnancy is abnormal and should be evaluated for its cause. When it occurs early in pregnancy, the most common causes are abortion, ectopic pregnancy, and hydatidiform mole. Bleeding that occurs late in pregnancy is most commonly caused by placenta previa and abruptio placentae. These two conditions involve the area of the uterus where the placenta is attached and the premature separation of the placenta from the uterus. Both complications can cause severe maternal blood loss and compromise the fetus (Table 21–6).

BLEEDING EARLY IN PREGNANCY

- Abortion
- Ectopic pregnancy
- Hydatidiform mole

BLEEDING LATE IN PREGNANCY

- Placenta previa
- Abruptio placentae

Spotting is relatively common during pregnancy. Because the cervix is highly vascular, strenuous activity can cause spotting. However, bleed-

---

KEY POINTS IN EDUCATION: PATIENT EDUCATION ON Rh FACTOR

- Explain the Rh factor to the woman.
- Explain how the Rh factor can affect the infant.
- Discuss the purpose of administration of RhoGAM during pregnancy and
after birth, abortion, and amniocentesis.
- Explain diagnostic tests.
- Discuss the possibility of an early delivery.

TABLE 21–6. DIFFERENTIATION BETWEEN PLACENTA PREVIA AND ABRUPTIO PLACENTAE[a]

SIGNS	PLACENTA PREVIA	ABRUPTIO PLACENTAE
Implantation	Lower ⅓ of uterus.	Normal
Onset	Frequently quiet for first episode of bleeding.	Stormy in moderate to severe abruptions.
Placenta	Palpable.	Nonpalpable.
Pain	None—painless bleeding (most significant sign).	May be cramp-like to severe.
Abdomen and uterus	Soft, not tender. May be contracting normally.	May or may not be tender to rigid.
Bleeding	External, bright red bleeding. Shock with excessive bleeding.	External and/or internal, either bright or dark blood. Woman may have signs of shock that are out of proportion to bleeding.
Blood pressure	Blood pressure usually normal. After excessive bleeding, hypovolemic shock can occur.	History of hypertension and toxemia. Postabruption hypovolemic shock can occur.
Fetal death	Depends on fetal maturity.	Fetal distress to fetal death may occur.
Coagulation defect	Not a problem.	Coagulation defect (DIC[b]) with moderate to severe abruption can be a complication.

[a]Several placental separations are mild and produce few or no symptoms; these separations are detected when the placenta is inspected after delivery.
[b]Disseminated intravascular coagulation.

ing also can be due to a life-threatening condition such as placenta previa. Therefore, every woman is asked to report bleeding during pregnancy so it can be assessed for its cause.

GOALS OF MEDICAL AND NURSING MANAGEMENT OF BLEEDING

- To prevent or control bleeding
- To establish the cause of bleeding
- To maintain the pregnancy and deliver a viable fetus, if possible
- To provide emergency care when necessary
- Replace blood loss
- Perform a cesarean birth when indicated
- Treat a compromised infant, whether premature or full term
- To provide psychological support to the woman and family for grief resulting from the loss of infant, loss of positive self-concept of the mother, or both

The major causes of bleeding during pregnancy are discussed in this chapter. Postpartum hemorrhage and interruption of pregnancy are discussed in Chapter 23.

ABORTION

Abortion is the termination of pregnancy before the fetus is viable (20 weeks' gestation or a weight of 500 g [1.1 lb]). Spontaneous abortions (miscarriages) occur because of natural causes. Induced abortion is a deliberate separation of the products of conception (fetus, placenta, and membranes) from the uterus for medical (therapeutic) or social (elective) reasons.

About 15% of all pregnancies terminate in spontaneous abortions. The majority of these abortions occur before the eighth week of gestation. A large number of abortions are due to fetal or placental developmental defects. Others are the result of maternal conditions or unknown causes.

Specific causes are as follows: defective ovum or sperm; defective implantation; maternal factors, including chronic conditions, acute infections, and nutritional deficiencies; abnormalities of maternal reproductive organs; and endocrine deficiencies. Blood group dyscrasias (ABO and Rh) can also cause an abortion. Psychological and physical trauma have been implicated, but there is little documented evidence that either is a major cause.

Counseling the woman and family after an abortion is very important. Once the woman has had a spontaneous abortion, she often asks, "What is my chance to carry a baby to term?" If this was a first abortion, her chances of abortion are 15%, or the same as a woman who has never had an abortion. Abortions are common obstetrical problems, and it is easy for caregivers to take them lightly. However, to the woman and to her family, regardless of whether the pregnancy was planned, the loss is often accompanied with some guilt. Many women go through the same grieving process as that caused by other types of personal loss.

When spontaneous abortion becomes a question, ultrasound scanning may be used to detect the presence of a gestational sac and to assess if there is a live embryo/fetus. The woman usually is asked to abstain from sexual intercourse. If the abortion (loss of the products of conception) appears to be imminent, the woman is hospitalized. Intravenous therapy is started to replace the fluid loss. Blood transfusions usually are not necessary and surgical intervention such as a dilatation and curettage (D&C) may be necessary to remove the remainder of the products of conception in order to stop the bleeding (fewer blood transfusions are now given to avoid the possibility of contamination with pathogens including HIV). If the pregnancy is beyond 12 weeks' gestation, an induction of labor may be done to expel a dead fetus.

Abortions are clinically defined according to symptoms and whether the products of conception are partially or completely retained or expelled (Table 21–7).

CLASSIFICATION OF SPONTANEOUS ABORTIONS

- Threatened abortion
- Inevitable (imminent) abortion
- Complete abortion
- Incomplete abortion
- Habitual abortion
- Missed abortion

Threatened Abortion

The clinical findings of a threatened abortion are bleeding and cramping. No cervical changes occur, and no products of conception are passed. The symptoms subside, and the pregnancy is carried to term. The patient management includes bed rest and close monitoring of the amount of bleeding (spotting to heavier amounts) and of passage of tissue. When the bleeding stops, the woman is usually allowed to begin physical and sexual activity. Progressive growth of the uterus is a favorable sign that pregnancy is continuing.

Inevitable (Imminent) Abortion

The clinical finding of the inevitable abortion is a progression in severity of symptoms. The bleeding becomes heavier, the uterine cramping is more pronounced, and the cervix becomes dilated. The pregnancy cannot be salvaged, and some or all of the products of conception are passed. Two of the chief concerns are the control of hemorrhage and the removal of retained tissue. A D&C is often necessary to remove the remaining tissue and thereby stop the bleeding.

There are two types of inevitable abortions: complete and incomplete abortions. Both end in the loss of the pregnancy.

Complete Abortion. When all the products of conception are expelled, the abortion is called *complete*. If the bleeding stops and if no other symptoms appear, usually no special treatment is necessary.

Incomplete Abortion. Symptoms of an incomplete abortion include bleeding, some discharge of tissue, and abdominal cramping. Hospitalization is necessary. Bed rest, assessment of the amount of bleeding, and observation for passage of tissue are an important part of care. A D&C is often needed to remove tissue and stop bleeding.

TABLE 21–7. COMPARISON OF TYPES AND MANAGEMENT OF SPONTANEOUS ABORTION (MISCARRIAGE)[a]

TYPE	CRAMPS	BLEEDING	TISSUE PASSED	CERVICAL OPENING	UTERINE SIZE	CARE AND MANAGEMENT
Threatened	Slight	Slight to moderate	None	Closed	Commensurate with date	Bed rest, sedation,[b] avoidance of coitus, ultrasound. Observe bleeding (save pads). Woman to gradually increase activity. Do pregnancy tests. Give Rh$_o$ (D) immune globulin within 72 hr if indicated.
Inevitable	Moderate	Moderate to severe	Placental or fetal tissue	Open with membranes or tissues bulging the ruptured membranes.	Commensurate with date	Bed rest, sedation. Transfusion often indicated. Observe bleeding (save pads). Give Rh$_o$ (D) immune globulin if indicated.
Incomplete	Severe	Severe and continuous	Placental or fetal tissue	Open with tissue in cervical canal or passage of tissue	Smaller than date	Bed rest, sedation. Observe to determine how much tissue is passed; save all available tissue. Carefully record vital signs. D&C as necessary. Give Rh$_o$ (D) immune globulin if indicated.
Complete	None	Minimal	Complete placenta and fetus	Closed with no tissue in cervical canal	Smaller than date	Observe to determine if all tissue passed (save pads). Give Rh$_o$ (D) immune globulin if indicated.
Missed	None; no life felt	Brownish discharge	None	Closed	Smaller than expected	No specific treatment available. Oxytocics may be used to induce labor and delivery. Check for coagulation defect (DIC[c]).
Habitual						Comprehensive and conservative care essential in early months. Shirodkar surgery done if necessary.

[a]Psychologically, many patients experience a grief period and have fears of inability and inadequacy as a woman. They express anxiety over next pregnancy or ability to conceive again.

[b]Drugs are kept to a minimum to safeguard the fetus.

[c]Disseminated intravascular coagulation.

Habitual Abortion

When the woman has had three or more spontaneous abortions, she is referred to as a *habitual aborter*. The most common reason for this condition is an incompetent cervix. The cervix dilates without perceivable contractions, and the products of conception are expelled. In other words, the internal os of the cervix dilates, making it incapable of supporting the increasing weight and pressure of the growing fetus. For the woman to carry a fetus to term, often the cervix is reinforced surgically, with a heavy ligature placed submucosally around the cervix. This procedure is called *Shirodkar surgery*. If a heavy silk purse-string suture is used, it is called *McDonald's procedure*. When the pregnancy reaches term or labor begins, the suture is cut and labor is allowed to progress. Shirodkar surgery should be done by 12 weeks' gestation, and there always is a chance of rupturing the membranes. Therefore, the best time for the surgical procedure is before the next pregnancy.

Missed Abortion

If the embryo dies, it is usually expelled from the uterus within weeks. If the fetus has not been expelled for 6 or more weeks, or even years, it is called a *missed abortion*. After the death of the fetus, there is a loss of the symptoms of pregnancy, such as breast tenderness and nausea. The uterus shrinks and returns to the nonpregnant state. If the fetus is retained, it can become calcified. The complication that can occur with missed abortion is disseminated intravascular coagulation (DIC) (see Coagulation Defects). A woman with a missed abortion needs a great deal of psychological support by caregivers.

The following nursing diagnoses are listed to assist the nurse in the assessment and care of a woman who has had an unexpected termination of pregnancy.

NURSING DIAGNOSES

• Fear related to potential loss of pregnancy
• Knowledge deficit related to the cause of abortion

• Pain related to abdominal cramping with contractions of uterine muscles
• Disturbance in self-esteem related to feelings of guilt and blame for abortion
• Potential for injury related to retention of tissue and surgery required to empty uterus
• Spiritual distress because couple's preference in religious rites is not carried out
• Potential for injury owing to possible isoimmunization of an Rh− mother

ECTOPIC (EXTRAUTERINE) PREGNANCY

Ectopic pregnancy is the abnormal implantation of the fertilized ovum outside the uterine cavity (Fig. 21–2). Most frequently, implantation occurs in some portion of the fallopian (uterine) tube. Other sites, although rare, include the ovary, the abdominal cavity, and the cervix. Because the uterine tube is not anatomically suited for implantation, the trophoblast cells erode the blood vessels and weaken the tissue, and the tube ruptures. The tubal rupture can cause a fatal hemorrhage. Predisposing conditions include any factor that affects tubal patency, ciliary action, and contractility. Two prominent causes are partial tubal occlusion secondary to pelvic infection and the use of an intrauterine contraceptive device.

The treatment of ectopic pregnancy consists of early recognition of the complication. The ruptured tube is surgically removed (salpingectomy) as soon as it is diagnosed to prevent a massive hemorrhage. Replacement of fluid loss and maintenance of electrolytes are essential aspects of treatment.

Characteristically, the woman misses one or two menstrual periods and then may have stabbing pain in either lower abdominal quadrant. These signs may or may not be followed by vaginal spotting. Shoulder pain caused by blood irritating the diaphragm is a common symptom. If a mass of old blood is found in the cul de sac of Douglas (pouch formed with fold of peritoneum in posterior wall of the uterus), the diagnosis of ectopic pregnancy is almost confirmed. The signs of shock that develop are out of proportion to the apparent blood loss, because most of the blood lost is hidden within the abdominal cavity. This is one

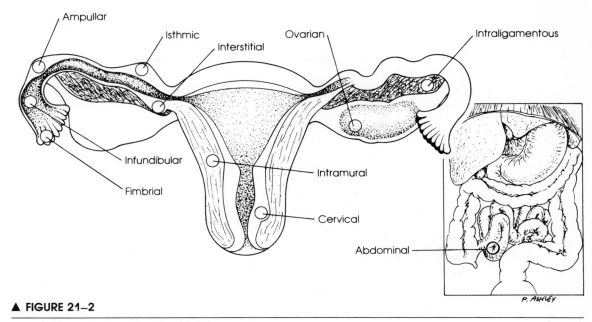

▲ **FIGURE 21–2**

Various implantation sites in ectopic pregnancy.

obstetrical complication in which rapid surgical treatment can save the woman's life. The incidence of ectopic pregnancy is approximately 1 in every 250 pregnancies. Fetal mortality is near 100%, and maternal mortality in the United States approaches 1 in 800 cases.

NURSING DIAGNOSES

- Potential for injury due to rupture of tube and maternal shock
- Potential for infection due to massive blood loss
- Pain related to bleeding into abdominal cavity
- Anticipatory grieving related to the loss of the pregnancy

HYDATIDIFORM MOLE (GESTATIONAL TROPHOBLASTIC DISEASE)

Hydatidiform mole (sometimes shortened to *hydatid mole*) is a developmental placental abnormality of trophoblastic cells that causes the chorionic villi to become swollen and to degenerate into grape-like clusters. This condition is a developmental anomaly of the placenta; there is no fetus. A retained, blighted ovum may sometimes be found (Fig. 21–3).

The cause is unknown, but the incidence increases with maternal age and parity. Women over 40 years of age who have had three or more pregnancies are at greater risk for molar pregnancy. In the United States, this condition is fairly rare, occurring in 1 in 2000 pregnancies. However, in parts of Asia and the South Pacific, the incidence can be as high as 1 in 500 pregnancies. Because of a high incidence (30%) of the extremely malignant *choriocarcinoma* following a molar pregnancy, a hysterectomy is often the treatment of choice. If the woman desires another pregnancy, the uterus is evacuated with a D&C, and the woman is closely monitored for the following year.

A hydatidiform mole should be suspected when there is severe nausea and vomiting in the first trimester; marked elevation in human chorionic gonadotropin (hCG) level; persistent vaginal bleeding, sometimes with passage of vesicles; signs of preeclampsia before the twentieth week of gestation; and absence of fetal parts or fetal heart tones.

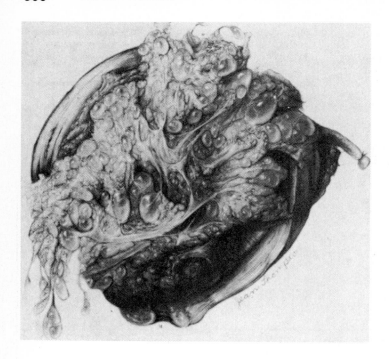

▲ FIGURE 21–3

A uterus containing a hydatidiform mole. (From Page, E. W., Villee, C. A., & Villee, D. B. (1981). *Human Reproduction*, 3rd ed. Phila- delphia, W. B. Saunders Company.)

Assessment and Management

Early diagnosis is often made by the use of ultrasonography, which reveals no fetus. Once the diagnosis is made, patient instruction becomes very important. The woman must understand the importance of close monitoring and the need for surgical intervention. She may need assistance in working through her grief over the loss of her pregnancy. Also, she needs to know the risk of choriocarcinoma and the importance of frequent assessment of hCG levels for the following year. HCG levels are monitored every month for 1 year. The woman is often placed on oral contraceptives to prevent another pregnancy and allow the hCG levels to return to normal. A pregnancy would make it impossible to monitor the decline in hCG, which is the significant part of follow-up care. If malignant cells are found, the woman is placed on chemotherapy. The drug methotrexate is often used. The woman should be instructed about the side effects of this drug. If the hCG levels remain normal for 1 year, another pregnancy can be attempted safely.

PLACENTA PREVIA

Placenta previa is the abnormal implantation of the placenta in the lower portion of the uterus instead of the upper portion. The placenta covers some portion of the cervical opening when the cervix is fully dilated. There are three types of placenta previa, classified according to the degree of coverage of the cervical os by the placenta either prior to or during labor. (The type of classification can change during labor.) The types of placenta previa are as follows (Fig. 21–4):

- Complete or total placental previa—The placenta totally covers the internal os.
- Partial placenta previa—The placenta covers only part of the internal os.
- Low-lying or marginal placenta previa—The placenta is near the cervical opening but does not cover it.

The cause is unknown; however, reduced vascularity or previous infection in the upper uterine segment appears to increase the risk. Because the lower uterine segment is not as vascular as the upper segment, the placenta must cover a larger area for adequate function. The surface area covered by the placenta may be 30% greater than when the placenta is normally implanted in the upper part of the uterus.

Placenta previa should be suspected when there is onset of *painless bleeding* in the last half of

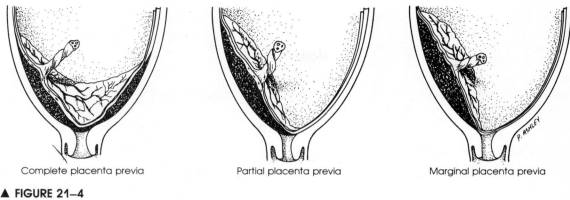

Complete placenta previa   Partial placenta previa   Marginal placenta previa

▲ **FIGURE 21–4**

Types of placenta previa.

pregnancy. Painless bleeding is due to the separation from the uterus of that part of the placenta that is near, or covering, the internal cervical os.

Clinical Findings

Painless bleeding is the most reliable sign of placenta previa. The bleeding is of maternal and not of fetal origin. Bleeding may be intermittent or in gushes. It is rarely continuous in the beginning. Also, the initial episode of vaginal bleeding is usually slight. Later, the bleeding can be extensive and can prove to be fatal. An abnormal fetal presentation may coexist in 15% to 20% of the cases. Therefore, a breech or transverse presentation should suggest the possibility of placenta previa. Ultrasonography can locate the attachment area of the placenta and can aid in the diagnosis.

Complications

The main complications are hemorrhage for the woman and prematurity for the infant. Immediate postpartum hemorrhage often accompanies this condition because the surface area of attachment is greater and the site of placental implantation in the lower uterine segment does not contract well after the placenta is expelled. Postpartum infection may also occur because of the closeness of the placental site to the cervix and vagina. Microorganisms may be introduced directly into the

uterus. Because of this, the woman is closely monitored postnatally for bleeding and infection.

Assessment and Intervention

Management is based on the amount of bleeding and the duration of pregnancy. The goal is to provide conservative treatment until the infant is mature enough to survive when born. No vaginal examinations should be done without a "double set-up" in a room where a cesarean birth can be done immediately if the bleeding becomes profuse. The infant's maturity should be assessed by evaluating the lecithin/sphingomyelin ratio for lung maturity (see Chapter 8). If premature labor begins, a drug such as betamethasone might be given to attempt to accelerate fetal pulmonary maturation. If bleeding is severe, a cesarean birth is done regardless of the number of gestational weeks to protect the mother's life. Laboratory blood tests, including type and cross-match, are carried out immediately on admission to the hospital, and usually one or two units of blood are made available for the woman. Psychological support is an important part of nursing care. An understanding of the management of this complication usually will decrease the woman's and family's anxiety.

Fetal Implications

The prognosis for the fetus depends on the type of placenta previa, the extent of bleeding, and the gestational age of the fetus. Fetal heart rate monitoring should be continuous during a bleeding episode. In profuse bleeding, the fetus is compromised and can suffer some hypoxia (lack of oxygen). After birth, blood sampling is done to determine whether the bleeding episode of the woman caused anemia in the newborn.

NURSING DIAGNOSES

- Potential fluid volume deficit due to blood loss
- Fear of loss of pregnancy
- Knowledge deficit related to lack of understanding of the measures involved in attempt to retain pregnancy for fetal lung development
- Anxiety related to procedures such as electronic fetal monitoring

ABRUPTIO PLACENTAE

Abruptio placentae is the premature (before the birth of the infant) separation of the normally implanted placenta from the wall of the uterus. Abruptio placentae may occur at any time after the twentieth week of gestation, but it is most common in the last trimester. The primary cause is unknown; however, several factors appear to increase its incidence. It is associated with maternal hypertension and is more common in multiparous, high-parity, and older women. Other predisposing factors are a short umbilical cord and a precipitous labor. Approximately one-third of all placental separations are mild and produce few or no symptoms. In many of these cases, the condition is not detected until the placenta is inspected after delivery. In other instances the bleeding is severe, and both fetal and maternal compromise may occur. The degree depends on the extent of the separation and the amount of blood loss (see Nursing Care Plan 21–2).

Abruptio placentae is subdivided into two types (Fig. 21–5):

- Marginal or partial separation of the placenta—This type usually has external drainage of blood through the cervix.
- Complete separation of the placenta—This

type allows blood to be trapped behind the placenta, and there may or may not be evidence of external bleeding.

Complications

If the blood is trapped behind the placenta (concealed bleeding), the woman experiences severe pain. Her uterus becomes irritable and is rigid on palpation. If the blood gets into the muscles of the uterus, it may be difficult for the uterus to contract after the delivery of the infant and placenta. Also, trapping of the blood may release thromboplastin into the maternal circulation. This event can cause the risk of DIC (discussed below).

Assessment and Intervention

Management includes early diagnosis of excessive bleeding. Continuous fetal monitoring is necessary, because the fetus can become distressed. Laboratory work-up should include blood type and cross-match and a coagulation profile. Usually two units of blood are made available. The woman should be prepared for a cesarean birth or an immediate vaginal delivery (whichever is quicker) if the hemorrhage is severe or if the infant becomes distressed (Table 21–8).

Continuous monitoring for DIC is part of the care. The caregiver should assess for signs of unusual bleeding from the gums, epistaxis, and petechiae. Psychological support should be given to the woman and family when possible.

NURSING DIAGNOSES

- Fluid volume deficit related to hemorrhage
- Altered tissue perfusion in fetus, related to the degree of placental separation
- Pain related to retroplacental bleeding
- Anxiety related to fear for self and infant

DISSEMINATED INTRAVASCULAR COAGULATION

DIC is the overstimulation of the normal coagulation process. Massive, rapid fibrin formation

NURSING CARE PLAN 21–2

MANAGEMENT OF THE WOMAN WITH BLEEDING LATE IN PREGNANCY DUE TO ABRUPTIO PLACENTAE

Potential Problems and Nursing Diagnoses	Nursing Interventions
1. Anxiety related to threat to self-esteem and loss of fetus.	Explain that the presence of vaginal bleeding does not mean the baby will not live.
2. Altered tissue perfusion related to blood loss.	Monitor vital signs for increase in pulse rate and decrease in blood pressure. Monitor for signs of shock (clammy skin, pallor). Assess need for oxygen.
3. Knowledge deficit related to degree of placental separation and where it occus.	Determine that signs and symptoms correlate with type and amount of placental separation.
4. Pain related to intensity of uterine contractions.	Recognize that increase in intensity of contractions causes pain or discomfort. Assess need for medication.
5. Fluid volume deficit related to blood loss.	Maintain an open intravenous infusion. Observe, record, and report amount of blood on pads, chux, and sheets. Observe skin color for pallor, faintness, and other signs of shock.
6. Potential for injury related to infection.	Monitor vital signs every 2 hours. Report significant change. Maintain open intravenous infusion for potential administration of antibiotics.
7. Spiritual distress related to baptismal rights for baby.	Determine woman's or couple's decision to see a member of the clergy.

Expected Outcomes

1. Woman verbalizes understanding that vaginal bleeding does not mean infant will die.
2. Woman recognizes need for close observation of vital signs and possible need for administration of oxygen.
3. Woman verbalizes understanding of placental separation before birth of baby.
4. Woman communicates level of discomfort and need for medication.
5. Woman recognizes need to assess amount of blood loss and will inform caregiver if she feels dizzy or faint.
6. Vital signs are within normal limits.
7. Woman communicates a desire to see a member of the clergy and discuss religious concerns.

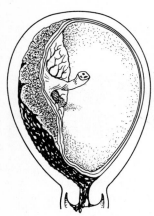
Partial separation

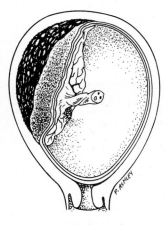
Complete separation

▲ FIGURE 21–5

Abruptio placentae.

results. This condition causes the widespread appearance of small thrombi in the small blood vessels.

Owing to the amount of clotting and to the rapidity with which DIC occurs, the blood platelets and clotting factors are depleted. The end product of the clot lysis can have an anticoagulant effect. The following clinical problems may occur:

- A tendency toward generalized bleeding (because the clotting factors are depleted)

TABLE 21–8. GENERAL CARE OF THE WOMAN WITH EXCESSIVE BLEEDING

Estimate blood loss.
Monitor vital signs frequently.
Assess presence and character of:
  Pain;
  Uterine tenderness;
  Abdominal and uterine rigidity.
Have woman's blood typed and cross-matched.
Start or maintain intravenous infusion.
Observe for signs of shock.
Prepare woman for surgery, as indicated.
If bleeding is late in pregnancy:
  Monitor fetal heart tones;
  Monitor labor contractions;
  Assess if woman's vaginal examination should be omitted;
  Order coagulation profile test studies;
  Prepare for infant resuscitation.

- Ischemia of the vital organs (owing to obstruction in the blood vessels)
- Severe anemia (owing to excessive bleeding)

DIC does not occur as the primary disorder but rather occurs secondary to some other complication. It can occur in abruptio placentae, PIH, retained products of conception, and septic abortions. In addition, infection can activate the coagulation pathway. This disorder is best resolved by correcting the underlying cause, which may require terminating the pregnancy or treating the infection.

The nurse can help in the early diagnosis of DIC by being alert to signs of bleeding and vascular occlusion. Bleeding from the gums or injection sites, epistaxis, and the presence of petechiae on the skin are signs of developing DIC. Providing emotional support for the woman and her family is an important part of nursing care.

Infections During Pregnancy

Sexually transmitted diseases, including syphilis, gonorrhea, chlamydia, herpes simplex, cytomegalovirus, hepatitis B, and acquired immune deficiency syndrome (AIDS) are discussed in Chapter 7. Rubella, tuberculosis, toxoplasmosis, and urinary tract infections are discussed in this section.

RUBELLA

Rubella, or German measles, is caused by a virus that usually produces a mild rash, which lasts for about 3 days. It may be so mild that many women may not know whether they have had it during their childhood. Estimates are that approximately 10% to 22% of all pregnant women are susceptible to rubella. The only accurate method of screening for rubella is performing a test for hemagglutination inhibition (HAI). The presence of a 1:16 HAI titer is evidence of immunity. A titer of less than 1:8 HAI indicates susceptibility. If a repeated test shows an elevated titer, the woman has recently acquired the infection.

If the woman has rubella during the first 3 months of pregnancy, there can be fetal damage. However, the most critical time of severe fetal damage is during the first 8 weeks of pregnancy, while the fetal organs are being formed. Routine, prenatal antigen-titer testing should be done. If the titer is 1:8 or less, every effort should be made to prevent the mother from exposure during the remainder of her pregnancy.

Immunization

The primary approach to rubella is immunization. This should protect the woman from the rubella infection. The vaccine should be given during childhood. Also, women who have a rubella titer of less than 1:10 are often given rubella vaccine in the postpartum period. Women of childbearing age should be instructed not to become pregnant for 3 months after vaccination. Of course, a woman who might be pregnant should *not* be given the vaccine.

Fetal Complications

If the woman is pregnant when she has rubella, the infant is likely to be born with a major abnormality. Rubella can cause a defect of major organs. The fetus can have defects in the heart, eyes, ears, brain, liver, and spleen. Also, the infant may be born with an active viral infection. The isolation of these infants is mandatory.

A therapeutic abortion is often suggested to the woman who has rubella during the first 3 months of pregnancy. Nursing support and understanding are essential at this time because such a decision is most difficult even for one with an unplanned pregnancy.

TOXOPLASMOSIS

Toxoplasmosis is caused by the parasite *Toxoplasma gondii*. It is innocuous in adults, but when contracted during pregnancy, it can be transmitted to the fetus with damaging effects. Toxoplasmosis can be contracted by eating raw or poorly cooked meat or by coming in contact with the feces of infected animals. In the United States, the most common carrier is the cat, which transmits the infection by way of its feces. Because cats serve as a reservoir of toxoplasmosis, the caregiver should inquire about their presence in the home. A pregnant woman who is exposed to cats should be alerted to the potential risk of *Toxoplasma* infection and should avoid close contact with cats.

Toxoplasmosis is important because the organism can produce clinically vague (flu-like) symptoms in the mother but can produce severe forms of congenital infection in the fetus. The risk to the fetus appears to be related to the timing of maternal infection during pregnancy. If the mother is infected early in pregnancy, the congenital infection is more severe. The incidence of abortions, stillbirths, and neonatal deaths is increased when the mother is infected. Other conditions seen in infants are neurological abnormalities, microcephaly, and hydrocephaly. Jaundice, seizures, and abnormal cerebrospinal fluid are manifestations in the newborn infant. Currently, there is no way to predict the outcome of subclinical or asymptomatic congenital *Toxoplasma* infection in an infant.

The diagnosis can be established by doing serological tests, such as the Sabin-Feldman dye test. When acute toxoplasmosis has been diagnosed during the first 20 weeks of pregnancy, an abortion may be considered. The use of drugs such as spiramycin and pyrimethamine in pregnant women with toxoplasmosis should be considered experimental; these drugs not indicated for general use.

TUBERCULOSIS

Tuberculosis is caused by the tubercle bacillus. It most commonly infects the lungs, but the bacillus may invade other organs. Pulmonary tuberculosis is characterized by a productive cough, low-grade fever, weight loss, and fatigue. As the disease progresses, large areas of lung tissue may become involved, and the woman may spit up bright red blood and become dyspneic on exertion. The disease is a problem for both the mother and the infant, because the disease may be worsened by pregnancy and postpartum demands, and it may be transmitted to the newborn infant.

A pregnant woman with tuberculosis should be under close medical supervision. Drug therapy with medications, such as ethambutol, streptomycin, and isoniazid, have made the outlook for treating tuberculosis much more optimistic. As a rule, general anesthetics are avoided at the time of birth. The woman should not care for her baby until she is noninfectious. Thus, breastfeeding is not recommended. The disease is said to be inactive when no bacilli are found in the sputum or gastric washes.

Because tuberculosis is still an ever-present health problem, especially among low-income groups, a skin test is used as an important case-finding tool. If the woman's history puts her at risk for potential tuberculosis, a skin test should be carried out during prenatal care.

URINARY TRACT INFECTIONS

Urinary tract infection (UTI) affects 5% to 20% of pregnant women. During pregnancy, anatomical changes in the urinary tract predispose women to infections. The growing uterus compresses both ureters, which decreases the flow to the bladder, thereby causing urinary stasis. Dilatation of the renal structures and a rotation of the uterus toward the right side cause compression of the right kidney and ureter, which accounts for increased infection on the right side. In addition, because of the alteration in the renal system during pregnancy, the incidence of glycosuria (glucose in the urine) is increased, which predisposes the woman to UTI. The organism most commonly found in UTI during pregnancy is *Escherichia coli (E. coli)* because in the female, the urinary meatus is near the rectum.

There are three clinical types of UTI during pregnancy: asymptomatic, lower tract (cystitis), and upper tract (pyelonephritis). Some of the asymptomatic women with UTI develop upper tract infections. It is important to inform patients of this so that they can practice preventive health care, because pyelonephritis is a serious problem to the mother and fetus. The symptoms and signs of UTI vary with the site and degree of infection. The significant symptoms are dysuria, increased frequency of urination, urgency, and hematuria (with cystitis). Backache, elevated temperature,

---

KEY POINTS IN EDUCATION: PATIENT EDUCATION ON URINARY TRACT INFECTION

- Explain to the woman the predisposing causes of UTI during pregnancy.
- Encourage an increase in fluid intake to decrease risk of infection.
- Explain the method of obtaining a "clean-catch," midstream-voided urine specimen.
- Instruct the woman to cleanse her perineal area from front to back to avoid vaginal contamination with *E. coli.*
- Suggest the following: (a) a source of vitamin C daily to promote healing, (b) a glass of cranberry juice at bedtime to acidify urine, (c) a list of foods high in iron, (d) avoidance of coffee, tea, alcohol, and spices, because they are potential bladder irritants
- Counsel the woman to empty her bladder frequently and never ignore her urge to void.
- If drugs are ordered, explain the importance of maintaining medication schedules to keep blood levels stable.
- Instruct the woman to keep all appointments with the clinic or physician.

and tenderness over the kidney area occur with pyelonephritis. Septic shock and death, though rare, can occur with upper tract infections.

Assessment and Intervention

The nurse or physician, or both, should ask the woman at each prenatal visit if she has any signs or symptoms of UTI. If symptoms are present, a "clean-catch" urine specimen for microanalysis, culture, and sensitivity tests should be ordered. If the urine shows infection, ampicillin is usually the drug of choice. Antibiotics cross the placenta, and some have adverse effects on the fetus. Tetracycline causes bone and infant tooth discoloration, chloramphenicol (Chloromycetin) can cause gray baby syndrome, and sulfonamides have the potential to bind to albumin and thereby displace bilirubin.

References

Auvenshine, M. A., & Enriquez, M. G. (1990). *Comprehensive Maternity Nursing: Perinatal and Women's Health,* 2nd ed. Boston: Jones and Bartlett.

Bokak, I. M., & Jensen, M. D. (1991). *Essentials of Maternity Nursing,* 3rd ed. St. Louis: Mosby Year Book.

Creasy, R. K., & Resnik, R. (1989). *Maternal-Fetal Medicine: Principles and Practice,* 2nd ed. Philadelphia: W. B. Saunders Company.

Dickason, E. J., Schult, M. O., & Silverman, B. L. (1990). *Maternal-Infant Nursing Care.* St. Louis: C. V. Mosby.

Hernandez, C., & Cunningham, F. (1990). Eclampsia. *Clinical Obstetrics and Gynecology* 33:460–472.

Ladewig, P. W., London, M. L., & Olds, S. B. (1990). *Essentials of Maternal-Newborn Nursing,* 2nd ed. Redwood City, CA: Addison-Wesley Nursing.

Lavery, J. P. (1990). Placenta previa. *Clinical Obstetrics and Gynecology* 33:414–421.

May, K. A., & Mahlmeister, L. R. (1990). *Comprehensive Maternity Nursing: Nursing Process and the Childbearing Family,* 2nd ed. Philadelphia: J. B. Lippincott.

Sherwen, L. N., Scoloveno, M. A., & Weingarten, C. T. (1991). *Nursing Care of the Childbearing Family.* Norwalk, CT: Appleton & Lange.

White, P. (1974). Diabetes mellitus in pregnancy. *Clinics in Perinatology* 1:331.

SUGGESTED ACTIVITIES

1. List the leading causes of high-risk pregnancies.
2. Describe the symptoms, prevention, and management of four common conditions that complicate pregnancy.
3. Explain the causes and management of infectious diseases that complicate pregnancy.

REVIEW QUESTIONS

A. Select the best answer to each multiple-choice question.

1. Mrs. A. comes to the emergency room complaining of abdominal cramps and vaginal spotting. A vaginal examination reveals that her cervix is 1 cm dilated with no tissue passed. The diagnosis likely is
   A. Threatened abortion
   B. Inevitable abortion
   C. Habitual abortion
   D. Complete abortion

2. In the third trimester of pregnancy, painless, vaginal bleeding is a classic symptom of
   A. Placenta previa
   B. Spontaneous abortion
   C. Hydatidiform mole
   D. Tubal pregnancy

3. Ms. B., 2 months pregnant, comes to the clinic complaining of severe cramps and vaginal bleeding. She mentions that she expelled "something" when she was voiding, after which her cramps increased in intensity. Because it is likely that Ms. B. expelled some of the products of conception and that some tissue is retained, the diagnosis probably is
   A. A complete abortion
   B. An incomplete abortion
   C. A threatened abortion
   D. A missed abortion

4. Gestational trophoblastic disease, known as hydatidiform mole, is suspected if
   A. Severe nausea and vomiting occur during   C. Vesicles are passed
      pregnancy   ✓D. All of the above
   B. Human chorionic gonadotropin is markedly
      elevated

5. Pregnancy-induced hypertension (PIH) is characterized by the following triad:
   A. Hypertension, glucosuria, and edema   C. Edema, excessive weight gain, and hypertension
   B. Hypertension, vomiting, and proteinuria   D. Edema, hypertension, and proteinuria

6. The nurse should withhold MgSO₄ if all of the following are found EXCEPT
   A. Respirations below 14/minute   C. Dull reflexes
   B. Urine output less than 30 mL/hour   ✓D. Increase in heart rate of 5 bpm

7. To avoid the possibility of contacting toxoplasmosis, the pregnant woman should be advised to
   ✓A. Avoid contact with cat feces   C. Avoid touching dog hair
   B. Avoid contact with any animals   D. Avoid exposure to the spirochete

8. PIH most often occurs after the
   A. 12th week of pregnancy   C. 20th week of pregnancy
   B. 16th week of pregnancy   ✓D. 34th week of pregnancy

9. The woman with PIH has a greater incidence of all of the following in her history EXCEPT
   A. Diabetes   ✓C. Member of middle socioeconomic group
   B. Chronic hypertension   D. Increased kidney function

10. The woman who has the beginning signs of PIH should be instructed to carry out all of the following
    EXCEPT
    A. Bed rest   ✓C. Reduction of protein in diet
    B. Side-lying position   D. Reduction of anxiety

11. Hyperemesis gravidarum—excessive nausea and vomiting—is influenced by all of the following EXCEPT
    A. Increased hormones   C. Psychological disturbances
    B. Metabolic disturbances   ✓D. Excessive eating

12. The most common causes of bleeding in early pregnancy are
    A. Abortion, incompetent cervix, and ectopic   C. Ectopic pregnancy, placenta previa, and
       pregnancy   hydatidiform mole
    ✓B. Abortion, ectopic pregnancy, and   D. Ectopic pregnancy, incompetent cervix, and
       hydatidiform mole   hydatidiform mole

13. When a woman experiences clinical signs of bleeding, with or without cramping, in early pregnancy, the
    condition is called
    A. A complete abortion   ✓C. A threatened abortion
    B. An incomplete abortion   D. A habitual abortion

14. When some of the products of conception are expelled and some retained, the type of abortion is referred
    to as
    A. A complete abortion   C. A threatened abortion
    ✓B. An incomplete abortion   D. A missed abortion

15. The most common causes of excessive bleeding in the last trimester are
    ✓A. Placenta previa, abruptio placentae, and   C. Abruptio placentae, excessive uterine contractions,
       rupture of uterus   and ectopic pregnancy
    B. Placenta previa, rupture of uterus and   D. Excessive uterine contractions, ectopic pregnancy,
       hydatidiform mole   and retained placenta

16. Disseminated intravascular coagulation (DIC) is a secondary complication following
    A. Abruptio placentae   C. Retained products of conception
    B. Septic abortion   ✓D. All of the above

17. The pregnant woman who is a diabetic will be at risk for the following:
    A. An infant with congenital anomalies   C. A stillborn infant
    B. A preterm infant   ✓ D. All of the above

18. Maternal insulin level instability during pregnancy is influenced by all of the following factors EXCEPT
    A. Increased placental and fetal use of glucose   C. Decreased hepatic production of glucose
    B. Nausea and vomiting   ✓ D. Decreased urinary output

19. It is important to achieve strict control of blood glucose levels in a diabetic during pregnancy in order to prevent
    A. Ketoacidosis   C. Stillbirth
    B. Large infant over 9 lb   ✓ D. All of the above

20. Malformations of the fetus that can result from maternal rubella are
    ✓ A. Congenital cataracts, heart defects, deafness   C. Heart defect, large size, and club foot
    B. Congenital cataracts, heart defects, large size   D. None of the above

21. A mother who is Rh − is likely to
    A. Have an Rh + infant, if the father is Rh +   C. Have an infant who becomes jaundiced
    B. Develop antibodies after an abortion if she does not receive RhoGam   D. All of the above

B. Choose from Column II the response that most accurately defines the word or words in Column I with regard to management of pregnancy-induced hypertension.

I

1. Epigastric pain _____
2. Decreased sensory stimulation _____
3. Increased tendon reflexes _____
4. Daily weighings _____
5. Bed rest _____
6. Increased anxiety _____
7. Frequent blood pressure readings _____
8. Protein in urine _____

II

A. Promotes diuresis and reduces blood pressure
B. Indicates reduced kidney function
C. Indicates amount of fluid retention
D. Reduces neuromuscular irritability
E. Indicates impending convulsion
F. Increases blood pressure
G. Increases muscle and nerve irritability
H. Vital sign that indicates response to treatment

C. Match the symptom in Column II with the complication it may indicate in Column I.

I

1. Ectopic pregnancy _____
2. Abruptio placentae _____
3. Hyperemesis gravidarum _____
4. Placenta previa _____
5. Eclampsia _____

II

A. Excessive vomiting
B. Convulsions
C. Painless bleeding
D. Severe pain in lower part of abdomen
E. Painful bleeding with shock symptoms

CHAPTER 22

Chapter Outline

Learning Objectives

Upon completion of Chapter 22, the student should be able to

- Explain the term *premature rupture of membranes.*
- List two complications of premature rupture of membranes.
- Name three signs of preterm labor.
- Define precipitate labor and describe two nursing actions that should be taken to safeguard the baby.
- Differentiate between hypotonic and hypertonic uterine dysfunction.
- Name the most common cause of rupture of the uterus during labor.
- Name and describe the three different types of breech presentation.
- List two potential complications of a breech birth.
- Explain the term *cephalopelvic disproportion* (CPD) and discuss the management of CPD.
- Explain why sacral counterpressure is appreciated when a woman labors with the fetus in a persistent occiput position.
- Describe umbilical cord prolapse and name two potential complications associated with it.
- Explain two basic types of episiotomies and at what stage of labor they are done.
- Define three types of lacerations that can occur during the birth process.
- List two indications for using forceps to deliver the baby.
- Describe vacuum extraction.
- List five indications for a cesarean birth.
- Name three types of incisions used for cesarean births.
- Describe the preoperative care of a woman who is going to have a cesarean birth.
- List three potential complications of multiple pregnancy.

COMPLICATIONS DURING LABOR AND BIRTH

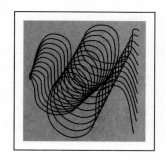

Labor and birth usually progress with few problems. The outcomes for the mother and infant are generally positive. However, when complications occur during labor, they can have devastating effects on the maternal/fetal outcome. Health care providers must quickly and accurately identify the nature of the problem and intervene to reduce or limit detrimental effects on the mother and infant. This chapter discusses high-risk intrapartal care.

Premature Rupture of Membranes

Premature rupture of the membranes (PROM) is the rupture of membranes at least 1 hour or more before the onset of labor. The cause is unknown in many cases. PROM is associated with both maternal and fetal factors.

MATERNAL RISK FACTORS FOR PROM

- Incompetent cervical os
- Intrauterine infections
- Placenta previa and abruptio placentae
- Damage of cervix by instrumentation
- Vitamin C deficiency
- Coitus with organisms attached to sperm

FETAL RISK FACTORS FOR PROM

- Fetal sepsis owing to introduction of pathogens
- Fetal malpresentation
- Prolapse of umbilical cord
- Increased intrauterine tension with multiple pregnancy

DIAGNOSIS

The direct visualization of amniotic fluid escaping from the cervical os is the most reliable method of diagnosing PROM and should be done under aseptic conditions. Nitrazine paper, which is sensitive to pH, will turn bright blue when applied to moist vaginal secretions if the membranes have ruptured. This is because of the slight alkalinity of amniotic fluid. If membranes have not ruptured, paper will remain unchanged, indicating the normal acidity of the vaginal fluid. Another test is to see if the amniotic fluid forms a ferning pattern when placed on a slide and allowed to dry. The fluid should be evaluated soon after it is placed on the slide to increase the accuracy. If vaginal secretions contain blood, urine, or antiseptic solutions, false-positive results may occur.

MANAGEMENT

Management of PROM in the absence of infection and at gestation of less than 37 weeks is usually conservative. The woman is hospitalized and prescribed bed rest. On admission, a complete blood-work profile is done and attention is directed toward assessing the gestational age of fetus. Ultrasound is useful for giving an estimate of fetal age as well as the position of the fetus and placenta. A prolapsed cord is a complication associated with PROM and is discussed later. External electronic fetal monitoring is used to detect signs of fetal distress. Assessment of the amniotic fluid for lung maturity is used in further management. If the fetus is at 32 weeks' gestation or less, betamethasone may be given prophylactically. This delays delivery for 24 to 48 hours to allow natural elevation of maternal–fetal blood glucocorticoids, thus contributing to fetal lung maturity. Betamethasone is contraindicated in the presence of uterine infection because the fetus will have a better chance of survival outside the infected environment of the uterus (Table 22–1).

MANAGEMENT OF WOMEN WITH PROM

Preterm Infant

- Determination of PROM
- Assessment for prolapsed cord
- Observation for infection
- Administration of corticosteroids, with or without delivery in 24 to 48 hours
- Delivery when the infant has the best chance for survival (that is, before fetal distress)

Full-Term Infant

- Induction of labor if spontaneous labor has not begun by approximately 12 hours after PROM
- Potential for cesarean birth
- Expectant management of maternal–fetal infection
- Increased chance of asphyxia and respiratory distress in infant after birth

NURSING ASSESSMENT

The nurse can assist in determining the duration of the rupture of membranes. The time of the rupture should be recorded when it occurs in the hospital. The nurse should record the woman's temperature and pulse rate every 4 hours, or more frequently if elevated. Elevation of temperature and/or pulse rate is indicative of infection. Also, the woman's hydration should be monitored. Usually intravenous fluids are given. The woman's coping ability should be evaluated, particularly when a preterm or cesarean birth is anticipated.

NURSING DIAGNOSES DURING PROM

- Potential for infection related to PROM
- Impaired gas exchange in fetus related to potential prolapse of umbilical cord

---

TABLE 22–1. DRUG ALERT: BETAMETHASONE (CELESTONE, SOLUPAN)—USED TO ACCELERATE FETAL LUNG MATURATION

Drug overview
Betamethasone is a glucocorticoid that acts to accelerate fetal lung maturation.
Best results are obtained when fetus is between 30 and 32 weeks' gestation.
Betamethasone is used as early as 26 weeks' and as late as 34 weeks' gestation.
Betamethasone is used for preterm labor. To obtain optimal results, delivery should be delayed 24 hours after end of treatment. Effect of drug disappears in about 1 week.

Route, dosage, and frequency
Prenatal maternal intramuscular administration of 12 mg once a day for 2 days.
Repeat therapy on weekly basis until 34 weeks' gestation (unless birth occurs).

Contraindications
Inability to delay birth for 48 hours.
L/S[a] ratio of 2/1.
Maternal condition that requires immediate delivery (e.g., maternal bleeding).
Presence of maternal infection, hypertension, or diabetes mellitus.
Gestational age greater than 34 weeks.

Maternal side effects
Increased risk of infection or pulmonary edema when used concurrently with tocolytic drugs (such as ritodrine).

Effects on fetus/infant
Hypoglycemia.
Increased risk of infant sepsis.
Possible suppression of aldosterone levels for 2 weeks postbirth.

Nursing considerations
Assess blood pressure, pulse, weight, and presence of edema.
Assess laboratory data for electrolytes.
Administer drug deep into maternal gluteal muscles; avoid injection into deltoid (high incidence of local atrophy).
Provide instruction regarding possible side effects.

---

[a]Lecithin/sphingomyelin.

- Anxiety related to unknown outcome of pregnancy

Preterm Labor

Preterm (premature) labor is labor that occurs between 20 and 38 weeks of pregnancy. The main risk is for the fetus, not for the mother; preterm labor is one of the leading causes of perinatal deaths worldwide. Because preterm infants are more likely to have birth trauma and respiratory distress, every effort is made to stop the labor until it becomes evident that the fetus is viable and birth is inevitable.

RISK FACTORS

The following are risk factors for preterm labor:

- Spontaneous rupture of membranes
- Maternal medical complications
- Fetal factors, such as multiple pregnancy and infection
- Preterm infant

SIGNS AND SYMPTOMS

Typically, women note uterine contractions that are frequently painless. They are often described as nothing more than tightening. The contractions may be accompanied by abdominal pain and back pain. Some women state that they experienced a sudden increase in mucoid discharge or vaginal spotting; these signs may reflect cervical change. If there is no vaginal bleeding, a vaginal examination is often done to evaluate the status of the cervix and to assess if the membranes are ruptured or intact. Ultrasound and electronic monitoring of fetal heart rate are done to see if there is a healthy fetus without distress. Tocolytic therapy (using drugs such as ritodrine, terbutaline, or magnesium sulfate) may be done when the fetus is healthy, cervical dilation is less than 4 cm, there is no significant vaginal bleeding, and gestational age is less than 36 weeks but more than 20 weeks. The woman is prescribed bed rest and carefully ob-

served in attempts to delay the labor. The goal is to relax the uterine muscle and to prevent ascending infection (Table 22–2).

SIGNS AND SYMPTOMS OF PRETERM LABOR

- Uterine contractions
- Abdominal pain
- Back pain
- Vaginal pressure
- Vaginal spotting
- Change in vaginal discharge

Women need to be instructed on the signs of premature labor because of their subtlety. If a woman experiences symptoms that appear to be preterm labor, she should notify her care provider. Home monitoring includes bed rest and timing uterine contractions that seem obvious and appear to be increasing in strength and/or frequency (Nursing Care Plan 22–1).

Induction of Labor

The induction of labor is the deliberate attempt to initiate uterine contractions before their spontaneous onset. Usually labor is induced because of maternal medical reasons, obstetrical complications, or the baby's health status. Labor should not be induced for the convenience of the woman or physician. The following are contraindications for doing an induction of labor:

- Previous cesarean birth
- Cephalopelvic disproportion
- Placenta previa
- Presence of herpesvirus 2
- Preterm fetus
- Fetal malposition (breech or transverse)

AMNIOTOMY

An amniotomy is the artificial rupturing of membranes (AROM). It has become a common procedure in medical management, most often done to shorten the labor. It does so by causing an increase in uterine contractions that causes the head to

TABLE 22–2. DRUG ALERT: RITODRINE (YUTOPAR)—USED IN THE TREATMENT OF PRETERM LABOR

Drug overview
Ritodrine is a tocolytic, uterine relaxant.
It reduces the frequency and intensity of uterine contractions by stimulation of the beta-adrenergic receptors in uterine smooth muscle.
Ritodrine also stimulates the beta receptors located in other smooth muscle organs, which accounts for the side effects of this drug.

Route, dosage, and frequency
Ritodrine hydrochloride is administered IV using the recommended FDA protocol. Maximum IV rate of 125 mL/hr should *not* be exceeded.
Infusion is maintained at maximum level for 12 hr (or until contractions have ceased).
Orally, initial dose of 10 mg is administered 30 min before stopping IV infusion.
Oral regimen is 10 mg every 2 hr for 24 hr. This dose is adjusted to 10–29 mg every 4–6 hr, depending on the response. The maximum daily oral dose should not exceed 120 mg.

Maternal contraindications
Cervical dilatation > 4 cm.
Excessive bleeding.
Chorioamnionitis.
Severe pregnancy-induced hypertension (PIH).
Fetal death.
Diabetes mellitus.
Cardiac disease.
Gestation < 20 wks.

Maternal side effects
Side effects related to cardiovascular system include tachycardia, hypotension, chest tightness or actual chest pain, and, in rare cases, pulmonary edema.
Ritodrine causes a shift in potassium which may cause hypokalemia and cardiac arrhythmias.

Effects on fetus/infant
Fetal tachycardia, cardiac arrhythmias.
Fetal hypoxia.
Fetal acidosis.
Neonatal hypoglycemia, hypocalcemia, and hypotension.
Neonatal irritability, tremors.

Nursing considerations
Position woman to lie on her left side to decrease incidence of hypotension and increase placental perfusion.
Explain procedure, which will include electronic fetal monitoring and frequent assessments of vital signs, fluid intake and urine output, daily weight.
Assess maternal blood pressure and pulse rate every 15 min while dosage is being increased and every 30 min during maintenance IV. Notify physician if maternal pulse is greater than 120 beats/min.
Assess respiratory rate and listen to breath sounds. Note signs of pulmonary edema (rales and rhonchi).
With oral therapy, assess vital signs with every dose given.
Assess hydration; evaluate fluid intake/urine output and concentration.
Observe weight at same time of day on same scale.
Observe woman closely for signs of dyspnea, wheezing, coughing, rales, fast pulse, muscle weakness, or cardiac arrhythmia.
Antiembolism stockings may be ordered to prevent pooling of blood in extremities.
Provide psychological support. The woman often continually fears losing her baby.
Discontinue ritodrine in presence of the following: maternal heart rate above 140 beats/min, fetal heart rate above 200 beats/min, maternal systolic pressure above 180 mm Hg or diastolic below 40 mm Hg, chest pain, or other cardiac symptoms. (Physician should be in close contact with patient receiving ritodrine.)
Monitor uterine activity (contractions) and fetal heart rate continuously with electronic monitor.

NURSING CARE PLAN 22–1

CARE OF THE WOMAN EXPERIENCING PRETERM LABOR

Potential Problems and Nursing Diagnoses	Nursing Interventions
1. Anxiety related to uncertain outcome of pregnancy.	Promote communication about hospitalization. Encourage woman to express fears and concerns. Explain procedures to decrease fear of unknown.
2. Ineffectual individual coping related to preterm labor with infant at 35 weeks' gestation.	Reinforce effective coping mechanisms; teach new ones as needed. Support woman by having someone stay with her (caregiver and/or significant other).
3. Potential fluid volume deficit related to dehydration.	Explain the need to increase fluid intake. Assess for hydration by observing status of skin and urine output.
4. Knowledge deficit related to preterm uterine contractions.	Explain care, including potential medication (ritodrine) to suppress the uterine smooth muscle activity.
5. Potential injury related to possible fetal tachycardia.	Explain need for continuous fetal heart rate monitoring due to possibility that prescribed drug will cause increased fetal heart rate.
6. Impaired physical mobility related to bed rest.	Instruct the woman about the need for bed rest to lessen or stop uterine contractions.
7. Potential for infection related to bathing and hygiene.	Frequently change bed linens; have woman practice adequate female hygiene and bathing.
8. Potential altered parenting related to impaired parent–infant attachment.	Provide opportunity for questions regarding care of premature infant, including holding and feeding infant.

Expected Outcomes

1. Woman verbalizes fears and concerns about the possibility that the baby will be born early.
2. Woman demonstrates breathing as a relaxing intervention. She states that she feels relieved to know she will not be left alone but someone will be with her.
3. Woman recognizes need for increased fluid intake.
4. Woman communicates understanding of prescribed drug and need to attempt to stop the uterine contractions to allow the baby to mature.
5. Woman verbalizes an understanding of the need for continuous fetal heart rate monitoring to safeguard the infant.
6. Woman recognizes that bed rest is part of the management to stop or lessen uterine contractions.
7. Woman demonstrates good hygiene after voiding.
8. Woman verbalizes understanding of care of premature infant including the possibility of breastfeeding, if desired.

descend more quickly into the pelvic canal. The risks of an amniotomy include potential maternal and fetal infection from pathogens introduced during prolonged rupture of membranes before birth of the infant. Also, there is an increased risk that the umbilical cord will prolapse when fluid flows from the vagina without the head (or other presenting part) engaged. Fetal heart rate should be assessed immediately after AROM.

The woman should be carefully monitored after the membranes are ruptured. Electronic fetal monitoring is done to closely assess the fetal heart rate pattern. The color of the amniotic fluid should be assessed frequently for signs of fetal distress (in which case the amniotic fluid would be stained with meconium).

The caregiver should explain the procedure to the woman. She should be told that she will be evaluated frequently. Nursing care includes frequent perineal cleansing and change of linen to reduce the introduction of organisms and thus decrease the risk of infection and to promote comfort. In addition, the number of vaginal examinations done during labor should be decreased. The woman's vital signs, especially temperature, should be taken frequently (every 2 hours).

OXYTOCIN INFUSION

An oxytocin infusion is used to stimulate labor or increase labor contractions that are ineffective. Because some women are extremely sensitive to oxytocins, these drugs are administered by an intravenous infusion pump that controls the rate of flow. The Food and Drug Administration now prohibits induction simply for convenience; it should be used only when there are maternal or fetal indications. The maternal indications include severe pregnancy-induced hypertension and fetal death. Fetal indications include fetal jeopardy by diabetes mellitus, postterm pregnancy, intrauterine growth retardation, hypertensive complications of pregnancy, isoimmunization, and PROM when fetal maturity is well established. It has been shown that an elective induction is associated with a higher rate of cesarean birth.

During an induction of labor with oxytocin, the woman should constantly be observed for excessive uterine contractions and fetal distress. Notations should be made on the electronic fetal monitor tracing regarding changes in uterine contraction frequency, intensity, and duration. When hyperstimulation of the uterus occurs, there is risk of decreased placental perfusion with decreased oxygen to the fetus.

In addition, labor and birth induced with oxytocin can be rapid, creating the danger of cervical or perineal lacerations. A ruptured uterus is also a potential complication. The nurse should report changes in uterine activity to the physician. Because the intensity of uterine contractions is increased in induced labor, comfort measures should be implemented (Table 22–3).

Precipitate Labor

A precipitate labor is one that lasts less than 3 hours from the time of the first contraction to the delivery of the baby. When the maternal soft tissues offer little resistance and the uterus contracts strongly and frequently, both maternal and fetal injury may result. If the uterus has little relaxation between contractions, the intervillous blood flow may be impaired enough to cause fetal hypoxia (lack of oxygen). Also, rapid passage of the fetal head through the birth canal may result in intracranial hemorrhage. The woman may have cervical, vaginal, and rectal lacerations.

Because a precipitate labor is often unexpected, the delivery may occur before the physician or nurse midwife arrives, and therefore the baby may not receive necessary resuscitation. If a nurse is present, she/he should not attempt to keep the baby from being born. Rather, the nurse should quickly put on sterile gloves and gently guide the baby's head and the rest of the body out. The head should be kept out of the amniotic fluid. The baby's face, mouth, and nose should be wiped at once, and a bulb syringe should be used orally to lessen the likelihood that the baby will aspirate amniotic fluid. The baby can be placed on the mother's abdomen or on a clean area of the bed. If the baby is in distress, a qualified caregiver (physician, midwife, or qualified neonatal nurse) should begin resuscitation measures immediately. The baby is taken to the delivery room or nursery

TABLE 22–3. DRUG ALERT: OXYTOCIN (PITOCIN)—USED FOR AUGMENTATION OR INDUCTION OF LABOR

Drug overview

Oxytocin (Pitocin) affects the myometrial cells of the uterus by increasing the excitability of the muscle and the strength of the muscle contraction.

The effects of oxytocin on the cardiovascular system can be pronounced. Initially the blood pressure may decrease, but with prolonged use a 30% increase in baseline blood pressure may be noted. The cardiac output and stroke volume are increased.

Oxytocin is used to induce labor at term and to augment uterine contractions in the first and second stages of labor.

Oxytocin is used immediately after delivery to stimulate uterine contractions, control uterine atony, and lessen blood loss.

Oxytocin has an antidiuretic effect.

Route, dosage, and frequency

For labor induction: Ten units of Pitocin are added to 1000 mL of IV solution (resulting in a dilute concentration). Preferably using an infusion pump, IV infusion is started at 0.5 mU/min to 1 mU/min, with very gradual increase every 30 to 50 min. Most patients (90%) respond with 16 mU/min or less.

For augmentation of labor: Ten units of Pitocin are added to 1000 mL of intravenous solution. The flow rate is gradually increased until labor contractions are of good quality.

Maternal and fetal contraindications

Severe preeclampsia–eclampsia.

Potential uterine rupture (overdistention of uterus, previous cesarean section, or major surgery).

Preterm infant.

Cephalopelvic disproportion.

Placenta previa.

Fetal distress.

Maternal side effects

Hyperstimulation of uterus may cause abruptio placentae; impaired uterine blood flow, causing fetal hypoxia; rapid labor and delivery, causing lacerations of cervix, vagina, perineum; or rapid delivery, causing fetal trauma.

Hypotension can occur with rapid IV administration.

Nausea, vomiting, tachycardia, and cardiac arrhythmia may occur.

Effects on fetus/infant

Increased, frequent uterine contractions can cause decrease in oxygen supply to fetus, which is reflected by decrease or irregularities in fetal heart rate (FHR).

Hyperbilirubinemia can also occur.

Nursing considerations

Explain procedure of either induction or augmentation to woman.

Nonstress test is done to assess FHR before starting IV Pitocin.

Monitor fetal status and uterine contractions continuously.

Assess FHR, maternal blood pressure, pulse, and uterine contractions (frequency, duration, intensity, and resting tone between contractions) before increasing IV infusion rate.

Record all assessments and IV rate on monitor strip.

Assess comfort measures.

Be aware of cervical dilatation.

Discontinue IV oxytocin infusion when the following is observed: fetal distress (bradycardia, late or variable decelerations, and meconium staining) occurs, uterine contractions are more frequent than every 2 min, or duration of contractions is more than 90 min.

where resuscitation equipment is available. If the baby is not in distress, there is no need to hurry to cut the cord. However, the nurse should keep the baby from getting chilled by drying the baby and keeping it warm with a blanket until the cord is clamped and cut and the baby is taken to the nursery.

If precipitate labor occurs in the hospital, usually a physician will be available to deliver the placenta. If the physician is not available, the nurse must deliver the placenta. This is done not by pulling on the cord but by simply guiding the placenta out after spontaneous separation. Once the placenta is expelled, the uterus should be massaged to keep it well contracted and to reduce the amount of blood loss. Some caregivers put the baby to the mother's breast to nurse, because suckling is a natural way of causing the uterus to contract.

Dysfunctional Labor

DYSTOCIA

Dystocia (dysfunctional or difficult labor) results from contractions that deviate from normal, failure of the baby to rotate properly, a large baby, or a contracted pelvis. The cause may be maternal, fetal, or a combination of both. A prolonged labor, with potential injury to the fetus, may result. Nursing assessment of the intensity, frequency, and duration of contractions is important. Electronic fetal monitoring is used to accurately assess uterine contractions and fetal well-being.

Increased intensity and little to no resting tone between contractions indicate possible fetal compromise. A dysfunctional labor can be associated with problems such as maternal dehydration, exhaustion, increased risk of infection, and fetal distress. Deviation of vital signs such as elevation of temperature or rise in pulse rate should be reported. Comfort measures should be implemented by the nursing personnel. The woman and significant other should be kept informed about the labor.

NURSING DIAGNOSES DURING DYSFUNCTIONAL LABOR
- Anxiety related to slow progress of labor
- Fatigue related to the length of labor
- Ineffective coping related to inability to relax
- Potential fluid volume deficit related to lack of fluid intake
- Potential for infection related to prolonged labor
- Sleep pattern disturbance related to maternal exhaustion and inability to relax
- Knowledge deficit related to potential fetal distress and fetal sepsis

HYPOTONIC UTERINE DYSFUNCTION

Hypotonic uterine dysfunction is the inability of the uterus to contract strongly enough to cause the cervix to dilate beyond 4 cm. Consequently, labor fails to progress. The contractions may become farther apart and irregular as well as decreased in intensity. A prolonged labor is the result, which can increase the risk of intrauterine infection, placing both the mother and infant at risk of infection.

Hypotonic contractions can occur as a result of fetopelvic disproportion, fetal malposition, prolonged maternal dehydration, and excessive maternal anxiety. The woman usually becomes very tired and in need of rest. The risks increase for fetal distress, infection, and postpartum hemorrhage.

The management of hypotonic uterine dysfunction consists of ultrasound and possibly x-rays to see if the fetus is in an abnormal position or is excessively large. If either of these findings is present, a cesarean birth is performed. If neither is present, labor is stimulated either by artificial rupture of the membranes or by an intravenous infusion of an oxytocin solution. If an oxytocin infusion is started, the labor and the fetal heart rate are monitored continuously by electronic monitoring. Oxytocin stimulation usually increases the intensity of uterine contractions. There is always risk that the contractions will become very intense and close, diminishing the fetus's oxygen supply. In addition, with strong, long, close contractions, there is a risk of uterine rupture. The physician or nurse midwife should be nearby or in the labor unit and kept informed about the changes in the patient's labor contraction pattern.

The woman should be encouraged to ambulate

TABLE 22–4. COMPARISON OF HYPOTONIC AND HYPERTONIC LABOR

WHEN OCCURS	CONTRACTIONS	IMPLICATIONS	MANAGEMENT
Hypotonic Labor			
Active phase; may occur in latent phase	Infrequent; poor intensity; low resting tone between contractions	Maternal—seldom painful; prolonged labor; PROM; risk of infection; anxiety Fetal—risk of subsequent sepsis	Rule out cephalopelvic disproportion; use IV oxytocin to stimulate contractions; cesarean birth is performed for abnormal fetal position or large infant Nursing interventions—assess contraction pattern; provide support; monitor vital signs; assess fetal status frequently; If considering cesarean birth, instruct mother about procedure
Hypertonic Labor			
Prolonged latent phase; may occur in active phase	Become more frequent; ineffective; painful; uterus does not relax between contractions	Maternal—exhaustion; discouragement; fatigue; anxiety Fetal—possible distress with decreased uterine perfusion	Analgesia for rest; hydration; oxytocin is *not* administered (discontinue IV oxytocin if infusing) Nursing interventions—assess uterine contraction pattern; provide rest (analgesia); provide comfort measures; monitor maternal vital signs; monitor fetal status frequently

if her membranes are intact. If her membranes have ruptured, she is kept on bed rest, and frequent position changes should be encouraged. Conscientious assessment of the woman's labor contractions by the nurse is essential for prompt identification of the abnormal labor pattern. Documentation of changes in the contraction pattern (for example, intensity) is important in the care. An explanation of the possible need for a cesarean birth and a report of the fetal condition are important parts of nursing care.

HYPERTONIC UTERINE DYSFUNCTION

Hypertonic uterine dysfunction refers to insufficient relaxation of the uterus between contractions. Contractions may become more frequent and painful but be unable to produce cervical dilation. The latent phase of labor is often prolonged, which may lead to severe discomfort, exhaustion, and anxiety (Table 22–4). The laboring woman may experience supine hypotensive syndrome when she lies on her back. If this happens she should immediately be turned on her left side (see Chapter 5). The risk of maternal infection and hemorrhage increases with a potential prolonged labor.

Prompt recognition of the abnormal uterine contractions is of great importance in the care of the woman with hypertonic uterine contractions. Often, the initial management is sedation or analgesia, causing the woman to sleep or rest for several hours. The woman may awaken with a normal labor pattern, and labor may progress appropriately. Because of the risk of fetal distress, continuous monitoring of the labor is important. If fetal distress develops, a cesarean birth may be indicated (Table 22–4).

Rupture of the Uterus

Rupture of the uterus is rare; however, it can present an emergency condition because it causes severe bleeding. It occurs most often during labor and delivery.

Uterine rupture is usually associated with a previous cesarean birth. In this case, the rupture occurs at the site of the surgical scar. Aggressive, poorly supervised induction of labor may be responsible for rupture of the uterus. A prolonged labor with fetopelvic disproportion is another cause.

A clue to a pending rupture is persistent localized pain or tenderness beneath the cesarean scar. As labor progresses, the woman might experience pain in the suprapubic area. With severe bleeding, symptoms of shock can occur. The major complications are maternal hemorrhage and fetal distress. Treatment of severe cases usually consists of an immediate laparotomy and possible hysterectomy. Often, blood transfusions are necessary.

Malpresentation of Fetus

A malpresentation refers to any presentation of the fetus other than the vertex presentation, in which the top of the head presents. Malpresentation may prolong labor and make it more uncomfortable.

FACE AND BROW PRESENTATION

The face and brow presentation, with the forces of labor, may convert to a vertex presentation, thereby decreasing the diameter of the head. Fetal anomalies or defects of the umbilical cord can contribute to the conversion. The face is a less effective dilating wedge than the top of the fetal head. The safest means of delivery of the baby in the posterior face position is a cesarean birth. A forceps delivery may be done, but there is always the risk of poor forceps application in a brow presentation.

BREECH PRESENTATION

In approximately 3% to 4% of all deliveries, the presentation is breech. The labor with a breech presentation is often longer because the buttocks,

legs, and feet are softer than the head and therefore exert less pressure on the cervix. Cord prolapse occurs more frequently during breech birth and increases the risk of birth trauma because the presenting part is smaller and does not fit as snugly into the pelvis. There is also the increased risk of postpartum hemorrhage. The three basic types of breech presentation are shown in Figure 22–1.

Breech presentations are frequently associated with preterm birth, multiple gestation, placenta previa, and multiparity. Also, fetuses that assume the breech presentation are at a greater risk for congenital anomalies than those in the cephalic presentation.

Ultrasound may be done later in pregnancy to identify fetal anomalies or the presence of a prolapsed cord. A cesarean birth may be indicated as a means of preventing fetal distress and birth injury of the infant. The woman and significant other need both psychological and physical support when there is a breech birth.

NURSING DIAGNOSES

- Knowledge deficit related to the complications of breech presentation to mother and fetus
- Impaired gas exchange in the fetus related to decreased blood flow caused by compression or prolapse of the cord

Cephalopelvic Disproportion

Cephalopelvic disproportion (CPD) is a condition in which the presenting part of the fetus (usually the head) is too large to pass through the woman's pelvis. Because of the disproportion, it becomes physically impossible for the fetus to be delivered, and a cesarean birth is necessary. CPD is suspected when the infant's head does not continue to descend even though the woman is having strong uterine contractions.

When one or more diameters (inlet, midpelvis, or outlet) of the maternal pelvis is shortened, the pelvis is said to be *contracted*. A contracted pelvis that is too narrow at some point is one of the

Footling breech   Frank breech   Complete breech

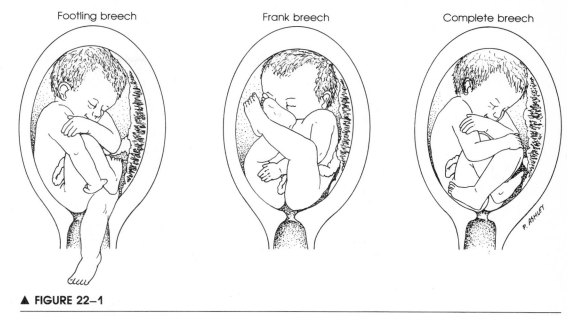

▲ **FIGURE 22–1**

Types of breech presentations.

major causes of CPD. Excessive fetal size is another significant cause.

Sometimes, the maternal pelvic measurements are believed to be marginal, and the woman is given a "trial of labor" for 4 to 6 hours. If there is no labor progress, a cesarean birth is performed.

The complications of CPD are exhaustion and hemorrhage for the woman. Anoxia and birth trauma are complications for the fetus.

Persistent Occiput Posterior Positions

Persistent occiput positions occur when the back of the fetal head (the occiput) enters the maternal pelvis and is directed toward the back of the pelvis instead of toward the front. When this position occurs, labor is usually prolonged, because, in the process of internal rotation, the head must rotate more. If the occiput remains posterior, the baby is born with the face upward. The woman usually experiences a great deal of back discomfort, because the baby's head presses against her sacrum during rotation. Sacral counterpressure and back rubs are appreciated by the woman during labor.

Sometimes, the woman is asked to push while lying on her side, which may help the fetus rotate to an anterior position.

Hydramnios

Hydramnios is an excessive amount of amniotic fluid. When hydramnios is present, congenital anomalies often exist, particularly those of the gastrointestinal tract. This condition is a complication of uncontrolled diabetes. When hydramnios develops, the uterus overdistends. This problem may cause a loss of uterine muscle tone, placing the woman at a greater risk for dysfunctional labor and postpartum hemorrhage.

Cord Compression or Prolapse

When the umbilical cord precedes the fetal presenting part, it is said to have prolapsed. The cord can be alongside or ahead of the presenting part (Fig. 22–2). It may be occult (not palpable on vaginal examination), inside the vagina, or even outside the vulva. Because compression of the

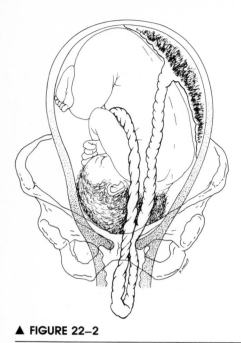

▲ **FIGURE 22–2**

Prolapsed umbilical cord.

cord between the presenting part and the bony pelvis greatly decreases the flow of oxygen to the fetus, prolapse of the cord causes great risk to the fetus. Factors that contribute to cord prolapse are rupture of membranes with excessive discharge of fluid at one time when the presenting part is not engaged, breech presentation, an unusually long cord, multiple pregnancy, hydramnios, and a contracted pelvis.

Prevention of cord prolapse is an important part of care. Bed rest is indicated for all women in labor with ROM until engagement has been documented. In addition, at the time of spontaneous rupture of membranes or amniotomy, the fetal heart rate should be taken for at least 1 full minute. If fetal bradycardia (decreased fetal heart rate) is found, the woman should be examined to rule out a cord prolapse. Electronic fetal monitoring should be started immediately. If the cord has prolapsed, the tracing will show moderately to severely variable decelerations with fetal bradycardia.

If the cord is felt by vaginal examination, the gloved fingers are left in the vagina, and attempts are made to lift the fetal head off the cord to relieve compression until the physician arrives.

Oxygen is begun, and, to assist the force of gravity, the woman is placed in the knee–chest position or a deep Trendelenburg (head-down) position. If the cord protrudes outside the vulva, it should be covered with a moist, sterile dressing. The fetal heart rate should be monitored continuously. Unless the cervix is completely dilated and a vaginal delivery can be done immediately, delivery of the baby is by cesarean birth.

NURSING DIAGNOSES DURING CORD PROLAPSE

- Impaired gas exchange related to the decrease in oxygen to the fetus caused by interruption of blood flow through the umbilical cord
- Potential for infection related to exposure of cord to pathogens
- Anxiety related to potential poor outcome of fetus
- Knowledge deficit related to lack of understanding of need for oxygen and position change
- Ineffectual individual coping related to potential fetal complications

Operative Procedures

EPISIOTOMY

An *episiotomy* is a clean cut made in the vagina to prevent tearing (laceration), shorten the second stage, decrease pressure on the fetal head, and facilitate manipulative delivery. There are two types of episiotomy: (a) the median (midline) episiotomy, which extends from the posterior fourchette of the vagina downward but not to the rectal sphincter, and (b) the mediolateral episiotomy, which is a cut on an angle to the woman's right or left side (Fig. 22–3). An episiotomy heals more satisfactorily than a laceration. A regional or local block is given before the episiotomy is done. Ideally, the episiotomy is performed just before the birth of the infant to reduce the blood loss.

If a laceration does occur, it is classified as one of four degrees: A *first-degree* laceration extends into the mucous membrane and the skin. A *second-*

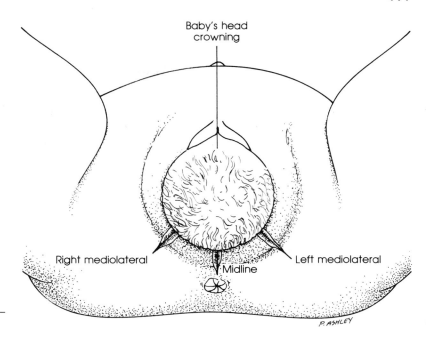

▲ **FIGURE 22–3**

Episiotomy. Three typical incisions.

degree laceration extends farther, reaching the muscles of the perineum. In a *third-degree* laceration, the anal sphincter muscles are torn as well as the muscles of the perineum. A *fourth-degree* laceration reaches into the anal sphincter muscles and into the anterior wall of the rectum. Because of the potential risk of a laceration, an episiotomy in the

perineum is common practice. A median episiotomy is considered to be less uncomfortable and heals more quickly than a mediolateral incision. However, a median incision can extend into the rectum.

Frequently, after episiotomy repair an ice bag is applied to the incision to reduce swelling. Other nursing measures for an episiotomy are discussed in Chapter 22.

FORCEPS DELIVERY

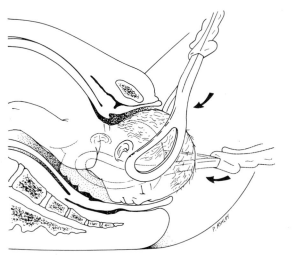

▲ **FIGURE 22–4**

Application of forceps (top arrow) and direction of traction (bottom arrow).

Forceps are instruments used by the physician to provide traction to deliver the baby's head, rotate the head, or both (Fig. 22–4). These instruments may be used to deliver preterm infants to prevent undue pressure's being placed on the fragile fetal skull by continued contractions. They are also used to shorten the second stage of labor when the mother is exhausted and cannot effectively bear down. Sometimes regional or general anesthesia has affected the motor innervation, and the mother cannot push effectively. Forceps are also employed to deliver the baby as soon as possible when fetal distress occurs and the cervix is completely dilated with the fetus's head low or visible on the perineum (this is called low forceps delivery). Forceps should be applied only by a skilled physician. There is always the risks of marks on the infant's face and potential injury from forceps.

Maternal complications may include lacerations of the birth canal and perineum, with increased blood loss. Fetal implications include bruising and edema of the fetal head. In a difficult forceps application, temporary or even permanent paralysis of the facial nerve may occur. For this reason, a cesarean delivery is frequently chosen over mid-forceps delivery when the head is higher than the perineum.

The nurse should explain the procedure to the woman, if she is awake during forceps application. After birth, the newborn should be assessed for bruising, edema, and potential paralysis.

VACUUM EXTRACTION

Vacuum extraction can be used as an alternative to forceps application in some cases. In vacuum extraction, a metal or plastic cup is applied to the fetal head, and suction is initiated by a pump that withdraws air between the head and the cup. The pump is used to create negative pressure inside the cup. Traction is applied during the uterine contractions, and the fetal head is delivered.

With vacuum extraction, risks to the fetus include cephalohematomas, edema, scalp lacerations, intracranial hemorrhage, and fetal distress. Further investigation is necessary to determine if vacuum extraction is an effective alternative to forceps.

During the procedure, the woman should be informed about the medical procedure. The fetal heart rate should be taken frequently or continuously. Parents need instruction that the caput (edema) will disappear in about 2 days. Assessment of the newborn should include continued observation for cerebral hemorrhage and injury.

CESAREAN BIRTH

A cesarean birth is the delivery of the baby through a surgical incision in the abdominal wall and the uterus (Fig. 22–5). The rate of cesarean births has increased dramatically in the last dec-

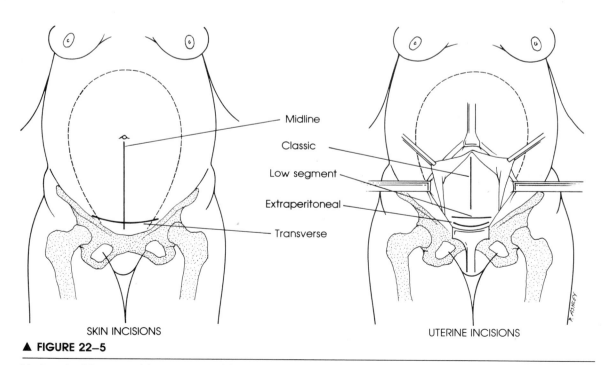

Midline
Classic
Low segment
Extraperitoneal
Transverse

SKIN INCISIONS

UTERINE INCISIONS

▲ **FIGURE 22–5**

Various incisions used for cesarean births.

ade. One reason for this is that the availability of antibiotics and whole blood has made cesarean birth less dangerous. Cesarean birth may be performed for either maternal or fetal reasons.

Indications for Cesarean Birth

Cesarean birth is indicated in the following conditions:

- Previous cesarean birth
- Fetal distress
- Uncontrollable third-trimester bleeding
- Placenta previa
- Abruptio placentae
- Fetopelvic disproportion
- Fetal malpresentation
- Prolapsed cord
- Medical complications of pregnancy, such as maternal heart disorder
- Failure of labor to progress
- History of herpes simplex virus infection
- Postmaturity (with failed induction)

Types of Cesarean Birth

There are three basic types of cesarean births. In the classic cesarean birth, the incision is made in the fundus at the midline. The advantage of a classic cesarean birth is the speed with which it can be done. Disadvantages include increased risks of hemorrhage, infection, and subsequent uterine rupture during the next labor experience. In the second and most common type of cesarean birth, a transverse incision is made in the lower segment of the uterus. The advantages of a transverse lower segment incision are easier repair, less blood loss, lower incidence of infection, and less risk of subsequent rupture. The disadvantages are that it takes more time and requires more surgical skill. The third type of cesarean birth, the extraperitoneal cesarean birth, is less frequently seen. In the extraperitoneal cesarean birth, the obstetrician exposes the uterus below the peritoneum by dissecting the bladder downward. Great surgical skill is required to avoid nicking the bladder (Fig. 22–6).

The types of anesthesia used during cesarean birth are general anesthesia for emergency procedures and an epidural or spinal block for the woman who wants to be awake and aware of the birth.

If the woman knows during her pregnancy that she is going to have a cesarean birth, she should be informed about the three different types available. Currently, some prenatal classes, such as the Lamaze classes, incorporate discussions on cesarean births. It is preferable that the nurse use the term *cesarean birth* rather than *cesarean section* because the former is more meaningful. Nurses need to be aware of some couples' feelings about cesarean birth and should attempt to relieve their anxiety, apprehension, guilt, anger, and confusion about having the baby in that manner.

Preoperative Care

The preoperative nursing care includes all the usual procedures for preparing a patient for surgery. The abdominal skin is prepared, and a Foley catheter is inserted into the bladder to ensure that it is empty. Elastic stockings are often put on the woman's legs to reduce peripheral blood pooling and hypotension. The fetal heart rate is recorded with electronic monitoring until the infant is delivered.

Newborn Care

Often, a nurse from the nursery and a pediatrician are present in the operating room to assist in the care of the infant when delivered. A heated crib and resuscitation equipment are readily available. In some hospitals, the father or significant other can be with the mother during the cesarean birth.

After the baby is born, he or she is brought to the transitional nursery for immediate postbirth care. Eye care, identification, placement of skin temperature probe, and placement of the infant in a radiant heat warmer to prevent chilling are done at this time. Frequently, the mother and significant other are given an early opportunity to see the infant.

A   B

E   F

I   J

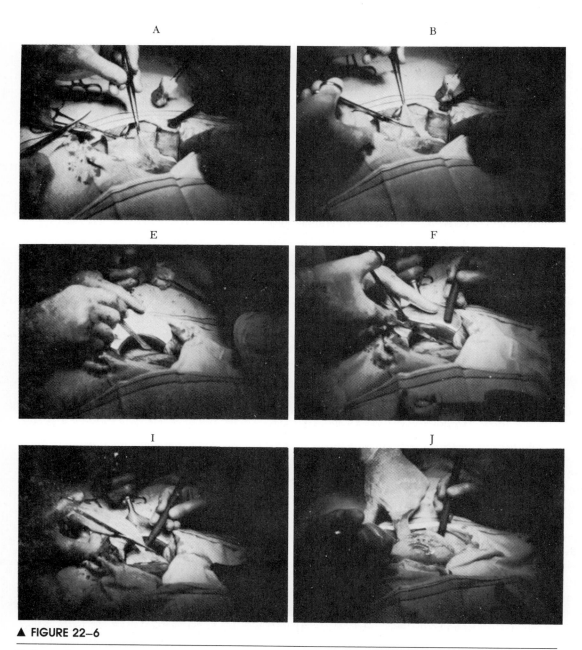

▲ FIGURE 22–6

Delivery by cesarean section. (From Danforth, D. N. (Ed.) (1971). *Textbook of Obstetrics and Gynecology*, 2nd ed., New York: Harper and Row.)

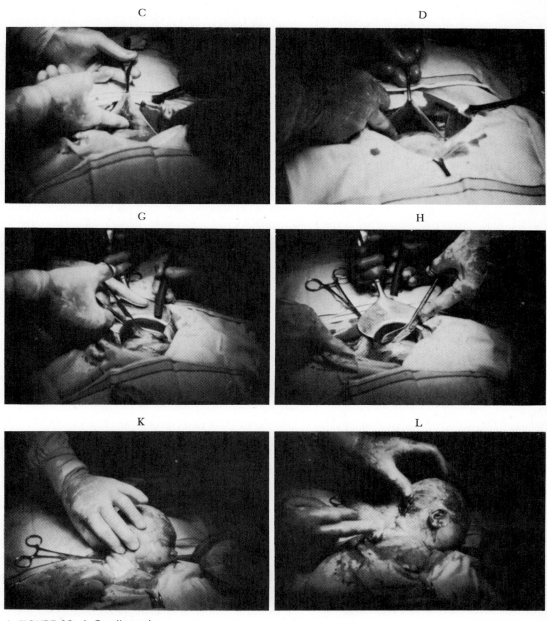

▲ **FIGURE 22–6** *Continued*

NURSING CARE PLAN 22–2

CARE OF THE WOMAN EXPERIENCING CESAREAN BIRTH

Potential Problems and Nursing Diagnoses	Nursing Interventions
1. Knowledge deficit related to cesarean birth.	Preparatory needs for cesarean birth. Explanation of pre- and postoperative measures, including deep breathing.
2. Anxiety related to increased risks in a cesarean birth.	Create a positive and relaxed atmosphere to prevent anxiety and make experience less negative.
3. Ineffectual individual coping related to unanticipated cesarean birth.	Allow woman and significant other to express their fears and concerns. Reinforce effective coping mechanisms; teach new ones as needed.
4. Potential for infection during surgery.	Use aseptic technique in inserting Foley catheter. Use elastic stockings to reduce the peripheral blood pooling and stasis. After surgery inspect the wound for drainage and apply sterile dressings to incision.
5. Altered tissue perfusion related to blood loss during surgery.	After surgery evaluate firmness and position of uterus. Monitor change in vital signs.
6. Potential alteration in self-esteem related to not having a vaginal birth.	Praise woman for her efforts in coping with unanticipated cesarean birth.
7. Ineffective airway clearance related to tracheobronchial secretions.	After surgery have patient cough and encourage deep breathing (to prevent pneumonia).
8. Pain related to abdominal incision.	Offer prescribed analgesics after surgery.
9. Potential fluid volume deficit related to dehydration.	Maintain an open intravenous infusion. Offer oral fluids as tolerated.

Expected Outcomes

1. Mother verbalizes understanding of reasons for interventions.
2. Mother demonstrates decrease in anxiety and states that explanations have decreased her fear of the unknown.
3. Mother verbalizes the significance of caregiver's support and of allowing significant other to be with her during surgery.
4. Wound is clean and dry with no evidence of infection.
5. Uterus remains firm and below umbilicus. Vital signs remain stable and within normal limits.
6. Mother recognizes a cesarean birth will not limit parent–infant interaction, which is more important than how the infant is born.
7. Chest is clear with normal breath sounds and respiratory rate.
8. Mother receives prescribed medications for pain.
9. Mother's intravenous line remains open, and she tolerates oral fluids.

Postsurgical and Postpartum Care

After surgery, the woman is taken to the recovery room. Recovery room care includes observing the firmness of the uterus and the amount of bleeding from the vagina and the abdominal incision. In addition, the woman receives the usual postoperative care. Usually the woman is given oxytocin intravenously to stimulate the uterus to contract and reduce the blood loss. She is given analgesic medications to promote comfort.

Early ambulation is encouraged to reduce respiratory and circulatory complications. Vital signs are taken frequently until the woman's condition has stabilized. The lochia is observed a minimum of every 8 hours (every shift). As a rule, the woman with a cesarean birth has less lochial flow, most likely because of the removal of some of the uterine decidua during the surgical procedure. She usually receives intravenous fluids during the first 24 to 48 hours. The first intravenous bag frequently contains an oxytocin (Pitocin) to keep the uterus well contracted. An in-dwelling Foley catheter is normally maintained for 12 to 24 hours or until the intravenous fluids are discontinued. Deep breathing and coughing are encouraged. In addition, the woman should be instructed to "splint" her abdomen with a pillow when she coughs or gets out of bed. She should receive the pain medication, as necessary, that the physician prescribed. Patient-controlled analgesics, administered by an intravenous pump with a preset safety limit dosage, may be used. If the woman plans to breastfeed her baby, she can begin as soon as she feels comfortable. The hospitalization period for a cesarean birth patient has shortened to an average of 4 days (see Nursing Care Plan 22–2).

Multiple Pregnancy

Although some women are happy to hear that they are carrying twins, most are overwhelmed.

A positive diagnosis of more than one fetus is made by ultrasound. Women who are pregnant with more than one fetus usually experience more discomfort during pregnancy, and premature labor is quite common. There is an increased frequency of anemia, hypertension, and hemorrhage. The woman is more likely to hemorrhage because the uterus frequently is distended with more than one fetus. Therefore, a multiple pregnancy is considered to pose greater risks than a single fetus.

Twins may be in various positions; one may be breech and the other vertex. The labor may be normal or prolonged. During the birth, the nurse should be prepared to identify each baby at the time it is born. A cesarean birth may be necessary if the cord has prolapsed or one baby is malpresenting. The nursing care of the woman after the babies are born is the same as for other women, except that the nurse is aware of the greater risk of postpartum hemorrhage.

References

Bobak, I. M., & Jensen, M. D. (1991). *Essentials of Maternity Nursing*, 3rd ed. St. Louis: Mosby Year Book.

Creasy, R. K., & Resnik, R. (1989). *Maternal-Fetal Medicine: Principles and Practice*, 2nd ed. Philadelphia: W. B. Saunders Company.

Dickason, E. J., Schult, M. O., & Silverman, B. L. (1990). *Maternal-Infant Nursing Care*. St. Louis: C. V. Mosby.

Gill, P., Smith, M., & McGregor, C. (1989). Terbutaline by pump to prevent recurrent preterm labor. *American Journal of Maternal/Child Nursing* 14(3):163–167.

Johnson, F. F. (1988). Assessment and education to prevent preterm labor. *American Journal of Maternal-Child Nursing* 14(3):157–160.

Ladewig, P. W., London, M. L., & Olds, S. B. (1990). *Essentials of Maternal-Newborn Nursing*, 2nd ed. Redwood City, CA: Addison-Wesley Nursing.

Sala, D. J., & Moise, K. (1990). The treatment of preterm labor using a portable subcutaneous terbutaline pump. *Journal of Obstetric, Gynecologic, and Neonatal Nursing* 19(2):108–115.

Wilkins, I., & Creasy, R. K. (1990). Preterm labor. *Clinical Obstetrics and Gynecology* 33:502–514.

SUGGESTED ACTIVITIES

1. Identify problems that can complicate labor and birth.
2. Describe the nursing actions in a precipitate labor if no physician is present.

REVIEW QUESTIONS

A. **Select the best answer to each multiple-choice question.**

1. Precipitate labor is often defined as lasting
   A. 3 hours or less
   B. 5 hours
   C. 7 hours
   D. 10 hours

2. Premature labor is defined as labor that
   A. Occurs before 38 weeks' gestation
   B. Begins 1 week before the expected date
   C. Is of short duration
   D. Has mild contractions

3. Dysfunctional labor may be caused by
   A. Insufficient intensity of uterine contractions
   B. Abnormally strong uterine contractions
   C. Fetal malposition
   D. All of the above

4. When the fetal head is directed toward the back of the maternal pelvis instead of the front, it is known as
   A. Face presentation
   B. Breech presentation
   C. Brow presentation
   D. Persistent occiput posterior position

5. A third-degree laceration extends into the
   A. Mucous membrane
   B. Muscles of the perineum
   C. Anal sphincter muscles
   D. Mediolateral incision

6. A cesarean birth is likely to be performed for all of the following reasons EXCEPT
   A. Fetal distress
   B. Fetopelvic disproportion
   C. Birth of seventh child
   D. Herpes simplex virus

7. Immediately after the cesarean surgery is completed, the woman should be assessed for all of the following EXCEPT
   A. Firmness of uterus
   B. Amount of vaginal bleeding
   C. Wound infection
   D. Amount of bleeding from abdominal incision

8. After the woman has delivered twins, she should be closely observed for
   A. Anxiety
   B. Hemorrhage
   C. Exhaustion
   D. Pain in her lower extremities

9. An abnormal fetal heart rate during late labor would show which characteristic?
   A. Rate between 120 and 160 bpm
   B. Acceleration with contraction or movement
   C. A beat-to-beat variability of two to five beats
   D. Deceleration in a mirror pattern with contraction

10. Cesarean birth is indicated for the woman infected with which one of the following at the *onset* of labor?
    A. Hepatitis
    B. Toxoplasmosis
    C. Syphilis
    D. Herpes virus 2

11. The nurse should be knowledgeable about tocolytic drugs used to stop preterm labor. One such drug is ritodrine. The side effects of ritodrine include
    A. Headache, nausea, and vomiting
    B. Restlessness and anxiety
    C. Tachycardia and palpitations
    D. All of the above

12. The nurse should be knowledgeable about the action of drugs used to augment or induce labor. The action of oxytocin (Pitocin), a drug commonly used to induce labor, includes all of the following EXCEPT
    A. Increases the excitability of the myometrial cells of the uterus
    B. Increases the strength of the muscle contraction
    C. Decreases the excitability of the uterine muscles
    D. Stimulates frequency of contractions

B. Choose from Column II the phrase that most accurately defines the term in Column I.

I

1. Cephalopelvic disproportion _____
2. Precipitate labor _____
3. Premature labor _____
4. Hypertonic uterine dysfunction _____
5. Malpresentation of fetus _____
6. Breech presentation _____
7. Prolapsed cord _____
8. Contracted pelvis _____
9. Occiput posterior position _____
10. Hydramnios _____

II

A. Shortened diameter of pelvis
B. Long labor with increased back discomfort
C. Face presentation
D. Fetus too large for maternal pelvis
E. Excessive amniotic fluid
F. Less than 3-hour labor
G. Birth before 38 weeks' gestation
H. Cord protruding from vagina
I. Head in fundus of uterus
J. Abnormally strong uterine activity

CHAPTER 23 _____

Chapter Outline

Postpartum Hemorrhage
    Uterine atony
    Lacerations
    Retained placental tissue
    Nursing assessment and intervention
Puerperal Infection
    Causes
    Symptoms
    Intervention
    Prevention or reduction
Thrombophlebitis
Mastitis
    Symptoms
    Intervention
    Prevention
Urinary Tract Infection
    Cystitis
    Pyelonephritis
Psychiatric Disorders
Surgical Procedures
    Cesarean birth
    Sterilization surgery
    Elective abortion

Learning Objectives

Upon completion of Chapter 23, the student should be able to
- Define postpartum hemorrhage.
- List three main causes of postpartum hemorrhage.
- Summarize the appropriate nursing interventions for hemorrhage during the postpartum period.
- Define puerperal infection and name the organisms that most commonly cause the infection.
- Name three symptoms that suggest puerperal infection.
- Describe two symptoms that suggest an infected episiotomy.
- Discuss the nursing care of a woman who has an infected episiotomy.
- Discuss the nursing care of a woman who has thrombophlebitis.
- Name the organism that most commonly causes mastitis.
- List three ways to prevent mastitis.
- Discuss discharge instructions regarding breast care for the woman who is breastfeeding her infant.
- List three causes of postpartum cystitis.
- Discuss the management of a woman who has cystitis.
- List four symptoms of pyelonephritis and describe the management of the infection.
- Compare "postpartum blues" with postpartum psychosis.
- Discuss the postpartum care of a woman who had a cesarean birth.
- Explain female sterilization surgery.

POSTPARTUM COMPLICATIONS AND SURGERY

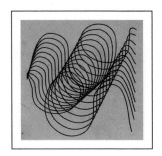

Complications of pregnancy, labor, and birth are discussed in Chapters 21 and 22. Some of the conditions described in those chapters, such as diabetes and hypertension, continue beyond birth. Other problems that occur during the postpartum period are discussed in this chapter, together with surgical procedures including cesarean birth, sterilization, and elective abortions.

Postpartum Hemorrhage

Postpartum hemorrhage is defined as the loss of 500 mL or more of blood during delivery or within the first 24 hours after delivery. Loss of 1000 mL (2 pints) of blood is considered a major hemorrhage and is an especially serious threat to the woman's life. When blood accumulates within the uterus or peritoneal cavity, even if vaginal bleeding is minimal, profound shock may develop. If vaginal bleeding is excessive over a period of time without intervention, the woman's life may be in danger. The ultimate effect of hemorrhage depends on the woman's general condition and, especially, her previous blood volume. The woman's blood volume reserve can be seriously depleted by anemia and dehydration.

The main causes of postpartum hemorrhage are uterine atony (the most common cause), lacerations of the cervix or birth canal, and retained placental fragments. Certain factors predispose the woman to hemorrhage: overdistention of the uterus due to multiple pregnancy; a large infant; hydramnios; prolonged labor, leading to muscle fatigue; relaxant-type anesthesia; high parity (more than five previous births), resulting in diminished muscle tone; trauma due to obstetric procedures (for example, use of forceps); abnormal third stage of labor; prior bleeding (placenta previa); general poor health; and rapid delivery (a slow delivery allows the uterus to contract firmly while it is decreasing in size). If any of these conditions exist, the woman should be carefully monitored for the first 24 hours (see Nursing Care Plan 23–1).

MAIN CAUSES OF POSTPARTUM HEMORRHAGE

- Uterine atony
- Lacerations of the cervix or birth canal
- Retained placental fragments

UTERINE ATONY

Uterine atony—failure of the uterine muscles to stay contracted after delivery—is the most common cause of postpartum hemorrhage. The first nursing action in uterine atony is to massage the uterus to stimulate it to contract (Fig. 23–1). If blood clots are present, they should be expelled so they do not hinder muscle contraction. In addition, oxytocin (Pitocin) is given in a slow intravenous drip to help the uterine muscles remain contracted.

LACERATIONS

Lacerations of the cervix, vagina, or perineum can significantly deplete blood volume. The uterus may be firm, and blood may be continuously trickling from unrepaired lacerations. No amount of uterine contraction will stop the bleeding. The

NURSING CARE PLAN 23–1

CARE OF THE WOMAN WITH POSTPARTUM HEMORRHAGE

Potential Problems and Nursing Diagnoses	Nursing Interventions
1. Potential fluid volume deficit related to loss of blood.	Assess amount of vaginal blood flow. Monitor vital signs; be alert to signs of hypovolemic shock (fast pulse, decreased blood pressure, restlessness, and stupor). Maintain open intravenous infusion. Encourage families to donate blood. Have blood available for woman. Instruct woman how to massage her own fundus.
2. Anxiety related to feelings of uncertainty and helplessness.	Help woman express feelings of anxiety. Provide information about potential interventions.
3. Potential for infection.	Use precautions in touching contaminated articles. Use proper handwashing before caring for woman. Recognize that large blood loss makes woman more susceptible to infection.
4. Altered comfort.	Recognize that the amount of discomfort is related to cause of hemorrhage and method of treatment.
5. Potential for altered tissue perfusion secondary to blood loss.	Monitor vital signs; compare present blood pressure with baseline blood pressure. Recognize that thready, rapid pulse and hypotension reflect decreased cardiac output.
6. Potential altered parenting due to delay in holding and possibly feeding infant.	Continue to give information about status of infant. Allow mother to see infant, even if she at that time feels unable to hold infant.

Expected Outcomes

1. Woman correctly massages her fundus. Caregiver maintains an open intravenous line.
2. Woman uses relaxation techniques to reduce anxiety.
3. Frequent handwashing is carried out by patient, significant others, and caregivers.
4. Woman appears comfortable.
5. Vital signs show normal blood pressure and pulse.
6. Mother is able to see and hold infant.

---

open vessels must be located and sutured. Usually, the physician or nurse midwife inspects the birth canal after delivery to immediately repair possible tears. However, it is possible for an open vessel to be overlooked and hemorrhage to result. Lacerations are more likely to be present after a forceps delivery. Sometimes a hematoma (bleeding into the tissues) occurs from open vessels after an episiotomy or laceration. This type of bleeding is usually slow and frequently involves the vulvar and vaginal mucosae. Bleeding from lacerations or an episiotomy incision should be reported immediately. Often, the woman is taken back to the delivery room for additional repair to stop the bleeding.

RETAINED PLACENTAL TISSUE

Retained placental fragments, regardless of size, can interfere with constriction of the uterine blood

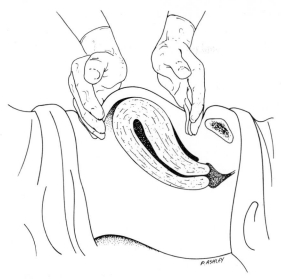

▲ FIGURE 23-1

Suggested method to palpate the fundus after birth. One hand is placed just above the symphysis pubis, and gentle pressure is exerted. The other hand is cupped around the uterine fundus. If the uterus does not feel firm, it can be massaged with the hands in the same position.

vessels, causing a hemorrhage. The placenta should always be inspected for completeness. Evidence of torn blood vessels is suggestive of retained placental tissue. Occasionally, a piece of the placenta is embedded in the uterine lining when the placenta is expelled. Retained placenta may be removed manually or surgically by curettage. A hysterectomy may be necessary in the case of placenta accreta or tumors.

NURSING DIAGNOSES

- Fluid volume deficit related to decrease in blood volume
- Altered tissue perfusion related to reduction in tissue oxygenation and rapidity of blood loss.
- Fluid volume deficit related to loss of extracellular fluid
- Anxiety related to feelings of uncertainty and apprehension
- Potential for infection related to retention of placental tissue and excessive blood loss

- Knowledge deficit related to the cause of the excessive bleeding

NURSING ASSESSMENT AND INTERVENTION

After delivery, the caregiver should be alert to signs of hemorrhage in the woman and report them immediately, so that prompt treatment can be started. The uterine assessment involves checking for sustained firmness, amount of blood flow, status of vital signs, and signs of shock.

If bleeding is excessive or the uterus is relaxed or boggy, the caregiver should massage the uterus until it is firm and press on the uterus to empty it of blood clots. Because a tremendous amount of blood can be lost in a short period of time, prompt reporting of hemorrhage may save the woman's life. Signs of hypovolemic shock include a rapid, weak pulse; pallor; excessive thirst; and restlessness followed by periods of unconsciousness and possible death. With excessive bleeding, hypovolemic shock may be difficult to correct despite adequate teamwork and treatment.

A necessary measure for excessive bleeding is ordering blood that is typed and cross-matched for transfusion. An intravenous infusion of a glucose solution would be started with an 18- to 19-gauge needle so that the blood transfusion can be added if necessary. Oxytocic agents may be added to the intravenous solution if the uterus does not remain contracted. A woman's coagulation profile is usually ordered, and heparin may be needed to stop an abnormal clotting and check the bleeding. The woman should be prepared for a dilatation and curettage (D&C) if retained tissue is the cause of bleeding. It is important for the caregiver to stay with the woman and support her until the bleeding is controlled.

Puerperal Infection

Puerperal morbidity is a term used to describe any infection of the reproductive tract during the puerperium. The woman is considered to have a puerperal infection if she has a temperature of 100.4° F (38° C) on two days during the first 10 postpartum days, excluding the first 24 hours, unless another source is determined. Puerperal sepsis involves the introduction of pathogenic organisms into susceptible tissues. The signs of puerperal infection are always considered serious. The infection may involve the perineum, the uterine lining (endometritis), or the pelvic area outside the uterus (parametritis). The infection may extend by means of blood vessels and the lymphatic system to areas relatively distant from the infection site, as in the case of septic thrombophlebitis of the leg. Such infections are most often localized, but they can become generalized to peritonitis or septicemia.

CAUSES

Puerperal infection can be caused by several organisms, but the most common are *Streptococcus* and *Staphylococcus*. *Escherichia coli* (colon bacillus) and *Neisseria gonorrhoeae* (gonococcus) may also be causes. The severity of the infection depends on the original invaders. Bacteria of the normal vaginal flora may increase in number and become virulent when tissues are traumatized. In addition, pathogens may be introduced by hospital personnel (through the nasopharynx, for example); failure of aseptic technique; or contamination by other sources, such as feces that gain access to the uterus during labor and delivery.

Before the onset of labor, the vaginal contents are slightly acidic because of the conversion of glycogen to lactic acid. This acid medium is unsuitable for the growth of many pathogens. However, in the puerperium, the lochial discharge contains blood that forms an ideal culture medium for many organisms and is more alkaline.

SYMPTOMS

The symptoms of puerperal infection depend somewhat on the area involved. The first and most obvious symptom is an elevated temperature (fever). Other symptoms include rapid pulse, malaise, chills, headache, and pain or tenderness in the area involved. If the episiotomy incision becomes infected, there often is local tenderness and purulent drainage around the sutures or a break-down of the incision. If the infection is endometritis, the uterus becomes tender, and a foul odor and a greenish color of the lochia are characteristic findings.

INTERVENTION

Culture samples of the drainage, blood, or both are taken for culture and sensitivity tests to determine which organisms have invaded the birth canal. The results will determine which drugs will be most effective in destroying the identified organisms. After culture and sensitivity tests, aggressive treatment with intravenous antibiotics is carried out. In addition, fluids are forced and temperature, pulse, and respirations monitored a minimum of every 4 hours. If the episiotomy area or perineum is infected, warm sitz baths are ordered. If the woman has endometritis, she may be asked to assume Fowler's position (lying down with the head and upper body elevated) to promote pelvic localization of the infection.

Because the infectious organisms may be transmitted to other patients and to the infant, isolation technique (Centers for Disease Control universal precautions) is instituted. This means that the woman may not be able to have as close contact with her infant as she would normally have.

If the woman is breastfeeding, she can continue to stimulate her breasts by expressing the milk manually or by breast pump. The milk is discarded because it may contain infectious organisms. The woman may feel depressed if she is separated from her infant. An explanation of the reasons for her plan of care and psychological support are essential.

PREVENTION OR REDUCTION

One of the most important preventive measures is frequent and thorough handwashing by all personnel who care for the woman during labor, birth, and early puerperium. Maintenance of strict asepsis in the delivery room is also important. If catheterization becomes necessary to correct urinary retention, strict aseptic technique should be used to reduce the likelihood that bacteria will be introduced into the bladder. Caregivers who have upper respiratory or skin infections should not be allowed to care for maternity patients. The nasopharynx of attendants is considered to be a major source of infections.

NURSING DIAGNOSES

- Knowledge deficit related to lack of understanding of prevention of infection
- Pain related to the presence of inflammation and discomfort
- Potential injury related to the spread of infection to other tissues

Thrombophlebitis

Thrombophlebitis is a venous inflammation and may cause an obstruction of venous return. The common symptoms and signs are pain, tenderness, and swelling of one or both legs. Elevated skin temperature and erythema may be observed over the involved vessel. Homans' sign (dorsiflexion of the foot) is usually positive, and the woman experiences pain when raising the leg.

Treatment depends on whether vein involvement is superficial or deep. Anticoagulant therapy is indicated because of the threat of embolism. If anticoagulant therapy is given, the patient needs to be closely monitored for bleeding. Nursing assessment includes taking the circumference of the calf and thigh. Antibiotics are given as in other infections. Doppler ultrasonography is done to assist in determining whether a clot formation exists, where it is located, and whether partial occlusion is present. Bed rest is required. When the symptoms have subsided, the woman may begin ambulation while wearing elastic support stockings.

Mastitis

Postpartum *mastitis* is an infection in the glandular tissue of the breasts. The most common infectious organism is *Staphylococcus aureus*, but mastitis may also be caused by a Group A *Streptococcus*. The pathogens enter the subcutaneous lymphatic system through nipple fissures or erosions, or a plugged duct can precipitate the infectious process. The source of infection can sometimes be traced to the infant, who may acquire the pathogen from the mother or from a health care provider. Proper handwashing is important to reduce this infection. Because mastitis usually affects only one breast and occurs several days postpartum or by the second or third postpartum week, the woman often is discharged before symptoms occur. Therefore adequate patient instruction about the symptoms of mastitis is an essential part of her discharge plan.

SYMPTOMS

The physical findings of mastitis are tenderness, warmth, localized erythema, and an elevated body temperature. Usually the infection is confined to a lobe or local area of the breast. If treatment is not begun immediately, the invading bacteria multiply rapidly and a breast abscess forms (Fig. 23–2).

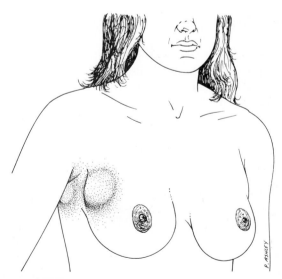

▲ **FIGURE 23—2**

Mastitis. Erythema and edema are present in the upper outer quadrant of the breast. By assessment, the axillary lymph nodes show enlargement and tenderness.

NURSING DIAGNOSES

- Knowledge deficit related to appropriate breastfeeding practices
- Potential for injury related to breast tissue damage
- Pain related to the development of mastitis
- Altered comfort related to tenderness of infected area of breast

INTERVENTION

The mother's milk is cultured for sensitivity tests, and antibiotics are started. A mother can continue to breastfeed her infant, if it is not too uncomfortable. Also, a breast pump may be used to mechanically empty the breasts. Ice packs, bed rest, and pain-relieving drugs are used to provide comfort. With prompt treatment the symptoms subside in 1 or 2 days, and abscess formation seldom occurs. If an abscess does form, it is incised to allow healing to take place. The mother's temperature should be checked every 4 hours. She may feel guilty, depressed, and frustrated and may need psychological support as well as physical comfort.

PREVENTION

Current literature suggests that the mother should nurse frequently while infected to prevent milk stasis and engorgement, both of which are associated with risk of infection and formation of breast abscess. Because mastitis usually does not occur until the mother is home, she should be instructed about the importance of complete emp-

tying of the breast, changing the infant's position while nursing (allowing different pressure points on the nipple), and breaking the infant suction before removing the infant from the breast. If the woman is having difficulty in breastfeeding, she may find it helpful to seek advice from a support group such as the La Leche League or a lactation consultant. Personal hygiene is important to reduce the incidence of mastitis and should be included in patient instruction.

Urinary Tract Infection

NURSING DIAGNOSES

- Knowledge deficit related to potential causes of urinary tract infection
- Altered urinary elimination secondary to cystitis
- Anxiety related to the outcome of the infection

CYSTITIS

The puerperal woman is a likely candidate for the development of urinary tract infections. Stretching of the bladder (overdistention) or the base of the bladder occurs to some extent in all vaginal deliveries and sometimes results in edema of the trigone that is great enough to obstruct the urethra and cause urinary retention. The symptoms of cystitis are urinary frequency and urgency, dysuria, and low-grade fever. Urine often remains in the bladder after the woman voids; this is called

---

KEY POINTS IN EDUCATION: PATIENT EDUCATION ON PERSONAL HYGIENE MEASURES RELATING TO BREAST CARE

- Wash hands frequently
- Keep breasts clean and avoid irritating cleansing agents
- Provide adequate support of breasts (24-hour nonconstricting support)
- Use gentleness in care

- Avoid decrusting the nipple
- Intermittently expose nipples to air
- Avoid exposure to known sources of infection
- Change breast pads frequently

residual urine. Residual urine is a medium for the development of the bacteria that cause cystitis.

As soon as symptoms of cystitis appear, a clean-catch midstream urine sample should be obtained for microscopic examination, culture, and antibiotic sensitivity tests. The management consists of high fluid intake, emptying the bladder, and administering antibiotics. A sulfisoxazole drug (Gantrisin) may be given. An indwelling catheter may be inserted to keep the bladder empty until the infection has subsided.

It is important for the woman to continue drinking fluids and to take the medication ordered until after the symptoms disappear, because this infection is tenacious and tends to recur.

PYELONEPHRITIS

Pyelonephritis (upper urinary tract infection) occurs less frequently than cystitis. In most cases, the infection has ascended from the lower urinary tract. When urinary tract infection progresses to pyelonephritis, systemic symptoms usually appear, including high fever, chills, nausea and vomiting, and pain over the kidney area. An additional symptom is costovertebral angle tenderness. Broad-spectrum antibiotics are prescribed immediately. The woman should be instructed about the seriousness of the condition and continue to take antibiotics for 2 to 4 weeks after clinical symptoms disappear.

Psychiatric Disorders

During pregnancy, it is not uncommon for a woman to experience feelings of inadequacy, even hostility, toward herself and the developing fetus. Moreover, fears about the outcome of pregnancy and childbirth may color her emotional responses and evoke defense reactions. Education and informed reassurance can do much to relieve her distress.

After delivery a woman must make profound adjustments to the new interactions among herself, the infant, the father, and siblings in the family. The new mother may display confusion, depression, resentment, and other ambivalent feelings. These reactions are within the normal range of behavior often referred to as the "postpartum blues."

Psychosis or mental illness after pregnancy is rare without a prior history of an emotional disorder. However, in rare cases the stress of labor may trigger bizarre behavior while the woman is in the hospital; such behavior should be reported immediately. A psychiatric consultation will help determine if the woman may harm herself or her infant. Appropriate steps should be taken to ensure the safety of the woman and her infant.

Surgical Procedures

CESAREAN BIRTH

A cesarean birth is the delivery of the infant through the abdominal wall and the uterus, as discussed in Chapter 22. The mother and the significant other will need additional postpartum care and discharge instructions, particularly because her hospitalization period is relatively short (average of 4 days).

STERILIZATION SURGERY

Sterilization surgery may be done during the postpartum period. Usually, a tubal ligation is performed to make the woman incapable of reproduction. A tubal ligation interrupts the passage of the ovum through the uterine tubes. A signed consent from the woman is required by the physician and the hospital.

Although some physicians are more inclined to do tubal ligations than others, the most common indications are the following:

- Serious complications of pregnancy
- Three or more cesarean births
- Multiparity (a woman with several children)
- Psychiatric problems

Tubal ligation is commonly performed through a small transverse subumbilical incision. The peritoneal cavity is entered, and a segment of each tube is ligated (see Fig. 15–7). Alternatively, a minilaparotomy technique may be used in which the tubes are crushed, ligated, or (in the newer, potentially reversible procedure) plugged. Pre- and postoperative care is the same as for any patient having abdominal surgery. The postoperative recovery is usually rapid and uneventful. It is important to meet the woman's postpartum, personal health care, and infant-caretaking needs. Some women experience guilt; the caregiver should recognize this feeling and support her.

ELECTIVE ABORTION

An elective, or induced, abortion is the purposeful termination of pregnancy. It is discussed in this chapter because the postabortion nursing care has some similarities to postpartum care. For example, the patient is assessed for vaginal bleeding and potential infection.

In the 1990s controversy over elective abortions is likely to continue in both the Congress and the state legislatures, as well as among the public. The United States Supreme Court has changed its membership in the last few years, and test cases are pending in the Court that might result in additional restrictions on or an overthrow of *Roe vs. Wade,* the landmark decision made in 1973 that legalized abortion in the United States. Since that time numerous controversies have arisen concerning funding of abortion; state regulation of abortion; and where, when, and how abortions can be performed. In 1989, the Supreme Court, in *Webster vs. Reproductive Health Services,* upheld a Missouri law in a decision that gave the states a much greater ability to restrict pregnancy termination. In 1991, Louisiana used its rights to impose the greatest restrictions on abortion in the United States.

The opponents of abortion, the "pro-life" group, support the moral principle that "the unborn fetus is a human being with a right to life." The proponents of abortion, the "pro-choice" group, believe any woman has the right to control her own body and reproductive activity.

The risks for elective abortions include hemorrhage, infection, disseminated intravascular coagulation, and possible sterility due to adhesions after an infection (Table 23–1). Also, with repeated abortions, a condition known as Asherman syndrome may exist. In Asherman syndrome, the

TABLE 23–1. RISKS WOMEN MAY ENCOUNTER IN AN ABORTION

Hemorrhage
Uterine perforation
Cervical lacerations
Sterility
Infection
Maternal death from disseminated intravascular coagulation (DIC), saline in maternal circulation, hemorrhage, cardiac failure, and septic shock
Guilt and depression

endometrium does not build up an adequate lining during the proliferative period of the menstrual cycle because of adhesions that are usually caused by infections. In addition, some women are known to experience guilt and depression.

Methods

EARLY ABORTION (UP TO 12 WEEKS)

Laminaria. The stem of the seaweed *laminaria,* is sterilized and packaged according to length. The length of the woman's cervical os is determined by the physician, and the laminaria of appropriate size is inserted past the tip of the internal os. Laminaria absorbs fluid from the tissues, and it increases in diameter, which gradually dilates the cervix. Frequently, within a few hours, the cervix is dilated sufficiently to allow the passage of a curette to remove the products of conception. Successful use of laminaria avoids cervical lacerations caused by the metal curette.

Dilatation and Curettage. In a D&C, the cervix is dilated with a metal dilator's sound, and the uterine lining is scraped with a curette or removed by suction evacuation. This procedure may be done on an outpatient basis. It is important to observe the woman for excessive bleeding and possible uterine cramps.

LATE ABORTION (12 TO 16 WEEKS)

If an abortion is performed late in pregnancy, it should be done in the hospital to safeguard the woman, and she should be encouraged to discuss her decision with the care provider. There is a greater risk of complications. Three methods used are saline instillation, prostaglandin injection, and hysterotomy.

Saline Instillation. A hypertonic solution is injected. The abdomen is cleansed, and a local anesthetic is injected at the site. A needle is inserted through the abdominal and uterine walls into the amniotic sac. About 100 to 200 mL of amniotic fluid is removed. This is followed by the infusion of 100 to 200 mL of 20% hypertonic saline. The onset of contractions usually occurs within 6 to 12 hours. A curettage may be necessary if the placenta is not spontaneously expelled. The death of the fetus usually occurs within 1 hour after the injection of saline.

Serious complications can occur with saline instillation: maternal death from entry of the hypertonic saline solution into the maternal circulation, septic shock, hemorrhage, infection, and disseminated intravascular coagulation.

Prostaglandin Injection. Prostaglandin is administered intravenously. It also can be administered transabdominally into the amniotic sac. As in the hypertonic saline injection, the abdomen is cleansed, and a local anesthetic is injected at the site before a needle containing prostaglandin is inserted into the amniotic sac. Labor usually begins, the cervix dilates, and the fetus aborts within 18 hours or less. Nausea, vomiting, and diarrhea may develop after the prostaglandin injection.

Hysterotomy. In a hysterotomy, the fetus is removed through an abdominal incision, as if it were a mini-cesarean birth. This procedure is done only when no other option is available, such as when the fetus is grossly deformed and large. The woman would need the same preoperative and postoperative preparation as for a cesarean birth (Table 23–2).

Postabortion Care

In the immediate postabortion period, vital signs, bleeding, and uterine cramps need to be monitored. An injection of Rh_o (D) immune globulin (RhoGAM) should be given to Rh− women. The woman should be instructed to call her physician or clinic if her temperature is above 102° F (over a period of 6 hours), if she has excessive bleeding, or if she has extreme uterine cramps. Because the cervix is usually dilated for 2 to 3 weeks, women should be instructed to avoid sexual intercourse, tampons, and douching for that interval. Regular activities, if not vigorous, can be resumed in 2 weeks. The woman should be instructed about contraceptive methods, because she can ovulate and become pregnant shortly after the abortion.

TABLE 23–2. METHODS USED FOR ELECTIVE ABORTIONS	
EARLY ABORTIONS (12 WEEKS OR LESS)	**LATE ABORTIONS (12 TO 16 WEEKS)**
Suction evacuation	Saline instillation
Dilatation and curettage (D&C)	Prostaglandin injection
Laminaria (seaweed "sticks")	Hysterotomy

References

Dickason, E. J., Schult, M. O., & Silverman, B. L. (1990). *Maternal-Infant Nursing Care.* St. Louis: C.V. Mosby.

Ladewig, P. W., London, M. L., & Olds, S. B. (1990). *Essentials of Maternal-Newborn Nursing,* 2nd ed. Redwood City, CA: Addison-Wesley Nursing.

Marieskind, H. I. (1989). Cesarean section in the United States: Has it changed since 1979? *Birth* 16(4):196–201.

Sherwen, L. M., Scoloveno, M. A., & Weingarten, C. T. (1991). *Nursing Care of the Childbearing Family.* Norwalk, CT: Appleton & Lange.

Unterman, R. R., Postner, N. A., & Williams, K. N. (1990). Postpartum depressive disorders: Changing trends. *Birth* 17(3):131–137.

SUGGESTED ACTIVITIES

1. Discuss nursing assessment and intervention regarding the care of a woman who has excessive postpartum bleeding.
2. List three common types of infection found during the postpartum period. Give the nursing intervention for each one.

REVIEW QUESTIONS

Select the best answer to each multiple-choice question.

1. A woman would be considered to have a postpartum hemorrhage if her blood loss was more than
   A. 150 mL
   B. 300 mL
   C. 400 mL
   D. 500 mL

2. If, by assessment, the postpartum woman's uterus feels soft and relaxed, the first thing the nurse should do is to
   A. Notify the physician
   B. Start an oxytocin infusion
   C. Massage the uterus until firm
   D. Change the woman's perineal pads

3. The most common cause of postpartum hemorrhage is
   A. Retained pieces of membranes
   B. Lacerations of the cervix
   C. Uterine atony
   D. None of the above

4. Pain, tenderness, and swelling of the leg are indicative of
   A. Endometritis
   B. Parametritis
   C. Thrombophlebitis
   D. Mastitis

5. The most common organism that causes mastitis is
   A. *Streptococcus*
   B. *Staphylococcus*
   C. *Escherichia coli*
   D. *Neisseria gonorrhoeae*

6. Symptoms of mastitis include all of the following EXCEPT
   A. Localized erythema
   B. Elevated temperature
   C. Pain in involved breast
   D. Shortness of breath

7. Cystitis can result from
   A. Trauma of bladder during delivery
   B. Urinary retention during labor
   C. Obstruction of urethra due to edema
   D. All of the above

8. Psychosis is uncommon during the postpartum period without a prior history of an emotional disorder. Emotional reactions within the normal range of behavior include
   A. Mild depression
   B. Initial resentment
   C. Ambivalent feelings
   D. All of the above

9. The assessment of a woman who had a cesarean birth includes all of the following EXCEPT
   A. Lochial flow
   B. Palpation of uterus
   C. Deep breathing and coughing
   D. Encouragement of complete bed rest

10. Risk(s) of an induced abortion is (are)
    A. Hemorrhage
    B. Uterine perforation
    C. Sterility
    D. All of the above

11. On her 3rd postpartum day, Mrs. A. complains of severe pain in the perineum. An appropriate nursing intervention would be
    A. Inspect perineum for discolored areas
    B. Give Tylenol orally
    C. Tell Mrs. A that this is normal during the postpartum period
    D. Suggest bed rest

12. Clinical symptoms associated with endometritis are
    A. Tender, boggy uterus and profuse lochia with foul odor
    B. Small, tender uterus and temperature of 99° F
    C. Decreased pulse rate and hard, tender fundus
    D. Anorexia and a large, firm uterus

13. It is important to recognize and report early signs and symptoms of puerperal infections so treatment may be started as soon as possible. One of the first signs usually observed is
    A. Nausea
    B. Rubra vaginal discharge
    C. Pelvic pain
    D. Temperature of 100.4° F (38° C) or higher on 2 of the first 10 days after the first 24 hours after delivery

CHAPTER 24 _____

Chapter Outline

Birth Injuries
    Forceps marks
    Cephalohematoma
    Intracranial hemorrhage
    Fractures
    Brachial plexus injury
Congenital Defects
    Heart defects
    Cleft palate and lip
    Clubfoot (talipes)
    Tracheoesophageal fistula
    Pyloric stenosis
    Omphalocele
    Imperforate anus
    Cryptorchidism (undescended testicles)
    Hypospadias and epispadias
    Hydrocephalus
    Spina bifida
    Down's syndrome
    Phenylketonuria
    Galactosemia
Disorders of the Blood
    Hyperbilirubinemia
    ABO incompatibility
Infection
    Diarrhea
    Umbilical cord (omphalitis)
    Impetigo contagiosa
    Conjunctivitis (ophthalmia neonatorum)
    Thrush
    Congenital syphilis
The Infant of a Diabetic Mother
Respiratory Distress
Drug Dependency

Learning Objectives

Upon completion of Chapter 24, the student should be able to

- Describe common birth injuries that occur in newborn infants and the nursing care for these injuries.
- Describe common congenital defects in newborns and the nursing care for these defects.
- Discuss the common neonatal blood disorders and the nursing care for these disorders.
- Identify the common types of infections of newborn infants and the nursing care of these infections.
- List the problems in the newborn infant of a diabetic mother.
- Explain the care of a newborn infant with respiratory distress.
- List five withdrawal symptoms in an infant of a drug-addicted mother.

PROBLEMS THAT MAY AFFECT THE NEWBORN INFANT

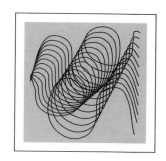

Although most newborn infants are born healthy and ready to meet the challenge of the outside world, some are not so fortunate. Some newborn infants have an abnormality that causes disfigurement for life, a mental handicap, or a complication that will shorten their life. Many of these problems can be noted at birth, and the prognosis is improved with an early diagnosis.

It is difficult for most parents to accept an infant who is not normal. Many times, the parents (especially the mother) experience anxiety, guilt, frustration, and anger when they are told about their infant's condition. Some parents become increasingly demanding of the caregiver because of their uncontrolled feelings. The caregiver should be very supportive and allow the parents to express their feelings about the infant. It is important that professional guidance, which would involve community resources, be given as necessary. In working with the parents (or mother), it is important that the caregiver know how much they have been told about the infant's condition. It is necessary that all the health providers work as a team in assisting the parents through their difficulty. Often, the nurse can be a vital liaison among the family, medical staff, clergy, and community resource personnel.

Birth Injuries

FORCEPS MARKS

Forceps marks are bruised tissue or a breakdown in the tissue made by the pressure of the forceps applied to the infant's head (Fig. 24–1). Usually, the marks will disappear in a few days; however, sometimes the fifth facial nerve is damaged, and this damage lasts longer. It is important to reassure the mother that the marks usually will disappear by approximately 2 weeks.

CEPHALOHEMATOMA

Cephalohematoma is a collection of blood between the periosteum and the skull. Its margins are well defined and usually extend to the parietal

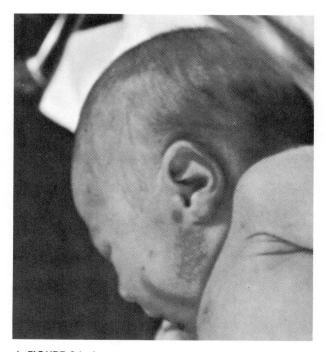

▲ FIGURE 24–1

Forceps marks on infant's face. (Courtesy of Mead Johnson Laboratories, Evansville, IN.)

bone. It does not cross the suture lines (a caput succedaneum does). The blood mass may increase during the first 2 to 3 days after birth. The blood is gradually absorbed, and no surgical intervention is necessary. It is important to assess the infant's bilirubin level during absorption of the blood. The bilirubin level will rise as the blood is absorbed, possibly beyond the arbitrary safe level.

INTRACRANIAL HEMORRHAGE

Intracranial hemorrhage is bleeding anywhere within the cranial vault. It can be a serious and fatal birth injury. The hemorrhage is most often seen in infants born during difficult deliveries or after prolonged labors. Intracranial hemorrhage may also occur as a result of a rapid, precipitate delivery due to excessive pressure on the fetal head. In addition, it is often observed in preterm infants because of the fragility of their blood vessels. The signs of intracranial hemorrhage may occur suddenly or gradually. The symptoms include a poor sucking reflex; irritability; listlessness; a sharp, shrill cry; poor color; grunt-like respirations; convulsions; unequally dilated pupils; and bulging fontanelles. Sometimes, the bleeding is mild and stops spontaneously, and the infant will recover with little or no damage. At other times, the pressure is so great that it must be relieved by aspiration of fluid from the subdural space or by surgery. In more severe hemorrhages, residual damage or death can occur. The residual damage can later cause mental retardation, cerebral palsy, or hydrocephalus.

The infant with intracranial hemorrhage may be positioned with the head slightly elevated to relieve the pressure. Vitamin K may be prescribed to decrease the bleeding. It is important that the caregiver accurately observe and describe the signs and symptoms that relate to intracranial hemorrhage to assist in the medical management and care of the infant.

FRACTURES

Fractures may occur during the birth of the infant. The most common bones affected are the clavicle, humerus, and femur. A breech delivery presents the greatest risk of infant fractures.

A fracture should be suspected if the infant has lack of movement, deformity in alignment, or a shrill cry when the bone is moved. It is important to recognize fractures for early and prompt treatment. The injured part is immobilized in the correct position by pinning the infant's sleeve to the shirt to stabilize the arm. In rare cases, a cast is applied. The injured tissues usually heal rapidly in the infant. Because the parents may be fearful of hurting their infants by handling them, instruction and encouragement to hold, fondle, and talk to the infants are important. Sometimes, the parents will be instructed to gently exercise the injured part after about 2 weeks.

BRACHIAL PLEXUS INJURY

Brachial plexus injury is damage to a network of cervical spinal nerves, which control upper extremity functions. Brachial plexus palsy (Erb's palsy) can occur with excessive stretching of the neck muscles during delivery. If the infant does not raise both arms when startled (Moro's reflex), a brachial plexus injury should be suspected, diagnosed, or ruled out as a cause (Fig. 24–2). As soon as the condition is diagnosed, the affected arm is usually immobilized by placing the arm in a brace or by pinning the arm to the shirt. This injury usually is temporary.

Congenital Defects

Some infants are born with defects that are developmental or hereditary, which may be present anywhere in the body. In addition to the defects that may be inherited, others may be caused by drugs, irradiation, and maternal disease. The first 12 weeks of gestation are the most critical time of development, because the organs and body systems are forming. In spite of the potential hazards, congenital defects are relatively uncommon. If the abnormalities are recognized and treated promptly, the chance of infant survival is greater. For this reason, the caregiver working with newborn infants should assess every one for defects. Once the defects are diagnosed, the pediatrician or pediatric team will begin the management of the infant. Some of the most common defects are described in this section.

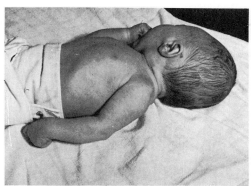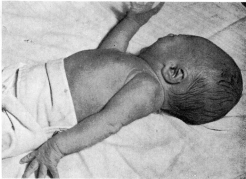

▲ FIGURE 24–2

Brachial plexus injury of the left arm (asymmetrical Moro reflex). (From Behrman, R. E., & Vaughan, V. C. III (1983). *Nelson Textbook of Pediatrics*, 12th ed. Philadelphia: W.B. Saunders Company.)

HEART DEFECTS

Major congenital anomalies can result in acyanotic heart disease. A common heart defect is the *patent ductus arteriosus,* in which a fetal shunt between the aorta and the pulmonary artery may fail to close at birth (Chapter 17). An arterial septal defect *(patent foramen ovale)* can also occur. *Coarctation of the aorta* is fairly common. It is a narrowing of the aorta after it leaves the heart. A group of four heart defects called the *tetralogy of Fallot,* if present, requires immediate attention. When cyanosis is present, a heart defect is always a potential cause. During the initial examination of the newborn, the heart's sounds and position are carefully observed.

CLEFT PALATE AND LIP

A cleft lip is a separation of the upper lip. It can be on one side only, which is called unilateral cleft lip, or it can be on both sides, which is called bilateral cleft lip. A cleft palate is an incomplete closure of the palate or roof of the mouth. How much a cleft palate interferes with suckling and breathing depends on the severity of the defect. This defect may affect the parental–infant attachment because of the infant's appearance (Fig. 24–3). Sometimes, the first surgical repair of the lip is made by 2 months of age. Repair of the palate is usually postponed until the facial tissues have grown.

The nursing care interventions are to maintain an open airway and to feed the infant in such a way as to avoid aspiration. The infant should be held in an upright position during feeding and burped frequently. It is sometimes helpful for the parents to see an infant who has had surgical correction to relieve their anxiety. Often the cosmetic repair leaves only a hairline incision.

CLUBFOOT (TALIPES)

Clubfoot is an abnormal turning of the foot either inward or outward (Fig. 24–4). It can be caused by intrauterine position. If this is the case,

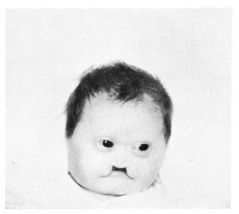

▲ FIGURE 24–3

Newborn with cleft lip and cleft palate.

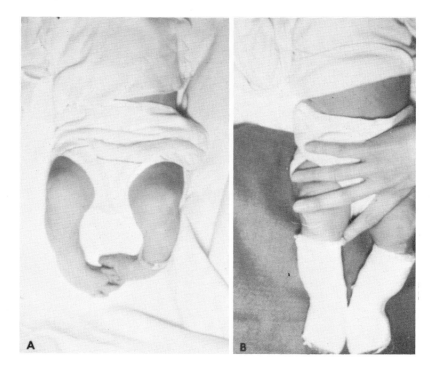

▲ **FIGURE 24—4**

A. Bilateral clubfoot. **B.** Same baby after casts have been applied. Note that toes have been left exposed to aid in ascertaining blood circulation.

the foot or feet can be passively put through the normal range of motion. If there is an unequal pull of muscles or a defect, however, the treatment may be passive overcorrection exercises or applying successive plaster casts during infancy.

If the infant is placed in a cast, the parents need to be instructed to observe the toes and thighs to detect signs of circulatory impairment, such as discoloration, swelling, or coldness. Sometimes, at a later date, special shoes are necessary, depending on the severity of the deformity and how early the treatment was started.

TRACHEOESOPHAGEAL FISTULA

In the most frequent condition, the esophagus ends in a blind pouch (atresia) with a fistula that connects it to the trachea. This arrangement causes choking, coughing, gagging, or cyanosis at the time of the first feeding. Usually the infant becomes cyanotic. It is important that all feeding be

stopped and the physician be notified about the infant's distress. Tracheoesophageal fistula channels oral fluids directly into the lungs, which can prove fatal to the infant. As soon as a positive diagnosis is made, surgery is performed. The infant is then cared for in the pediatric unit.

PYLORIC STENOSIS

The pylorus is the lower opening of the stomach (pyloric sphincter), which forms the exit of the stomach. In pyloric stenosis, there is an abnormal narrowing of the pyloric sphincter. The common symptom is projectile vomiting (forceful vomiting). When the stomach becomes distended, the pyloric sphincter forcefully ejects the fluids given to the infant. Sometimes, this type of vomiting does not appear until the infant is about 3 to 4 weeks old. However, if forceful vomiting is present, it should be reported immediately.

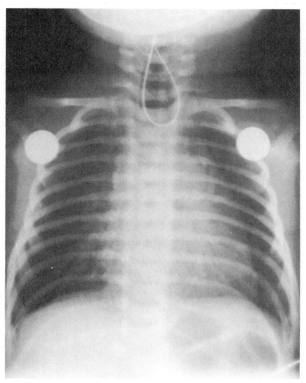

▲ FIGURE 24–5

X-ray of a newborn infant with an esophageal fistula. The esophagus ends in a blind pouch (as shown by the coiled catheter) instead of forming a continuous tube to the stomach. (From Behrman, R. E., & Vaughan, V. C. III (1987). *Nelson Textbook of Pediatrics*, 13th ed. Philadelphia: W.B. Saunders Company.)

OMPHALOCELE

An omphalocele is a defect or a herniation of the abdominal viscera, where the umbilical cord connects to the abdomen (Fig. 24–5). The defect is caused by a failure of the abdominal wall to develop properly. The infant, at birth, has the abdominal viscera exposed and covered only by a thin transparent membrane. At delivery, the exposed contents should be protected immediately with a sterile, moist gauze to reduce the chance of infection. Surgery is done immediately if possible. When the infant's condition is critical, surgery may be postponed until the condition is stable.

IMPERFORATE ANUS

An imperforate anus is the absence of an anal opening. The opening may simply be blocked by a thin membrane, in which case perforation is all that is necessary. However, if the colon ends in a blind pouch, surgical treatment is necessary to join the colon to the anus. Often, a temporary colostomy is made as the initial surgical repair.

The lack of an anal opening may first be observed by the nursery caregiver when an attempt to take the rectal temperature is impossible. If the newborn infant does not have a stool within 24 hours, an imperforate anus is one possible reason.

CRYPTORCHIDISM (UNDESCENDED TESTICLES)

Usually, the testicles descend into the scrotum during the eighth month of fetal life. Therefore, it is common to have undescended testicles in the preterm infant. Failure of the testes to descend in the full-term infant may be due to trauma, tumor formation, or a developmental failure. An inguinal hernia or hydrocele (water in the scrotum) may be present.

Because spontaneous descent sometimes occurs during the first year of life, surgical intervention is not performed until then, or it may be delayed until the child is of preschool age.

HYPOSPADIAS AND EPISPADIAS

In hypospadias, the male uretheral opening is on the under surface of the penis; in epispadias, it is on the upper surface (Fig. 24–6). In most cases, surgery is not necessary for either condition unless the defect is extensive and requires urethroplasty. Epispadias is often associated with other genitourinary anomalies. The main concern is to prevent embarrassment and to have a normal urethral opening, so that, when he is older, the boy can stand to urinate like other boys.

HYDROCEPHALUS

Hydrocephalus is a defect that results from the accumulation of abnormal amounts of cerebrospi-

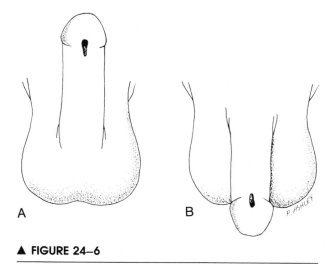

▲ FIGURE 24–6

Anomalies of genitalia. **A.** Hypospadias—urethral opening on under surface of penis. **B.** Epispadias—urethral opening on upper surface.

nal fluid within the skull. A congenital defect in fluid drainage may exist, preventing the flow of fluid from the ventricles of the brain, where it is produced, into the subarachnoid space. The fluid is then reabsorbed by the venous system. In hydrocephalus, there is some type of blockage of the cerebrospinal fluid pathway. It may result from a tumor or the defective absorption of the fluid.

Hydrocephalus may be present at birth, causing the infant's head to be significantly enlarged. The accumulation of fluid in the brain's ventricles easily enlarges the infant's head, because the bones are not yet ossified or closed. Serial measurement of the circumference of the head, indicating continual enlargement, is helpful in the diagnosis of the less obvious cases. The infant's eyes exhibit the setting-sun sign and often the infant has a high-pitched cry.

Treatment of hydrocephalus should begin as soon as the diagnosis is made to prevent further brain damage. The treatment usually consists of inserting a shunting device that by-passes the obstruction and drains the excess fluid into a body cavity (Fig. 24–7). It is important to remember that the infant with hydrocephalus has the same need to be touched, held, and loved as any other infant. The surgical treatment (shunting) and nursing care are described in detail in most pediatric texts.

SPINA BIFIDA

Spina bifida is a spinal defect in which the bony part of the spinal cord fails to close (Fig. 24–8). It can occur in any area of the spine but is most common in the lumbosacral region. The defect may vary in type and severity. *Spina bifida occulta* is a defect only of the vertebrae. There is no need for treatment unless neurological symptoms are present. A *meningocele* is protrusion of the meninges through the opening of the spinal cavity. A *meningomyelocele* occurs when the spinal cord and the meninges protrude through the defect of the spinal column. With meningomyelocele, there may be a range of conditions from muscle weakness to paralysis of the lower extremities.

The caregiver should prevent the rupture and infection of a protruding sac. The infant's position is usually on the side, with rolled towels placed to prevent pressure or injury to the defect, thereby reducing the chance of infection. The position should be changed frequently to avoid pressure areas. In addition, skin care is important to prevent breakdown, which would establish a portal of entry for infectious agents.

Surgical repair often can be done in the neonatal period. The prognosis is guarded. The parents will need considerable support and instruction in their infant's care.

DOWN'S SYNDROME

Down's syndrome, formerly called *mongolism*, results from an abnormal number of chromosomes in most cases. Most commonly, it is caused by trisomy of chromosome 21, which increases the chromosome count to 47 instead of the normal 46. The infants of older women are at greater risk for Down's syndrome. Another type of chromosomal defect, which is not as common, results from translocation of a chromosome during cell division. In this type of defect, the chromosome count is 46, but two chromosomes are misplaced (Figs. 24–9 to 24–13).

The infant with Down's syndrome is mentally retarded (sometimes severely). Characteristically, the infant has slanted eyes that are close together;

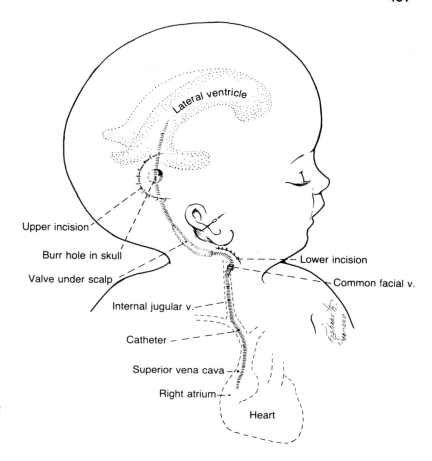

▲ FIGURE 24—7

Hydrocephalus. Operative procedure in which a catheter drains the ventricular system into the right atrium. (From Jacob, S. W., et al. (1982). *Structure and Function in Man*, 5th ed. Philadelphia: W.B. Saunders Company.)

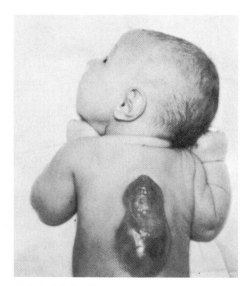

▲ FIGURE 24—8

Newborn with spina bifida.

a flat nose; a thick neck; and flabby, underdeveloped muscles and relaxed joints. The infant's tongue appears large and protrudes from the mouth (Fig. 24–14). Often, the infant with Down's syndrome has an unusually noticeable single transverse crease (simian crease) in the palms of the hands. Many of these infants have heart defects or digestive tract abnormalities. The infants often have very little resistance to infection; thus, they may die as a result of some infection during childhood.

It is difficult for many parents to learn that their child has Down's syndrome. The parents need a great deal of support and understanding about their feelings. The caregiver can help the parents by allowing them to express themselves. Some communities have parent groups that get together to discuss their similar problems. The parents should be informed about the available resources to assist in caring for the child.

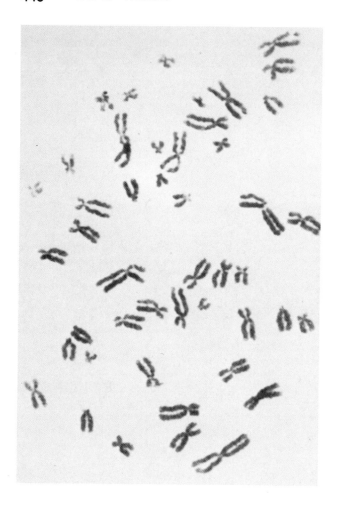

▲ FIGURE 24–9

Photograph of the chromosomes of a normal male. This cell has been stopped in the middle of cell division and chemically treated to make the chromosomes spread apart for easier counting.

PHENYLKETONURIA

Phenylketonuria (PKU) is an inherited error in the metabolism of a certain essential amino acid, or protein, called *phenylalanine*. When phenylalanine is taken into the body, it cannot be metabolized. Therefore, it accumulates in the tissues and blood and eventually is excreted in the urine as phenylketone bodies. Thus the name *phenylketonuria*.

It is important to detect this problem early and treat it to prevent mental retardation. The treatment consists of placing the infant on a special diet that limits the intake of phenylalanine.

Many states require a PKU blood test before the baby is sent home from the hospital or before the infant is 2 weeks old. The PKU test can be done after the infant is 2 days old and has been fed milk for at least 24 hours. Many physicians wait until the 3rd day to test breastfed infants. A simple blood test can be used to detect PKU, after the infant has had protein, by obtaining a couple of drops of blood from the infant's heel to determine the PKU level. Early discharge practices necessitate conscientious follow-up. The infant can be tested at home by a public health nurse or at the clinic or physician's office during the 4th to 6th week's check-up.

GALACTOSEMIA

Galactosemia, another metabolic error that can produce mental retardation, involves the metabolism of sugar (galactose). It is usually found after the infant is discharged from the hospital.

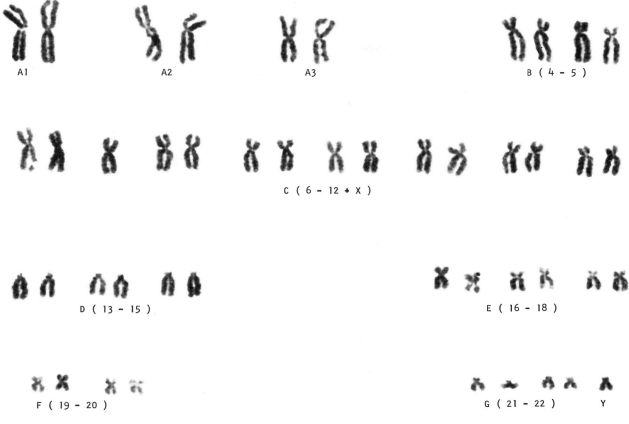

▲ FIGURE 24–10

Karyotype of the chromosomes of a normal male. These are the same chromosomes shown in Figure 24–9, but they were cut apart and arranged in pairs for easier analysis. The 22 paired chromosomes (the autosomes) are arranged in descending order, according to size and shape. The X chromosome appears between the first and second pair in the second row.

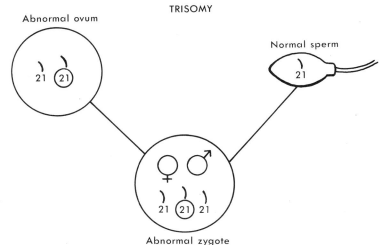

▲ FIGURE 24–11

In trisomy 21, the abnormal zygote has an extra chromosome (21), which results in a total chromosome count of 47, causing Down's syndrome. This type usually occurs in infants born to older women.

TRANSLOCATION

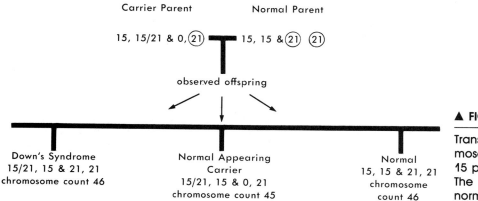

Carrier Parent   Normal Parent

15, 15/21 & 0, (21)   15, 15 & (21) (21)

observed offspring

Down's Syndrome
15/21, 15 & 21, 21
chromosome count 46

Normal Appearing
Carrier
15/21, 15 & 0, 21
chromosome count 45

Normal
15, 15 & 21, 21
chromosome
count 46

▲ FIGURE 24–12

Translocation of the extra chromosome 21 into chromosome 15 produces Down's syndrome. The chromosome count is the normal 46.

Disorders of the Blood

The most common problems of the blood in newborn infants are Rh incompatibility and ABO incompatibility. The mechanisms that are known to be responsible for both conditions are discussed in Chapter 21. The following discussion primarily concerns the symptoms, treatment, and care of infants with these disorders.

HYPERBILIRUBINEMIA

Hyperbilirubinemia is the presence of an abnormally high level of bilirubin. This occurs when normal pathways of bilirubin metabolism and excretion are altered. A primary cause of hyperbili-

rubinemia is hemolytic disease of the newborn, secondary to Rh incompatibility. A hemolytic disease caused by the development of antibodies in the mother's blood against antigens from the infant occurs when the mother is Rh− and the infant is Rh+. Simply stated, the newborn infant's red blood cells are destroyed. As a result, the infant produces an increased number of red blood cells called *erythroblasts*. As these cells are destroyed, they increase the level of bilirubin, which causes hyperbilirubinemia. In addition, with the breakdown of the red blood cells, the infant develops anemia and edema. The amount of elevated bilirubin and the severity of anemia and edema vary. Infants may require no treatment, or they may develop *kernicterus* (bilirubin in brain tissue), cardiac failure, and death.

It is necessary to assess the infant closely for

MOSAICISM

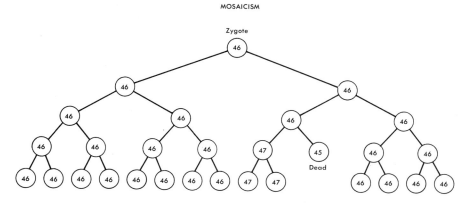

Zygote

Dead

▲ FIGURE 24–13

Mosaicism in Down's syndrome is the coexistence, in one individual, of cells with different chromosome counts. It is the result of an error in division of an early embryonic cell.

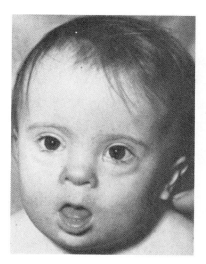

▲ FIGURE 24–14

An infant with trisomy 21 (Down's syndrome). (From Smith, D. W. (1988). *Recognizable Patterns of Human Malformation*, 4th ed. Philadelphia: W.B. Saunders Company.)

jaundice and obtain blood bilirubin levels when an Rh− mother gives birth. Immediately after delivery, an umbilical cord blood sample is sent to the laboratory. If the infant has a positive Coombs test result (infant's red blood cells are coated with antibodies). A total serum bilirubin concentration exceeding 12 mg/dL in term infants or 15 mg/dL in preterm infants indicates that further treatment is necessary. These laboratory findings are suggestive of erythroblastosis. It is important to reduce the bilirubin level, because it has an affinity for brain tissue and can produce brain damage.

Unlike physiological jaundice, discussed in Chapter 17, which appears on the third or fourth day of life, jaundice of Rh incompatibility usually appears within the first or second day. The caregiver's assessment of the presence of jaundice is significant. In addition, the infant should be observed for lethargy and poor sucking reflex.

The treatment will largely depend on the level of bilirubin present. If the bilirubin continues to rise to a dangerous level, an exchange transfusion is done. This transfusion consists of replacing the infant's blood with Rh− blood. It is a sterile procedure, and the amount of the infant's blood withdrawn is equal to the amount of Rh− blood injected.

In some cases, phototherapy is prescribed to reduce the bilirubin levels in the infant's blood and thus prevent brain damage due to kernicterus. Phototherapy consists of exposing the infant to a blue fluorescent light to reduce the amount of circulating bilirubin. The light is placed over the infant's crib or incubator at a distance of 15 to 24 inches from the infant. The infant's eyes are covered during the therapy as a precaution against possible retinal damage from irradiation. The infant's eyes are covered with eye pads, which are held in place with a piece of stockinette. It is important to make sure that the eyelids are closed when covering them so that a corneal abrasion cannot occur.

Because photooxidation (reduction of serum bilirubin by oxidation of bilirubin into water-soluble compound by use of light) of bilirubin occurs in the skin and not in the plasma, the maximum amount of skin is exposed during therapy. The infant is kept undressed except for a "bikini" diaper. The diaper is protective for the male infant, in particular, because it reduces a possible side effect of continued erection of the penis (priapism). Other side effects from phototherapy are dilation of the skin's capillaries, which can result in temperature regulation problems and increased water loss. When the infant does not excrete the photooxidation products adequately, the skin can turn a bronze color; hence the term *bronze baby*.

The caregiver needs to observe closely the infant receiving phototherapy (Fig. 24–15). The infant's temperature must be monitored. Any elevation of temperature during phototherapy must be reported and the infant must be removed from phototherapy. Because infants often have loose stools and lose fluid excessively, they should frequently receive water to replace this loss. The infant's eyes should be checked frequently to make sure that they are covered. The infant's position should be changed every 1 or 2 hours (see Nursing Care Plan 24–1).

ABO INCOMPATIBILITY

If the mother's blood type is O, and the infant's blood type is A or B, an ABO incompatibility may develop (Chapter 21). This condition can produce hyperbilirubinemia (elevated bilirubin levels) in

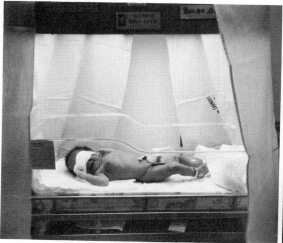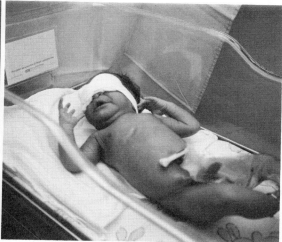

▲ **FIGURE 24–15**

Infant receiving phototherapy. Infant's eyes are covered to protect them from possible retinal damage. A urine specimen is being collected, so the bikini diaper is off. Note the penile erection caused by the light stimulus.

the infant. ABO incompatibility occurs more often than Rh incompatibility. The clinical problems of ABO incompatibility in the infant are usually less severe than those of Rh incompatibility. ABO incompatibility can appear with the first pregnancy. The infant with ABO incompatibility may become jaundiced during the first 24 hours after birth. Usually, anemia is not severe and no pallor or cardiac stress is observed. The treatment is the same as that for hyperbilirubinemia due to Rh incompatibility; however, an exchange transfusion is rarely necessary.

Infection

See Nursing Care Plan 24–2 for the care of a newborn who has an infection.

DIARRHEA

Diarrhea of the newborn infant is a viral gastroenteritis that is highly contagious and may be widespread. It can be responsible for infant death; thus, it is always dreaded. Infants suspected of having diarrhea are isolated immediately until it is proved that they are noninfectious. The care-

giver in the nursery is the key person to observe and report this condition to the physician and the infectious disease control committee of the hospital.

Infectious diarrhea can be caused by a variety of pathogenic organisms. *Escherichia coli* is commonly found in the stool. As soon as diarrhea is suspected, a warm stool specimen is sent to the laboratory for culture to identify the causative organisms.

The infant with infectious diarrhea has frequent, loose, watery, and green stools. As a result, the newborn becomes dehydrated and loses weight very quickly. Broad-spectrum antibiotics or other specified drugs are started at once. Intravenous fluids and an oral electrolyte solution (Pedialyte) may be started to replace fluid loss and maintain electrolyte balance. As the infant's condition improves, formula feedings are resumed.

UMBILICAL CORD INFECTION (OMPHALITIS)

Normally, the umbilical cord dries in a few days. It falls off in about 5 to 7 days. Pathogenic bacteria sometimes invade the cord stump, and an infection occurs. The signs of infection are moistness of the cord, a foul odor, and a purulent discharge.

NURSING CARE PLAN 24–1

NURSING CARE FOR THE INFANT WITH INCREASED BILIRUBIN LEVEL

Potential Problems and Nursing Diagnoses	Nursing Interventions
1. Potential for injury related to increase in bilirubin level.	Monitor infant for developing jaundice. Assess sclera, skin color by blanching. Assess oral mucosa for yellow color. Recognize that excessive bilirubin is damaging to central nervous system.
2. Knowledge deficit related to early identification of elevated bilirubin level.	Monitor infant and recognize signs for early identification and treatment to ensure infant safety.
3. Potential for injury related to phototherapy.	Maintain coverage of eyes to prevent possible retinal damage. Phototherapy causes loose stools, which can be irritating to infant's skin. Recognize that phototherapy reduces bilirubin by changing its form so that it can be excreted through urine and feces.
4. Potential fluid volume deficit related to phototherapy.	Recognize that phototherapy can increase insensible water loss. Observe for dehydration, diarrhea, and elevated temperature.
5. Sensory perceptual alteration related to eye shields.	Allow eye shields to be removed during feeding.
6. Diarrhea related to phototherapy.	Monitor number and consistency of stools, skin turgor, and temperature.
7. Potential altered parenting related to impaired parent-infant attachment.	Provide opportunity for mother to hold and feed infant.

Expected Outcomes

1. Presence of jaundice is promptly recognized.
2. Infant's bilirubin level is maintained in the normal ranges.
3. Infant has an intact skin with no diaper rash.
4. Infant remains well hydrated.
5. Infant is stimulated by massage, and eye shields are removed when the infant is held or fed.
6. Skin turgor and temperature are normal.
7. Mother is allowed to hold and feed infant with eye shields removed.

NURSING CARE PLAN 24–2

NURSING CARE OF THE NEWBORN WITH INFECTION

Potential Problems and Nursing Diagnoses	Nursing Interventions
1. Potential for infection related to immature immune system.	Monitor for development of sepsis. Monitor temperature and hydration. Observe open sites (umbilical cord and cracks in skin) for redness and purulent discharge.
2. Knowledge deficit related to susceptibility of newborn to infection from invasive procedures and caregivers with upper respiratory infections.	Recognize that infants are in a sterile environment before birth. After birth, they come in contact with varous pathogens. Protect infant by washing hands properly. Safeguard infant from other infants and persons with infections by taking appropriate precautions.
3. Ineffective thermoregulation related to chilling and infection.	Recognize that infant's thermoregulation is unstable and chilling, and infection can disrupt process, causing hypothermia.
4. Ineffective breathing pattern related to infection.	Recognize that septic infants may experience varying degrees of respiratory distress.
5. Altered family process related to hospitalization.	Recognize that infants are frequently kept in radiant heat beds for warmth. Allow mother to breastfeed if infant is stable. Provide opportunity for siblings to visit, if hospital policy permits.
6. Potential fluid volume deficit related to poor feeding during infection.	Provide more feeding opportunities to infants with poor sucking response and inadequate intake.
7. Diarrhea related to gastrointestinal irritation.	Monitor for diarrhea and vomiting; if present, electrolyte imbalance could be present.

Expected Outcomes

1. Infant with potential infection is promptly identified.
2. Mother verbalizes understanding of protection against infection by proper handwashing and need to take necessary precautions around individuals with infections.
3. Infant maintains normal temperature.
4. Infant maintains normal breathing pattern.
5. Mother holds and feeds infant.
6. Provision is made for more frequent feedings, and infant is given water between feedings.
7. Infant's stools are normal, and no vomiting is noted.

In addition, the area around the cord often becomes red and edematous. Frequently, the infant will develop a fever.

The treatment will depend on the extent of the infection. Signs of a cord infection should be reported to the physician immediately. A sample is sent to the laboratory for culturing to identify the organisms involved, and antibiotics are usually started.

Cord infection is more apt to occur after the infant is discharged; therefore, the mother should receive instructions to keep the navel (umbilicus) dry. The mother is also often instructed to apply 70% alcohol on the cord daily until the cord is fully healed. The mother should be told to bring the infant to the physician's office or clinic if the navel becomes red or swollen.

IMPETIGO CONTAGIOSA

Impetigo is a skin infection usually caused by staphylococci (Fig. 24–16). The infant who is thought to have impetigo should be isolated from other infants until the skin lesions disappear.

CONJUNCTIVITIS (OPHTHALMIA NEONATORUM)

Newborn infants can have conjunctivitis as a result of the silver nitrate drops placed in their eyes. This type of conjunctivitis is of no clinical importance. If the infant has profuse purulent discharge from the eyes, it is important to rule out the possibility of gonorrheal infection.

Gonorrheal conjunctivitis can be acquired as the infant passes through the birth canal of the infected mother. The infant should be isolated and treated immediately. Large doses of penicillin are given to combat the infection. If only one eye is infected, the uninvolved eye should be protected with an eye patch. Without treatment, ulcers of the cornea may develop with permanent damage to the eyeball. It is possible for the infant to become blind as a result of this infection. Therefore, all states require prophylactic instillation of 1% silver nitrate or erythromycin ophthalmic ointment into the eyes shortly after birth.

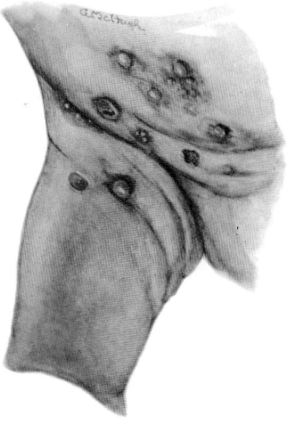

▲ FIGURE 24–16

Impetigo of the newborn. (Courtesy of Mead Johnson Laboratories, Evansville, IN.)

THRUSH

Thrush is an infection caused by *Candida albicans (Monilia)*, a fungus. This organism may be picked up during the birth, and it can cause the mucous membranes of the infant's mouth to become infected. Also, it is possible for mothers with fungal vaginitis to infect their infants by touching them, if they do not wash their hands properly.

The infection is characterized by white patches that resemble milk curds. If the patches are thrush, they will not wipe off but will leave a raw, bleeding surface.

The infant with thrush should be isolated from the other infants, and both the infant and the mother should be treated (if the mother is infected). This infection can spread into the esophagus and cause feeding problems. Thrush responds very well to a local application of nystatin (Mycostatin), an antibiotic. Usually, the infant's mouth is swabbed with the prescribed drug several times a day. The caregiver and mother should wash their hands frequently and meticulously so the infants can rid themselves of the infections. In addition, caregivers should be extremely careful to avoid infecting other infants.

CONGENITAL SYPHILIS

Syphilis, a venereal disease, is becoming more prevalent in the pregnant population. The disease is discussed in Chapter 7. The caregiver should be familiar with the typical signs of congenital syphilis in order to promptly report them, so the infant can receive immediate treatment. Penicillin is given to the infant in large doses after a diagnosis is established.

The Infant of a Diabetic Mother

Diabetes in the pregnant woman is discussed in detail in Chapter 21. The infants of these mothers will have various problems after birth. Factors that will influence the infant's status at birth include the duration and severity of the mother's diabetes, the degree of control of the diabetes, and the gestational age of the infant, especially if the infant is premature.

Many infants of diabetic mothers have serious complications, such as respiratory distress, hypoglycemia, hyperbilirubinemia, and hypocalcemia. In addition, they may have congenital abnormalities, and they are more prone to infection. Most of the infants are preterm but are large for their gestational age. In other words, the infant born of a diabetic mother should be treated as a "sick infant" and carefully observed for the common potential problems.

At birth, the infant may be hypoglycemic, with a blood glucose level of less than 35 mg/dL during the first 72 hours. This clinical finding is common because of the abrupt end to the excessive supply of maternal glucose. Dextrostix tests (blood tests using reagent strips) are done frequently during the first several hours after birth for the presence of glucose. If necessary, the infant is started on intravenous glucose until the glucose level has stabilized.

These newborns need careful assessment for respiratory distress, which may not be present at birth but often is present later. Arterial blood gases are monitored frequently to evaluate the infant's condition. Oxygen may be needed for the first few hours of life. If the infants are large (more than 8 lb), they are likely to have additional problems, such as intracranial hemorrhage from a prolonged or difficult labor.

Respiratory Distress

Respiratory distress syndrome (RDS) is a common disorder of preterm infants. The most frequent cause of RDS is a condition called *hyaline membrane disease*, in which a hyaline membrane forms in the lining of the infant's alveoli (air sacs) of the lungs. This membrane prevents the normal exchange of oxygen and carbon dioxide. As a result, some part of the lung may collapse, or atelectasis occurs, forcing the unaffected part of the lung to work harder to provide sufficient oxygen for the infant's needs. For this reason, the newborn with RDS has rapid and labored breathing (40 to 60 respirations/minute in quiet state). A grunt-like sound, flaring of the nostrils, and retraction ("sucking-in") of the chest may be observed during the infant's respirations. Seesaw breathing (Fig. 24–17) is observed, with the abdomen rising and the chest sinking on inspiration and the reverse occurring on expiration. It is important to note the color of the newborn. When unable to get enough oxygen, the infant will become cyanotic (turn blue).

Frequently, the infant with RDS is transferred to a neonatal intensive care unit for close observation and specialized attention (Fig. 24–18). At this time, the infant is placed in an incubator or radiantly heated bed and is administered humidified oxygen. More severely affected infants will require continuous positive airway pressure to

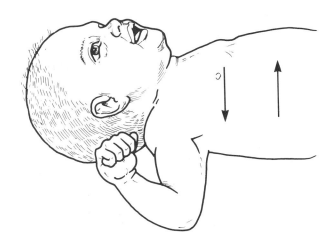

▲ **FIGURE 24–17**

Seesaw respirations found in the infant with respiratory distress syndrome.

make breathing easier. Some newborns with RDS improve fairly rapidly, but for others the condition is fatal.

Drug Dependency

The number of infants born to drug-dependent mothers is increasing. Caregivers should be alert to subtle as well as obvious signs of withdrawal. Tremors, started by minimal tactile stimulation, may be the first sign of withdrawal. Rigidity, irritability, wakefulness with interference of deep sleep, and a shrill, high-pitched cry are other signs

that may be due to drug withdrawal. The infant often frantically sucks on the fists. The infant frequently has a poor appetite and loose stools and may have convulsions.

Treatment and care consist of supportive measures, increasing fluid intake, and decreasing doses of sedatives or anticonvulsant drugs (Table 24–1). If the mother is still taking drugs, she should not breastfeed her infant, because her milk will contain the drugs. The infant should be given a pacifier to meet the greater need to suck.

Some drugs increase the risk of congenital malformations. Therefore, the newborn should be carefully examined for any abnormalities.

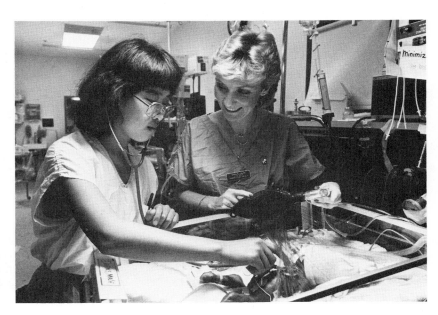

▲ **FIGURE 24–18**

This infant is on a ventilator in a high-risk nursery. (Courtesy of University of Illinois Hospital.)

TABLE 24–1. NURSING CARE OF THE DRUG-DEPENDENT INFANT

INFANT BEHAVIOR	NURSING OBSERVATIONS	NURSING INTERVENTION
High-pitched cry	Note onset. Note length of time cry persists. Is it continuous? Is it high pitched and piercing as though infant were in pain? Observe infant for other causes of abnormal crying patterns (meningitis, intracranial bleeding, and so forth). Is anterior fontanelle full or bulging? Are cranial sutures widely separated? Is head circumference increased? Does infant stare without blinking? Is cry aggravated or alleviated when infant is picked up?	Soothe infant by wrapping infant tightly in blankets (swaddling) or holding infant tightly and close to one's body, or both. Decrease feeding intervals or implement a demand-feeding schedule, or both. Reduce environmental stimuli.
Inability to sleep	Note how long infant sleeps after feeding. Note general sleep and wake patterns. If drug therapy has been initiated, note changes in sleep patterns, ability to rest, and whether there is decreased activity that may indicate drug overdose.	Decrease environmental stimuli. Swaddle. Feed small amounts at frequent intervals.
Frantic sucking of fists	Note onset and amount of sucking. Observe for blisters on fingertips and knuckles. If blistering occurs, observe sites for signs of infection.	Use infant shirts with sewn-in sleeves or mitts to prevent skin trauma. Keep skin area clean; use aseptic technique.
Yawning	Note onset and frequency.	None
Sneezing, nasal stuffiness	Observe onset and frequency. Note severity of nasal stuffiness and determine whether it hinders feeding. If mucus is excessive, consider possibility of other underlying problems, such as esophageal atresia, tracheoesophageal fistula, and congenital syphilis.	Aspirate nasopharynx. Give frequent nose care. Allow more time for feeding with rest between sucking. Aspirate trachea if tracheal mucus is increased. Check rate and character of respirations frequently.
Poor feeding	Note sucking pattern—is infant uncoordinated in the attempt to suck? Observe for other possible causes of poor feeding (sepsis, hypoglycemia, immaturity, bowel obstruction, pyloric stenosis).	Feed small amounts at close intervals. Maintain fluid and caloric intake required for infant's weight
Regurgitation, vomiting	Note when regurgitation or vomiting occurs—is there a precipitating factor (medication, handling, manipulation, position and so forth)?	Measure intake and output closely and correlate with infant's general condition, progress, and therapy.

TABLE 24–1. NURSING CARE OF THE DRUG-DEPENDENT INFANT *Continued*

INFANT BEHAVIOR	NURSING OBSERVATIONS	NURSING INTERVENTION
Loose stools	Observe for signs of dehydration: Poor skin turgor Sunken anterior fontanelle Sunken orbits around eyes Marked weight loss Note time, color, consistency, and quantity of vomitus and stool. When stools are loose, estimate amount of water lost with stools. Note whether vomiting is nonforceful or forceful. Observe for electrolyte imbalance.	Offer supplementary fluids if signs of dehydration appear. Weigh frequently if weight loss, vomiting, and diarrhea persist. Maintain intravenous flow at prescribed rate. Maintain infant on side to prevent aspiration of vomitus. Give skin care to prevent excoriation of neck folds, buttocks, and perineum.
Tachypnea, mottling	Note onset of respirations over 60/min. If tachypnea worsens, note heart rate and report if more than 180/min. Note retractions, their severity (mild, moderate, severe), and location (subcostal, intercostal, sternal, suprasternal, supraclavicular). Note presence of nasal flaring. Note infant's color—is there pallor? Cyanosis? If cyanosis is present, note location (extremities, circumoral, generalized) and degree (mild, moderate, severe). Observe for other possible underlying pathophysiological causes (anemia, aspiration pneumonia, congenital heart disease and so forth). Is mottling precipitated by factors such as handling, hypothermia? Watch closely for apnea.	Maintain infant in semi-Fowler's position. Hyperextend head slightly to ensure patent airway. Minimize handling and manipulation. Correlate respiration rate, heart rate, retractions, and color with infant's progress, general condition, and blood gas values. If infant is receiving O_2 and is premature, observe color closely, correlate with blood gases, and reduce O_2 if PO_2 exceeds 85–90. Maintain warmth, since hypothermia or hyperthermia increases O_2 consumption. Place infant on cardiac-apnea monitor. If apnea occurs, resuscitate.
Hyperactive Moro reflex	Is reflex moderately or markedly exaggerated? If drug therapy has been started, note a diminished or absent Moro reflex. Is there asymmetry of the reflex? Asymmetry may indicate underlying pathophysiology: Erb's palsy, fractured clavicle, intracranial hemorrhage.	

Table continued on following page

TABLE 24–1. NURSING CARE OF THE DRUG-DEPENDENT INFANT *Continued*

INFANT BEHAVIOR	NURSING OBSERVATIONS	NURSING INTERVENTION
Hypertonicity	Note degree (mild, moderate, or severe) of increased muscle tone by (a) attempting to straighten arms and legs and recording degree of resistance; (b) picking infant up by hands and noting body rigidity with degree of head lag (withdrawing infant often exhibits trunk rigidity and holds the head on a plane with the body for a prolonged time); and (c) raising infant by arms and letting him or her stand (withdrawing neonate exhibits marked leg rigidity and can support the body's weight for considerable periods). Correlate mother's obstetrical history and delivery with infant's condition and observe baby for other pathophysiology: hypocalcemia, hypoglycemia, meningitis, asphyxia neonatorum, and intracranial hemorrhage. Observe for reddened areas over heels, occiput, sacrum, and knees. Check temperature frequently; increased activity may cause pyrexia.	Change infant's position often, because prolonged or marked rigidity predisposes to pressure areas. Decrease environmental temperature if infant's temperature goes above 99° F.
Tremors, convulsions	Note if tremors occur when infant is disturbed or undisturbed. Note location of tremors: upper extremities, lower extremities, or generalized. Note whether degree of tremor is mild, moderate, or severe. Observe skin over nose, elbows, fingers, toes, knees, heels for excoriation. Observe face for scratches. Check temperature often for pyrexia. Observe for seizures; if they occur, note onset; length; origin; body involvement; whether tonic, clonic, or both; eye deviation; and infant's color.	Change position frequently to prevent excoriation. Give frequent skin care (cleansing, ointment, and exposure to air or a heat lamp, or both). Use sheepskin. Observe excoriation for healing, worsening, infection. Decrease environmental temperature if infant exhibits pyrexia. If infant convulses, maintain patent airway and prevent self-trauma. If infant is apneic after seizure, begin resuscitation. Decrease environmental stimuli.

Adapted from Finnegan, L. P., & Macnew, B. A. (1974). Care of the drug addicted infant. *American Journal of Nursing* 74:685. Copyright 1974 American Journal of Nursing Company. Used with permission. All right reserved.

References

Auvenshine, M. A., & Enriquez, M. G. (1990). *Comprehensive Maternity Nursing: Perinatal and Women's Health,* 2nd ed. Boston: Jones and Bartlett.

Brucker, M. C., & MacMuller, N. J. (1987). Neonatal jaundice in the home: Assessment with a noninvasive device. *Journal of Obstetric, Gynecologic, and Neonatal Nursing* 16(5):355–358.

Dickason, E. J., Schult, M. O., & Silverman, B. L. (1990). *Maternal-Infant Nursing Care.* St. Louis: C.V. Mosby.

Finnegan, L., Macnew, B. (1974). Care of the drug addicted infant. *American Journal of Nursing* 74:685–686.

Ladewig, P. W., London, M. L., & Olds, S. B. (1990). *Essentials of Maternal-Newborn Nursing,* 2nd ed. Redwood City, CA: Addison-Wesley Nursing.

Lewis, K. D., Bennett, B., & Schneder, N. H. (1989). The care of infants menaced by cocaine abuse. *American Journal of Maternal-Child Nursing* 14(5):324–329.

Lieber, M. T., & Taub, A. S. (1988). Common foot deformities and what they mean for parents. *American Journal of Maternal-Child Nursing* 13(1):47–50.

Wilkerson, N. N. (1989). Treating hyperbilirubinemia. *American Journal of Maternal-Child Nursing* 14(1):32–36.

SUGGESTED ACTIVITIES

1. Identify five common birth defects. Discuss the nursing care for each one.
2. Explain how parents may react when informed they have a deformed infant. Identify ways to encourage parent participation in infant care.

REVIEW QUESTIONS

A. Select the best answer to each multiple-choice question.

1. The difference between a cephalohematoma and a caput succedaneum is that a cephalohematoma
   - A. Does not cross the suture line and usually is over the parietal bone
   - B. Always crosses suture lines of the skull
   - C. Cannot be felt on palpation
   - D. None of the above

2. Symptoms of intracranial hemorrhage include
   - A. Shrill cry, irritability, and bulging fontanelles
   - B. Shrill cry, irritability, and irregular respirations
   - C. Irregular respirations, listlessness, and sunken fontanelles
   - D. Irregular respirations, poor sucking reflex, and sunken fontanelles

3. Nursing care of the infant with intracranial hemorrhage would include
   - A. Assessment of the sucking reflex
   - B. Close monitoring of the infant
   - C. Gentle handling
   - D. All of the above

4. The nursing care of an infant with a cleft palate and lip includes all of the following EXCEPT
   - A. Avoiding aspiration of fluid during feeding
   - B. Holding infant in upright position during feeding
   - C. Burping infant frequently during feeding
   - D. Allowing infant to eat in a prone position

5. Hydrocephalus causes
   - A. An abnormally large head
   - B. An abnormally small head
   - C. Enlargement of the heart
   - D. A defect in the heart

6. Down's syndrome results from
   - A. An abnormal number of chromosomes
   - B. Trisomy of chromosome 21
   - C. Translocation of a chromosome
   - D. All of the above

7. The characteristics of an infant with Down's syndrome include all of the following EXCEPT
   - A. Slanted eyes
   - B. Transverse palm crease
   - C. Well-developed muscle tone
   - D. Protruding tongue

8. Jaundice due to Rh incompatibility usually appears
   - A. Within 1st or 2nd day
   - B. On the 3rd or 4th day
   - C. On the 5th to 7th day
   - D. After the first 2 weeks

9. The purpose of phototherapy is to
    A. Increase red blood cell number
    B. Reduce bilirubin levels in the blood
    C. Destroy antibodies in the blood
    D. Decrease the infant's temperature

10. Nursing measures taken when caring for an infant receiving phototherapy include
    A. Changing the infant's position frequently
    B. Keeping the infant's eyes covered
    C. Taking the infant's temperature frequently
    D. All of the above

11. If white, curd-like patches are found in the infant's mouth and bleeding occurs when they are removed, one would suspect
    A. Impetigo
    B. Thrush
    C. Syphilis
    D. Conjunctivitis

12. Symptoms that may be indicative of infant drug dependency include
    A. Rigidity and irritability
    B. Wakefulness
    C. Tremors and shrill cry
    D. All of the above

13. An infant suspected to have RDS should be closely monitored. Which of the following is NOT a symptom of RDS?
    A. Seesaw respirations
    B. Irregular, abdominal respirations
    C. Rapid, labored breathing with a retraction of the chest wall
    D. Grunt-like respirations accompanied by flaring of the nostrils

14. Symptom(s) associated with RDS in a newborn infant is (are)
    A. Respiratory rate over 60/minute while quiet
    B. Nasal flaring
    C. Sternal retractions
    D. All of the above

15. Baby Susan's posture and movements are observed. Which one of the following should be reported?
    A. Occasional jittery movements
    B. Flexion of all four extremities
    C. Repetitive blinking
    D. None of the above

16. The infant delivered from a woman with untreated gonorrhea is at risk for
    A. Ophthalmia neonatorum
    B. Pneumonia
    C. Convulsions
    D. Large weight loss

17. After a cephalic birth, an infant does not move the right arm. The diagnostic possibility is
    A. Facial paralysis
    B. Fractured right clavicle
    C. Cephalohematoma
    D. Erythema toxicum neonatorum

B. Choose from Column II the phrase that most accurately defines the term in Column I.

I

1. Forceps marks _____
2. Coarctation of aorta _____
3. Pyloric stenosis _____
4. Hydrocephalus _____
5. Spina bifida _____
6. Phenylketonuria _____
7. Hypoglycemia _____
8. Atelectasis _____
9. Cleft palate _____
10. Kernicterus _____
11. Tracheoesophageal fistula _____
12. Meningocele _____
13. Clubfoot _____
14. Phototherapy _____
15. Impetigo contagiosa _____

II

A. Treatment to reduce bilirubin levels
B. Separation in roof of mouth
C. Forceful, projectile vomiting
D. Brain damage caused by accumulation of bilirubin in brain
E. Bruised tissue on sides of infant's face
F. Narrowing of aorta
G. Collapsed part of lung
H. Skin lesions
I. Condition in which meninges protrude through spinal canal
J. Accumulation of cerebrospinal fluid
K. Hereditary problem in which body is unable to metabolize the protein phenylalanine
L. Spinal cord defect in which portion of bony part of spinal cord fails to close
M. Common in infants of diabetic mothers
N. Deformity in which there is an abnormal inward or outward turning of foot
O. Defect in which esophagus ends in a blind pouch

CHAPTER 25 _____

Chapter Outline

Vaginitis
Toxic Shock Syndrome
Endometriosis
    Symptoms
    Consequences
    Management
    Teaching and counseling
Premenstrual Syndrome
Dysmenorrhea
Disturbance in Blood Flow
Fibrocystic Breast Disorder
Breast Cancer
    Diagnosis
    Treatment options
    Breast reconstruction

Learning Objectives

Upon completion of Chapter 25, the student should be able to

- Name two types of vaginitis commonly found during pregnancy.
- Explain four ways to decrease the incidence of vaginitis during pregnancy.
- Describe toxic shock syndrome and list four of its symptoms.
- Name the pathogenic organisms most commonly found in toxic shock syndrome.
- Explain three measures that women should be taught to prevent toxic shock syndrome.
- Define endometriosis and give one common symptom of it.
- Describe premenstrual syndrome and list potential ways to reduce it.
- Identify potential causes of dysmenorrhea and explain how it can be relieved.
- Explain fibrocystic breast disorder.
- State the frequency of breast cancer in women in the United States.
- Explain the importance of teaching women how to properly conduct a breast self-examination.
- Recall when women should begin having an annual mammography and why it is important.
- Provide a profile of the woman who is at high risk for cancer of the breast.
- Describe three surgical options in the treatment of breast cancer.
- Name two major postoperative complications of a mastectomy.

WOMEN'S HEALTH CARE

The nurse caring for a pregnant woman is in an ideal position to assess, and provide instruction on, the common gynecological disorders. These include vaginitis, toxic shock syndrome, endometriosis, premenstrual syndrome, dysmenorrhea, disturbance in blood flow, and breast cancer. One of these problems may be discovered when a woman requests contraceptives, prenatal or postpartum care, or treatment for infection. These complaints are often ignored by the woman. Some women are intimidated by the sexuality of the menstrual process and hesitate to discuss this intimate issue with their physician. Other women accept their discomfort as natural or think their complaints are unimportant. Finally, a knowledge deficit related to the occurrence of breast cancer and methods for early detection is prevalent; thus, health care providers should emphasize this problem, particularly in women age 35 and over.

NURSING DIAGNOSES

- Knowledge deficit related to the disease process and prevention of disease
- Potential for impaired tissue integrity related to irritation and inflammation
- Altered family processes related to the effects of the diagnosis on the couple's relationship
- Pain related to coitus
- Anxiety related to the diagnosis and subsequent health problems

Vaginitis

The vagina is a warm, moist vault in which organisms flourish. The vagina's main line of defense against infection is the normally occurring Doderlein's bacilli, which require a slightly acidic environment (pH of 3.8 to 4.2) to multiply. Anything that decreases acidity or destroys the vaginal flora decreases the number and effectiveness of the Doderlein's bacilli. When this happens, vaginitis can result.

Vaginitis is a common problem of women in general. It is encouraged by antibiotics, by tight clothing that holds moisture, by an alkaline vaginal pH caused by frequent douching, by diabetes mellitus, and by mechanical irritation.

Physiological changes that occur during pregnancy also predispose a woman to vaginitis. Increased estrogen secretions cause an increased production of cervical mucus, which is alkaline and favors growth of organisms (inflammation of the vagina). In addition, during pregnancy, many women have glucose in their urine owing to alterations in the renal system. Urine that contains glucose is a good medium for the growth of bacteria.

Two infections in particular, *Candidiasis* and *trichomoniasis,* appear frequently during pregnancy and in general (Table 25–1). Candidiasis, a yeast infection caused by *Candida albicans,* may cause a profuse, cheesy, white, irritating discharge. The symptoms are leukorrhea, pruritus, white patches on the vulva, and a reddened vaginal mucosa. A variety of antifungal vaginal creams, suppositories, or tablets are available to treat candidiasis. The fungicide nystatin (Mycostatin) and miconazole cream are often used. The woman with candidiasis should avoid coitus during therapy or have the man use a condom and also be treated until they both are cured.

Trichomoniasis, an infection caused by the protozoan *Trichomonas vaginalis,* is characterized by a

KEY POINTS IN EDUCATION: PREVENTION OF VAGINITIS

- Maintain proper feminine hygiene (cleanse from front to back to avoid contamination of vagina by feces).
- Bathe daily (use clean linen each day; use separate washcloth for perineum).
- Avoid sharing washcloths, towels, and underwear.
- Wear absorbent underpants, preferably 100% cotton or cotton crotch (nylon panty hose hold warmth and moisture, facilitating the growth of organisms).
- Avoid using vaginal douches and feminine sprays, which shift pH toward alkaline (douches and sprays encourage growth of bacteria).
- Avoid mechanical sources of irritation to vaginal tissue, such as deodorant sprays, perfumed soaps, and leaving tampons in for extended periods of time.
- Change positions frequently (avoid sitting in same position and/or crossing legs for long periods of time).

- Recognize that antibiotics cause destruction of vaginal flora (by changing the vaginal pH).
- Obtain adequate nutrition.
- Change sanitary napkins and tampons frequently during menstruation.
- Encourage the use of condoms to provide some protection.
- Inspect the sexual partner for discharge or reddened areas of penis.
- Realize the importance of taking prescribed medications.
- Recognize chronic infection can be avoided by obtaining vigorous treatment.
- If coitus is painful, avoid coitus during infection and treatment until culture results are negative.
- Have the sexual partner obtain treatment to avoid reinfections.

yellowish-white, green to gray foamy discharge, causing irritation and pruritus (Fig. 25–1). Typical symptoms are leukorrhea, vaginal soreness, burning, itching, dyspareunia (painful coitus), vulvar redness, and urinary frequency. Trichomoniasis may also cause dysuria (painful urination). This infection is treated by the use of local medications such as sulfanilamide (AVC Cream) and metronidazole (Flagyl). Flagyl is very effective; however, it should *not* be used during early pregnancy because of the potential harm to the fetus (even by topical application). Symptomatic relief may be achieved with a gentle, dilute vinegar douche; however, the douche should be given at low pressure during pregnancy. The woman should avoid sexual intercourse, or the sexual partner should use a condom until the infection disappears. If the sexual partner is not treated, the woman can become reinfected.

It is important for a woman to have healthy tissue in the cervix before she goes into labor. Because infections such as vaginitis make the tissue more fragile, the cervix will tear more readily during labor and delivery. Thus women with vaginitis are often treated rather vigorously near the end of pregnancy.

Toxic Shock Syndrome

Toxic shock syndrome (TSS) is a disease of reproductive-age women. Although it has been reported in young adolescents and postmenopausal women, it appears most frequently in women age 24 and younger.

TSS is apparently triggered by *Staphylococcus aureus*, a bacterium that can produce a toxin that enters the bloodstream. Passage of the toxin, containing blood, into the tissues typically causes the woman to exhibit shock symptoms or shock itself; hence the name.

The Centers for Disease Control (CDC) has defined TSS as the following: fever; hypotension;

TABLE 25–1. GYNECOLOGICAL CONDITIONS THAT OCCUR IN WOMEN

INFECTION	PREDISPOSING FACTORS	ORGANISM	CLINICAL FINDINGS	SYMPTOMS	TREATMENT
Nonspecific vaginitis	↑ pH Trauma to birth canal Altered physiology of vagina	Mixed bacteria Flora Streptococcus Staphylococcus Colon bacilli	↑ Cervical mucus Reddened vaginal wall ↑ discharge: creamy yellow → thick → watery Edema of cervix Ulceration of cervix and vagina Abnormal Pap test	Leukorrhea Pruritus Reddening of vulva Burning Urethritis	Mild antiseptic douche (limited use) Triple sulfacream Furazolidone (Tricofuron) suppository Cauterization Avoid coitus or use condom Lactose suppository Nitrofurazone (Furacin) or ampicillin
Candidiasis	Pregnancy Diabetes Oral contraceptives Postmenopause ↓ estrogen	Yeast-like fungi *Candida albicans* (identify hyphae)	Discharge (thin → thick, watery → curdy) Exudate, patches on vaginal mucosa Reddened vaginal mucosa Small ulcers on vagina Abnormal Pap test	Leukorrhea Pruritus Reddening of vulva Thrush-like patches on vulva Large gray and white areas of exudate Asymptomatic	Antifungal gel Nystatin (Mycostatin) Mycolog Baking soda douche (can be applied in clinic to relieve symptoms) Avoid coitus during therapy or use condom and have partner treated
Trichomoniasis	Antibiotics Pregnancy ↑ pH of vaginal flora Contamination from coitus, feces, etc.	Protozoan (highly motile flagellate, 2× size of leukocyte) *Trichomonas vaginalis* (identify flagella)	Discharge (thin, gray, foamy, greenish white) Strawberry spots on cervix and vaginal mucosa Cervical erosion Reddened vaginal mucosa Abnormal Pap test	Leukorrhea Vaginal soreness Burning Itching Dyspareunia Labial and vaginal excoriation Reddening of vulva Urinary frequency Dysuria (sometimes noticed)	Sulfanilamide (AVC Cream) Pregnancy May be necessary to treat sexual partner (to prevent reinfection) Metronidazole (Flagyl)—during pregnancy use topical *only;* do not use systemic route during pregnancy Avoid coitus or use condom, and have partner treated
Gonorrhea	Immature, thin mucous membrane susceptibility Contact with infected person Alkaline pH of 7.2–7.6 Menstruation Pregnancy	Gram-negative diplococcus *Neisseria gonorrhoeae*	Bartholinitis, skenitis Urethral discharge Cervical pus Vaginal discharge (green, yellow, usually thin) Reddening of vulva and vaginal mucosa Inflammation of meatus Mushroom-like odor Abnormal Pap test	Leukorrhea Pruritus Reddening vulva Low back pain Abdominal discharge Frequent urination Dysuria Asymptomatic	Penicillin Tetracycline Erythromycin Avoid coitus

Table continued on following page

	TABLE 25–1. GYNECOLOGICAL CONDITIONS THAT OCCUR IN WOMEN *Continued*				
INFECTION	**PREDISPOSING FACTORS**	**ORGANISM**	**CLINICAL FINDINGS**	**SYMPTOMS**	**TREATMENT**
Herpes genitalis	Contact with infected person Emotional stress Drug therapy Sunlight exposure Temperature changes	Herpes virus Herpes simplex type 2	Vesicular rash Vaginal pain Vaginal discharge Vesicles followed by ulcers on cervix and vulva	Pain Dysuria Sudden onset of vaginal discharge Dyspareunia Itching Paresthesia and anesthesia of perineum Systemic: fever, chills, head-ache, general malaise	Photosensitive proflavine (red dye) Exposure to fluorescent light If present at time of delivery, cesarean to protect infant from serious jeopardy (infant can die from viremia) Cytologic smears Avoid coitus
Haemophilus vaginalis	Contamination during coitus	Gram-negative bacillus	Gray discharge (profuse, offensive odor)	Heavy vaginal discharge Itching Burning	Triple sulfacream Antibiotics Avoid coitus or use condom
Condylomata acuminata (venereal warts)	Contamination during coitus	Virus	Pink, elongated, soft, moist lesions Growth may become exuberant during pregnancy Ulcers may develop Secondary infection common Usually regress markedly during puerperium	Vaginal discharge and bleeding may occur Warts may regress or be persistent	Fluorouracil (effective drug, but noxious to fetus, therefore, contraindicated during pregnancy) Excision of lesions may be necessary Avoid coitus Biopsy for persistent warts because of association with cancer

rash; desquamation; and involvement of organ systems, such as the hematological (blood), gastrointestinal, muscular, and renal systems. Early diagnosis and treatment are important in preventing a fatal outcome.

The typical symptoms of TSS are sudden onset of fever (usually over 102° F); vomiting or diarrhea, or both; headache; sore throat or aching muscles; rash that is noticed on the hands and feet and that later peels; and a rapid drop in blood pressure (below 90 mm Hg systolic). This drop in blood pressure can cause dizziness, disorientation, and possibly vital organ damage. The acute phase of TSS lasts 4 to 5 days. The convalescent period typically takes 1 to 2 weeks.

Staphylococcus aureus is known to grow faster (or produce its toxins more quickly) in the presence of vaginal tampons and menstrual fluid. The superabsorbent tampons possibly dry out the vaginal walls, causing microulcerations. Bacterial toxin may escape into the woman's bloodstream through these wounds. Although the reason is unclear, the facts indicate that the use of high-absorbency tampons carries the greatest risk for TSS. Occluding the cervical os with a diaphragm or contraceptive sponge, especially if it is left in place for a long period of time (more than 24 hours), may also increase the risk of TSS.

Women with TSS are often treated with large volumes of intravenous fluids and medications to

KEY POINTS IN EDUCATION: REDUCING THE RISK OF TOXIC SHOCK SYNDROME

Women should be instructed that they can reduce their risk of TSS by adhering to the following practices:

- Do not leave high-absorbency tampons in the vagina for extended periods of time. Change tampons frequently.
- Alternate the use of tampons with sanitary napkins. Use napkins during sleeping hours.
- Remove diaphragms or contraceptive sponges no later than 6 hours after sexual intercourse.
- Postpartal women should avoid the use of tampons for 6 to 8 weeks after childbirth.

- Women with a history of TSS should cease using tampons altogether.
- Women should thoroughly wash their hands before inserting a vaginal sponge or tampon and should change tampons frequently.
- Women should avoid using tampons if they have staphylococcal infections of skin, such as infected pimples.
- Women should practice good perineal cleansing during menses.
- Women should be aware of the signs and symptoms of TSS and seek treatment promptly if signs occur.

raise the blood pressure. Many physicians use beta-lactamase–resistant antibiotics after taking a bacterial culture for the specific organism. It appears that antibiotics only reduce the present infection and do not prevent a recurrence of TSS.

TSS can be fatal. Some women have lost fingers or toes as a result of gangrene caused by decreased blood flow. Damage to vital organs has occurred in some women during the period of shock. Other women have developed aneurysms that place

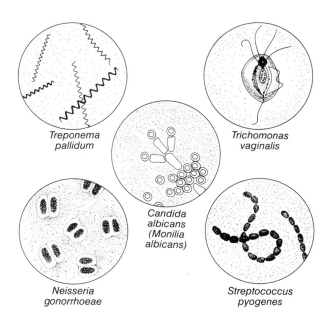

▲ **FIGURE 25–1**

Pathogenic organisms that commonly invade the female reproductive organs.

them at risk for possible cardiovascular problems. Cases have been reported in which muscle damage has resulted in some partial paralysis.

Endometriosis

Endometriosis is characterized by the presence of endometrial tissue outside the uterus (endometrial cells make up the lining of the uterus). Endometrial tissue has been found in the ovary, cul de sac of Douglas, uterine ligaments, pelvic peritoneum, rectovaginal septum, cervix, and inguinal area. About 12% of women with endometriosis have lesions in the gastrointestinal tract, most often in the rectosigmoid area and less often in the appendix and ileum. The most common site for endometrial tissue outside the uterus is the ovary. The sequelae of endometriosis may include bleeding from lesions, adhesions, and anatomic obstructions.

SYMPTOMS

The severity of symptoms of endometriosis is not always related to the severity of the disease. Generally, women present symptoms such as dysmenorrhea, dyspareunia, and/or pelvic pain. Some women describe "deep-seated aching pain" in the lower abdomen, posterior pelvis, vagina, and back. The pain may radiate to the bowel and perineum, even the thighs. The pain gradually subsides and ends just before the end of menstruation or shortly afterward; however, over time both the intensity and duration of pain can progress. Although symptoms vary, they often include premenstrual spotting, dysfunctional uterine bleeding, and dysuria. Urinary frequency and rectal bleeding may occur. Women may have an infertility problem with or without other signs or symptoms.

CONSEQUENCES

Endometriosis has been found to be strongly associated with infertility, which is caused by the formation of adhesions in the endometrial tissue in the uterine tubes. Spontaneous abortion is also increased with endometriosis. Occasionally, endometrial tissue undergoes malignant transformation; this is usually accompanied by an abrupt increase in the severity of pain. Enlargement of a pelvic mass or rupture of an endometrioma may be indicative of cancer.

MANAGEMENT

The definitive diagnosis of endometriosis is made operatively, usually by laparoscopy. A biopsy is often taken for histological analysis. The goals of treatment include prevention of disease progression, alleviation of pain, and establishment or restoration of fertility (for women who want to bear children). For women who do not desire to maintain their reproductive capacity, a hysterectomy and bilateral salpingo-oophorectomy constitute the only cure. Surgery may be performed, with conventional or laser techniques, to remove endometrial implants, break up adhesions, yet conserve the reproductive organs. Medical management includes use of oral contraceptives, androgens, and, most recently, Danazol (a testosterone derivative). The goal of medical treatment is the suppression of ovarian function.

TEACHING AND COUNSELING

Women in whom there is a high suspicion of endometriosis need to be referred to a gynecologist. Each woman, depending on the severity of the disease, must make an individualized and informed decision. Psychological support should be given to women who experience severe, disabling pain; sexual difficulties; and infertility.

Premenstrual Syndrome

Many women experience varying degrees of physical discomfort in relation to their menstrual cycle. Premenstrual syndrome (PMS) is defined as the presence of symptoms in the premenstrual period or the early menstrual period. In some women, symptoms begin as early as ovulation then disappear before the onset of menstrual flow. PMS often causes emotional distress.

This syndrome appears to be most prominent in women in their 30s, although it may occur well before and after. The onset and symptoms may increase during periods in which the woman experiences rapid hormonal changes, such as puberty, after pregnancy, discontinuation of oral contraceptives, or after a period of menstrual irregularity.

Women with PMS should be encouraged to acknowledge the condition and attempt to avoid stress at the time of the premenstrual period. Fatigue seems to exaggerate PMS symptoms; therefore, the woman should plan for extra sleep, rest, and relaxation. Dietary changes may decrease irritability and mood swings. A modified hypoglycemic diet with adequate protein (limit red meats) and decreased simple sugars might be helpful. A greater intake of whole grains, vegetables, and natural sources of vitamin B with modified intake of dairy products and animal fats may provide relief. Using natural diuretics such as water, celery, cucumber, watermelon, and herbal teas to reduce fluid retention is recommended. Restriction of caffeine, tobacco, and alcohol may be helpful.

Exercise has been suggested to reduce PMS. Several possible mechanisms may explain the positive effects of exercise on PMS. Exercise improves the circulatory system. Exercise has also been found to increase the blood levels of beta-endorphin (an opiate-like substance produced by the human body). Drugs are prescribed only for temporary symptomatic relief.

Dysmenorrhea

One of the most common menstrual disturbances is *dysmenorrhea*, painful menstruation. Although many women observe some discomfort from pelvic congestion, incapacitating symptoms are experienced by about 5% to 10% of women during menses. Repeated experiences of dysmenorrhea should be evaluated by a physician. In some cases, a physical cause may be found, such as endometriosis, pelvic inflammatory disease, adhesions, genital tract abnormalities, poor uter-

ine position, presence of uterine tumors, or possible endocrine imbalances.

Dysmenorrhea may be aggravated by constipation and fatigue. Also, it may be worsened by the woman's being emotionally upset. The maintenance of good hygiene, a proper diet, and good emotional health is very important. Application of heat to the pelvic region and mild sedatives or muscle relaxants often help lessen the discomfort. Medications ordered by the physician may be necessary in severe cases of discomfort.

Disturbance in Blood Flow

Other types of menstrual disorders that should be evaluated by a physician include *amenorrhea*, the abnormal absence of menses; *menorrhagia*, excessive flow during the menses; and *metrorrhagia*, the presence of bloody vaginal discharge between periods. All three conditions should be assessed to determine the cause.

It is important that menstrual disorders be explained to the woman in terms that she can understand. The caregiver needs to remember that menstruation remains an emotional issue for most women. Sexuality and self-image can be influenced by myths and misinformation. Therefore, education and counseling are important in the health history.

Fibrocystic Breast Disorder

Fibrocystic breast disorder is a common benign breast problem. It is most prevalent in women 35 to 50 years of age. This condition is probably caused by an imbalance in estrogen and progesterone, which distorts the normal changes of the menstrual cycle. Generally the condition improves after menopause. Women with fibrocystic breast disorder have an increased risk of developing breast cancer.

Women with fibrocystic disorder may complain of breast lumpiness or breast pain, usually increasing before menstruation. Masses may be generalized or localized. Mammography, palpation, and fine-needle aspiration are used to confirm fibro-

KEY POINTS IN EDUCATION: RELIEVING MILD SYMPTOMS OF FIBROCYSTIC BREAST DISORDER

- Mild analgesics
- Warm compresses
- Nighttime supportive bra
- Restriction of sodium intake the week before the onset of menses
- Mild diuretic the week before menses
- Restriction of methylxanthines, including caffeine found in coffee, tea, cola, and chocolate
- Vitamins B (thiamine), E, and C

cystic breast disease. Invasive procedures such as a biopsy are used when the diagnosis is questionable and to rule out breast cancer.

Breast Cancer

Breast cancer is a major public health problem. Approximately ONE IN TEN women in the United States will develop this disease. This greatly ex-

ceeds the rate of cancer in other organs. On a positive note, the survival rate for localized breast cancer has improved from 78% in the 1940s to 90% today.

Early detection is the most important factor in greatly increasing the survival rate. Breast self-examination should be performed on a regular, monthly basis approximately 1 week after menstruation and also each month after menopause. The woman should be taught by the caregiver how to do a breast self-examination (Fig. 25–2).

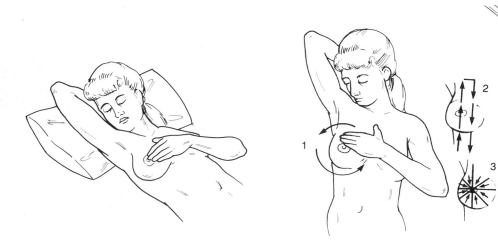

▲ FIGURE 25–2

Breast self-examination (BSE). *WHEN TO DO BSE:* Monthly assessment will increase chances of identifying changes in breasts. Do BSE about 1 week after menstrual period and on the same day every month. *HOW TO DO BSE:* **A.** Lie down. Place a pillow under your shoulder on the side being examined. Put one hand behind your head. Use pads of three middle fingers to feel for lumps. Press firmly enough to know how your breast feels. **B.** Move around the breasts in a set way. You can choose (1) the circle, (2) the up and down line, or (3) the wedge. Do the BSE the same way each time. It will help you to be sure that you have gone over the entire breast area. Assess the other breast using the same technique. **C.** In the shower, soapy hands will glide over the wet skin, making it easy to check your breasts.
Note: Visually assess your breasts while standing in front of a mirror, right after your BSE. See if there are any skin changes, dimpling of the skin, or changes in the nipples. Redness or swelling should also be observed. If you find any changes, see your physician immediately. (Adapted from The Nurse and Breast Self-Examination. American Cancer Society, Inc., 1989.)

Although the year a woman should begin having annual routine mammographies is decided by the woman's physician, a baseline mammogram is important to assess breast changes. The American Cancer Society suggests "a baseline mammogram between the ages of 35 and 40, followed by annual or biennial mammograms from 40 to 49, and annual mammograms from 50 years of age onward." Abnormal breast tissue can be detected by a mammogram that cannot be palpated during the self-examination.

FACTORS THAT INCREASE THE RISK OF BREAST CANCER

- Sex—Breast cancer is more than 100 times more common in females than males.
- Age—Incidence rises steadily until 59 years of age, which implies that increased exposure to endogenous sex hormones may play a role.
- Early menarche (before age 12) or late menopause (after age 50)—Both imply that increased time exposure to endogenous sex hormones may play a role.
- Nulliparity—A woman who does not have a child before age 30 is at a greater risk for breast cancer.
- Family history—A maternal history of breast cancer increases the risk threefold (especially if mother or sister have had breast cancer).

TABLE 25–2. CLINICAL CLASSIFICATION FOR THE STAGING OF BREAST CANCER

STAGE I: Tumor < 2 cm without skin involvement and with no clinically suspicious axillary nodes.
STAGE II: Tumor < 2 cm with clinically suspicious nodes; any tumor 2–5 cm with or without clinically suspicious nodes.
STAGE III: Any tumor > 5 cm; skin involvement; solid fixation of tumor to chest wall; axillary lymph nodes ≥2.5 cm in transverse diameter; edema of arm; nodes overlying or in surrounding tissue
STAGE IV: More advanced breast cancer; metastatic disease.

- Race—Incidence is highest among white Jewish women.
- Nutrition and obesity—A high-fat diet and obesity are thought to affect the storage and metabolism of estrogens. Although not conclusive, high-fiber diets, high intake of vegetables (especially yellow ones containing carotene), and vitamins A, C, and E may reduce the risk of breast cancer.
- Stress—Stress has been cited to increase the risk for breast cancer.

FACTORS THAT MAY DECREASE THE RISK OF BREAST CANCER

- Multiparity—Especially with parity beginning before 20 years of age.
- Sterilization before the age of 40—Implies decreased exposure to endogenous sex hormones.
- Prolonged lactation—Probably related to suppression of ovulation.

The clinical manifestations are important in the prognosis of breast cancer. Unfavorable prognostic signs include skin involvement, inflammatory signs, fixation to the chest wall, tumor size in excess of 5 cm, palpable axillary nodes, and nipple involvement. A malignant breast neoplasm may originate either in the duct or in the lobular epithelium. It may or may not have infiltrated the surrounding tissue. All forms of breast cancer can spread locally by invasion. About 50% of all breast cancers originate in the upper outside quadrant and metastasize to the axillary nodes. The tumor that adheres to the chest wall causes a skin dimpling and retraction in the later stages of the disease.

The clinical staging system for breast cancer is shown in Table 25–2.

DIAGNOSIS

Biopsy is the definitive way to diagnose breast cancer. A fine-needle biopsy is used when a mass is most likely a fluid-filled cyst. Disappearance of the mass after withdrawal of fluid usually indicates the mass is cystic and needs to be followed closely for recurrence. In a wide-needle biopsy, a cutting needle is used to remove tissue for diagnosis. Needle biopsies can be done under local anesthesia on an outpatient basis.

Surgical biopsies are used for solid masses, although in 75% of cases, the tumors turn out to be benign. A removal of the entire lump is called a *lumpectomy*. When the mass is larger than 3 cm or is a nonpalpable lesion detected by mammography, anesthesia will be required and the procedure is usually done in the hospital.

A *hormonal receptor assay* is performed on all breast cancer biopsy specimens to determine the tumor's response to estrogen and progesterone. This gives prognostic information and is helpful in choosing appropriate therapy.

Surgical alternatives are available to the woman with breast cancer. The patient should be involved in deciding the type of therapy that is done. Patients who are offered a choice among treatments show better overall adjustment and seem to be less concerned about recurrence of the disease than those who are not offered a choice. Patients who choose immediate breast reconstruction with the mastectomy tend to be younger and more concerned about their appearance, and more frightened by alteration in their body image.

TREATMENT OPTIONS

Local Regional Treatment (Lumpectomy). The lumpectomy is breast-preserving surgery in which the tumor mass along with a margin of tissue and the axillary lymph nodes are removed. In early breast cancer, this method followed with definitive radiation with or without chemotherapy yields survival rates that compare favorably with those of other treatments. This procedure is done for cosmetic effect in women who are highly motivated to preserve their breast. However, many women are not suitable candidates for excision and radiation because of the stage of their cancer.

Partial (Segmented) Mastectomy. In the partial mastectomy, the tumor and 2 to 3 cm of surrounding tissue are removed. Some of the breast remains. Axillary nodes are removed. Current trends support the use of both radiation and chemotherapy in women who have positive nodes.

Modified Mastectomy. In the modified mastec-

tomy, the breast, but not the pectoral muscle, is surgically removed. This procedure is used for early-stage breast cancer and is usually followed by postoperative radiation of the regional nodes and often chemotherapy. Breast reconstruction can be performed during the mastectomy or at a later time.

Radical Mastectomy. In the radical mastectomy, the breast, the axillary nodes, and the pectoralis major muscle are removed. Radiotherapy and chemotherapy are given if the disease has advanced to the point that a radical mastectomy is done.

The potential postoperative complications of a mastectomy include infection, nerve trauma causing numbness, edema of the arm, weakness, impaired functioning of the shoulder, heightened sensitivity of the skin, itching, and "pins and needles" and "phantom breast" sensations. These symptoms may persist for several months or even up to a year after surgery.

BREAST RECONSTRUCTION

Breast reconstruction entails either a flap reconstruction using the patient's own transplanted tissue and skin or, more commonly, a prosthesis implanted under the musculofascial layer of the chest wall. The implant usually is a permanent silicone prosthesis, sized to match the opposite breast, or a temporary tissue expander. The expander is a sac filled with 75 to 200 mL of normal saline solution. Postoperatively, the sac is injected with saline every week to 3 weeks until the breast tissue stretches enough to enclose a prosthesis of the desired size. Recent controversy over silicone prostheses includes two risk factors: first, the silicone material can irritate the tissues, and second, if the prosthesis ruptures, a mammogram may be difficult to interpret.

Several published studies have found the psychological adjustment of women who had modified mastectomies to be similar to that of women who had conservative surgery (lumpectomies). Also outcomes related to sexuality and body image seem similar among women who have breast reconstruction and women who opt for conservative surgery.

The drugs used for chemotherapy include methotrexate, 5-fluorouracil, and cyclophosphamide.

An assay of the breast cancer can determine whether the malignant cells were estrogen and progesterone receptor positive or negative. Women with estrogen-receptor–positive tumors have been found to respond better to adjuvant therapy and have an overall improved survival rate. Additive hormonal therapy involves administering large doses of estrogen, androgen, or progestin in postmenopausal women. High doses of these hormones have been observed to cause tumor regression.

Hospitalization for breast surgery is 3 to 4 days. The usual postoperative nursing care is given. Psychological support is very important at this time. In addition, the woman must be instructed about exercises necessary for rehabilitation to gain proper arm and shoulder function. A Reach to Recovery volunteer from the American Cancer Society will visit the patient during her hospitalization to inform her of exercises, give educational materials, and discuss the patient's personal feelings about her disease. The volunteer is able to closely identify with the patient's present and future emotional feelings because she has had a mastectomy herself. Thus she can serve as a role model. The patient will be invited to a local discussion group formed by women who have had breast cancer.

DISCHARGE PLANNING

- Assist the woman to understand her diagnosis, therapy, and long-term prognosis.
- Instruct the woman to participate in her recovery program.

- Instruct the woman to recognize complications that may occur.
- Instruct the woman about planned exercises, activities, and follow-up care.
- Encourage the woman to attend Reach to Recovery group discussions.

References

Aiken, M. M. (1990). Documenting sexual abuse in prepubertal girls. *American Journal of Maternal-Child Nursing,* 15(3):176–177.

American Cancer Society (1989). *The Nurse and Breast Self-Examination* (No. 3408PE). New York: American Cancer Society.

Brown-Daniels, C. J., & Blasdell, A. (1990). Early-stage breast cancer: Adjuvant drug therapy. *American Journal of Nursing* 90(11):32–33.

Deitch, K. V., & Smith, J. E. (1990). Symptoms of chronic vaginal infection and microscopic condyloma in women. *Journal of Obstetric, Gynecologic, and Neonatal Nursing* 19(2):133–138.

Dulaney, P. (1990). A comprehensive education and support program for women experiencing hysterectomies. *Journal of Obstetric, Gynecologic, and Neonatal Nursing* 19(4):319–325.

Ginsberg, C. K. (1991). Exfoliative cytologic screening: The Papanicolaou test. *Journal of Obstetric, Gynecologic, and Neonatal Nursing* 20(1):39–46.

Hale, M. (1990). Current and former smokers have approximately twice the risk of PID as women who have never smoked. *American Journal of Nursing* 90(6):77.

Knobf, M. T. (1990). Early-stage breast cancer: The options. *American Journal of Nursing* 90(11):28–30.

Ladewig, P. W., London, M. L., & Olds, S. B. (1990). *Essentials of Maternal-Newborn Nursing,* 2nd ed. Redwood City, CA: Addison-Wesley Nursing.

Lichtman, R., & Papera, S. (1990). *Gynecology: Well-Woman Care.* Norwalk, CT: Appleton & Lange.

Murata, J. M. (1990). Abnormal genital bleeding and secondary amenorrhea: Common gynecological problems. *Journal of Obstetric, Gynecologic, and Neonatal Nursing* 19(1):26–36.

SUGGESTED ACTIVITIES

1. Review the symptoms, treatment, and prevention of the types of vaginitis that commonly occur during pregnancy.
2. Explain how to conduct a breast self-examination.
3. Recall when and how often a mammogram should be done.

REVIEW QUESTIONS

A. Select the best answer to each multiple-choice question.

1. Vaginitis caused by the yeast infection candidiasis is manifested by
   A. Profuse, cheesy, white vaginal discharge
   B. Leukorrhea
   C. White patches on the vulva
   D. All of the above

2. Vaginitis caused by a trichomonal protozoan is characterized by all of the following EXCEPT
   A. Leukorrhea
   B. Greenish-white, foamy vaginal discharge
   C. Vulva redness
   D. Watery, curd-like patches

3. The woman with a history of vaginitis should be instructed to do all of the following EXCEPT
   A. Avoid tight clothing in the genital area
   B. Use feminine sprays to make the vaginal secretion more alkaline
   C. Have the sexual partner treated, if he is infected
   D. Change sitting positions frequently

4. Which of the following is the most common site of endometriosis?
   A. Uterosacral ligament
   B. Broad ligament
   C. Ovary
   D. Bowel

5. Which one of the following types of cancer causes the most deaths in women?
   A. Cervical
   B. Uterine
   C. Lung
   D. Breast

6. Which one of the following carcinomas is more frequent in women who have not had children?
   A. Breast
   B. Ovarian
   C. Cervical
   D. Endometrial

7. Toxic shock syndrome is primarily a disease of women during their reproductive years. The typical signs of toxic shock syndrome are
   A. Elevated temperature over 102° F
   B. Sore throat or aching muscles
   C. Rapid drop in blood pressure
   D. All of the above

8. Endometriosis is characterized by the presence of endometrial tissue outside the uterus. The symptoms of endometriosis include
   A. Dysmenorrhea, dyspareunia, and nausea and vomiting
   B. Dysmenorrhea, dyspareunia, and pelvic pain
   C. Dyspareunia, pelvic pain, and nausea and vomiting
   D. Dysuria, pelvic pain, and elevated temperature

9. Dysmenorrhea is one of the most common menstrual disturbances. It can be aggravated by the following:
   A. Diet, stress, and muscle relaxants
   B. Diet, poor hygiene, and emotional stress
   C. Application of heat and pelvic adhesions
   D. Application of heat and muscle relaxants

APPENDIX A

Glossary

Abortion. Termination of pregnancy before viability of fetus (approximately 20 weeks' gestation). *Miscarriage* is lay term for spontaneous abortion.

Abruptio placentae. Premature separation of a normally implanted placenta from the uterine wall.

Acceleration. Periodic increase in the baseline fetal heart rate.

Acidosis. Depletion of alkaline reserves in the blood and body tissues.

Acini cells. Secretory cells of the alveoli of the breasts that produce milk.

Acrocyanosis. Sluggish peripheral cyanosis of hands and feet. Common after birth.

Adolescence. Time between puberty and adulthood.

Afterbirth. Placenta and membranes that are expelled after the birth of an infant.

Afterpains. Cramp-like uterine contractions after the birth of the baby.

AIDS. Acquired immune deficiency syndrome, a sexually transmitted viral disease that is fatal.

Albuminuria. Presence of albumin, a protein, in the urine.

Alveoli. Small air sacs present in the lungs.

Amenorrhea. Absence of menstruation.

Amniocentesis. Removal of amniotic fluid by insertion of a needle into the amniotic sac. Amniotic fluid is obtained to assess fetal health and maturity.

Amnion. The inner of the two membranes that form a sac containing the fetus and the amniotic fluid. (The outer membrane is the chorion.)

Amnionitis. Infection of the amniotic fluid.

Amniotic fluid. Fluid that surrounds the fetus within the amniotic sac which permits fetal movement, absorbs shocks, and prevents heat loss.

Analgesic. Drug used to relieve pain.

Androgen. Substance that stimulates development of secondary male characteristics, such as the male hormone testosterone.

Anemia. Condition caused by a decrease in erythrocytes or hemoglobin or both.

Anoxia. Lack of oxygen.

Antepartum. Occurring before birth; prenatal.

Antibody. Protein substance formed by the body in response to an antigen.

Antigen. Foreign substance introduced into the body that stimulates the immune system to form antibodies.

Anuria. Failure of the kidney to produce urine.

Apnea. A transitory cessation of respirations.

Areola. Pigmented ring surrounding the nipple of the breast.

Asphyxia. Life-threatening condition caused by lack of oxygen and accumulation of carbon dioxide in the blood.

Asphyxia neonatorum. Delayed onset of breathing at the time of birth.

Atelectasis. Incomplete expansion of the lung or portion of the lung.

Atony. Lack of normal muscle tone or strength.

Attachment. A bond or relationship of affection between persons.

Attitude (of fetus). The relationship of the fetal parts to one another.

Autosome. A chromosome that is not a sex chromosome.

Bag of water (BOW). The membranes containing the amniotic fluid and the fetus.

Bartholin's glands. Small, mucus-secreting glands located on either side of the base of the vagina.

Baseline fetal heart rate (FHR). Average fetal heart rate observed within a 10-minute period of monitoring.

Bilirubin. Yellowish pigment of bile produced from the hemoglobin of the red blood cells.

Bilirubinemia. Presence of an abnormal amount of bilirubin in the blood when red blood cells are broken down or destroyed from a pathological cause.

Birth. The process of being born.

Blastocyst. The inner solid mass of cells within the morula.

Blastula. Stage of the fertilized ovum in which the cells are arranged in a hollow ball.

Bradycardia. Slow heart rate.

Braxton-Hicks contractions. Intermittent painless contractions of the uterus. These are more noticeable toward the end of pregnancy and are sometimes mistaken for true labor signs.

Breasts. Mammary glands.

Breech birth. Birth in which the buttocks or feet are presented first instead of the head.

Brown adipose tissue (BAT). Fat deposits in neonates (infants) that generate more heat than usual fat. Found around the neck, between the scapulas; around the kidneys; around the adrenals; and behind the sternum. Also called *brown fat.*

Caput succedaneum. Edema formed under the fetal scalp (or presenting part) during labor.

Cephalic. Pertaining to the head.

Cephalohematoma. Accumulation of blood under the periosteum of the newborn's skull caused by trauma to blood vessels during birth.

Cephalopelvic disproportion (CPD). A condition in which the fetal head is of a shape, size, or position that prevents it from passing through the maternal pelvis.

Cervix. Lower portion of the uterus extending into the vagina.

Cesarean birth. Extraction of the fetus, placenta, and membranes through an incision into the abdominal wall and the uterus.

Chorion. Outer membrane of the amniotic sac.

Chorionic villi. Slender, branching projections of the chorion containing capillaries that are the means by which substances (gases, nutrients, and waste products) are exchanged between the maternal and fetal circulation.

Chromosomes. Rod-shaped bodies within cells on which the genes are located.

Circumcision. Surgical removal of part or all of the prepuce (foreskin) of the penis.

Cleft lip. Separation of one or both sides of the upper lip.

Cleft palate. Deformity caused by the failure of the bones of the roof of the mouth to fuse in the midline.

Clitoris. A female organ that is made of erectile tissue and situated at the anterior junction of the vulva.

Coitus. Sexual intercourse.

Colostrum. Yellowish secretion from the breasts before the onset of true lactation.

Conception. Union of the sperm and ovum; fertilization.

Conceptus. Products of fertilization.

Condom. Thin, flexible sheath worn over the penis during sexual intercourse to prevent sperm from entering the vagina and prevent disease.

Condyloma. Sexually transmitted, viral, wart-like growth on the skin of genitals.

Congenital. Present at birth.

Conjunctivitis. Inflammation of the mucous membrane lining of the eyelids.

Coombs test. Test used to detect sensitized red blood cells. The indirect test determines the presence of Rh+ antibodies in maternal blood; the direct test determines the presence of maternal Rh+ antibodies in fetal cord blood.

Corpus luteum. Solid yellow body that develops within a ruptured follicle; an endocrine structure that primarily secretes progesterone.

Cotyledon. Segment or subdivision of the uterine surface of the placenta.

Crowning. Visibility of the fetal head in the birth canal before delivery.

Cyanosis. Blueness of the skin due to a lack of oxygenation of the blood.

Deceleration. Periodic decrease in the baseline fetal heart rate.

Decidua. Endometrium, or lining of the uterus, that thickens during pregnancy and is shed after delivery.

Decrement. Decline or decrease of uterine contraction.

Delivery. Expulsion of the fetus at birth.

Dilation of cervix. Stretching of cervical canal to size of opening large enough to allow the passage of infant.

Disproportion. Lack of normal relationship between fetus and maternal pelvis. Fetus is too large or pelvis too small for normal vaginal birth.

Ductus arteriosus. A fetal vessel connecting the pulmonary artery with the aorta.

Ductus venosus. A fetal vessel that connects the umbilical vein and the inferior vena cava.

Dysmenorrhea. Painful menstruation.

Dyspareunia. Painful intercourse.

Dyspnea. Difficult or labored breathing.

Dystocia. Difficult or slow labor or delivery or both.

Early deceleration. Periodic change in fetal heart rate pattern caused by head compression. Deceleration has a uniform appearance and early onset in relation to the maternal contraction.

Eclampsia. Severe form of toxemia or pregnancy-induced hypertension; accompanied by convulsions.

Ectopic pregnancy. Implantation of the fertilized ovum outside the uterus.

Effacement. Thinning and shortening of the cervix before and during labor.

Embryo. Stage of human development occurring between the ovum and fetal stages, or from 2 to 8 weeks' gestation.

Endometriosis. Endometrium located outside the uterus.

Endometrium. Mucous membrane lining of the uterus (during pregnancy it is called decidua).

Engagement. Largest diameter of the fetal presenting part (head) passing through the pelvic inlet.

Engorgement. Vascular congestion and distention causing breast engorgement.

Epidural block. Injection of local anesthetic into the epidural space of the spinal column.

Episiotomy. Surgical incision of the perineum before birth to permit delivery of infant without lacerations to the area.

Erythema. Inflammation of the skin or mucous membrane.

Erythroblastosis fetalis. Hemolytic disease of the newborn caused by isoimmunization due to Rh incompatibility or ABO incompatibility.

Estrogen. Female sex hormone secreted by ovaries and placenta.

Expulsion. Pushing out or expelling.

Extension. Stretching out of fetal part; opposite of flexion.

Fallopian tube (uterine tube). An oviduct or tube extending laterally from each side of the uterus to the ovary.

Fertilization. Penetration of one ovum (single pregnancy) by a sperm.

Fetal heart rate (FHR). Number of fetal heartbeats in a given time. Normal FHR is 120 to 160 beats per minute.

Fetal heart rate fluctuations. Tachycardia, bradycardia, accelerations, decelerations, or changes in FHR variability.

Fetoscope. A stethoscope especially adapted for listening to fetal heart tones.

Fetus. Baby after the embryonic period of development and before delivery.

Fibrinogen. A blood constituent necessary for the formation of clots.

Fibrocystic breast disease. Benign breast disorder characterized by the formation of cysts.

Follicle-stimulating hormone (FSH). Hormone produced by the anterior pituitary gland during the first half of the menstrual cycle, stimulating development of the graafian follicle.

Fontanelle. Unfused area between fetal skull bones covered with strong connective tissue; allows for movement of bones and molding during birth.

Foramen ovale. Opening between the right and then the left atrium in fetus.

Foreskin (prepuce). Fold of skin covering the glans penis. Removed during circumcision.

Fundus. Upper portion of the uterus.

Gavage. Feeding of liquid nutrients through a tube passed into the stomach through the nose or mouth.

Gene. Structure within the chromosome that transmits the parents' hereditary traits.

Gestation. Time from conception to birth, approximately 280 days.

Gestational age. Estimated age of the fetus calculated in weeks from the first day of the last normal menstrual period.

Glomerular filtration rate (GFR). Amount of plasma filtered by the glomeruli of both kidneys per minute.

Glucosuria. Presence of glucose in the urine.

Gonads. Male and female sex organs (testes and ovaries).

Graafian follicle. Ovarian cyst containing the ripe ovum to be released; it secretes hormones.

Gravid. Pregnant.

Gravida. A pregnant woman; called primigravida during the first pregnancy and multigravida during the second and subsequent pregnancies.

Gynecoid pelvis. A female-type pelvis in which the inlet is round.

Gynecology. Care of disorders of the female reproductive tract and associated structures.

Homans' sign. Pain or tenderness in the calf of the leg on dorsiflexion of the foot; an indicator of thrombosis or thrombophlebitis.

Hormone. Chemical substance originating in a gland or organ that is carried by the blood or lymph to another organ or tissue where it acts as a stimulator or accelerator.

Hydramnios. Excessive amount of amniotic fluid.

Hydrocephalus. Abnormal condition in which there is an excessive amount of cerebral fluid within the brain cavities or surrounding the brain or both.

Hydrops fetalis. Massive edema of the fetus due to hyperbilirubinemia

Hyperbilirubinemia. Excessive amount of bilirubin in the blood; indicative of hemolytic disorder due to blood incompatibility, intrauterine infection, septicemia, and other disorders.

Hyperemesis gravidarum. Excessive vomiting during pregnancy.

Hyperventilation. Decrease of carbon dioxide in the blood as result of rapid and deep breathing; symptoms may include dizziness and confusion.

Hypocalcemia. Decrease of calcium in the blood.

Hypoglycemia. Decreased level of blood glucose.

Hypotension. Low blood pressure.

Hypothermia. Below-normal body temperature.

Hypoxia. Lack of available oxygen to the body tissues.

Hysterectomy. Surgical removal of uterus.

Icterus neonatorum. Jaundice of newborn; a clinical form of hemolytic disease.

Immune response. Reaction of the body to foreign substances or substances body interprets as being foreign.

Implantation. Process by which the conceptus attaches to the uterine wall.

Impotence. Inability of the male to achieve or maintain an erection.

Inborn error of metabolism. A hereditary deficiency of a specific enzyme needed for normal metabolism of specific chemicals.

Increment. Increased intensity of a uterine contraction.

Internal os. An inside opening; the opening between the cervix and the uterus.

Intrauterine growth retardation (IUGR). Fetal condition characterized by failure to grow at the expected rate.

Involution. Return of the uterus to its prepregnant size and function.

Jaundice. Yellow pigmentation of body tissues caused by excessive bilirubin in the blood.

Kegel exercise. Conscious tightening and relaxing of the pubococcygeal muscles to strength the vagina and perineum.

Kilogram (kg). 1000 g, or 2.2 lb.

Labor. Process by which the fetus, placenta, and membranes are expelled from the body.

Laceration. Tearing of tissue; during labor, tearing of vulvar, vaginal, and possibly rectal tissue as infant is born.

Lactation. Process of producing and supplying breast milk.

Lanugo. Fine, downy hair found on the fetus and parts of the infant after birth.

Large-for-gestational age infant. Infant of any weight who falls above the 90th percentile on the intrauterine growth curve.

Leopold's maneuvers. A series of four maneuvers (abdominal palpation) designed to provide a systematic approach to determine fetal presentation and position.

Libido. Sexual drive.

Lie. Relationship of the long axis of the fetus to the long axis of the mother.

Lightening. Moving of the fetus and uterus downward into the pelvic cavity; engagement.

Lochia. Uterine (vaginal) discharge following delivery, lasting 3 to 6 weeks.

Lunar month. A period of 28 days (4 weeks).

Luteinizing hormone (LH). One of the gonadotropic hormones produced by the anterior pituitary gland that stimulates development of the corpus luteum.

Mastitis. Acute inflammation of the breast.

Mechanism of labor. A series of passive movements undergone by the fetus in passing through the birth canal.

Meconium. First stool of newborn; greenish-black, viscid. Contains mucus, bile, and epithelial shreds.

Menstruation. A periodic vaginal discharge.

Midwife, certified nurse. A registered nurse who has passed a national certification examination, cares for normal maternity patients, and conducts a normal delivery.

Milia. Tiny white papules or cysts commonly over the bridge of the nose, chin, and cheeks of newborn infants; disappear within a few weeks.

Miscarriage. A lay term used for spontaneous abortion.

Molding. Shaping the fetal head by overlapping of the cranial bones to facilitate movement through the birth canal during labor.

Mongolian spots. Benign bluish pigmentation over the lower back and buttocks that may be present at birth, especially in dark-skinned races.

Montgomery's tubercles. Small glands situated on the areola around the nipple.

Morbidity. The state of being sick or diseased.

Mortality. Pertains to the death rate.

Morula. Development stage of the fertilized ovum in which there is a solid mass of cells.

Multigravida. A woman during her second or subsequent pregnancies.

Multipara. A woman who has delivered two or more babies after the period of viability, regardless of whether they were alive or stillborn.

Multiple pregnancy. Pregnancy involving more than one fetus, for example, twins.

Nagele's rule. Method used to calculate the expected date of confinement; count back 3 months from the first day of the last menstrual period and add 7 days.

Nares. Nostrils.

Neonate. Infant from birth through the first 28 days of life.

Obstetrics. The art and science of caring for a pregnant women.

Occiput. The back part of the head.

Ophthalmia neonatorum. Purulent infection of the eyes or conjunctiva of the newborn, most often caused by gonococci or chlamydia.

Ovulation. The maturation and release of the ovum from the ovary.

Ovum. Female reproductive cell; egg.

Oxytocic. A drug that stimulates uterine contractions.

Palpation. Examination performed by touching and exploring with the hands.

Papanicolaou (Pap) smear. Cytological test of cervical cells used as a screening test for cervical cancer.

Paracervical block. Injection of local anesthetic into the paracervical nerve to relieve pain during active labor.

Parity (para). Number of pregnancies reaching viability. It does not refer to number of fetuses delivered.

Parturition. Childbirth.

Patent ductus arteriosus. Congenital abnormal opening between the pulmonary artery and the aorta that does not close after birth.

Penis. The male organ of copulation and reproduction.

Perineum. Floor of the pelvis; area of tissue between the anus and vagina in the female and the anus and scrotum in the male.

Peristalsis. Wave-like progression of muscular contraction and relaxation propelling the contents through a tubular organ.

Phototherapy. Treatment of jaundice by exposure to light rays; used to aid bilirubin clearance.

Placenta. Flat, vascular structure that connects the fetus to the uterine wall for gas exchange and nutrient exchange. Also known as the *afterbirth*.

Placenta previa. Abnormal implantation of the placenta in the lower uterine segment.

Polyhydramnios. Excessive amount of amniotic fluid.

Position. Relation of the fetal presenting part to the maternal pelvis.

Postpartum. After childbirth.

Postpartum hemorrhage. Loss of 500 mL or more of blood from the uterus after delivery.

Preeclampsia. Disorder of pregnancy or the puerperium, characterized by hypertension, proteinuria, and edema.

Premature infant. Infant born before the end of the thirty-seventh week of gestation (also called *preterm infant*).

Prenatal. Occurring before birth.

Primigravida. A woman who is pregnant for the first time.

Primipara. A woman who is giving birth to her first child at viability stage.

Prolactin. A hormone secreted by the anterior pituitary that stimulates and sustains lactation.

Prolapsed cord. Umbilical cord that becomes trapped in the vagina before the fetus is delivered; cord is beside or ahead of the presenting part.

Prolonged rupture of membranes. Rupture of amniotic sac that occurs 6 to 12 hours or more before the onset of labor.

Prophylaxis. Protection from or prevention of a disease.

Proteinuria. Presence of protein in the urine.

Puerperal morbidity. A maternal temperature of 100.4°F (38.0°C) or higher on any 2 of the first 10 postpartum days, excluding the first 24 hours.

Puerperium. The period of time after delivery to complete involution of organs (such as uterus), usually 6 weeks.

Quickening. Perception of the first fetal movement by the mother; usually between eighteenth and twentieth weeks of pregnancy.

Radioimmunoassay. Test for pregnancy based on an antigen–antibody reaction and measured by a sensitive radioisotope technique.

Rh factor. An inherited antigen in the blood. Blood that contains this factor is called Rh + and that which does not is called Rh − .

RhoGAM. $Rh_o(D)$ Immune globulin given after delivery to an Rh − mother of an Rh + fetus to prevent the maternal Rh immune response.

Rhythm method. Timing of sexual intercourse to avoid the fertile period associated with ovulation.

Rubella (German measles). An acute infection that can cause serious anomalies in the developing fetus.

Semen. Thick, whitish fluid ejaculated by the male during orgasm and containing the spermatozoa.

Sex chromosomes. Chromosomes responsible for sex determination. Females have two X chromosomes, and males have one X and one Y.

Skene's glands. Two glands opening near the meatus of the female urethra.

Small-for-gestation age (SGA) infant. Infant of any weight who falls below the tenth percentile on the intrauterine growth curve.

Spermatozoon. The male reproductive cell, consisting of a nucleus (head) and a flagellum (tail).

Spina bifida. A congenital defect involving failure in closure of the spinal cord.

Spinnbarkeit. Demonstrates the elasticity of the cervical mucus that is present at time of ovulation.

Station. Relationship of the presenting fetal part to the pelvic ischial spines of the birth canal.

Sterility. Inability to conceive.

Stillbirth. The delivery of a dead infant.

Subinvolution. Delay in the return of pelvic organs and structures to their prepregnant state.

Supine hypotension syndrome. Lowered blood pressure and decreased pulse when in the supine position. Due to compression of the inferior vena cava by pressure from the gravid uterus.

Surfactant. A substance formed in the lungs that, by reducing surface tension, helps to prevent the air sacs from collapsing.

Suture. Junction of the cranial bones.

Tachycardia (fetal). Rapid fetal heart rate of 160 beats or more per minute.

Tachypnea. Rapid respiration.

Teratogen. An agent that can cause damage in the developing fetus.

Thrombosis. Formation of a blood clot.

Tocolytic agent. Drug that alters the force of uterine contractions. Is used with labors involving preterm infants.

Transplacental. Across the placenta, such as exchange of nutrients, waste products, and hormones between mother and fetus. Also, refers to passing of drugs or harmful agents to fetus.

Trimester. A 3-month period of time in pregnancy. Pregnancy has three distinct trimesters.

Ultrasound. Use of high-frequency sound waves that may be directed through a transducer, into the maternal abdomen. Used in fetal assessment.

Umbilical cord. Cord containing two arteries and one vein that connects the fetus with the placenta.

Umbilicus. The navel.

Uterine dysfunction. A labor pattern that interferes with the normal progress of cervical dilatation.

Vagina. The canal from the vulva to the cervix of the uterus.

Vasectomy. Surgical removal of a portion of the vas deferens to produce male infertility.

Vernix caseosa. A protective cheese-like, whitish coating found in varying quantities on the skin of the newborn.

Vertex. The top of the fetal head, between the anterior and posterior fontanelles.

Viability. Ability to live outside the uterus.

Vulva. The external female genitalia, lying below the mons veneris.

Wharton's jelly. Yellow-white gelatinous material surrounding the vessels in the umbilical cord.

Womb. Lay term for the uterus.

Zygote. A fertilized ovum (egg).

APPENDIX B

DRUGS USED DURING PREGNANCY, LABOR, BIRTH, AND THE POSTPARTUM PERIOD

During pregnancy, drugs can be absorbed, enter the mother's bloodstream, and cross the placenta. Therefore, drugs taken by the mother during pregnancy can affect the fetus. In addition, after the infant is born, drugs can get into the mother's breast milk. Careful attention must be given to the mother's and infant's health status, in relation to the drugs taken by the mother. Long-term drug therapy, rather than single-dose therapy, may influence fetal cell growth during early and late periods of development. Drugs may act as *teratogenic agents* (substances causing birth defects) and cause problems such as abortions, malformations, altered fetal growth, functional deficits, cancer, and mutagenesis.

The blood flow is proportionally greater in the fetus than in the adult. Blood in the fetus is preferentially circulated to the essential organs, such as the brain and heart, and then the blood becomes diffused. Some drugs have a greater "liking" (affinity) for specific target tissues. The excretion of most drugs is slower in the fetus than in the adult.

At the end of pregnancy, some drugs must be used with caution because of their effect on the infant. When birth is imminent, administration of some drugs may cause respiratory distress of the infant at the critical time of adjustment to extrauterine life. Many of the analgesics and sedatives are in this group. The drugs, which are easily metabolized by the mother, may be difficult to metabolize by the infant, who has an immature and not fully functioning liver. In fact, it may take several days for the infant to rid his or her system of the drugs given to the mother and present in her circulation at birth.

Some chemicals, not usually considered to be drugs, have been shown to have an effect on the fetus. Studies have shown that caffeine (found in coffee, tea, cocoa, and cola) may increase fetal activity and, in high amounts, may cause chromosome breakdown. Cigarette smoking has been shown to increase fetal risks.

Many women are not aware that over-the-counter drugs (for example, Tums, Dristan, and Dramamine) should be taken with the same caution as drugs prescribed by the physician. The caregiver should encourage the pregnant woman to tell her physician or clinic staff about any drugs she is taking during the pregnancy.

TABLE B–1. DRUGS AND CHEMICALS USED DURING PREGNANCY, LABOR, BIRTH, AND THE POSTPARTUM PERIOD

DRUGS	CLASSIFICATION	INDICATIONS/ACTION	DOSAGE/ROUTE	NURSING CONSIDERATIONS	
				Assess: Maternal Side Effects	Assess: Fetal/Neonatal Side Effects
Acetaminophen Tylenol Datril	Analgesic, antipyretic	Acts on hypothalamic heat-regulating center Produces analgesia by ill-defined effect on hypothalamus	325–650 mg PO q 4 hr, prn	CNS (drowsiness, dizziness, stimulation, euphoria, lightheadedness) Skin rash, elevated temperature Hemolytic anemia Hypoglycemia Myocardial damage Coma with overdose Liver toxicity	In large doses, renal damage
Acetylsalicylic acid Aspirin	Analgesic Antipyretic Antiinflammatory	Elevates pain threshold Inhibits histamine release During pregnancy, use is limited to antiinflammatory effect of arthritis	325–650 mg PO q 4 hr, prn	Sensitivity to salicylates Bleeding disorders Peptic ulcer Prolonged bleeding time Prolonged labor GI irritation and bleeding Vomiting, sweating, tinnitus Thirst, drowsiness Toxic doses may cause renal damage and CNS disturbances	Teratogenicity is suspected but not proved Prolonged bleeding or hemorrhage at birth
Adrenalin (see epinephrine)					
Ethyl alcohol Social drinking	Tocolytic agent	Used in treatment of preterm labor (can inhibit labor) Inhibits release of oxytocin from posterior pituitary gland	No safe amount for fetus, oral	Tachycardia, CNS depression, headache, hypoglycemia, mood swings, mild hypotension, slurred speech, nausea and vomiting Chronic excessive intake can cause alcoholic hepatitis and cirrhosis Diuresis, vasodilation, and stimulation of gastric secretions	Fetal alcohol syndrome (craniofacial abnormalities) Growth retardation Maxillary hypoplasia Microcephaly
Alphaprodine hydrochloride Nisentil	Narcotic Analgesic	Decreases pain (more rapid onset of action and shorter duration than other narcotics) Used to decrease discomfort of labor	40–50 mg IM 15–20 mg IV (during labor)	Allergic reactions	Respiratory depression Narcotic withdrawal Effects during early pregnancy unknown
Aluminum hydroxide (should not be administered with tetracycline) Gelusil Maalox	Antacid Antiflatulent	Relief of heartburn, "acid indigestion," and flatulence	2 tsp or 2 tablets, PO, 1 hr after meals and at bedtime	Renal disease Hypersensitivity to some contents	Unknown

Drug	Classification	Action	Dosage	Precautions/Nursing Considerations	Side Effects
Americaine spray (benzocaine)	Local anesthetic	Produces surface anesthesia of skin and mucous membranes	20% aerosol 5% ointment Topical 200–600 mg Suppositories	Hypersensitivity reactions Avoid contact with eye Watch for allergic reaction such as swelling or redness If using spray hold can 6–12 inches from affected area	Unknown
Aminophylline	Bronchodilator	Relaxes smooth muscle while stimulating cardiac muscle Increases rate and depth of respirations Stimulates CNS Increases blood flow	0.9 mg/kg/hr (100–200 mg PO tid or q 6–8 hr when not pregnant)	Nausea and vomiting Heart palpitations, tachycardia, anxiety Fever, diuresis, abdominal distention Tremors, convulsions Insomnia, restlessness Fast administration can cause hypotension	Vomiting, jitteriness Tachycardia, cardiac arrhythmias Transient hyperglycemia Teratogenesis not proved
Ampicillin Omnipen Polycillin	Broad-spectrum antibiotic Effective for Gram-positive and -negative organisms	Interferes with bacterial cell-wall production Particularly effective for treatment of urinary tract infection, because it is unchanged in the urine	250–500 mg, q 6 hr, PO, IM, or IV	Allergic reactions (rash, diarrhea, nausea and vomiting, epigastric pain) Vaginitis flare up Hypersensitivity may cause hemolytic anemia, thrombocytopenia, nephritis, or anaphylactic reaction *Always check for allergy before administering*	Unknown
Antacids (see Gelusil)					
Anusol suppository	Analgesic (rectal)	Provides symptomatic relief of pain and itching of hemorrhoids or anal fissures	Insert suppository rectally bid or after each bowel movement	Burning, irritation	Unknown
Apresoline (see hydralazine hydrochloride)					
AquaMEPHYTON (see vitamin K)					
Aspirin (see acetylsalicylic acid)					
AVC Cream	Antibiotic (contains sulfanilamide, aminacrine hydrochloride)	Interferes with growth and enzyme systems of susceptible organisms Used for vaginal infection when specific organism cannot be found	1 application or 1 suppository inserted vaginally q a day or bid for 14 days	Hypersensitivity reactions Skin rashes, local burning or itching of vagina	Systemic absorption appears minimal Hemolytic anemia is possible
Benadryl (see diphenhydramine hydrochloride)					
Benzocaine (see Americaine spray)					
Betadine (povidone-iodine)		Germicide for skin preparation for wound (used during labor and birth)	Apply to skin	Prolonged use may lead to systematic absorption and toxicity Discontinue if redness or rash occurs Contraindicated if skin is hypersensitive Do not use with alcohol or hydrogen peroxide	Unknown

Table continued on following page

479

TABLE B–1. DRUGS AND CHEMICALS USED DURING PREGNANCY, LABOR, BIRTH, AND THE POSTPARTUM PERIOD *Continued*

| | | | | NURSING CONSIDERATIONS | |
| | | | | Assess: Maternal Side Effects | Assess: Fetal/Neonatal Side Effects |
DRUGS	CLASSIFICATION	INDICATIONS/ACTION	DOSAGE/ROUTE		
Betamethasone Celestone	Corticosteroid	Promotes fetal lung maturation (mechanism unknown) Prevents respiratory distress in preterm infant Antiinflammatory agent	12 mg IM q 24 hr before delivery	Contraindicated in cases of hypertension, diabetes, bleeding, skin reactions, systemic fungal infections Causes fluid and electrolyte imbalances, hypertension, dizziness, headache, GI irritation, bleeding	Transient adrenal insufficiency
Bisacodyl Dulcolax *(should not be used in acute abdominal pain)*	Stimulating laxative	Increases fluid and electrolyte secretion into intestinal mucosa, stimulating peristalsis Used for postpartum constipation	5–15 mg PO or 1 rectal suppository	Abdominal cramps Diarrhea Rectal burning (suppositories) Nausea and vomiting Do not take within 1 hr of other drugs Do not take during pregnancy Give postpartum	
Brethine (see terbutaline sulfate)					
Bricanyl (see terbutaline sulfate)					
Bromocriptine mesylate Parlodel	Lactation inhibitor Nonestrogenic and nonhormonal drug	Direct effect on the anterior pituitary gland, resulting in inhibition of prolactin secretion	2.5 mg PO with meals, bid for 5–14 days	Hypotension, dizziness, nausea, headache, diarrhea, abdominal cramps, constipation (appears safe since does not include estrogen—not cancerous)	None known (given to nonnursing mothers after delivery)
Butorphanol tartrate Stadol	Nonnarcotic analgesic	Inhibits ascending pain pathways in limbic system, thalamus, midbrain, hypothalamus	2 mg IM or 0.5 mg IV q 3–4 hr	Drowsiness Dizziness Confusion Headache Euphoria Diaphoresis Flushing Nausea and vomiting Respiratory dysfunction Palpitations Bradycardia Monitor intake and output (I & O) for decreased output Report CNS change (for overdose, give Narcan)	Decreases fetal beat-to-beat variability Newborn respiratory distress (Narcan should be available)

Drug	Classification	Action/Use	Dosage	Side Effects	Effects on Fetus/Newborn
Caffeine (principal alkaloid of several plants; kola) Coffee Tea Cola NoDoz Excedrin Anacin Vanquish	Cerebral stimulant Mild analgesic	CNS stimulation ↑ Heart rate ↑ Respiratory rate ↑ Wakefulness ↑ Vasoconstriction ↓ Muscle fatigue	<600 mg PO per day advisable	Insomnia Nervousness Tachycardia Cardiac arrhythmias GI irritation Tremors Psychological dependency Diuresis Excess of 600 mg/day associated with higher incidence of abortions, stillbirths, and preterm infants Sudden discontinuation of caffeine may cause headache and instability	Abortions, stillbirths, preterm births Potential teratogenic agent Caffeine in breast milk can make infant hyperactive and wakeful
Calcium gluconate	Mineral	Antidote to combat hypermagnesemia (magnesium sulfate toxicity)	IV (IM is very irritating to tissues) PO	Bradycardia Cardiac arrhythmias Carpal spasm Tetany Kidney stones	Respiratory distress
Carbocaine (mepivacaine hydrochloride)	Local anesthetic	Nerve block used for regional anesthesia	1–2% parenteral solution	Toxic potential of local anesthetics	Fetal bradycardia Neonatal depression
Celestone (see betamethasone)					
Cephalexin Keflex	Antibiotic (cephalosporin)	For Streptococcus pneumoniae and hemolytic streptococcal respiratory infections For soft tissue, staphylococcal infections For Escherichia coli urinary tract infections	250–500 mg PO q 6 hr daily	Possible cross-sensitivity to penicillin Allergic reactions (fever, rash, nausea and vomiting, dizziness, headache) Take with food or milk to lessen GI discomfort Store in refrigerator after using	Infant of woman taking drug during pregnancy may have a positive Coombs test result
Chloramphenicol Chloromycetin	Antibiotic	Useful in certain urinary infections Rapidly absorbed	50–250 mg PO q 6 hr daily	Can cause blood dyscrasias Bone marrow depression GI effects (nausea and vomiting, diarrhea, enterocolitis) Reserved for serious infections	Gray spinal syndrome or fetal death, since drug readily crosses placental barrier
Chlorotrianisene Tace	Lactation suppressant Estrogen	Prevention of breast engorgement, pain, and lactation	72 mg PO bid for 2 days 12 mg PO qid for 7 days	Can cause hyperplasia of endometrium Contraindicated in estrogen-induced cancer; hepatic, cardiac, and renal diseases Similar to those of oral contraceptives (skin rash, nausea, vomiting, edema) Increases risk of endometrial cancer Teach woman how to perform BSE	Unknown

Table continued on following page

TABLE B–1. DRUGS AND CHEMICALS USED DURING PREGNANCY, LABOR, BIRTH, AND THE POSTPARTUM PERIOD *Continued*

DRUGS	CLASSIFICATION	INDICATIONS/ACTION	DOSAGE/ROUTE	NURSING CONSIDERATIONS	
				Assess: Maternal Side Effects	Assess: Fetal/Neonatal Side Effects
Clindamycin Cleocin	Antibiotic	Bacteriostatic (interferes with protein synthesis) Well absorbed after oral administration For beta-hemolytic streptococcal infections For *Bacteroides fragilis* infection	150–450 mg PO 150–600 mg IM or IV q 6 hr	Abdominal cramps, diarrhea, colitis Allergic reactions Altered liver function Leukocytosis Pain or abscess of site of injection	Unknown
Clomiphene citrate Clomid	Fertility drug	Acts on the hypothalamus receptors to produce low estrogen levels Induces ovulation in anovulatory women (appears to stimulate release of pituitary gonadotropins, follicle-stimulating hormone, and luteinizing hormone)	50–100 mg PO daily for 5 days	Visual symptoms Ovarian enlargement Abdominal discomfort "Hot flashes" Multiple births Contraindicated in pregnancy, liver disease, abnormal vaginal bleeding	Prematurity (with multiple births)
Clotrimazole Gyne-Lotrimin Mycelex	Antibiotic	Antifungal Treatment of vaginal candidiasis (vaginitis)	1 tablet or 1 applicator vaginally daily for 7 days	Redness, burning, itching, irritation, lower abdominal cramps Urinary frequency	Unknown
Colace (see dioctyl sodium sulfosuccinate)					
Coumadin (see warfarin)					
Darvon (see propoxyphene hydrochloride)					
Datril (see acetaminophen)					
Deladumone OB (see testosterone enanthate and estradiol valerate)					
Demerol (see meperidine hydrochloride)					
Diazepam Valium	Antianxiety agent	Reduces mild anxiety Relieves alcohol withdrawal Controls epilepsy	2.5–10 mg PO tid or qid	Drowsiness, lethargy, skin rashes, nausea, ataxia, paradoxical anxiety Contraindicated during labor Potential abuse and addiction Warn patients to avoid activities requiring alertness and to not combine drug with alcohol or other depressants	Fetal tachycardia Decreased fetal heart rate Respiratory depression Increased bilirubin level Associated with cleft lip Breastfed infant may be lethargic, poor sucking reflex

Dilantin (see phenytoin sodium)

Drug	Classification	Action/Use	Dosage	Side Effects	Notes
Dinoprostone Prostaglandin E₂	Uterine stimulant	Stimulates uterine contractions to terminate pregnancy (second trimester abortion)	Vaginal suppositories IV infusion	Nausea and vomiting, diarrhea Headache, chills, shivering (10% of cases) Transient hypotension Cardiac arrhythmias Bronchospasm	*Not used for induction of labor because of potential fetal side effects*
Dioctyl sodium sulfosuccinate Colace	Stool softener	Relieves constipation (does not stimulate peristalsis)	50–200 mg PO daily	Nausea and vomiting Abdominal cramps Rash	Unknown
Diphenhydramine hydrochloride Benadryl	Antihistamine	Symptomatic relief of allergies Used in anaphylaxis as adjunct to epinephrine	25–50 mg PO qid	CNS reactions (drowsiness, dizziness, headache, fatigue, restlessness, insomnia) Palpitations, tachycardia Blurred vision, skin rash Hypersensitivity reactions (anaphylactic shock)	Unknown
Dulcolax (see bisacodyl)					
Empirin (see phenacetin)					
Epinephrine Adrenaline	Antipyretic Analgesic Antispasmodic		300–600 mg PO q 4 hr (no more than 3 g in 24 hr)	Heartburn, nausea, gastritis, gastric hemorrhage, dizziness, tinnitus, sweating	Unknown
Ergonovine maleate Ergotrate (methergine is a semisynthetic preparation)	Oxytocic Uterine stimulant (stimulates uterine contractions)	Sustains uterine contractions Prevents or lessens risk of postpartum hemorrhage Constricts smooth muscle, cranial blood vessels (used for vascular-migraine headaches)	0.2 mg IM or PO q 4–6 hr for 2–7 days	Hypertension Nausea and vomiting, dizziness, palpitations, tinnitus, diaphoresis Contraindicated before delivery of placenta and in hypertension, renal disease, and cardiac disease Monitor BP, pulse, and respiratory rate and depth Have crash cart available	Fetal compromise can occur if used during labor owing to potential, sustained contractions that are not correctable Secreted in breast milk; breastfed infant may experience vomiting, diarrhea
Erythromycin	Antibiotic against gram-negative and gram-positive bacteria	Alternative to penicillin when patient is allergic For respiratory infections For syphilis, gonorrhea	250–500 mg PO q 6 hr	Parenteral use is limited because of frequency of thrombophlebitis Oral use for epigastric pain, nausea and vomiting, diarrhea	Unknown
Erythromycin ophthalmic ointment	Antiinfective	Inhibits bacterial cell wall in organisms Prophylaxis for ophthalmic neonatorum caused by gonorrhea or chlamydia infections	Conjunctival sacs, ribbon of ointment 0.5–1 cm long, 0.5%		For prophylaxis of ophthalmic neonatorum, ointment must be applied no later than 1 hr after birth
Estradiol valerate	Ovarian hormone	Used for primary ovarian failure	1–2 mg PO daily in 21-day cycles	Headache, dizziness, depression, libido changes, hypertension, edema, nausea, weight changes	Possibly teratogenic

Table continued on following page

483

TABLE B–1. DRUGS AND CHEMICALS USED DURING PREGNANCY, LABOR, BIRTH, AND THE POSTPARTUM PERIOD *Continued*

DRUGS	CLASSIFICATION	INDICATIONS/ACTION	DOSAGE/ROUTE	NURSING CONSIDERATIONS	
				Assess: Maternal Side Effects	Assess: Fetal/Neonatal Side Effects
Ferro-Sequels (see iron preparations)					
Ferrous sulfate (see iron preparations)					
Filibon (see vitamins, prenatal)					
Flagyl (see metronidazole)					
Folic acid Folacine	Vitamin (member of vitamin B complex) Hematinic	Required for normoblastic bone marrow formation Prevention or treatment of folate-deficiency anemia or macrocytic anemia	400 µg	Allergic reactions May lower phenytoin sodium levels	Deficiency may cause congenital malformation
Furosemide Lasix	Diuretic	Inhibits reabsorption of sodium and chloride from proximal distal tubules of loop of Henle Used in congestive heart failure (not used for physiological edema of preeclampsia)	40 mg PO bid 20–40 mg IV	Weakness, dizziness, nausea and vomiting Anuria, leg cramps Hypovolemia, hyponatremia, hypokalemia, hypochloremia Alkalosis	Decreased placental perfusion causing fetal distress Possible teratogenic effects Increased fetal urine output
Gelusil, Maalox, Mylanta	Antacid Antiflatulent (contains magnesium and aluminum hydroxide)	Relief of heartburn, "acid indigestion," and flatulence	2 tablets or 2 tsp PO 1 hr after meals and at bedtime	Sodium is present in preparations; avoid overloading with sodium	Unknown
Milk of magnesia *(should be taken with physician's approval)*	Contains only magnesium hydroxide				
Guaifenesin Robitussin	Expectorant	Relief of cough of common cold	2 tsp PO q 4 hr	Hypersensitivity reactions No serious side effects reported	Unknown
Gyne-Lotrimin (see clotrimazole)					
Heparin	Anticoagulant	Inhibits the thrombin-induced aggregation of platelets Treatment or prevention of pulmonary embolism and thromboembolic disease Accelerates formation of antithrombin III complex Inactivates thrombin and prevents conversion of fibrinogen to fibrin	Varies depending on condition and blood test results IV with infusion pump	Any condition with increased bleeding Urticaria, fever, chills, conjunctival itching, alopecia Excessive dose may cause bleeding from body orifices, petechiae, bruises Aspirin should not be taken with heparin	Prolonged bleeding possible at birth; however, large molecule has difficulty crossing placenta

Drug	Classification	Action/Use	Dosage	Side Effects	Fetal Effects
Hydralazine hydrochloride Apresoline	Antihypertensive	Relaxes smooth muscle of arterioles, particularly in the coronary, cerebral, renal, and uterine circulations Controls moderate to severe hypertension of preeclampsia (lowers blood pressure) Controls chronic hypertension in pregnancy	10 mg PO qid 5–20 mg IM or IV Gradually increase to 50 mg qid (lower dose given during pregnancy, when possible)	Tachycardia, palpiations Angina Nausea and vomiting, headaches, dizziness, perspiration, nasal congestion, flushing Long-term use may cause blood dyscrasias	Fetal side effects not proved, although animal studies show teratogenicity Fetal distress
Hydroxyzine pamoate Vistaril	Ataractic Antihistamine Antiemetic Mild sedative	Relief of anxiety Prevention of nausea and vomiting Reduces dose of narcotics, if needed	25–100 mg IM only (deep injection because irritating to tissues)	Drowsiness, dry mouth Pain and irritation of injection site Tremors, convulsions with excess use	Sedation of infant Animal studies indicate teratogenicity Quickly crosses placenta, stimulates fetal pancreas, and hyperinsulinemia can result
Hypoglycemic agents (oral) Tolazamide (Tolinase) Tolbutamide (Orinase)	Antidiabetic agent	Contraindicated during pregnancy			
Inderal (see propranolol hydrochloride)					
Insulin Lente (insulin zinc suspension) Isophane insulin suspension (NPH)	Hormone Hypoglycemic agent	Controls faulty pancreatic activity (hyperglycemia) due to disturbance in insulin release and carbohydrate metabolism Only fast-acting (regular) and intermediate-acting (Lente and NPH) are used during pregnancy Insulin by injection is rapidly degraded before reaching fetal circulation	Varies according to individual's needs (injection only during pregnancy) Accuracy in measurement is very important	Hypoglycemia and insulin shock Rigid control to avoid ketoacidosis during pregnancy Nausea and vomiting Hypoglycemia Assess accurate dosage Instruct how to self-monitor blood glucose level Emphasize meals not to be omitted Cigarette smoking decreases the amount and absorption of insulin	Maternal hyperglycemia stimulates fetal insulin secretion, causing macrosomia and infant hypoglycemia
Iron preparations Ferrous sulfate Ferro-Sequels Mol-Iron	Mineral	Reduces iron-deficiency anemia Iron supplementation (average diet is poor in iron in United States) Provides for increased need for iron of maternal tissues and growing fetus Absorption enhanced with vitamin C	300–600 mg PO tid	Nausea, vomiting, constipation, diarrhea, GI irritation, black stools	None known (fetus will obtain iron needs at mother's expense)
Isoxsuprine hydrochloride Vasodilan	Tocolytic agent Beta-receptor stimulant	Inhibits premature labor Inhibits uterine contractions	0.25 mg IV infusion pump q 8–12 hr, followed by 5–20 mg IM or PO q 3–6 hr	Hypotension, tachycardia, hyperglycemia, palpitations, tremors, restlessness, nausea and vomiting, allergic skin reactions Contraindicated in hypotension, diabetes, heart disease	Accelerated fetal lung maturity May cause infant hypotension, hypoglycemia

Table continued on following page

TABLE B–1. DRUGS AND CHEMICALS USED DURING PREGNANCY, LABOR, BIRTH, AND THE POSTPARTUM PERIOD *Continued*

					NURSING CONSIDERATIONS	
DRUGS	CLASSIFICATION	INDICATIONS/ACTION	DOSAGE/ROUTE		Assess: Maternal Side Effects	Assess: Fetal/Neonatal Side Effects
Keflex (see cephalexin)						
Lasix (see furosemide)						
Lidocaine hydrochloride Xylocaine	Local anesthetic	Blocks nerve impulses at sensory nerve endings	1% solution for local infiltration (paracervical, pudendal, spinal, caudal, or epidural block)		Hypotension, bradycardia, tremors, dizziness, respiratory/cardiac arrest	Fetal bradycardia when administered paracervically Possible fetal distress
Magnesium hydroxide (see Gelusil)						
Magnesium sulfate	CNS depressant Tocolytic agent	Anticonvulsant activity when given parenterally Depresses CNS; blocks neuromuscular transmission, producing anticonvulsant effect Reduces risk of convulsion in severe preeclampsia	4 g in 250 ml D5W IV followed by IM injection (5 g in each buttock)		Decreased frequency and intensity of uterine contractions Flushing, nausea and vomiting, hypotension With overdose diminished reflexes, respiratory rate, and urinary output Cardiac and respiratory arrest Magnesium may accumulate in renal insufficiency Assess I&O Contraindicated in abdominal pain, rectal bleeding	Decreased fetal heart rate Decreased muscle tone Low Apgar score Fetal distress Hypermagnesemia
	Laxative	Draws fluid from colon (takes 12–24 hr) Exact mechanism unknown, however, excessive magnesium appears to decrease amount of acetylcholine liberated by motor nerve impulses Acts peripherally, producing vasodilation Excreted by kidneys				
Meperidine hydrochloride Demerol	Narcotic analgesic	Reduces pain of active labor with full-term infant	50–100 mg IM 25–50 mg IV		Hypersensitivity, preterm labor Nausea and vomiting, dizziness, urinary retention, euphoria, dry mouth, flushing	Decreased fetal heart rate Respiratory depression
Mepivacaine hydrochloride (see Carbocaine)						
Metamucil (see psyllium hydrophilic mucilloid)						
Methadone hydrochloride *Should not be used in pregnancy unless benefits outweigh risks; safe use during pregnancy not established*	Narcotic analgesic	Detoxification and maintenance of narcotic addict	Usually PO with dose adjusted to patient's need		Respiratory depression Shock, circulatory depression, cardiac arrest Nausea and vomiting, dysphoria, light-headedness Urinary retention	Infant undergoes withdrawal symptoms

Drug	Classification	Dosage	Action	Side Effects and Contraindications	Effect on Fetus or Newborn
Methylergonovine maleate Methergine	Oxytocic	0.2 mg IM or PO q 4 hr for 6 doses (may be used IV after third stage of labor)	Stimulates contractions of uterine, vascular smooth muscle Hastens uterine involution Lessens postpartum hemorrhage	Hypertension Administered IV can cause acute hypertension and cardiac crises Nausea and vomiting, dizziness, headache, dyspnea, diaphoresis, palpitations, tinnitus Pain from uterine muscle cramps	None (administered after birth)
Metronidazole Flagyl (used in pregnancy only if other agents are not effective)	Antibiotic	250 mg PO tid for 7 days	Possesses direct trichomonacidal and amebacidal activity Used for Trichomonas vaginalis (vaginitis)	Contraindicated during pregnancy Not given to women with histories of blood dyscrasias Carcinogenic (animal studies) Metallic taste, abdominal cramps, nausea, dizziness, insomnia, weakness, depression Allergic reactions	Animal studies indicate genetic mutations
Miconazole nitrate Monistat	Antifungal agent	1 applicator of cream inserted into vagina at bedtime for 7 days	Used for vaginal candidiasis (vaginitis)	Vaginal burning, itching, pruritus Abdominal cramps Headache Hives, skin rash	Unknown
Milk of magnesia (magnesium hydroxide)	Laxative Antacid	2–4 tsp PO with glass of water As antacid, 1–3 tsp PO up to qid	Reacts with hydrochloric acid in stomach to form magnesium chloride, which distends colon and increases peristaltic activity	Dehydration Contraindicated with impaired renal function or cardiac disease	Unknown
Mineral oil	Laxative Lubricant	15–30 ml PO or rectally for retention enema	Lubricates and softens feces Retards water absorption from feces Eases passage of stool	Contraindicated in hypertension and cardiac disorders (due to straining at stool) Prolonged use (more than 2 wks) can reduce absorption of fat-soluble vitamins A, D, E, and K plus calcium and phosphate Contraindicated during pregnancy	May reduce nutrients needed by fetus
Mol-Iron (see iron preparations)					
Monistat (see miconazole nitrate)					
Morphine sulfate	Narcotic analgesic	5–45 mg IV diluted and injected slowly	Reduces hypertonic uterine dysfunction during early labor (used in emergency situations because of fetal effects)	Respiratory depression CNS depression Nausea and vomiting, euphoria, dizziness, itching, urinary retention Orthostatic hypotension Allergic reactions	Decreased fetal heart rate Neonatal respiratory depression (have antagonist available to combat severe respiratory depression)

Table continued on following page

487

TABLE B–1. DRUGS AND CHEMICALS USED DURING PREGNANCY, LABOR, BIRTH, AND THE POSTPARTUM PERIOD Continued

DRUGS	CLASSIFICATION	INDICATIONS/ACTION	DOSAGE/ROUTE	NURSING CONSIDERATIONS	
				Assess: Maternal Side Effects	Assess: Fetal/Neonatal Side Effects
Mycelex (see clotrimazole)					
Mycostatin (see nystatin)					
Mylanta (see Gelusil)					
Naloxone hydrochloride Narcan	Narcotic antagonist	Reverses respiratory depression induced by narcotics	Neonatal dose of 0.01 mg/kg IV or IM Owing to short-lasting action may be repeated in 2–3 min (preferable to administer to infant after birth so drug effects can be monitored)	Will produce withdrawal symptoms of narcotic addiction (nausea and vomiting, sweating, tachycardia, tremors, hypertension)	Narcotic-induced respiratory depression Can precipitate withdrawal, if mother is drug addict Respiratory rate may change drastically Monitor for 4 hr Have oxygen available
Natalins (see vitamins, prenatal)					
Neo-Synephrine hydrochloride (see phenylephrine hydrochloride)					
Nicotine Cigarettes	Chemical in cigarettes	May impair maternal nutrients to fetus (depletes vitamin C levels) Causes sympathetic stimulation of epinephrine, which increases metabolic rate	None recommended	Potentially carcinogenic Two cigarettes in succession can increase fetal heart rate	Teratogenic effect (human studies) Intrauterine growth retardation (decreased birth weight, length, and head circumference) Increased risk for minimal brain dysfunction
Carbon monoxide	Chemical in cigarettes	Binds to sites available for hemoglobin; therefore, decreases available oxygen to fetus Places fetus at risk for impaired growth and asphyxia			
Benzo[a]pyrene	Chemical in cigarettes	Readily crosses placental barrier and stimulates production of enzymes, which compete with nutrients and oxygen for developing fetus			
Nisentil (see alphaprodine hydrochloride)					
Nystatin Mycostatin Nilstat	Antifungal agent	Alters fungal cell permeability Used for monilial infections of skin, mucous membranes (thrush)	Vaginal suppository (100,000 units), 1 applicator or suppository bid for 14 days 400,000–600,000 PO tid	Hypersensitivity reactions Occasional diarrhea, irritation, nausea and vomiting	Unknown

Drug	Classification	Action	Dosage	Contraindications	Side effects / Nursing considerations
Omnipen (see ampicillin)					
Oral contraceptives (estrogen-dominant) Enovid-E Ovulen Ortho-Novum (2 mg) Norinyl (2 mg)	Hormone	Prevents ovulation Inhibits secretion of pituitary gonadotropins by high blood levels of estrogen and progesterone Estrogen suppresses secretion of follicle-stimulating hormone	1 pill daily PO for 21 days (28-day regimen contains 7 placebo pills) Dosage varies in amount of estrogen and progesterone	Contraindicated in thromboembolic disease, thrombophlebitis, confirmed or suspected cancer, hepatic disorders, suspected estrogen-dependent neoplasia, undiagnosed vaginal bleeding, hypertension, cerebral vascular or coronary disease, history of depression Given with caution to women with histories of migraine, epilepsy, asthma, renal disorders; women over 40 years of age; and women who smoke excessively	Estrogen excess: nausea, bloating, edema, dizziness, leukorrhea, chloasma, migraine headache, hypertension, breast fullness and tenderness, cystic breast changes, thrombophlebitis, uterine cramps, irritability, increased fat deposition, and cerebrovascular accident Estrogen deficiency: early and midcycle breakthrough bleeding, increased spotting, hypomenorrhea, "hot flashes," irritability, nervousness, decreased libido, dry vaginal mucosa, headaches, and depression Progestin excess: increased appetite and weight gain, tiredness and fatigue, oily scalp, acne, loss of hair, cholestatic jaundice, hirsutism, hypertension, monilial vaginitis, and cervicitis Progestin deficiency: late breakthrough bleeding, amenorrhea Instruct woman to take pill at same time each day; night dosing may reduce nausea and headaches Documentation not clear Some physicians ask woman to delay pregnancy for 2 mo after discontinuing the pill.
Oral contraceptives (progestin-dominant) Ortho-Novum (10 mg) Ovral Loestrin 21 1/20		Progesterone suppresses luteinizing hormone secretion so ovulation cannot occur even if follicle develops Causes endometrial changes that prevent implantation of fertilized ovum			

Table continued on following page

TABLE B–1. DRUGS AND CHEMICALS USED DURING PREGNANCY, LABOR, BIRTH, AND THE POSTPARTUM PERIOD *Continued*

| | | | | NURSING CONSIDERATIONS | |
DRUGS	CLASSIFICATION	INDICATIONS/ACTION	DOSAGE/ROUTE	Assess: Maternal Side Effects	Assess: Fetal/Neonatal Side Effects
Ornade	Nasal decongestant Antihistamine	Relieves upper respiratory tract congestion (sneezing, runny nose)	1 capsule PO q 12 hr	Hypersensitivity to some ingredients (chlorpheniramine maleate, phenylpropanolamine hydrochloride, isopropamide) Contraindicated in hypertension, bronchial asthma, and heart disease	Safely to fetus not established
Oxytocin Pitocin Syntocinon	Oxytocic	Stimulates or induces uterine contractions	IV infusion pump adusted to uterine and fetal responses	Intense labor Hyperstimulation may cause uterine rupture, cervical lacerations, amniotic fluid embolism Hypotension Cardiovascular ventricular contractions	Fetal distress due to decreased placental perfusion Fetal hypoxia
		Used immediately after birth to decrease postpartum blood loss Rapidly degraded in the GI tract, therefore not given orally	10 U/mL in each ampule 10–20 U/mL IV postpartum	Abdominal cramps	
Parlodel (see bromocriptine mesylate)					
Penicillin G	Antibiotic	Bacteriostatic, bactericidal Treatment of infections caused by alphahemolytic streptococci, hemolytic streptococci, pneumonococci, gonococci, meningococci, susceptible strains of staphylococci Drug of choice for treatment of gonorrhea and syphilis	50,000–500,000 U q 2–3 hr PO, IM, or IV	Found in breast milk Allergic reactions (rash to anaphylactic shock) Nausea and vomiting, diarrhea Discolored tongue (black, hairy tongue) Nephritis Vaginal candidiasis (vaginitis) after treatment	Infant can become sensitized through breast milk May cause thrush (candidiasis) Diarrhea
Phenacetin Empirin	Analgesic Antipyretic	Inhibits transmission of pain impulse Decreases fever	300–600 mg PO q 4 hr (not more than 3 g in 24 hr)	Heartburn, nausea, gastritis, gastric hemorrhage, dizziness, tinnitus, sweating	Unknown
Phenylephrine hydrochloride Neo-Synephrine	Nasal decongestant Vasoconstrictor	Produces vasoconstriction Relieves symptoms of common cold	0.25% solution (nose drops) q 3–4 hr pm	Tremors, insomnia, palpitations	Unknown

Drug	Classification	Action	Dosage	Side effects	Fetal/neonatal effects
Phenytoin sodium / Dilantin	Anticonvulsant	Affects only motor centers of brain (cerebral cortex) / Controls seizures of epilepsy	100–600 mg PO daily	Drowsiness, irritability, confusion, ataxia, rash, nystagmus, nausea and vomiting, fever, hyperglycemia, hematopoietic abnormalities	Teratogenic in animals / Potential orofacial, neural tube, congenital heart, and limb defects / Intrauterine growth retardation
Pitocin (see oxytocin)					
Polycillin (see ampicillin)					
Povidone-iodine (see Betadine)					
Promethazine hydrochloride / Phenergan	Antihistamine / Antiemetic / Anticholinergic / Sedative (tranquilizer)	Relieves anxiety / Reduces the dose of narcotics without increasing the risk of neonatal depression / Treatment of severe nausea and vomiting during pregnancy	25–50 mg IM or IV	Hypersensitivity reactions / CNS depressant / Transient hypotension / Drowsiness, dizziness, blurred vision, nervousness, incoordination, insomnia, nausea and vomiting, tinnitus	Platelet aggregation may be impaired
Propoxyphene hydrochloride / Darvon	Analgesic (nonnarcotic)	Relieves pain	65 mg PO q 4 hr pm	Nausea and vomiting / Drowsiness, dizziness, headache, weakness, abdominal pain, constipation, euphoria	Possible teratogenic effect / Neonatal withdrawal
Propranolol hydrochloride / Inderal	Beta-adrenergic blocking agent	Reduces angina and cardiac arrhythmias	10–40 mg PO tid	Nausea and vomiting / Lightheadedness / Mental depression / Visual disturbances	Unknown
Psyllium hydrophilic mucilloid / Metamucil	Laxative	Provides bland bulk / Used for treatment of constipation and hemorrhoids	1 tsp stirred into glass of liquid PO daily	Contraindicated in fecal impaction or intestinal obstruction	Unknown
Rh₀(D) immune globulin / RhoGAM	Immunoglobulin	By preventing development of Rh-antibodies in Rh– mothers delivering Rh+ infants, prevents active immunization of mother	300 μg (1 vial) IM / Administered within 72 hr after delivery or abortion, amniocentesis, ectopic pregnancy, or birth of an Rh+ infant / May be administered to Rh– negative woman prophylactically between 28th and 32nd weeks of gestation	Fever, lethargy / Contraindicated in Rh-positive mothers, since the product is incompatible with their red blood cells and would cause their destruction / Must be cross-matched by the laboratory staff before administration	Unknown
Ritodrine hydrochloride / Yutopar	Tocolytic agent	Inhibits contractility of uterine muscle, decreasing uterine activity and prolonging gestation / Treatment of premature labor	100 μg/min IV (infusion pump), increased by 50 μg/min up to 350 μg/min	Tachycardia, hyperglycemia / Abnormal cardiac response / Pulmonary edema / Alterations in blood pressure	Tachycardia / Neonatal hypoglycemia

Table continued on following page

491

TABLE B–1. DRUGS AND CHEMICALS USED DURING PREGNANCY, LABOR, BIRTH, AND THE POSTPARTUM PERIOD *Continued*

DRUGS	CLASSIFICATION	INDICATIONS/ACTION	DOSAGE/ROUTE	NURSING CONSIDERATIONS	
				Assess: Maternal Side Effects	Assess: Fetal/Neonatal Side Effects
Silver nitrate	Antiinfective Bactericide	Prevention of ophthalmia neonatorum Prophylaxis for gonococcal conjunctivitis	1–2 drops 1% silver nitrate instilled into conjunctival sac of each eye (close eye to help spread medication)		Chemical conjunctivitis (given within 1 hr after birth)
Simethicone (see Gelusil)					
Stuart prenatal (see vitamins, prenatal)					
Sulfonamides	Antiinfectives	Effective against Gram-positive bacteria, such as streptococci, pneumococci, and staphylococci Effective against Gram-negative organisms, such as *Neisseria* (gonococci), *Escherichia coli* Primarily for treatment of lower urinary tract infections and vaginitis	0.5–1.0 g q 4–8 hr PO	Contraindicated during third trimester of pregnancy GI disturbances such as nausea and vomiting, stomatitis Blood dyscrasias Headache, confusion Hepatic and renal damage (encourage large fluid intake)	Neonatal kernicterus as a result of competition with bilirubin for binding Hemolytic anemia in infants who breastfeed
Syntocinon (see oxytocin)					
Tace (see chlorotrianisene)					
Terbutaline sulfate Bricanyl Brethine	Tocolytic agent Bronchodilator	Inhibits uterine contractions and stops labor	2.5–5 mg PO q 8 hr IV infusion (rate individualized)	Contraindicated in severe hyperfusion, third trimester bleeding, gestation of less than 20 wks Hypersensitivity reactions Nervousness, tremors, headaches, drowsiness, tachycardia, palpitations, cardiac arrhythmias, sweating, nausea and vomiting Bronchospasm (aminophylline should be available for relief of bronchospasm)	

Drug	Classification	Action and Use	Dosage	Side Effects	Additional Effects
Testosterone enanthate and estradiol valerate Deladumone OB	Lactation suppressant (contains both estrogen and androgen)	Lactation suppression of non-nursing mothers	2 ml IM at second stage of labor	Pain of injection site Virilization Slight increase of blood clot formation and thrombophlebitis Higher incidence of carcinoma in later life (when exposed to estrogens) Because of adverse effects, nonestrogenic drug is usually given	Teratogenic effect on fetus, if given during pregnancy
Tetracyclines (*should not be given during pregnancy because of fetal side effects*)	Antibiotics	Broad-spectrum antimicrobials against Gram-negative and -positive bacteria, rickettsia, and protozoa	Dose depends on infection 50–500 mg q 6 hr PO, IM, or IV	Nausea, vomiting, diarrhea, rash, stomatitis, pharyngitis, fever Vaginitis Pericarditis	Decreased skeletal growth Brown coloration of teeth later in child (permanent)
Tucks	Astringent cleansing agent (contains witch hazel and glycerin)	Pads applied to perineum for relief of discomfort of episiotomy incision or hemorrhoids Used as a "wipe" after bowel movement	PRN	Irritation due to sensitivity	
Tylenol (see acetaminophen)					
Valium (see diazepam)					
Vasodilan (see isoxsuprine hydrochloride)					
Vistaril (see hydroxyzine)					
Vitamin K AquaMEPHYTON Mephyton Konakion	Vitamin	Prevention of hemorrhagic disorder of newborn Correct prolonged prothrombin time (hypoprothrombinemia)	0.5–1 mg IM immediately after birth to infant		Neonatal hyperbilirubinemia with high doses Inflammation of injection site
Vitamins, prenatal Stuart Prenatal Filibon Natalins	Vitamins	Source of folic acid, iron, and other vitamins Meets increased nutritional requirements during pregnancy and lactation	1 tablet or capsule PO daily	Nausea and vomiting as a result of swallowing large capsule Folic acid may mask symptoms of pernicious anemia	Fetal anomalies secondary to overdose of vitamins A and D
Warfarin Coumadin	Anticoagulant	Prolongs clotting time of blood by preventing production of prothrombin in liver Used in treatment of inflammation of veins (thrombophlebitis)	2–25 mg (dosage adjusted to prothrombin time)	Excessive bleeding may occur in one or a number of smaller areas	Teratogenic effect Infant may have small nose as a result 2–3% have risk of brain damage and blindness, if mother takes drug during first trimester

Table continued on following page

TABLE B–1. DRUGS AND CHEMICALS USED DURING PREGNANCY, LABOR, BIRTH, AND THE POSTPARTUM PERIOD *Continued*

DRUGS	CLASSIFICATION	INDICATIONS/ACTION	DOSAGE/ROUTE	NURSING CONSIDERATIONS	
				Assess: Maternal Side Effects	Assess: Fetal/Neonatal Side Effects
Xylocaine (see lidocaine hydrochloride)					
Yutopar (see ritodrine hydrochloride)					
Zidovudine (formerly AZT) Retrovir	Antiviral	Prevents replication of the human immunodeficiency virus (HIV) by interfering with transcription of RNA and DNA Used in HIV infections Carinii pneumonia or T4 lymphocyte count below 200/mm	Adults: 200 mg PO q 4 hr around the clock	CNS: fever, headache, malaise, diaphoresis, dizziness, insomnia, paresthesia, chills, depression, tremors GI: nausea, vomiting, diarrhea, anorexia, rectal bleeding, mouth ulcer INTEG: Rash, acne, urticaria MS: Muscle spasm, arthralgia GU: Dysuria, polyuria Precautions: Severe bone marrow depression can occur Blood studies q 2 wks Patient education: Drug controls symptoms; does not cure AIDS. Even with drug administration, patient is still infective. Suggest ways to avoid missing doses, such as the use of alarm clock	

TABLE B–2. REPORTED EFFECTS OF DRUG EXPOSURE TO FETUS

DRUG	EFFECT ON FETUS OR INFANT
Alcohol	Fetal alcohol syndrome, growth retardation, increase in anomalies
Androgens	Masculinization of female fetus
Antihistamines	Anomalies
Caffeine	Jitteriness, growth retardation
Chloramphenicol (Chloromycetin)	Gray syndrome (anemia), death
Cortisone	Anomalies, cleft palates
Coumarin	Fetal death, hemorrhage
Dicumarol	Nasal hypoplasia, optic atrophy
Diethylstilbestrol	Vaginal adenosis, carcinogenesis
Estrogen	Masculinization of female fetus
Erythromycin	Liver damage
Heparin	Infant hemorrhage, death
Heroin	Possible fetal death
Meprobamate (Equanil, Miltown)	Retarded development
Metronidazole (Flagyl)	Possible fetal anomalies
Morphine	Possible fetal death
Narcotics (Demerol)	Respiratory depression, withdrawal symptoms
Nicotine (cigarette smoking)	Growth retardation
Nitrofurantoin (Furadantin)	Hemolysis
Phenobarbital (in excess)	Infant hemorrhage, death
Phenytoin (Dilantin)	Growth retardation, craniofacial abnormalities
Reserpin (Serpasil)	Respiratory distress, lethargy
Salicylate (aspirin)	Infant hemorrhage
Sulfonamides	Kernicterus, thrombocytopenia
Sulfonylureas (oral hypoglycemic agents)	Anomalies
Thalidomide	Phocomelia, hearing loss, death
Vitamin K preparations	Hyperbilirubinemia

Advisory

The drugs and chemicals (including oral contraceptives, alcohol, nicotine, and caffeine) listed in this appendix are taken before pregnancy and during pregnancy, labor, and birth. Some of the drugs are given to the infant and mother after delivery. These drugs may be prescribed by the physician or purchased by the woman as over-the-counter drugs.

The most common dosage prescribed during maternity care is given. For several drugs, the dosage is lower when the woman is pregnant or suckling her infant. The side effects to both mother and infant are delineated. It is important that both the caregiver and the mother know these side effects.

APPENDIX C

APPROVED NURSING DIAGNOSES FROM THE NINTH CONFERENCE OF THE NORTH AMERICAN NURSING DIAGNOSIS ASSOCIATION, 1990

Activity Intolerance
Activity Intolerance, Potential
Adjustment, Impaired
Airway Clearance, Ineffective
Anxiety
Aspiration, Potential for
Body Image Disturbance
Body Temperature, Potential Altered
Breastfeeding, Effective
Breastfeeding, Ineffective
Breathing Pattern, Ineffective
Communication, Impaired Verbal
Constipation
Constipation, Colonic
Constipation, Perceived
Decisional Conflict (Specify)
Decreased Cardiac Output
Defensive Coping
Denial, Ineffective
Diarrhea
Disuse Syndrome, Potential for
Diversional Activity Deficit
Dysreflexia
Family Coping: Compromised, Ineffective
Family Coping: Disabling, Ineffective
Family Coping: Potential for Growth
Family Processes, Altered
Fatigue
Fear
Fluid Volume Deficit
Fluid Volume Deficit, Potential
Fluid Volume Excess
Gas Exchange, Impaired
Grieving, Anticipatory
Grieving, Dysfunctional
Growth and Development, Altered

Health Maintenance, Altered
Health Seeking Behaviors (Specify)
Home Maintenance Management, Impaired
Hopelessness
Hyperthermia
Hypothermia
Incontinence, Bowel
Incontinence, Functional
Incontinence, Reflex
Incontinence, Stress
Incontinence, Total
Incontinence, Urge
Individual Coping, Ineffective
Infection, Potential for
Injury, Potential for
Knowledge Deficit (Specify)
Noncompliance (Specify)
Nutrition: Less than Body Requirements, Altered
Nutrition: More than Body Requirements, Altered
Nutrition: Potential for More than Body Requirements, Altered
Oral Mucous Membrane, Altered
Pain
Pain, Chronic
Parental Role Conflict
Parenting, Altered
Parenting, Potential Altered
Personal Identity Disturbance
Physical Mobility, Impaired
Poisoning, Potential for
Post-Trauma Response
Powerlessness
Protection, Altered
Rape-Trauma Syndrome
Rape-Trauma Syndrome: Compound Reaction
Rape-Trauma Syndrome: Silent Reaction
Role Performance, Altered
Self Care Deficit
   Bathing/Hygiene
   Feeding
   Dressing/Grooming
   Toileting
Self Esteem, Chronic Low
Self Esteem, Situational Low
Self Esteem Disturbance
Sensory/Perceptual Alterations (Specify)
   (visual, auditory, kinesthetic, gustatory, tactile, olfactory)
Sexual Dysfunction
Sexuality Patterns, Altered
Skin Integrity, Impaired
Skin Integrity, Potential Impaired
Sleep Pattern Disturbance

Social Interaction, Impaired
Social Isolation
Spiritual Distress
Suffocation, Potential for
Swallowing, Impaired
Thermoregulation, Ineffective
Thought Processes, Altered
Tissue Integrity, Impaired
Tissue Perfusion, Altered (Specify Type)
   (renal, cerebral, cardiopulmonary, gastrointestinal, peripheral)
Trauma, Potential for
Unilateral Neglect
Urinary Elimination, Altered
Urinary Retention
Violence, Potential for: Self-directed or Directed at Others

ANSWER KEY TO REVIEW QUESTIONS

CHAPTER 1

A.

1. C
2. D
3. D
4. B
5. C
6. A, B, C, D
7. A
8. B

CHAPTER 2

A.

1. D
2. A
3. A
4. D
5. D
6. B
7. B
8. C
9. B
10. B
11. B
12. B
13. C
14. D
15. A
16. B

17. C
18. A
19. C

B.

1. J
2. C
3. E
4. A
5. K
6. H
7. I
8. G
9. D
10. F
11. B

CHAPTER 3

A.

1. B
2. A
3. A
4. D

B.

1. B
2. A
3. E
4. D
5. F
6. C

C.

1. D
2. B
3. C
4. A

D.

1. C
2. D
3. B
4. A

CHAPTER 4

A.

1. D
2. A
3. C
4. C
5. B
6. B
7. B
8. D
9. A
10. B
11. D
12. C
13. B

B.

1. E
2. D

3. B
4. F
5. C
6. A

C.

1. D
2. C
3. A
4. B

CHAPTER 5

A.

1. C
2. B
3. C
4. A
5. D
6. D
7. B
8. A
9. B
10. B
11. C
12. B
13. B
14. D
15. D
16. A

B.

1. C
2. A
3. B
4. D

C.

1. C
2. D
3. E
4. B
5. A
6. G
7. H
8. F

D.

1. C
2. A
3. B

CHAPTER 6

A.

1. A
2. D
3. A
4. D
5. D
6. D
7. A
8. B
9. D
10. D
11. D
12. D

13. C
14. D
15. D
16. B
17. D
18. D
19. B
20. D
21. D
22. D

CHAPTER 7

A.

1. B
2. D
3. D
4. D
5. D
6. E

B.

1. D
2. A
3. E
4. B
5. C

CHAPTER 8

A.

1. D
2. C
3. D
4. D

5. C
6. A
7. D
8. B
9. A
10. C
11. D
12. C
13. D
14. E
15. B

B.

1. D
2. A
3. C
4. B
5. H
6. I
7. K
8. E
9. G
10. J
11. F

CHAPTER 9

A.

1. D
2. D
3. A
4. D
5. D
6. D
7. D

B.

1. D
2. E
3. F
4. A
5. C
6. B

CHAPTER 10

A.

1. C
2. D
3. B, C, D
4. C
5. D
6. A
7. B
8. A
9. C
10. A
11. A
12. D
13. A
14. B
15. C
16. C
17. B
18. C
19. D
20. C

B.

1. B
2. C

3. D

4. A

5. F

6. E

CHAPTER 11

1. D

2. B

3. A

4. B or C

5. A or B

6. D

7. B

8. A

9. E

10. A

11. B

CHAPTER 12

A.

1. A

2. D

3. C

4. D

5. D

6. D

7. C

8. C

9. A

10. D

11. B

12. A

13. B

14. B

15. B

B.

1. B

2. D

3. H

4. E

5. C

6. A

7. G

8. F

CHAPTER 13

A.

1. C

2. D

3. D

4. A

5. C

6. B

7. C

8. B

9. D

10. D

11. A

12. D

13. A

B.

1. D

2. K

3. B

4. A

5. E

6. C

7. F

8. G

9. J

10. H

CHAPTER 14

A.

1. D

2. C

3. B

4. B

5. A

6. B

7. D

8. D

9. D

10. A

11. D

12. A

13. D

B.

1. H

2. D

3. B

4. M

5. A

6. C

7. J

8. K

9. E

10. F

11. A

12. G

13. L or N

14. I

CHAPTER 15

A.

1. A

2. D

3. A

4. D

5. C

6. A

7. B

8. C

9. D

B.

1. C

2. H

3. G

4. F

5. A

6. E

7. B

8. D

CHAPTER 16

A.

1. D

2. D

3. D

4. B

5. A

6. C

B.

1. E

2. F

3. D

4. A

5. B

6. C

CHAPTER 17

A.

1. D

2. D

3. D

4. B

5. A

6. C

7. D

8. B

B.

1. D

2. B

3. F

4. C

5. E

6. A

7. G

8. J

9. K

10. H

11. I

CHAPTER 18

A.

1. C

2. D

3. A

4. D

5. D

6. A

7. B

8. A

9. C

10. D

11. B

12. D

13. B

14. D

15. C

16. D

17. D

18. C

19. C

20. C

B.

1. I

2. H

3. G

4. A

5. C

6. B

7. J

8. D

9. E

10. F

11. K

CHAPTER 19

A.

1. D

2. B

3. C

4. A, B, C

5. C

6. D

7. C

8. D

9. B

10. C

11. B

12. A

13. B

14. C

15. C

16. D

17. C

18. C

19. C

20. D

21. D

22. B

B.

1. B

2. D

3. G

4. C

5. A

6. E

7. F

CHAPTER 20

A.

1. B

2. A

3. D

4. B

5. B

6. C

7. B

8. D

9. D

10. D

B.

1. D

2. B

3. C

4. A

5. G

6. H

7. F

8. I

9. J

10. E

CHAPTER 21

A.

1. A

2. A

3. B
4. D
5. D
6. D
7. A
8. D
9. C
10. C
11. D
12. B
13. C
14. B
15. A
16. D
17. D
18. D
19. D
20. A
21. D

B.

1. E
2. D
3. G
4. C
5. A
6. F
7. H
8. B

C.

1. D
2. E
3. A

4. C
5. B

CHAPTER 22

A.

1. A
2. A
3. D
4. D
5. C
6. C
7. C
8. B
9. C
10. D
11. D
12. C

B.

1. D
2. F
3. G
4. J
5. C
6. I
7. H
8. A
9. B
10. E

CHAPTER 23

1. D
2. C
3. C

4. C
5. B
6. D
7. D
8. D
9. D
10. D
11. A
12. A
13. D

CHAPTER 24

A.

1. A
2. A
3. D
4. D
5. A
6. D
7. C
8. A
9. B
10. D
11. B
12. D
13. B
14. D
15. C
16. A
17. B

B.

1. E
2. F

3. C
4. J
5. L
6. K
7. M
8. G
9. B
10. D
11. O
12. I
13. N
14. A
15. H

CHAPTER 25

1. A
2. B
3. B
4. C
5. D
6. A
7. D
8. B
9. B

Unit Opening Credits

Unit I: From Dennis, L. B, and Hassol, J. (1983). *Introduction to Human Development and Health Issues*. Philadelphia: W. B. Saunders Company.

Unit II: From Moore, K. L. (1989). *Before We Are Born: Basic Embryology and Birth Defects,* 3rd ed. Philadelphia, W. B. Saunders Company.

Unit III: Photograph by Arlene Burroughs, MEd, RN

Unit IV: Courtesy of Nancy Fleming, CNM, PhD

Unit V: Courtesy of Nancy Fleming, CNM, PhD

Unit VI: From Dennis, L. B., and Hassol, J. (1983). *Introduction to Human Development and Health Issues*. Philadelphia, W. B. Saunders Company.

Unit VII: Photograph by Arlene Burroughs, MEd, RN

INDEX

Note: Page numbers in *italics* indicate illustrations; those followed by a t indicate tables.

Abdomen, in newborn, 315–316, 316t
  palpation of, for fetal position, 90–92, *93*
  in labor, 204–205, *205*
Abdominal breathing exercises, postpartum, 238, *239*
Abdominal muscles, postpartum, 234
ABO incompatibility, 382, 443–444
Abortion, elective, 428t, 428–429, 429t
  spontaneous, 383–386, 385t
Abruptio placentae, 382, 383t, 390, *392*
  nursing care plan for, 391
Accelerations, in fetal heart rate monitoring, 144–145, *147*
Acetaminophen (Tylenol), 478t
Acetylsalicylic acid, 478t
Acidosis, metabolic, in neonatal cold stress, 297
Acini, mammary, 14–15, *15*
Acoustic stimulation test, 141
Acquired immunodeficiency syndrome (AIDS), 125–128
Acrocyanosis, 307t, 309
Active-alert state, 325
Activity, in newborn, 319–325
  postpartum resumption of, 253–254
Admission, to labor suite, nursing care and interventions in, 203–206
Adolescent, as parent, 8
  contraception for, 34
  sexuality of, 33–34
Adrenaline (epinephrine), 483t
Afterpains, 232
Age, gestational, determination of, 353, 354t, *354–360*
  by ultrasonography, 133
Aging, sexuality and, 37
AIDS, 125–128
Air pocketing, in newborn, 293
Airway clearance, in newborn, 221, *221*, 329, *331*

Alcohol, in pregnancy, 108–110, *109*, 478t
  fetal/neonatal effects of, 478t
Aldosterone, in pregnancy, 69
Alphaprodine (Nisentil), 478t
Alternative birth settings, 3–4
Aluminum hydroxide (Gelusil, Maalox, Mylanta), 478t, 484t
Alveoli, mammary, 14–15
Ambulation, postpartum, 252–253
Amenorrhea, 463
  in pregnancy, 64
Americaine (benzocaine) spray, 479t
Aminophylline, 479t
Amniocentesis, 134–135, *136*
Amnion, 49, *49*, 50
Amniotic cavity, 48
Amniotic fluid, 49–50
  assessment of, in labor, 208
    in pregnancy, 134–135
  bilirubin in, 135
  creatinine in, 135
  functions of, 50
  meconium in, 56, 293
  tests for, 399
Amniotic membranes, 49–50, *50*
  rupture of, 168
    artificial, 401–404
    premature, 399–401
Amniotomy, 401–404
Ampicillin (Omnipen, Polycillin), 479t
Analgesia. See *Pain relief.*
Analysis, in nursing process, 9–10
Android pelvis, 22, *22*
Anemia, in pregnancy, 73
Anesthesia. See also *Pain relief.*
  in childbirth, 194–198, 195t, *196*, *198*
  topical, for episiotomy, 250–251
Ankle, edema of, in pregnancy, 103
Anovulation, 38
Antepartum, definition of, 63

Anterior fontanelle, 310, 311t
Anthropoid pelvis, 22, *22*
Anus, in newborn, 317, 317t
  imperforate, 437
Anusol suppository, 479t
Aortic coarctation, 435
Apgar score, 221, 221t, 331
Apnea, in preterm infants, 363–365
Apresoline (hydralazine), 485t
AquaMEPHYTON (vitamin K), 493t
Areola, 15, *15*
Arm raising, postpartum, 239
Arm recoil, gestational age and, 354t, *355*, *357*
Arrhythmias, fetal, monitoring of, 138–149, 139t. See also *Fetal heart rate monitoring.*
Arterial blood gas values, for newborn, 292t
Ascorbic acid, in pregnancy, 96t, 98
Asherman's syndrome, 428
Aspiration, in labor, prevention of, 209
Aspirin, 478t
Assessment, in nursing process, 9
Atonic uterus, postpartum hemorrhage and, 421, *422*
Attitude, fetal, 173
Auscultation, of fetal heart, 138
AVC Cream, 479t
Awareness, in newborn, 319–325
Axillary temperature, 305, 338

Babinski's reflex, 320t
Baby. See *Infant; Newborn.*
Backache, in pregnancy, 102
Ballard score, for gestational age, 354t, *355*
Ballottement, 65
Barbiturates, in labor, 192, 193t

505